Williams
Manual of Hematology

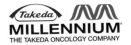

NOTICE

Medicine is an ever-changing science. As new research and clinical experience broaden our knowledge, changes in treatment and drug therapy are required. The authors and the publisher of this work have checked with sources believed to be reliable in their efforts to provide information that is complete and generally in accord with the standards accepted at the time of publication. However, in view of the possibility of human error or changes in medical sciences, neither the authors nor the publisher nor any other party who has been involved in the preparation or publication of this work warrants that the information contained herein is in every respect accurate or complete, and they disclaim all responsibility for any errors or omissions or for the results obtained from use of the information contained in this work. Readers are encouraged to confirm the information contained herein with other sources. For example and in particular, readers are advised to check the product information sheet included in the package of each drug they plan to administer to be certain that the information contained in this work is accurate and that changes have not been made in the recommended dose or in the contraindications for administration. This recommendation is of particular importance in connection with new or infrequently used drugs.

C. Hoogstede ARNP

Williams
Manual of Hematology

Eighth Edition

Marshall A. Lichtman, MD
Professor of Medicine and of Biochemistry and Biophysics
University of Rochester Medical Center
Rochester, New York

Kenneth Kaushansky, MD
Senior Vice President, Health Sciences
Dean, School of Medicine
Stony Brook University
Stony Brook, NY

Thomas J. Kipps, MD, PhD
Evelyn and Edwin Tasch Chair in Cancer Research
Professor of Medicine
Division of Hematology/Oncology
Deputy Director for Research Operations
Moores UCSD Cancer Center
University of California, San Diego
La Jolla, California

Josef T. Prchal, MD
Professor of Medicine, Pathology, and Genetics
Hematology Division
University of Utah
Salt Lake City, Utah
Department of Pathophysiology
First Faculty of Medicine
Charles University in Prague
Czech Republic

Marcel M. Levi, MD, PhD
Chairman, Department of Medicine
Academic Medical Center
University of Amsterdam
Amsterdam, The Netherlands

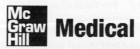 **Medical**

New York Chicago San Francisco Lisbon London Madrid Mexico City
Milan New Delhi San Juan Seoul Singapore Sydney Toronto

Williams Manual of Hematology, Eighth Edition

Copyright © 2011 by The McGraw-Hill Companies, Inc. All rights reserved. Printed in China. Except as permitted under the United States Copyright Act of 1976, no part of this publication may be reproduced or distributed in any form or by an means, or stored in a data base or retrieval system, without the prior written permission of the publisher.

3 4 5 6 7 8 9   CTP/CTP   14 13

ISBN 978-0-07-162242-4
MHID 0-07-162242-X

This book was set in Times Roman by Aptara, Inc.
The editors were James Shanahan and Harriet Lebowitz.
The production supervisor was Sherri Souffrance.
Project management was provided by Saima Ghaffar Aptara, Inc.
The cover designer was Margaret Webster-Shapiro.
China Translation & Printing, Ltd. was printer and binder.

Library of Congress Cataloging-in-Publication Data
Williams manual of hematology. — Eighth Edition / [edited by] Marshall A. Lichtman . . . [et al.].
    p. ; cm.
  Manual of hematology
  Includes bibliographical references and index.
  ISBN-13: 978-0-07-162242-4 (pbk. : alk. paper)
  ISBN-10: 0-07-162242-X (pbk. : alk. paper)
  1. Blood--Diseases. 2. Hematology. I. Lichtman, Marshall A., 1934- editor. II. Kaushansky, Kenneth, editor. III. Kipps, Thomas J., editor. IV. Prchal, Josef T., editor. V. Levi, Marcel, 1964- editor. VI. Williams, William J. (William Joseph), 1926- VII. Williams hematology. Companion to (work): VIII. Title: Manual of hematology.
  [DNLM: 1. Hematologic Diseases. WH 100]
  RC633.H43 2011 Suppl.
  616.1'5—dc22

                                                                        2010052298

International Edition ISBN 978-0-07-176730-9; MHID 0-07-1767304
Copyright © 2011. Exclusive rights by The McGraw-Hill Companies, Inc., for the manufacture and export. This book cannot be re-exported from the country to which it is consigned by McGraw-Hill. The International Edition is not available in North America.

McGraw-Hill books are available at special quantity discounts to use as premiums and sales promotions, or for use in corporate training programs. To contact a representative, please e-mail us at bulksales@mcgraw-hill.com.

CONTENTS

PART III   **DISORDERS OF GRANULOCYTES**

PART IV   **DISORDERS OF MONOCYTES AND MACROPHAGES**

PART V   **PRINCIPLES OF THERAPY FOR NEOPLASTIC HEMATOLOGIC
DISORDERS**

PART VI   **THE CLONAL MYELOID DISORDERS**

PREFACE

The purpose of the *Manual of Hematology* is to provide a convenient and easily navigable précis of the pathogenetic, diagnostic, and therapeutic essentials of blood cell and coagulation protein disorders. This handbook is comprehensive and clearly organized and, at the same time, its portable size allows it to serve as a companion to the physician in the hospital or clinic. We have included chapters on the classification of red cell, neutrophil, monocyte, platelet disorders, and diseases of coagulation proteins to provide a framework for considering the differential diagnosis of syndromes that are not readily apparent. We have incorporated numerous tables that include diagnostic and therapeutic information relevant to the diseases discussed.

Unlike the previous *Manual*, there are eight chapters on specific types of non-Hodgkin lymphoma, rather than a single chapter encompassing all lymphomas. Chapters on hereditary and acquired thrombophilia and their management respond to the increased role hematologists have in diagnosing and managing this important mechanism of disease.

For many tables, reproduced here, the reader can find explicit citations giving more detailed information for the Table entries in the 8th edition of *Williams Hematology*. The chapter and page of the more detailed information in the 8th edition of *Williams Hematology* is provided for easy cross-reference.

Each chapter ends with an acknowledgment of the authors of the relevant chapter in the 8th edition of Williams Hematology, including the chapter title and the page number. The publisher prints a caution in the Manual that admonishes readers to verify doses, routes, timing, and duration of administration and to check the contraindications and adverse effects of drugs used to treat the diseases described. The authors reemphasize that these often complex diseases require direct participation and close supervision of an experienced diagnostician and therapist. This oversight should be provided by a person who is able to individualize therapy depending on the nature of the expression of the primary hematological disease, the patients age, and the presence of coincidental medical conditions, among other factors.

The authors acknowledge the valuable assistance of Monica Gudea and Carolina Bump, at the University of California in San Diego, Susan Madden at the University of Utah, Petra Speek at the University of Amsterdam, The Netherlands, and, notably, Susan Daley at the University of Rochester who managed all administrative requirements in the preparation of the Manual.

We also acknowledge the encouragement and support of James F. Shanahan, Editor-in-Chief, Internal Medicine, and Harriet Lebowitz, our editor, both at McGraw-Hill Professional Publishing. Jennifer Bernstein provided the copyediting of the manuscript.

Marshall A. Lichtman, Rochester, NY
Kenneth Kaushansky, Stony Brook, NY
Thomas J. Kipps, San Diego, CA
Josef T. Prchal, Salt Lake City, UT
Marcel M. Levi, Amsterdam, The Netherlands

PART I

INITIAL CLINICAL EVALUATION

CHAPTER 1
Approach to the Patient

FINDINGS THAT MAY LEAD TO A HEMATOLOGY CONSULTATION

Table 1–1 lists abnormalities that often require an evaluation by a hematologist.

The care of a patient with a hematologic disorder begins with eliciting a medical history and performing a thorough physical examination. Certain parts of the history and physical examination that are of particular interest to the hematologist are presented here.

HISTORY OF THE PRESENT ILLNESS

- Estimation of the "performance status" helps establish the degree of disability and permits assessment of the effects of therapy (Tables 1–2 and 1–3).
- Drugs and chemicals often induce or aggravate hematologic diseases; drug use or chemical exposure, intentional or inadvertent, should be evaluated. One should inquire about professionally prescribed and self-prescribed drugs, such as herbal remedies. Occupational exposures should be defined.
- Fever may result from hematologic disease or, more often, from an associated infection. Night sweats suggest the presence of fever. It is especially prevalent in lymphomas.
- Weight loss may occur in some hematologic diseases.
- Fatigue, malaise, lassitude, and weakness are common but are nonspecific symptoms and may be the result of anemia, fever, or muscle wasting associated with hematologic malignancy or neurologic complications of hematologic disease.
- Symptoms related to specific organ systems or regions of the body may arise because of involvement in the basic disease process, such as spinal cord compression from a plasmacytoma, ureteral or intestinal obstruction from abdominal lymphoma, or stupor from exaggerated hyperleukocytosis in chronic myelogenous leukemia.

FAMILY HISTORY

- Hematologic disorders may be inherited as autosomal dominant, autosomal recessive, or X chromosome–linked traits (see *Williams Hematology,* 8th ed, Chap. 9, p. 129). The family history is crucial in such cases and should include information relevant to the disease in question in grandparents, parents, siblings,

TABLE 1–1	FINDINGS THAT MAY LEAD TO A HEMATOLOGY CONSULTATION

Decreased hemoglobin concentration (anemia) and/or abnormal red cell indexes
Increased hemoglobin concentration (polycythemia)
Elevated serum ferritin level
Accelerated sedimentation rate
Leukopenia or neutropenia
Immature granulocytes or nucleated red cells in the blood
Pancytopenia
Granulocytosis: neutrophilia, eosinophilia, basophilia, or mastocytosis
Monocytosis
Lymphocytosis
Lymphadenopathy
Splenomegaly
Hypergammaglobulinemia: monoclonal or polyclonal
Purpura
Thrombocytopenia
Thrombocytosis
Exaggerated bleeding: spontaneous or trauma related
Prolonged partial thromboplastin or prothrombin coagulation times
Venous thromboembolism
Thrombophilia
Obstetrical adverse events (e.g., recurrent fetal loss, stillbirth, and HELLP *
   syndrome).

*Hemolytic anemia, elevated liver enzymes, and low platelet count.
Source: *Williams Hematology,* 8th ed, Chap. 1, Table 1–1, p. 4.

children, maternal uncles and aunts, and nephews. Careful and repeated questioning is often necessary because some important details, such as the death of a sibling in infancy, may be forgotten years later.

- Absence of a family history in a dominantly inherited disease may indicate a *de novo* mutation or non-paternity.
- Deviations from mendelian inheritance may result from uniparental disomy (patient receives two copies of a chromosome, or part of a chromosome,

TABLE 1–2	CRITERIA OF PERFORMANCE STATUS (KARNOVSKY SCALE)

Able to carry on normal activity; no special care is needed.
100%   Normal; no complaints, no evidence of disease
90%   Able to carry on normal activity; minor signs or symptoms of disease
80%   Normal activity with effort; some signs or symptoms of disease

Unable to work; able to live at home, care for most personal needs; a varying amount of assistance is needed.
70%   Cares for self; unable to carry on normal activity or to do active work
60%   Requires occasional assistance but is able to care for most personal needs
50%   Requires considerable assistance and frequent medical care

Unable to care for self; requires equivalent of institutional or hospital care; disease may be progressing rapidly.
40%   Disabled; requires special care and assistance
30%   Severely disabled; hospitalization is indicated though death not imminent
20%   Very sick; hospitalization necessary; active supportive treatment necessary
10%   Moribund; fatal processes progressing rapidly
0%   Dead

Source: *Williams Hematology,* 8th ed, Chap. 1, Table 1–2, p. 4.

TABLE 1–3	EASTERN COOPERATIVE ONCOLOGY GROUP PERFORMANCE STATUS
Grade	Activity
0	Fully active, able to carry on all pre-disease performance without restriction
1	Restricted in physically strenuous activity but ambulatory and able to carry out work of a light or sedentary nature, e.g., light housework, office work
2	Ambulatory and capable of all self-care but unable to carry out any work activities; up and about more than 50% of waking hours
3	Capable of only limited self-care, confined to bed or chair more than 50% of waking hours
4	Completely disabled; cannot carry on any self-care; totally confined to bed or chair
5	Dead

Source: *Williams Hematology,* 8th ed, Chap. 1, Table 1–3, p. 4.

containing a mutation from one parent and no copies from the other parent) or genetic imprinting (same abnormal gene inherited from mother has a different phenotype than that inherited from father as a result of silencing or imprinting of one parent's portion of DNA) (see *Williams Hematology,* 8th ed, Chap. 10, p.141).

SEXUAL HISTORY

• One should obtain the history of the sexual preferences and practices of the patient.

PHYSICAL EXAMINATION

Special attention should be paid to the following aspects of the physical examination.

• *Skin:* cyanosis, ecchymoses, excoriation, flushing, jaundice, leg ulcers, nail changes, pallor, petechiae, telangiectases, rashes (e.g., lupus erythematosus, leukemia cutis, cutaneous T-cell lymphoma).
• *Eyes:* jaundice, pallor, plethora, retinal hemorrhages, exudates, or engorgement and segmentation of retinal veins.
• *Mouth:* bleeding, jaundice, mucosal ulceration, pallor, smooth tongue.
• *Lymph nodes:* slight enlargement may occur in the inguinal region in healthy adults, and in the cervical region in children. Enlargement elsewhere, or moderate to marked enlargement in these regions, should be considered abnormal.
• *Chest:* sternal and/or rib tenderness.
• *Liver:* enlargement.
• *Spleen:* enlargement, splenic rub.
• *Joints:* swelling, deformities.
• *Neurologic:* abnormal mental state, cranial nerve abnormalities, peripheral nerve abnormalities, spinal cord signs.

LABORATORY EVALUATION

The blood should be evaluated, both quantitatively and qualitatively. This is frequently achieved using automated equipment.
• Normal blood cell values are presented in **Table 1–4.**

TABLE 1–4	**BLOOD CELL VALUES IN A NORMAL POPULATION**		
	Men	Women	Either
White cell count,* × 10^9/L blood			7.8 (4.4–11.3)$^+$
Red cell count, × 10^{12}/L blood	5.21 (4.52–5.90)	4.60 (4.10–5.10)	
Hemoglobin, g/dL blood	15.7 (14.0–17.5)$^{++}$	13.8 (12.3–15.3)$^{++}$	
Hematocrit (Volume of packed red cells as a ratio to a volume of blood)	0.46 (0.42–0.50)	0.40 (0.36–0.45)	
Mean cell volume, fL/red cell			88.0 (80.0–96.1)
Mean cell hemoglobin, pg/red cell			30.4 (27.5–33.2)
Mean cell hemoglobin concentration, g/dL red cell			34.4 (33.4–35.5)
Red cell distribution width, CV(%)			13.1 (11.5–14.5)
Platelet count, × 10^9/L blood			311 (172–450)

*The International Committee for Standardization in Hematology recommends that SI units be used as follows: white cell count, number × 10^9/L; red cell count, number × 10^{12}/L; and hemoglobin, g/dL (dL = deciliter). The hematocrit (packed cell volume) is given as a numerical proportion, for example, 0.41, without designated units. Units of liter (of red cells) per liter (of blood) are implied. Mean cell volume is given as femtoliters (fL), mean cell hemoglobin as picograms (pg), and mean corpuscular hemoglobin concentration as g/dL. Platelets are reported as number × 10^9/L. CV = coefficient of variation.
$^+$ The mean and reference intervals (normal range) are given. Because the distribution curves may be non-Gaussian, the reference interval is the nonparametric central 95 percent confidence interval. Results are based on 426 normal adult men and 212 normal adult women, with studies performed on the Coulter Model S-Plus IV. The normal intervals in this table may vary somewhat in different laboratories and in populations with varying ethnic distributions. For example,
The mean neutrophil count in persons of African descent is approximately 1.5 × 10^9/L below that for individuals of European descent of similar sex and age. This difference also decreases the total leukocyte count in Americans of African descent by a similar concentration.
$^{++}$ The hemoglobin level of individuals of African descent is approximately 1.0 g/dL below that for individuals of European descent of similar sex and age.
Source: *Williams Hematology*, 8th ed, Chap. 2, Table 2–2, p. 17.

The normal total leukocyte and differential leukocyte counts are presented in Table 1–5.
• Hemoglobin concentration is measured photometrically after conversion to a stable derivative, usually cyanmethemoglobin.
• Packed cell volume (*hematocrit*) may be measured directly by high-speed centrifugation of anticoagulated blood. Automated instruments derive the hematocrit from the product of erythrocyte count and the mean red cell volume.

TABLE 1–6   DISEASES IN WHICH EXAMINATION OF THE BLOOD FILM CAN SUGGEST OR CONFIRM THE DISORDER

Disease	Findings on blood film
Immune hemolytic anemia	Spherocytes, polychromatophilia, erythrocyte agglutination, erythrophagocytosis
Hereditary spherocytosis	Spherocytes, polychromatophilia
Hereditary elliptocytosis	Elliptocytes
Hereditary ovalocytosis	Ovalocytes
Hemoglobin C disease	Target cells, spherocytes
Hemoglobin S disease	Sickle cells
Hemoglobin SC	Target cells, sickle cells
Thalassemia minor (alpha or beta)	Microcytosis, target cells, teardrop cells, basophilic stippling, other misshapen cells
Thalassemia major (alpha or beta)	Microcytosis, target cells, basophilic stippling, teardrop cells, other misshapen cells (often more exaggerated than minor form)
Iron deficiency	Microcytosis, hypochromia, absence of basophilic stippling
Lead poisoning	Basophilic stippling
Vitamin B 12 or folic acid deficiency	Macrocytosis, with oval macrocytes, hypersegmented neutrophils
Myeloma, macroglobulinemia	Pathologic rouleaux formation
Malaria, babesiosis	Parasites in the erythrocytes
Consumptive coagulopathy	Schistocytes
Mechanical hemolysis	Schistocytes
Severe infection	Increase in neutrophils; increased band forms, Döhle bodies, neutrophil vacuoles
Infectious mononucleosis	Reactive lymphocytes
Agranulocytosis	Decreased neutrophils
Allergic reactions	Eosinophilia
Chronic lymphocytic leukemia	Absolute small cell lymphocytosis
Chronic myelogenous leukemia	Promyelocytes, myelocytes, basophils, hypersegmented neutrophils
Oligoblastic myelogenous leukemia (refractory anemia with excess blast cells)	Blast forms, Pelger-Hüet cells, anisocytosis, poikilocytosis, abnormal platelets
Acute leukemia	Blast forms
Thrombocytopenia	Decreased platelets
Thrombocytosis or thrombocythemia	Increased platelets

- Leukocyte function may be depressed in normal infants in the newborn period.
- Reference values for coagulation factors in neonates and infants may be found in *Williams Hematology*, 8th ed, Chap. 6, Table 6–6, p. 98, and for coagulation factor inhibitors in neonates and infants in Table 6–7, p. 99.

Effects of Aging

- See *Williams Hematology*, 8th ed, Chap. 8, p. 115.
- Blood count and cell function may also vary with advanced age.
- The hemoglobin levels of men older than 60 years of age are statistically lower than those of younger men, even in the absence of a demonstrable cause for anemia, but are not sufficiently low to warrant use of specific normal values for older men. Anemia in an older person warrants careful evaluation before concluding it is the anemia of aging.

- The hemoglobin level in women does not change significantly with advancing age.
- Total and differential leukocyte counts also do not change significantly with advancing age.
- Leukocytosis in response to infection (e.g., appendicitis or pneumonia) is the same in older individuals as in people younger than age 60, but special studies indicate that the marrow granulocyte reserve may be reduced in the older person.
- Both cellular and humoral immune responses are reduced in older patients.
- The erythrocyte sedimentation rate increases significantly with age.
- Aging is associated with a net proagulant propensity and an increased risk of venous thrombosis.

Utility of the Blood Film in Diagnosis
- The blood film is invaluable in developing the differential diagnosis or the specific diagnosis of a blood cell disorder. Table 1–6 lists several situations in which the blood film can be important or decisive.

The Marrow
- Examination of the marrow is important in the diagnosis and management of a variety of hematologic disorders.
- All bones contain hematopoietic marrow at birth.
- Fat cells begin to replace hematopoietic marrow in the extremities in the fifth to sixth year of life.
- In adults, hematopoietic marrow is limited to the axial skeleton and the proximal quarter of the humeri and femora.
- Hematopoietic marrow cellularity is reduced in the elderly, falling after age 65 from about 50 percent to 30 percent, roughly in inverse proportion to age.
- Marrow is obtained by aspiration and/or needle biopsy. The most frequently utilized site is the iliac crest at the posterior superior iliac spine. The Jamshidi needle is most often used for biopsy and provides excellent material for study.
- Aspirated marrow may be evaluated after preparation of thin or thick films on glass slides and appropriate staining.
- Marrow biopsies are examined after fixation, sectioning, and staining. Touch preparations provide useful information and should be made at the time of biopsy.
- Interpretation of marrow films and biopsy sections is discussed in *Williams Hematology* 8th ed, Chap. 3, p. 25 and under specific diseases for which a marrow is usually performed. *Williams Hematology*, 8th ed, Table 3–1, p. 30 contains the normal differential count of cells in the marrow.

For a more detailed discussion, see Marshall A. Lichtman and Ernest Beutler: Approach to the Patient, Chap. 1, p. 1; Daniel H. Ryan: Examination of Blood Cells, Chap. 2, p. 11; Daniel H. Ryan: Examination of the Marrow, Chap. 3, p. 25; James Palis and George B. Segel: Hematology of the Fetus and Newborn, Chap. 6, p. 87; William B. Ershler and Dan L. Longo: Hematology in Older Persons, Chap. 8, p. 115; C. Wayne Smith: Morphology of Neutrophils, Eosinophils, and Basophils, Chap. 59, p. 875; Steven D. Douglas and Florin Tuluc: Morphology of Monocytes and Macrophages, Chap. 67, p. 989; H. Elizabeth Broome: Morphology of Lymphocytes and Plasma Cells, Chap. 74, p. 1079 in *Williams Hematology,* 8th ed.

PART II

DISORDERS OF RED CELLS

CHAPTER 2
Classification of Anemias and Polycythemias

- Clinically significant red cell disorders can be classified into:
  — Disorders in which the red cell mass is decreased (anemias). The principal effect is decreased oxygen-carrying capacity of the blood. They are best expressed in terms of hemoglobin concentration.
  — Disorders in which the red cell mass is increased (polycythemias). The principal effect is related to an increased viscosity of the blood (see Fig. 2–1). In addition to their specific effects, they are best expressed in terms of packed red cell volume (hematocrit).
- The red cell mass is the volume of red cells in the circulation.
  — The normal red cell mass of women is 23–29 mL/kg.
  — The normal red cell mass of men is 26–32 mL/kg.
  — More accurate formulas based on body surface have been recommended.
- Because the red cells are measured either as a concentration in the blood as the red cell count, the hemoglobin content of the blood, or the hematocrit (packed red cell volume per 100 mL of blood), rather than the volume of red cells in the total circulation, the anemias and polycythemias can each be subclassified as:
  — Relative, where the red cell mass is normal but the amount of plasma is decreased (relative polycythemia) or increased (relative anemia).
  — Absolute, where the red cell mass is increased (in true polycythemia) or decreased (in true anemia).
- It is essential that the specific cause of anemia be determined. The initial laboratory approach to the diagnosis of anemia follows. (Table 2–1).
  — Hematocrit, hemoglobin, or red cell count to determine degree of anemia. In most cases, these three variables are closely correlated. Hemoglobin concentration is the most direct measure of oxygen-carrying capacity.
  — Red cell indices (MCV, MCH, MCHC) to determine whether normocytic, macrocytic, or microcytic and normochromic or hypochromic red cells are present on average.
  — Exaggerated red cell distribution width (RDW) is a measure of anisocytosis.

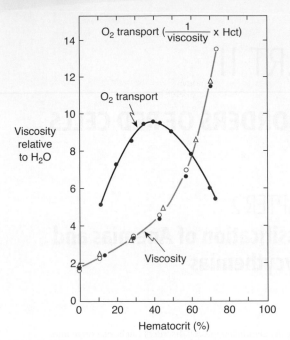

FIGURE 2–1 Viscosity of heparinized normal human blood related to hematocrit (Hct). Viscosity is measured with an Ostwald viscosimeter at 37°C (98.6°F) and expressed in relation to viscosity of saline solution. Oxygen transport is computed from hct and O_2 flow (1/viscosity) and is recorded in arbitrary units. Oxygen transport varies, however, with increases or decreases in blood volume. (Source: *Williams Hematology,* 8th ed, Chap. 33, Fig. 33–6, p. 460.).

TABLE 2–1   CLASSIFICATION OF ANEMIA

I. Absolute anemia (decreased red cell volume)
   A. Decreased red cell production
      1. Acquired
         a. Pluripotential stem cell failure
            (1) Aplastic anemia (see Chap. 3)
               (a) Radiation induced
               (b) Drugs and chemicals (chloramphenicol, benzene, etc.)
               (c) Viruses (hepatitis, Epstein-Barr virus, etc.)
               (d) Idiopathic
            (2) Anemia of leukemia and of myelodysplastic syndromes (see Chaps. 42, 46, and 55)
            (3) Anemia associated with marrow infiltration (see Chap. 12)
            (4) Postchemotherapy (see Chap. 39)
         b. Erythroid progenitor cell failure
            (1) Pure red cell aplasia (parvovirus B19 infection, drugs, associated with thymoma, autoantibodies, etc. [see Chap. 4])
            (2) Endocrine disorders (see Chap. 6)
            (3) Acquired sideroblastic anemia (drugs, copper deficiency, etc. [see Chaps. 11 and 42])

    c. Functional impairment of erythroid and other progenitors due to nutritional and other causes
      (1) Megaloblastic anemias (see Chap. 8)
        (a) Vitamin B_{12} deficiency
        (b) Folate deficiency
        (c) Acute megaloblastic anemia because of nitrous oxide (N_2O)
        (d) Drug-induced megaloblastic anemia (pemetrexed, methotrexate, phenytoin toxicity, etc.)
      (2) Iron-deficiency anemia (see Chap. 9)
      (3) Anemia resulting from other nutritional deficiencies (see Chap. 10)
      (4) Anemia of chronic disease and inflammation (see Chap. 13)
      (5) Anemia of renal disease (see Chap. 5)
      (6) Anemia caused by chemical agents (lead toxicity [see Chap. 22])
      (7) Acquired thalassemias (seen in some clonal hematopoietic disorders [see Chaps. 16 and 42])
      (8) Erythropoietin antibodies (see Chap. 4)
  2. Hereditary
    a. Pluripotential stem cell failure (see Chap. 3)
      (1) Fanconi anemia
      (2) Shwachman syndrome
      (3) Dyskeratosis congenita
    b. Erythroid progenitor cell failure
      (1) Diamond-Blackfan syndrome (see Chap. 3)
      (2) Congenital dyserythropoietic syndromes (see Chap. 7)
    c. Functional impairment of erythroid and other progenitors from nutritional and other causes
      (1) Megaloblastic anemias (see Chap. 8)
        (a) Selective malabsorption of vitamin B_{12} (Imerslund-Gräsbeck disease)
        (b) Congenital intrinsic factor deficiency
        (c) Transcobalamin II deficiency
        (d) Inborn errors of cobalamin metabolism (methylmalonic aciduria, homocystinuria, etc.)
        (e) Inborn errors of folate metabolism (congenital folate malabsorption, dihydrofolate deficiency, methyltransferase deficiency, etc.)
      (2) Inborn purine and pyrimidine metabolism defects (Lesch-Nyhan syndrome, hereditary orotic aciduria, etc.)
      (3) Disorders of iron metabolism (see Chap. 9)
        (a) Hereditary atransferrinemia
        (b) Hypochromic anemia caused by divalent metal transporter (DMT)-1 mutation
      (4) Hereditary sideroblastic anemia (see Chap. 11)
      (5) Thalassemias (see Chap. 16)
B. Increased red cell destruction
  1. Acquired
    a. Mechanical
      (1) Macroangiopathic (march hemoglobinuria, artificial heart valves [see Chap. 21])
      (2) Microangiopathic (disseminated intravascular coagulation [DIC]; thrombotic thrombocytopenic purpura [TTP]; vasculitis [see Chaps. 21, 78, and 86])
      (3) Parasites and microorganisms (malaria, bartonellosis, babesiosis, *Clostridium perfringens*, etc. (see Chap. 23)

(continued)

TABLE 2–1 **(CONTINUED)**

    b. Antibody mediated
       (1) Warm-type autoimmune hemolytic anemia (see Chap. 24)
       (2) Cryopathic syndromes (cold agglutinin disease, paroxysmal cold hemoglobinuria, cryoglobulinemia [see Chap. 24])
       (3) Transfusion reactions (immediate and delayed [see Chap. 24])
    c. Hypersplenism (see Chap. 28)
    d. Red cell membrane disorders (see Chap. 14)
       (1) Spur cell hemolysis
       (2) Acquired acanthocytosis and acquired stomatocytosis, etc.
    e. Chemical injury and complex chemicals (arsenic, copper, chlorate, spider, scorpion, and snake venoms, etc. [see Chap. 22])
    f. Physical injury (heat, oxygen, radiation [see Chap. 22])
  2. Hereditary
    a. Hemoglobinopathies (see Chap. 17)
       (1) Sickle cell disease
       (2) Unstable hemoglobins
    b. Red cell membrane disorders (see Chap. 14)
       (1) Cytoskeletal membrane disorders (hereditary spherocytosis, elliptocytosis, pyropoikilocytosis)
       (2) Lipid membrane disorders (hereditary abetalipoproteinemia, hereditary stomatocytosis, etc.)
       (3) Membrane disorders associated with abnormalities of erythrocyte antigens (McLeod syndrome, Rh deficiency syndromes, etc.)
       (4) Membrane disorders associated with abnormal transport (hereditary xerocytosis)
    c. Red cell enzyme defects (pyruvate kinase, 5′ nucleotidase, glucose-6-phosphate dehydrogenase deficiencies, other red cell membrane disorders [see Chap. 15])
    d. Porphyrias (congenital erythropoietic and hepatoerythropoietic porphyrias, rarely congenital erythropoietic protoporphyria [see Chap. 30])

  C. Blood loss and blood redistribution
    1. Acute blood loss
    2. Splenic sequestration crisis (see Chap. 28)

II. Relative (increased plasma volume)

  A. Macroglobulinemia (see Chap. 70)
  B. Pregnancy
  C. Athletes (see Chap. 20)
  D. Postflight astronauts

Source: *Williams Hematology*, 8th ed, Chap. 33, Table 33–1, p. 458.

— Reticulocyte count or index to estimate whether marrow response suggests inadequacy of red cell production or an appropriate erythropoietic response to hemolysis (or acute bleeding). The latter is usually readily apparent clinically.
— Examination of the blood film to determine red cell shape, hemoglobin content, presence of red cell inclusions, and accompanying abnormalities of white cells and platelets.
— These five studies should be the prelude to guide further specific testing.
• Important caveats:
— Red cell size and hemoglobin content is best determined from their indices because the blood film will usually make evident only gross deviations (e.g., the need to estimate red cell volume from a two-dimensional area). Moreover, the blood in macrocytic anemia usually contains many microcytic cells

TABLE 2–2	**CLASSIFICATION OF POLYCYTHEMIA**

I. **Absolute (true) polycythemia (increased red cell volume) (see Chap. 29)**
  A. **Primary polycythemias Chap. 29)**
      1. Acquired
          a. Polycythemia vera (see Chap. 43)
          b. Postrenal transplant (probable abnormal angiotensin II signaling)
      2. Hereditary
          a. Primary familial and congenital polycythemia (see Chap. 29)
          b. Unknown gene mutations
  B. **Secondary polycythemias**
      1. Acquired (see Chap. 29)
          a. Chronic lung disease
          b. Sleep apnea
          c. Right-to-left cardiac shunts
          d. High altitude
          e. Smoking
          f. Carboxyhemoglobinemia (see Chap. 19)
          g. Autonomous erythropoietin production (see Chap. 29)
              (1) Hepatocellular carcinoma
              (2) Renal cell carcinoma
              (3) Cerebellar hemangioblastoma
              (4) Pheochromocytoma
              (5) Parathyroid carcinoma
              (6) Meningioma
              (7) Uterine leiomyoma
              (8) Polycystic kidney disease
              (9) Exogenous erythropoietin administration ("EPO doping")
      2. Hereditary
          a. High-oxygen affinity hemoglobins (see Chap. 17)
          b. 2,3-Bisphosphoglycerate deficiency (see Chap. 15)
          c. Congenital methemoglobinemias (recessive, i.e., cytochrome b5 reductase deficiency [see Chap. 19])
  C. **Mixed primary and secondary polycythemia (see Chap. 29)**
      1. Proven or suspected congenital disorders of hypoxia sensing
          a. Chuvash polycythemia and other von Hippel-Lindau gene mutations (see Chap. 29)
          b. HIF-2 α mutations

II. **Relative (spurious) polycythemia (normal red cell volume) (see Chap. 29)**
  A. Dehydration
  B. Diuretics
  C. Smoking
  D. Gaisböck syndrome

Source: *Williams Hematology*, 8th ed, Chap. 33, Table 33–2, p. 461.

and in microcytic anemias, many normocytic cells, which make determination of the average red cell volume from a blood film difficult.

— In general, the abnormalities in size, hemoglobin content, and shape are approximately correlated with severity of anemia. If the anemia is slight, the other changes are often subtle.

— Anemia classically categorized as macrocytic or microcytic may be present in the face of red cell volumes that are in the normal range. This may be the case because the anemia is so mild that red cell volumes have not yet deviated beyond the normal range, or may be the case with more severe anemias because of confounding effects of two causal factors (e.g., iron deficiency and folate deficiency), or for unexplained reasons (e.g., well-established megaloblastic anemia may have normocytic index).

- A classification of the major causes of anemia is shown in Table 2–1.
- A classification of the major causes of polycythemia is shown in Table 2–2.
- Polycythemias are discussed in Chap. 29. It is important to search for the specific cause of polycythemia.

For a more detailed discussion, see Josef T. Prchal: Clinical Manifestations and Classification of Erythrocyte Disorders. Chap. 33, p. 455; Josef T. Prchal: Production of Erythrocytes. Chap. 31, p. 435; Josef T. Prchal: Primary and Secondary Polycythemia (Erythrocytosis). Chap. 56, p. 823; Brian S. Bull and Paul C. Herrmann: Morphology of the Erythron. Chap. 29, p. 409 in *Williams Hematology*, 8th ed.

CHAPTER 3
Aplastic Anemia: Acquired and Inherited

DEFINITION

- Pancytopenia with markedly hypocellular marrow and normal marrow cell cytogenetics.
- Incidence worldwide is 2 to 5 cases/million population per year and 5 to 12 cases/million population per year in the United States (and in other industrialized countries). Incidence is approximately twice as high in Asian countries.
- Peak incidence between ages 15 and 25 and 65 to 69 years.
- The definitions for range of severity of aplastic anemia are shown in Table 3–1.

ETIOLOGY AND PATHOGENESIS

Pathogenesis

- Immune suppression of marrow by autoreactive T lymphocytes.
- Toxic injury to stem and/or progenitor cells (e.g., certain chemotherapy or drugs) (see Table 3–2).
- Inherited intrinsic stem cell defect (e.g., Fanconi anemia).

Etiologic Classification

Acquired

- Acquired T lymphocyte mediated autoimmune suppression of hematopoietic stem cells and/or progenitor cells in most cases (~70%).
- Paroxysmal nocturnal hemoglobinuria (PNH) (frequently associated with hypoplastic marrow).
- Chemicals, e.g., benzene. Rare today in countries with workplace regulations limiting exposure.
- Drugs, e.g., chloramphenicol (see Table 3–2 for most frequent offenders; see also *Williams Hematology*, 8th ed, Chap. 34, Table 34–3, p. 467 for a more complete list).
- Viruses, e.g., Epstein-Barr; non-A,-B,-C,-D,-E, or G hepatitis; HIV.
- Immune and connective tissue diseases: e.g., eosinophilic fasciitis, Hashimoto thyroiditis, Graves disease, systemic lupus erythematosus.
- Pregnancy.
- Iatrogenic or accidental, e.g., intensive radiation to marrow-bearing bones, intensive marrow-suppressive chemotherapy.

Inherited

- Fanconi anemia
  - Autosomal recessive.
  - Any of 13 gene mutations, FANCA through FANCN, account for about 95 percent of cases.
  - Macrocytosis and poikilocytosis may precede cytopenias.
  - Cytopenias, sometimes starting with thrombocytopenia, develop after age 5 to 10 years.
  - Marrow hypocellularity explains cytopenias.

TABLE 3–1 DEGREE OF SEVERITY OF ACQUIRED APLASTIC ANEMIA

Diagnostic Categories	Hemoglobin	Reticulocyte Concentration	Reticulocyte Count	Neutrophil Count	Platelet Count	Marrow Biopsy	Comments
Moderately severe	<100 g/L	<40 × 10⁹/L		<1.5 × 10⁹/L	<50 × 10⁹/L	Decrease of hematopoietic cells.	At the time of diagnosis at least 2 of 3 blood counts should meet these criteria.
Severe	<90 g/L	<30.0 × 10⁹/L		<0.5 × 10⁹/L	<30.0 × 10⁹/L	Marked decrease of hematopoietic cells.	Search for a histocompatible sibling should be made if age permits.
Very Severe	<80 g/L	<20.0 × 10⁹/L		<0.2 × 10⁹/L	<20.0 × 10⁹/L	Marked decrease or absence of hematopoietic cells.	Search for a histocompatible sibling should be made if age permits.

These values are approximations and must be considered in the context of an individual patient's circumstances. (In some clinical trials, the blood count thresholds for moderately severe aplastic anemia are higher, e.g., platelet count <100 × 10⁹/L and absolute reticulocyte count <100 × 10⁹/L.) The marrow biopsy may contain the usual number of lymphocytes and plasma cells; Rare "hot spots," focal areas of erythroid cells, may be seen. No fibrosis, abnormal cells, or malignant cells should be evident in the marrow. Dysmorphic features of blood or marrow cells are not features of acquired aplastic anemia. Ethnic differences in the lower limit of the absolute neutrophil count should be considered (see Chap. 1).

Source: *Williams Hematology*, 8th ed, Chap. 34, Table 34–1, p. 464.

TABLE 3–2	**SOME DRUGS ASSOCIATED WITH MODERATE RISK OF APLASTIC ANEMIA***
Acetazolamide	
Carbamazepine	
Chloramphenicol	
Gold salts	
Hydantoins	
Oxyphenbutazone	
Penicillamine	
Phenylbutazone	
Quinacrine	

*Drugs with 30 or more reported cases.

Source: *Williams Hematology*, 8th ed, Chap. 34, Table 34–3, p. 467.

— Short stature; abnormal skin pigmentation (café-au-lait spots); skeletal abnormalities (e.g., dysplastic radii and thumbs); heart, kidney, and eye anomalies; microcephaly; and hypogonadism in different combinations often noted.

— Chromosome fragility, especially after exposure to DNA cross-linking agents such as diepoxybutane (used as a diagnostic test).

— Androgens occasionally may improve hematopoiesis.

— Allogeneic hematopoietic stem cell transplantation can be curative.

— Risk of acute myelogenous leukemia and other cancers.

• Dyskeratosis congenita

— Autosomal dominant, autosomal recessive, and X-linked inheritance patterns may be present (see *Williams Hematology* 8th ed, Chap. 34, Table 34–9, p. 478).

— Gene mutations identified in 60 percent of cases.

— Mutations involving genes encoding proteins in the telomerase complex.

— Resulting abnormalities in telomere length.

— Mucocutaneous (e.g., skin hyperpigmentation or hypopigmentation, alopecia leukoplakia) and finger and toenail abnormalities (ridging and longitudinal splitting, atrophy) in childhood.

— Pulmonary (e.g., fibrosis), gastrointestinal (e.g., esophageal webs), urogenital (e.g., hypospadius), neurologic (e.g., learning impairment), skeletal (e.g., hypoplasia of mandible) findings.

— Aplastic anemia in early adulthood. Principal cause of death.

— Increased incidence of various mucosal cancers (e.g., squamous cell carcinoma of mouth, nasopharynx, esophagus, rectum, vagina, others).

• Shwachman-Diamond syndrome

— Caused by mutation in *SBDS* gene (Shwachman-Bodian-Diamond syndrome) on chromosome 7.

— Exocrine pancreatic insufficiency and neutropenia. Pancreatic endocrine function (insulin secretion) generally remains intact (see Chap. 33).

— Neutropenia with functionally abnormal neutrophils (defective chemotaxis) present in virtually all patients.

— Anemia and thrombocytopenia less common.

— Elevated hemoglobin F in most patients.

— Pancytopenia in about 20 percent of patients.

— Patients usually present in early infancy with malabsorption; steatorrhea; failure to thrive; and deficiencies of fat-soluble vitamins A, D, E, and K.

— Approximately 50 percent of patients regain exocrine pancreatic function during later childhood.

— Skeletal anomalies are present in about 75 percent of patients. Short stature, osteochondrodysplasia (cartilage and bone anomalies), osteoporosis.

— Recurrent bacterial infections (e.g., upper respiratory tract infections, otitis media, sinusitis, pneumonia, paronychia, osteomyelitis, bacteremia) occur.
— Enzyme replacement therapy for exocrine pancreatic insufficiency.
— Progression to multicytopenia, hypoplastic marrow, myelodysplasia, or acute myelogenous leukemia can occur.
— Allogeneic hematopoietic stem cell transplantation can be curative.

For other rare causes of aplastic anemia see *Williams Hematology* 8th ed, Chap. 34, Table 34–8, p. 477.

CLINICAL FEATURES

- Fatigue, pallor, dyspnea on exertion, bleeding, or infections as a consequence of the cytopenias.
- Physical examination generally is unrevealing except for signs of anemia, bleeding, or infection.

LABORATORY FEATURES

- Pancytopenia.
- Red cells may be macrocytic.
- Markedly hypocellular marrow (see Fig. 3–1).
- Abnormal clonal cytogenetic findings suggest hypoplastic myelodysplastic syndrome (clonal myeloid disease) rather than aplastic anemia.
- Infrequent blast cells in marrow suggest hypoplastic acute myelogenous leukemia.
- Flow cytometry of CD55, CD59 on blood cells to rule out PNH.

Table 3–3 indicates important diagnostic procedures.

DIFFERENTIAL DIAGNOSIS OF PANCYTOPENIA AND HYPOPLASTIC MARROW

- Aplastic anemia.
- Hypoplastic myelodysplastic syndrome or hypoplastic acute myelogenous leukemia.
- PNH.
- Hypoplastic antecedent phase of acute lymphocytic leukemia (especially in children).
- Hypoplastic antecedent of hairy cell leukemia, lymphoma, large granular lymphocytic leukemia (rare).

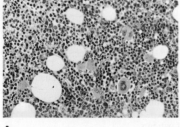 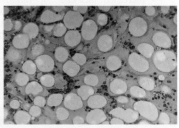

A   **B**

FIGURE 3–1 Marrow biopsy in aplastic anemia. **A.** Normal marrow biopsy section of a young adult. **B.** Marrow biopsy section of a young adult with very severe aplastic anemia. The specimen is devoid of hematopoietic cells and contains only scattered lymphocytes and stromal cells. The hematopoietic space is replaced by reticular cells (pre-adipocytic fibroblasts) converted to adipocytes.
(Source: *Williams Hematology,* 8th ed, Fig. 34–2, p. 472.)

TABLE 3-3 APPROACH TO DIAGNOSIS

- History and physical examination
- Complete blood counts, reticulocyte count, and examination of the blood film
- Marrow aspiration and biopsy
- Marrow cell cytogenetics to evaluate presence of a clonal myeloid disease
- Fetal hemoglobin level and DNA stability test as markers of Fanconi anemia
- Immunophenotyping of red and white cells, especially for CD55, CD59 to exclude PNH
- Coombs test to rule out antibody-mediated, immune multicytopenia (hypercellular marrow expected in this case)
- Serum lactate dehydrogenase (LDH) and uric acid that if increased may reflect neoplastic cell turnover
- Liver function tests to assess evidence of any recent hepatitis virus exposure
- Screening tests for hepatitis viruses A, B, and C
- Screening tests for EBV, cytomegalovirus (CMV), and HIV
- Serum B_{12} and red cell folic acid levels to rule out megaloblastic pancytopenia (hypercellular marrow expected in this case)
- Serum iron, iron-binding capacity, and ferritin as a baseline prior to chronic transfusion therapy

Source: *Williams Hematology*, 8th ed, Chap. 34, Table 34–4, p. 469.

TREATMENT

Table 3–4 lists important initial steps in management.
- Allogeneic hematopoietic stem cell transplantation is often curative.
- Indicated in patients < 55 years with a suitable donor and without serious comorbid conditions. Age for transplantation may increase with advances in transplantation.
- Less than one-third of patients in United States have a matched sibling donor.
- Success of transplantation is a function of age and whether related donor is used. Best results in patients < 20 years with a related donor.

Immunosuppressive Therapy
- Is the most successful therapy in patients unsuitable for allogeneic hematopoietic stem cell transplantation.
- Antithymocyte globulin (ATG) or antilymphocyte globulin (ALG)
  — ATG prepared in horses or rabbits from human thymocytes and ALG prepared in horses or rabbits from human thoracic duct lymphocytes.
  — Fifty percent response rate when used as single agent.
  — Dose: 15 to 40 mg/kg daily intravenously for 4 to 10 days.
  — Fever, chills common on first day of treatment.
  — Accelerated platelet destruction with thrombocytopenia frequent.
  — Serum sickness can occur with fever, rash, and arthralgias 7 to 10 days after beginning treatment.
  — Moderate dose of methylprednisolone is usually used to decrease allergic reactions.
- Cyclosporine
  — Treatment in patients if refractory to ATG.
  — Dose: 3 to 7 mg/kg daily orally for at least 4 to 6 months.
  — Dose adjusted to maintain appropriate blood levels (trough blood levels of 300 to 500 ng/mL).
  — Renal impairment is common side effect.
  — Twenty-five percent of patients respond overall.

TABLE 3–4	**INITIAL MANAGEMENT OF APLASTIC ANEMIA**

- Discontinue any potential offending drug and use an alternative class of agents if essential.
- Anemia: transfusion of leukocyte-depleted, irradiated red cells as required for very severe anemia.
- Very severe thrombocytopenia or thrombocytopenic bleeding: consider ϵ-aminocaproic acid or tranexamic acid; transfusion of platelets as required; thrombopoietin receptor agonists under study.
- Severe neutropenia; use infection precautions; granulocyte-colony stimulating factor usually ineffective.
- Fever (suspected infection): microbial cultures; broad-spectrum antibiotics if specific organism not identified, granulocyte colony-stimulating factor (G-CSF) in dire cases. If child or small adult with profound and prolonged infection (e.g., gram-negative bacteria, fungus, persistent positive blood cultures) can consider neutrophil transfusion from a G-CSF pretreated donor.
- Immediate assessment for allogeneic stem cell transplantation: Histocompatibility testing of patient, parents, and siblings. Search databases for unrelated donor, if appropriate (see Chap. 40).

Source: *Williams Hematology*, 8th ed, Chap. 34, Table 34–5, p. 471.

- High-dose glucocorticoids
  — For example, 5 to 10 mg/kg methylprednisolone for 3 to 14 days.
  — Very severe side effects: glycosuria, gastric distress, insomnia, psychosis, infection, aseptic necrosis of the femoral head.
  — Little evidence for efficacy of glucocorticoids used alone.
  — Usually used in lower doses (2 mg/kg and then taper) as adjunct to ATG.
- High-dose cyclophosphamide (e.g., 45 mg/kg per day for 4 doses).
- Androgen therapy
  — Danazol, 5 mg/kg per day for 6 months, as primary therapy has not been efficacious in severe or moderate aplastic anemia.
  — Androgen therapy combined with ALG and cyclosporine is being assessed.
  — Androgens can induce severe masculinization and liver damage.
- G-CSF as primary therapy not efficacious.
  — Transient improvement in neutrophil counts has been observed with GM-CSF or — G-CSF treatment in some patients but not sustained.
  — G-CSF used in combined therapy with ATG and cyclosporine has not improved remission or survival rates in most studies.
- IL-3 or IL-1 is not effective as primary treatment.
- Combination therapy: ATG and cyclosporine yield an improved response rate over either alone.
- Results of immunosuppressive therapy
  — Sixty to 80 percent of patients get marked hematologic improvement.
  — Long-term problems after immunosuppressive therapy may occur, such as continued moderate anemia and thrombocytopenia, recurrent aplasia, PNH, acute myelogenous leukemia, or myelodysplastic syndrome.

Supportive Care
- Immediate HLA typing of patient and siblings as possible stem cell donors.
- Minimal or no transfusions in potential transplant recipients, if possible.
- If transfusions are needed, do not use family donors in a potential transplant recipient.
- Transfuse platelets based on assessment of risk of bleeding and not solely on platelet count.

- Leukocyte-depleted, ABO blood group-compatible single-donor platelets should be used, if possible, to minimize HLA sensitization, subsequent refractoriness, and other problems.
- ε-Aminocaproic acid, 4 to 12 g/d, may decrease thrombocytopenic bleeding.
- Transfuse packed RBCs (irradiated, leukocyte-depleted) when hemoglobin level is less than 8 g/dL. Use a higher threshold if comorbid conditions require.
- Obtain CMV serology for prospective transplant recipients; transfuse only CMV-negative blood products until these results are known. If the patient is CMV-positive, can discontinue these precautions. Use of leukocyte depletion filters also decreases risk of CMV acquisition.
- Neutropenic precautions for hospitalized patients with absolute neutrophil counts of less than 500/μL.
- Prompt institution of broad-spectrum intravenous antibiotics for fever after appropriate cultures have been obtained.

CLINICAL COURSE

- Median survival of untreated severe aplastic anemia is 3 to 6 months (20% survive longer than 1 year). Allogeneic hematopoietic transplantation can cure a very large proportion of patients depending on their age at transplantation and the immunologic similarity of the donor (see Figure 3–2). Combined immunotherapy with ATG and cyclosporine can result in 10-year survival rate of 70 to 80 percent.

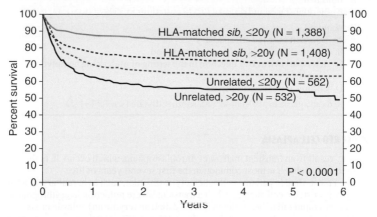

FIGURE 3-2 Probability of survival after hematopoietic stem cell transplantation for severe aplastic anemia by donor type and age, 1998–2008. Patients receiving marrow from a matched sibling had better outcomes if they were equal to or less than 20 years of age, compared to those older than 20 years of age. Patients receiving marrow from a matched sibling fared better than those who received marrow from a matched unrelated donor, at any age. Patients younger than 20 or older than 20 years of age did not have a significant difference in outcome if they received marrow from an unrelated matched donor. *sib*, sibling.

(Reproduced with permission from the Center for International Transplant Research data on the National Marrow Donor Program website. http://www.marrow.org/PATIENT/Undrstnd_Disease_Treat/Lrn_about_Disease/Aplastic_Anemia/AA_Tx_Outcomes/index.html.)

(Source: *Williams Hematology*, 8th ed, Fig. 34–3, p. 472.)

For a more detailed discussion, see George B. Segel and Marshall A. Lichtman: Aplastic Anemia: Acquired and Inherited. Chapter 34, p. 463 in *Williams Hematology*, 8th ed.

CHAPTER 4
Pure Red Cell Aplasia

DEFINITION

- *Pure red cell aplasia* describes anemia caused by an isolated depletion of erythroblasts characterized by severe reticulocytopenia and absent or markedly diminished marrow erythroid progenitors (erythroblasts).

CLASSIFICATION

- See Table 4–1.

TABLE 4–1	CLASSIFICATION OF PURE ERYTHROID APLASIA

I. Fetal Red Cell Aplasia (non-immune hydrops fetalis, parvovirus 19 infection *in utero*)

II. Inherited
   A. Blackfan-Diamond disease (*RPS19* mutations in 25% of cases)

III. Acquired
   A. Transient pure red cell aplasia
   B. Transient erythroblastopenia of childhood
   C. Acute parvovirus B19 infection in the setting of underlying hemolytic anemia
   D. Chronic pure red cell aplasia

IV. Red cell aplasia in association with another disease (see Table 4–3)

ACUTE RED CELL APLASIA

- May result from transient marrow erythroblastopenia, which occurs in both children and adults. It is most common in the first several years of life.
- Seen most often in patients with a hemolytic disorder, such as hereditary spherocytosis or sickle cell anemia, when a transient severe reduction in erythropoiesis causes a rapid fall in hemoglobin level—called an (erythroid) aplastic crisis.
- May also be seen in patients who are hematologically normal.
- True prevalence is unknown, and it is assumed that many mild cases are not detected.

Etiology

- Most patients with aplastic crises are infected with B19 parvovirus, but occasionally another viral infection may be responsible.
- IgG inhibitors of erythroid colony formation *in vitro* have been found in some patients with a condition called transient erythroblastopenia of childhood.
- Drugs may induce aplastic crises, either by an immunologic mechanism or by direct toxicity. Commonly implicated drugs are listed in Table 4–2.

Clinical Features

- Frequently, the patient has had a recent febrile illness, often with upper respiratory symptoms, gastrointestinal symptoms, or headache.
- Listlessness, increasing pallor, and tachycardia are characteristic.
- Usually no other significant changes are found on physical examination.

TABLE 4–2	**SOME DRUGS ASSOCIATED WITH THE DEVELOPMENT OF ERYTHROID APLASTIC CRISIS**

Generic Name
Alpha-Methyldopa (Aldomet)
Azathioprine
Aztreonam
Sulfobromophthalein sodium (bromsulphthalein)
Carbamazepine
Cephalothin
Chloramphenicol
Chlorpropamide
Co-trimoxazole
D-Penicillamine
Diphenylhydantoin
Fenoprofen
Lindane (gamma benzene hexachloride)
Gold
Indomethacin
Isoniazid
Dapsone
Methazolamide
Pentachlorophenol
Procainamide
Rifampicin
Sulfasalazine
Thiamphenicol
Valproic acid

Laboratory Features

- Evidence of an underlying hematologic disorder, such as hereditary spherocytosis or sickle cell anemia, may be present.
- Anemia and reticulocytopenia are characteristic. They are often severe.
- Granulocyte and platelet counts are usually normal.
- Erythroid cells are depleted in the marrow early in the illness, but reappear just before recovery; thus, if the marrow is tested during recovery, the erythroblastopenia may be missed.
- Reticulocytosis is the first sign of recovery, and some nucleated red cells may appear in the blood.
- Serum iron levels are high and serum iron-binding capacity is saturated during the aplastic phase because of markedly decreased iron utilization for erythropoiesis. Serum iron levels fall during recovery.

Differential Diagnosis

- Reduction in hemoglobin level with reticulocytopenia distinguishes red cell aplasia from acute bleeding in which reticulocyte count is mildly elevated and bleeding often apparent.

- Absence of involvement of neutrophils, monocytes, and platelets differentiates these disorders from aplastic anemia.
- Transient erythroblastopenia of childhood is differentiated from chronic forms of red cell aplasia by rapid recovery (days to weeks).

Therapy, Course, and Prognosis
- Discontinuation of potentially offending drugs when possible. Restitution of hematopoiesis may follow rapidly.
- Treatment of any associated illnesses.
- Maintenance of hemoglobin level by transfusion, as necessary.
- Recovery occurs spontaneously in days or weeks as neutralizing antibodies to B19 parvovirus ensues unless a chronic immunodeficiency state is present.

INHERITED PURE RED CELL APLASIA

- A form of pure red cell aplasia occurring early in childhood. Also known as the Diamond-Blackfan syndrome.
- Familial occurrence. Usually autosomal dominant or occasionally autosomal recessive inheritance if familial pattern. Sporadic cases are most frequent.
- A disease of abnormal ribosomal biogenesis. Mutations involve the *RPS19* gene in about 25 percent of cases; several other genes that regulate ribosome assembly have been implicated.
- The pathophysiology that leads to an isolated failure of erythropoiesis from ribosomal assembly abnormalities is unclear.

Clinical Features
- One-third of patients are diagnosed at birth or in the early neonatal period, but the disease may appear at any time into adulthood.
- Physical abnormalities occur in one-third of patients (e.g., craniofacial dysmorphism, short stature, abnormalities of the thumb, web-neck and urogenital and cardiac abnormalities).
- Onset in infancy with pallor, listlessness, poor appetite, failure to thrive.
- May progress to severe anemia, with cardiac failure, dyspnea, and hepatosplenomegaly.
- Signs of iron overload or glucocorticoid excess may develop after treatment with transfusions or prednisone, respectively.

Laboratory Features
- Normocytic, occasionally macrocytic, normochromic anemia.
- Leukocyte count is normal or slightly decreased. Neutropenia may develop over several years.
- Absolute severe reticulocytopenia in all cases.
- Platelet count is normal or mildly increased.
- Marrow is cellular but with marked erythroid hypoplasia. The few erythroid cells present may have megaloblastic changes. Other marrow cells are normal.
- Serum iron levels are elevated, and transferrin saturation is increased.
- In most cases, the fetal hemoglobin level is elevated, the density of i antigen on the erythrocyte surface is increased, and erythrocyte adenosine deaminase activity is elevated.
- Erythropoietin levels are elevated.

Differential Diagnosis
- Reticulocytopenia and the absence of erythroblasts in an otherwise normal marrow are characteristic of this disorder.
- Acute red cell aplasia is characterized by sudden onset and prompt resolution and is not characterized by dysmorphic physical findings.

Therapy, Course, and Prognosis

- Transfusions relieve symptoms of anemia but can lead to iron overload. Iron chelation therapy should be initiated promptly (see Chap. 19).
- Glucocorticoid therapy may be beneficial, although its mechanism of action is unclear.
- Glucocorticoid therapy should be initiated with prednisone at a daily dose of 1 to 2 mg/kg per day, orally, in two divided doses, than once each day, than once every other day, if feasible. A response is usually seen within 4 weeks. Initial dose is reduced very slowly to a maintenance level when the hemoglobin concentration exceeds 90 g/L. The goal is to get to low, alternate day therapy. Withdrawal of glucocorticoids is often, but not always, accompanied by relapse. Therapy should be continued for 4 to 6 weeks if no response occurs sooner. A trial of high doses of methylprednisolone may then be considered.
- Continuous glucocorticoid therapy is often required, and severe side effects frequently develop (e.g., Cushing syndrome). Long-term transfusions with iron chelation may be preferable to long-term higher dose glucocorticoids and resultant side effects.
- Allogeneic hematopoietic stem cell transplantation from a histocompatible sibling has been used but usually late in the disease. Timing is a function of balancing the serious side effects of therapy against the risk of stem cell transplantation.
- High-dose methylprednisolone, immunosuppressive agents, and IL-3 have been reported to ameliorate the disease but are not standard therapies.
- Most deaths are a result of therapeutic complications, such as chronic iron-overload, hypercorticism, or unsuccessful stem cell transplantation.
- Patients have developed acute myelogenous leukemia at a higher rate than expected.

ACQUIRED CHRONIC PURE RED CELL APLASIA

- An uncommon disorder of adults characterized by markedly diminished red cell production.
- May be associated with thymoma, but the true prevalence of this combination is unknown, and it appears to be less common than believed previously.
- May also be found in association with other diseases, such as chronic lymphocytic leukemia or large granular lymphocytic leukemia. See Table 4–3.
- An antibody or cellular immune mechanism is believed responsible in about one-half of patients. Persistent B19 parvovirus infection may be responsible in some immunocompromised patients.

Clinical Features

- Pallor, lassitude, and other signs and symptoms of anemia are usual.
- Side effects of multiple transfusions and prolonged glucocorticoid therapy can lead to additional clinical findings.
- May occur in the absence of an underlying disease.
- Coexisting immune (e.g., systemic lupus erythematosus) or clonal lymphoid disorder (chronic lymphocytic leukemia) is frequent.

Laboratory Features

- Blood shows normochromic, normocytic or macrocytic anemia with severe reticulocytopenia and a normal leukocyte and platelet count.
- The marrow is normocellular, with normal granulocytes and megakaryocytes, but with severe erythroid hypoplasia or aplasia.
- The serum iron level is elevated, and the iron-binding capacity almost fully saturated.
- The disorder is frequently associated with serum antibodies, such as antinuclear antibodies, cold and warm hemagglutinins, and heterophile antibodies.

TABLE 4–3	SOME DISEASES ASSOCIATED WITH OCCURRENCE OF PURE RED CELL APLASIA

I. Immune disorders
  A. Myasthenia gravis
  B. Autoimmune polyglandular syndrome
  C. Autoimmune hemolytic anemia
  D. Acquired hypogammaglobulinemia
  E. Anti-erythropoietin antibodies

II. Collagen vascular diseases
  A. Systemic lupus erythematosus
  B. Rheumatoid arthritis

III. Clonal lymphoid disorders
  A. Chronic lymphocytic leukemia
  B. Large granular lymphocytic leukemia
  C. Hodgkin lymphoma
  D. Thymoma

IV. Persistent B19 parvovirus in immune deficient individuals

V. Posthematopoietic stem cell transplantation (anti-ABO antibodies)

VI. Drug-induced (see Table 4–2)

VII. Pregnancy

VIII. 5q-syndrome (myelodysplasia)

- Thymic enlargement, if present, may be detected as an anterior mediastinal mass on routine chest films. If not, computed tomography may be required to determine if a thymoma is present (uncommon, perhaps 5% to 10% of patients).

Differential Diagnosis
- The disorder is suggested by evidence of isolated marked erythroid hypoplasia. In some cases, nuclear abnormalities in myeloid and platelet precursors may raise the possibility of a myelodysplastic syndrome.

Therapy, Course, and Prognosis
- Red cell transfusion can be used to prevent or treat symptoms of anemia, but iron overload is a predictable complication, and acquired red cell antibodies often make it difficult to obtain compatible blood and this diminishes the effectiveness of transfusion. Two units of red cells every 2 weeks may keep nadir hemoglobin above 70 g/L. Higher nadir may be required if comorbidities exist.
- Erythropoietin administration is sometimes of benefit.
- Thymectomy should be considered if thymic enlargement (thymoma) is present or evidence of invasiveness.
- Glucocorticoids may be effective in low doses for long-term maintenance, but often large doses are required for protracted periods, with consequent severe side effects.
- Cyclosporine has been used successfully.
- Daclizumab, a monoclonal antibody against the IL-2 receptor, has been effective in a significant proportion of cases.
- Immunosuppressive drugs, such as cyclophosphamide, 6-mercaptopurine, fludarabine, or cladrabine may induce a partial or very good response, obviating a transfusion requirement.
- Intravenous gamma globulin has also been effective and may eradicate B19 parvovirus infection in some patients.

- Antithymocyte and antilymphocyte sera have also been used successfully.
- Plasmapheresis may be helpful.
- With current therapy, about 50 percent of patients enter remission.
- The very low incidence of acquired red cell aplasia has made clinical trials difficult, so therapy is based on sequential trials of agents.
- Median survival of patients with idiopathic disease is greater than 10 years and a normal life expectancy can be achieved. Common causes of death have been iron overload (now decreased in frequency by good iron chelator options) and glucocorticoid-induced hemorrhage or infection (now decreased in frequency by alternative therapeutic options).

For a more detailed discussion, see Neal S. Young: Pure Red Cell Aplasia, Chap. 35, p. 485 in *Williams Hematology*, 8th ed.

CHAPTER 5
Anemia of Chronic Renal Disease

ETIOLOGY AND PATHOGENESIS

- Reduced production of erythropoietin (EPO) is the most significant factor in the development of anemia in renal insufficiency.
- A modest reduction in red cell life span occurs in uremia, probably as a result of metabolic impairment of red cells.
- Iron deficiency occurs from blood loss in dialysis tubing, laboratory testing, or external bleeding, sometimes as a result of uremia-induced platelet dysfunction. Further, increased hepcidin blocks iron absorption in the gut and iron release from macrophage stores (ameliorated by EPO therapy).
- The plasma volume varies widely in renal failure, with consequent variations in the hemoglobin concentration.

CLINICAL AND LABORATORY FEATURES

- The anemia is normocytic and normochromic with a reduced number of reticulocytes relative to the degree of anemia (result of EPO deficiency). Gastrointestinal and gynecologic bleeding occurs in one-third to one-half of all patients with chronic renal failure.
- Acanthocytes or schistocytes may be seen on the blood film.
- Total and differential leukocyte count and platelet count are usually normal.
- Platelet function is abnormal, in relationship to the degree of uremia and effectiveness of dialysis. Dialysis corrects, and EPO-therapy and or red cell transfusions ameliorate both the laboratory and clinical manifestations of abnormal platelet function.
- Cellularity and blood cell maturation sequences in the marrow are normal. Despite the anemia, there is no erythroid hyperplasia.

THERAPY, COURSE, AND PROGNOSIS

- Replacement therapy with EPO corrects the anemia in nearly all patients. Amelioration of the anemia improves the quality of life for uremic patients and leads to a decrease in bleeding time and to favorable endocrine changes.
- EPO is usually given intravenously in dialysis patients. A target hemoglobin level of 11 to 12 g/dL is recommended.
- Adequate iron and folate supply should be maintained to achieve an optimal response with EPO therapy.
- Long-acting preparations (darbepoietin) given subcutaneously may be more convenient for patients not undergoing dialysis because no peaks are observed and plasma levels are lower but more sustained.
- The National Kidney Foundation recommends subcutaneous EPO administration as the preferred route and, if needed, intravenous (rather than oral) iron supplementation to optimize response.
- Complications of EPO therapy include hypertension, seizures, and thrombosis of shunts; hemoglobin levels of >12 g/dL should be avoided. Blood pressure should be carefully monitored throughout the treatment.
- A small number of patients do not respond to EPO, most often because of iron deficiency but also because of aluminum toxicity or marrow fibrosis secondary to hyperparathyroidism or other causes (see Table 5–1). Common causes of EPO hyporesponsiveness are listed in Table 5–1.

TABLE 5–1	**COMMON CAUSES OF ERYTHROPOIETIN HYPORESPONSIVENESS**
Infection	
Cancer, administration of chemotherapy or radiotherapy	
Severe secondary hyperparathyroidism	
Iron deficiency	
Folate deficiency	
Sickle cell anemia	
Thalassemia	
Other hemolytic anemia	
Myelodysplastic syndrome	

Source: *Williams Hematology*, 8th ed, Chap. 36, Table 36–1, p. 500.

For a more detailed discussion, see Jaime Caro and Ubaldo Martinez Outschoorn: Anemia of Chronic Renal Disease. Chap. 36, p. 495 in Williams Hematology, 8th ed.

CHAPTER 6
Anemia of Endocrine Disorders

- Anemia due to endocrine disease is generally mild to moderate; however, a decreased plasma volume in some of these disorders may mask the severity of the decrease in red cell mass.
- The pathophysiologic basis of the anemia seen in endocrine disorders is often not fully understood.

THYROID DYSFUNCTION

- Anemia in hypothyroidism may be normocytic, macrocytic, or microcytic; coexisting deficiencies of iron, B_{12}, and folate may explain some of this heterogeneity.
- Iron deficiency often occurs in hypothyroidism as a result of increased predisposition to menorrhagia, an associated achlorhydria, or because a deficit of thyroid hormone may decrease iron absorption.
- In patients with coexisting iron-deficiency anemia and subclinical hypothyroidism, the anemia often does not adequately respond to oral iron therapy. Many cases of hypothyroidism and all cases of pernicious anemia are autoimmune states and the concurrence may reflect a type of autoimmune polyendocrine state.
- Anemia is also a direct consequence of thyroid hormone deficiency; thyroid hormones have been shown to potentiate the effect of erythropoietin on erythroid colony formation.
- Patients with hyperthyroidism have increased red cell mass but the hematocrit and hemoglobin concentration are usually not elevated because the plasma volume is also increased.
- Autoimmune hemolytic anemia and pancytopenia responsive to treatment of hyperthyroidism have also been reported.

ADRENAL INSUFFICIENCY AND CUSHING SYNDROME

- A normocytic normochromic anemia may be seen in primary adrenal insufficiency (Addison disease) but the anemia (decrease in red cell mass) is not reflected in the hematocrit or hemoglobin measurements because of a concomitant reduction in plasma volume.
- The pathophysiologic basis of the anemia and any influence of adrenal cortical hormones on erythropoiesis are not well defined.
- Some patients with Addison disease develop a transient fall in hematocrit and hemoglobin concentration after initiation of hormone replacement therapy (presumably secondary to an increased plasma volume).
- Polycythemia has been reported in Cushing syndrome, primary aldosteronism, Bartter syndrome, and congenital adrenal hyperplasia secondary to 21--hydroxylase deficiency.
- Pernicious anemia occurs in patients with autoimmune adrenal insufficiency, but is seen primarily in patients with type I polyglandular autoimmune syndrome, whose other manifestations include mucocutaneous candidiasis and hypoparathyroidism.

ANDROGEN DEFICIENCY

- Decrease in androgen production due to orchiectomy or medical androgen blockade causes anemia.

- Androgen therapy has been used for the treatment of various anemias, especially before the development of recombinant erythropoietin; in some patients, polycythemia can ensue and promptly subsides with discontinuation of androgen therapy.
- The mechanism of androgen action appears to be complex, with evidence for stimulation of erythropoietin secretion and a direct effect on the marrow erythroid progenitors.
- Estrogens in large doses cause moderately severe anemia by a mechanism not clearly defined.

PITUITARY INSUFFICIENCY

- Hypopituitarism results in a moderately severe normochromic normocytic anemia, with an average hemoglobin of 10 g/dL.
- Anemia of hypopituitarism results from the absence of the anterior lobe hormones, adrenocorticotropic hormone, thyroid-stimulating hormone, folliclestimulating hormone, luteinizing hormone, growth hormone, and prolactin; the resulting deficiencies of thyroid hormones, adrenal hormones and androgens are likely the major contributors to anemia.
- Red cell survival is normal in hypopituitarism, but the marrow is hypoplastic.
- In addition to anemia, leukopenia or pancytopenia can occur.
- Replacement therapy with a combination of thyroid, adrenal, and gonadal hormones usually corrects the anemia and other cytopenias.
- Erythropoietin therapy may be effective in postoperative hypopituitarism refractory to hormone replacement therapy.

HYPERPARATHYROIDISM

- A normochromic and normocytic anemia not attributable to other causes is present in 3 to 5 percent of patients with primary hyperparathyroidism.
- The cause of the anemia is unknown, but marrow fibrosis has been described in a few patients.
- Secondary hyperparathyroidism in patients with renal failure may contribute to refractoriness to erythropoietin therapy.

 For a more detailed discussion see Xylina T. Gregg and Josef T. Prchal: Anemia of Endocrine Disorders. Chap. 38, p. 509 in *Williams Hematology*, 8th ed.

CHAPTER 7
Congenital Dyserythropoietic Anemias

- Congenital dyserythropoietic anemias (CDA) are a heterogeneous group of disorders characterized by anemia, the presence of multinuclear erythroid precursors in the marrow, ineffective erythropoiesis, and iron overload.
- Although rare, uncovering the molecular basis of CDA has helped unravel novel aspects of the cell biology of erythropoiesis.
- Three types of CDA have been distinguished. In addition, a number of patients with forms of congenital dyserythropoietic anemia that do not fit these categories have been described.

CDA TYPE I

Clinical and Laboratory Features

- Presents in infancy or adolescence.
- Autosomal recessive inheritance, caused by mutations of the *CDAN1* gene (codanin-1), encoding a cell-cycle-regulated protein of yet unknown function; homozygosity is often associated with consanguinity. In a number of patients, only one *CDAN1* allele is identified with a mutation; other causative genes suspected because in rare CDA I families, no mutations of the *CDAN1* gene found.
- Moderately severe macrocytic anemia (approximately 9.0 g/dL).
- Hepatomegaly and cholelithiasis are common.
- Splenomegaly increases with age.
- Specific morphologic findings of CDA type I are summarized in Table 7–1 and exemplified in Fig. 7–1.
- Dysmorphologic features may be present, the most common involve the bones of the hand and the foot. Other, less common features are small stature, almond-shaped blue eyes, hypertelorism (increased distance between two body parts or organs), and micrognathism.

Differential Diagnosis

- May be confused with the thalassemia syndromes because of similar blood findings and evidence of ineffective erythropoiesis.
- Megaloblastoid marrow findings may suggest folic acid or vitamin B_{12} deficiency.

Treatment

- Severe forms may present with hydrops fetalis. In some cases, intrauterine red cell transfusions are warranted by the severity of the anemia.
- Red cell transfusions for long-term therapy should be avoided whenever possible because of the risk of iron overload.
- In compensated moderate anemia, small volume, regular phlebotomies, if tolerable, or chelating agents may be beneficial for iron overload.

CDA TYPE II (HEMPAS)

- Type II CDA is also known by its acronym HEMPAS for *H*ereditary *E*rythroblastic *M*ultinuclearity associated with a *P*ositive *A*cidified *S*erum test.

TABLE 7–1   MAIN FEATURES OF TYPES I, II, AND III CONGENITAL DYSERYTHROPOIETIC ANEMIAS

CDA Type	Light Microscopy	Electron Microscopy	Serology	Inheritance
I	Most erythroid cells abnormal: double nuclei, internuclear chromatin bridges (Fig. 7–1)	Widened nuclear pores, spongy appearance of the heterochromatin, invasion by the cytoplasm containing various organelles	No serologic abnormalities	Autosomal recessive
II	Mature stage erythroblasts with two or more nuclei, lobulated nuclei, karyorrhexis, pseudo-Gaucher cells (Fig. 7–1)	Endoplasmic reticulum cisternae lining the inner surface of the red cell plasma membrane	Cells containing the HEMPAS antigen are lysed by 30% of acidified normal sera; strong reactivity with anti-"i" autoantibodies	Autosomal recessive
III	Giant erythroblasts, up to 50 μm in diameter, with up to 12 nuclei, basophilic stippling	Clefts and blebs within nuclear areas, some iron-filled mitochondria, autophagic vacuoles and myelin figures in the cytoplasm	No clearly defined abnormalities	Autosomal dominant (not all cases)

Source: *Williams Hematology*, 8th ed, Chap. 39, Table 39–1, p. 514.

Clinical and Laboratory Features

- Autosomal recessive inheritance, due to mutations in *SEC23B*, the gene encoding a protein component of the coat protein complex II (COPII). COPII is responsible for the biogenesis of endoplasmic reticulum-derived vesicles destined for the *cis*-Golgi compartment. These protein complexes are thought to be the primary determinants underlying deformation of membranes into vesicles.
- Anemia varies from mild to severe.
- Moderate-to-marked anisocytosis and poikilocytosis, anisochromia, and contracted spherocytes are present in the blood film. Gaucher-like cells and ring sideroblasts may be present in the marrow (Table 7–1). Multinuclearity of red cell precursors is a morphologic hallmark (Fig. 7–1).
- Body iron stores are increased and frank hemochromatosis may occur even in the absence of transfusions.

Treatment

- Red cell transfusions may be necessary; iron chelation should be instituted when the ferritin level exceeds 500 to 1000 μg/L.
- Partial benefit may be obtained with splenectomy.
- Marrow transplantation has been used in few patients.

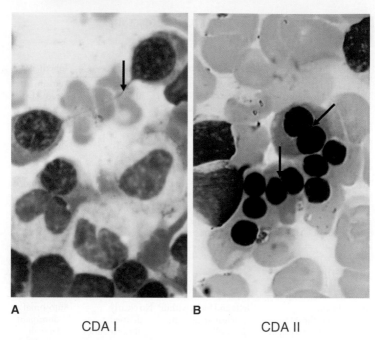

A   B

CDA I   CDA II

FIGURE 7-1 Light microscopy of marrow. **A.** Congenital dyserythropietic anemia type I. Note the intranuclear chromatin bridge marked by an arrow. This bridge is unusually long. **B.** Congenital dyserythropietic anemia type II. The two arrows point to binucleate erythroblasts, characteristic of this type. (Used with permission from Dr. Odile Fenneteau.)
(Source: *Williams Hematology*, 8th ed, Chap. 39, Fig. 39–2, p. 515.)

CDA TYPE III

Clinical and Laboratory Features

- Autosomal dominant inheritance due to an as yet unidentified mutation that maps to chromosome 15q22-25.
- Most patients are asymptomatic with mild to moderate anemia, mild jaundice and, commonly, cholelithiasis.
- Some macrocytes may be extremely large ("gigantocytes"), and poikilocytes are present; the marrow has marked erythroid hyperplasia, with large multinucleate erythroblasts with big lobulated nuclei, and giant multinucleate erythroblasts (Table 7–1).

Treatment

- Generally, none is needed. One symptomatic patient benefited from splenectomy.

For a more detailed discussion, see Jean Delaunay: The Congenital Dyserythropoietic Anemias. Chap. 39, p. 513 in *Williams Hematology*, 8th ed.

CHAPTER 8
The Megaloblastic Anemias

DEFINITION

- Disorders caused by impaired synthesis of DNA.
- Prototype is pernicious anemia, a deficiency of vitamin B_{12} (cobalamin) caused by lack of intrinsic factor, required for its absorption.
- Characteristics are megaloblastic cells, typically present in the erythroid series as large cells with immature-appearing nuclei but with increasing hemoglobinization of the cytoplasm—often referred to as *nuclear-cytoplasmic asynchrony*.
- Megaloblastic granulocytic cells have large size, giant band neutrophils are a feature in the marrow and hypersegmented neutrophils in the marrow and blood. Megakaryocytes may be abnormally large with nuclear abnormalities.
- Other rapidly dividing tissue cells, such as intestinal epithelium and uterine cervical epithelium may also show cytologic abnormalities. A uterine cervical smear when megaloblastic cytopoiesis is present may be strikingly dysplastic.

ETIOLOGY AND PATHOGENESIS

- Table 8–1 lists causes of megaloblastic anemia.
- Underlying defect is impaired DNA synthesis because of failure of conversion of dUMP to dTMP.
- Intramedullary destruction of red cell precursors (*ineffective erythropoiesis*) is a major feature of megaloblastic anemia. Ineffective granulopoiesis and thrombopoiesis are also present and can result in neutropenia and thrombocytopenia. Ineffective hematopoiesis is characterized by marked hyperplasia of precursor cells (hypercellular marrow) but exaggerated apoptosis of late precursors, which results in blood cytopenias.
- Mild hemolysis also occurs; the red cell life span is reduced by about 40 percent.

TABLE 8–1 **CAUSES OF MEGALOBLASTIC ANEMIAS**

I. Folate Deficiency
   A. Decreased intake
      1. Poor nutrition
      2. Old age, poverty, alcoholism
      3. Hyperalimentation
      4. Hemodialysis
      5. Premature infants
      6. Spinal cord injury
      7. Children on synthetic diets
      8. Goat's milk anemia
   B. Impaired absorption
      1. Nontropical sprue
      2. Tropical sprue
      3. Other disease of the small intestine
   C. Increased requirements
      1. Pregnancy
      2. Increased cell turnover
      3. Chronic hemolytic anemia
      4. Exfoliative dermatitis

(continued)

TABLE 8–1 **(CONTINUED)**

II. Cobalamin Deficiency

  A. Impaired absorption
1. Gastric causes
2. Pernicious anemia
3. Gastrectomy
4. Zollinger-Ellison syndrome
5. Intestinal causes
    a. Ileal resection or disease
    b. Blind loop syndrome
    c. Fish tapeworm
6. Pancreatic insufficiency

  B. Decreased intake
1. Vegans

III. Acute Megaloblastic Anemia

  A. Nitrous oxide exposure

  B. Severe illness with
1. Extensive transfusion
2. Dialysis
3. Total parenteral nutrition

IV. Drugs

  A. Dihydrofolate reductase inhibitors

  B. Antimetabolites

  C. Inhibitors of deoxynucleotide synthesis

  D. Anticonvulsants

  E. Oral contraceptives

  F. Others

V. Inborn errors

  A. Cobalamin deficiency
1. Imerslund-Graesbeck disease
2. Congenital deficiency of intrinsic factor
3. Transcobalamin deficiency

  B. Errors of cobalamin metabolism
1. "Cobalamin mutant" syndromes with homocystinuria and/or methylmalonic acidemia

  C. Errors of folate metabolism
1. Congenital folate malabsorption
2. Dihydrofolate reductase deficiency
3. N^5-methyl FH$_4$ homocysteine-methyltransferase deficiency

  D. Other errors
1. Hereditary orotic aciduria
2. Lesch-Nyhan syndrome
3. Thiamine-responsive megaloblastic anemia

VI. Unexplained

  A. Congenital dyserythropoietic anemia

  B. Refractory megaloblastic anemia

  C. Erythroleukemia

Source: *Williams Hematology,* 8th ed, Chap. 41, Table 41–5, p. 545.

CLINICAL FEATURES

- Anemia develops gradually and patients can adapt to very low hemoglobin levels. Eventually, as it progresses, the presenting symptoms are those of anemia with weakness, palpitation, fatigue, light-headedness, and shortness of breath.
- May present initially with neurologic manifestations without anemia.
- Folic acid deficiency and cobalamin deficiency have indistinguishable blood and marrow changes (megaloblastosis), but the former deficiency is not associated with neuropathology and the latter characteristically is (see below "*Pernicious Anemia*").

LABORATORY FEATURES

- Erythrocytes show marked anisocytosis and poikilocytosis, with many oval macrocytes and, in severe cases, basophilic stippling, Howell-Jolly bodies, and Cabot rings. Erythrocytes with megaloblastic nuclei may be present in the blood (Fig. 8-1).
- Absolute reticulocyte count is low.
- Anemia is usually macrocytic, with MCV of 100 to 150 fL or more, but coexisting iron deficiency, thalassemia trait, or inflammation may prevent macrocytosis.

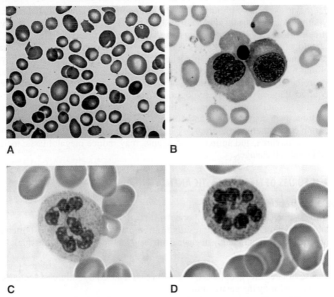

A   **B**

C   **D**

FIGURE 8-1 **A.** Pernicious anemia. Blood film. Note the striking oval macrocytes, wide variation in red cell size, and poikilocytes. Despite the anisocytosis and microcytes, the mean red cell volume is usually elevated, as in this case (MCV = 121 fL). **B.** Marrow precursors in pernicious anemia. Note very large size of erythroblasts (megaloblasts) and asynchronous maturation. Cell on *right* is a polychromatophilic megaloblast with an immature nucleus for that stage of maturation. Cell on *left* is an orthochromatic megaloblast with a lobulated immature nucleus. An orthochromatic megaloblast with a condensed nucleus is between and above those two cells. **C** and **D.** Two examples of hypersegmented neutrophils characteristic of megaloblastic anemia. The morphology of blood and marrow cells in folate-deficient and vitamin B_{12}-deficient patients is identical. The extent of the morphologic changes in each case is related to the severity of the vitamin deficiency. (Reproduced with permission from *Lichtman's Atlas of Hematology*, www.accessmedicine.com.) (Source: *Williams Hematology*, 8th ed, Chapter 41, Figure 41–12, p. 543.)

- Leukopenia and thrombocytopenia are frequently present.
- Hypersegmented neutrophils are an early sign of megaloblastosis. Typically, the nuclei of more than 5 percent of the cells have more than five lobes. Normal blood has less than 1 percent of five-lobed neutrophils.
- Platelets are smaller than usual and vary more widely in size. Platelets are functionally abnormal in severe megaloblastic anemia.
- Marrow cells show erythroid hyperplasia with striking megaloblastic changes. Promegaloblasts with mitotic figures are abundant in severe cases. The number of sideroblasts is increased, and macrophage iron content may also be increased.
- Coexisting iron deficiency may reduce the megaloblastic erythroid morphologic changes, but hypersegmented neutrophils are still present in the blood, and giant metamyelocytes and bands persist in the marrow.
- Treatment of a patient with folic acid or cobalamin more than 12 hours before marrow biopsy may mask the megaloblastic changes.
- Serum bilirubin, iron, and ferritin levels are somewhat elevated.
- Serum lactic dehydrogenase-1 and -2 and muramidase activities are markedly elevated.
- See below, "Laboratory Diagnosis of Tissue Cobalamin Deficiency" and "Folic Acid Deficiency," for measurement of B_{12} and folate tissue deficiency.

DIFFERENTIAL DIAGNOSIS

- Macrocytosis occurs without megaloblastic anemia in patients with liver disease, hypothyroidism, aplastic anemia, myelodysplasia, pregnancy, and anemias with reticulocytosis, but in these settings, the MCV rarely exceeds 110 fL.
- Pancytopenia with reticulocytopenia, which is often present in severe megaloblastic anemia, should be distinguished from aplastic anemia (markedly hypocellular marrow without megaloblastic morphologic changes), myelodysplastic syndrome (often blasts in blood or marrow, dysmorphic neutrophils (e.g., acquired Pelger-Huet cells, hypogranular cells) and platelets (e.g., abnormal size and granulation)), and acute myelogenous leukemia (evident leukemic myeloblasts in marrow and usually blood).
- Certain chemotherapeutic drugs, especially folate antagonists (e.g., methotrexate), hydroxyurea, and antiretroviral agents, may induce megaloblastic marrow and blood cell changes.

SPECIFIC FORMS OF MEGALOBLASTIC ANEMIA

Cobalamin Deficiency
- Table 8–1 presents the causes of cobalamin deficiency.
- Cobalamin deficiency usually results from impaired absorption, most often as a consequence of a deficiency in gastric intrinsic factor (pernicious anemia).

Pernicious Anemia
- Disease of later life, usually after age 40 years, caused by failure of secretion of intrinsic factor by the gastric mucosa.
- Autoimmune disease in which there is immune destruction of the acid- and pepsin-secreting cells of the stomach.
- Concordance with several other autoimmune diseases (e.g., immune thyroid diseases, type 1 diabetes mellitus, Addison disease, and others).
- A family history is common, and dominant inheritance with low penetrance has been proposed. More common in persons of Northern European or African descent. Less common in those of Asian descent.
- Gastric atrophy and achlorhydria occur in all patients. Absence of achlorhydria is incompatible with diagnosis of pernicious anemia.
- The skin often assumes a lemon-yellow hue because of pallor combined with slight hyperbilirubinemia.

- Lingual papillary atrophy (smooth, beefy red tongue) is seen in advanced disease.
- The clinical features of cobalamin deficiency are those of megaloblastic anemia generally, plus neurologic abnormalities specifically caused by cobalamin deficiency.
- Neurologic abnormalities may occur before the onset of anemia and may be irreversible.
- The neurologic disorder usually begins with paresthesias of the fingers and toes and disturbances of vibration and position sense.
- The earliest signs may be loss of position sense in the second toe and loss of vibration sense to 256 Hz but not to 128 Hz.
- If untreated, the disorder progresses to spastic ataxia because of demyelination of the posterior and lateral columns of the spinal cord, referred to as *combined system disease*.
- Cobalamin deficiency also affects the brain, and patients may develop somnolence and perversion of taste, smell, and vision, sometimes with optic atrophy.
- Dementia or frank psychosis may occur, the latter sometimes referred to as "*megaloblastic madness.*" Magnetic resonance imaging can confirm cobalamin deficiency affecting the brain by detecting demyelinization as T2-weighted hyperintensity of the white matter.
- There is a twofold increase in the incidence of gastric cancer.

Diagnostic laboratory findings include:
- Evidence of serum and tissue cobalamin deficiency (see below "Laboratory Diagnosis of Tissue Cobalamin Deficiency").
- Serum parietal cell antibodies (present in 90% of patients but not specific).
- Serum intrinsic factor antibodies are present in 70 percent of patients and specific for pernicious anemia. Their elevation is definitive evidence for pernicious anemia in patients with megaloblastic anemia and is an underutilized test.
- Elevated serum gastrin levels.

Gastrectomy and Ileal Resection Syndromes
- Cobalamin deficiency develops within 5 to 6 years of total gastrectomy or resection of the terminal ileum, as a result of loss of secretion of intrinsic factor from the stomach or failure to absorb cobalamin-intrinsic factor complexes in the ileum. The delay in onset of the anemia reflects the time required to exhaust cobalamin stores after absorption ceases. Diseases or injury to the terminal ileum may also lead to impaired cobalamin absorption and megaloblastic anemia (e.g., regional ileitis, radiation, sprue).
- Cobalamin absorption may also be impaired after subtotal gastrectomy.

Zollinger-Ellison Syndrome
- Gastrin-secreting tumor, usually in the pancreas, stimulates gastric mucosa to elaborate immense amounts of hydrochloric acid.
- Sufficient acid may be secreted to inactivate pancreatic proteases and to prevent release of cobalamin from its binder, preventing its attachment to intrinsic factor; both are necessary for cobalamin absorption.

"Blind Loop" Syndrome
- Intestinal stasis from anatomic lesions or impaired motility may lead to intestinal colonization with bacteria that bind cobalamin before it can be absorbed.

Diphyllobothrium latum Infestation
- These intestinal parasites, usually ingested in raw fish, bind cobalamin and prevent absorption. Only about 3 percent of people infested with the parasites become anemic. It is most prevalent in the Baltic Sea region, Canada, and Alaska where raw or undercooked fish is consumed. Diagnosis is made by identification of tape worm ova in the feces.

Pancreatic Disease

- Pancreatic exocrine insufficiency leads to deficiency of pancreatic proteases necessary for cobalamin absorption. Clinically significant deficiency of cobalamin is rare. The disorder can be ameliorated by oral trypsin therapy.

Dietary Cobalamin Deficiency

- Occurs rarely, usually in strict vegetarians who also avoid dairy products and eggs ("vegans").
- Symptomatic cobalamin deficiency can take decades to appear because of enterohepatic reabsorption of cobalamin conserving body stores.
- Breast-fed infants of vegan mothers may also develop cobalamin deficiency.

Acute Megaloblastic Anemia

- Acute megaloblastic anemia refers to a syndrome of rapidly developing thrombocytopenia and/or leukopenia, with very little change in the hemoglobin level. The marrow is floridly megaloblastic.
- The most common cause is nitrous oxide anesthesia. Nitrous oxide destroys methylcobalamin, inducing cobalamin deficiency. The marrow becomes megaloblastic within 12 to 24 hours. Hypersegmented neutrophils appear in the blood after 5 days.
- Serum cobalamin levels are low in most affected patients but may be normal in cobalamin deficiency because of nitrous oxide inhalation and, in some of the inherited abnormalities, of cobalamin metabolism (see below).
- The effects of nitrous oxide disappear in a few days. Administration of folinic acid or vitamin B_{12} accelerates recovery.
- Fatal megaloblastic anemia has occurred in patients with tetanus who were treated with nitrous oxide for weeks.
- Acute megaloblastic anemia may occur in seriously ill patients in intensive care units, patients transfused extensively, patients on dialysis or total parenteral nutrition, or patients receiving weak folic acid antagonists. The diagnosis is made from finding a megaloblastic marrow. Treatment is with parenteral folic acid (5 mg) and cobalamin (1 mg).

Megaloblastic Anemia Caused by Drugs

- Table 8–2 presents a partial list of drugs that cause megaloblastic anemia.
- Methotrexate acts by inhibiting dihydrofolate reductase, the enzyme which reduces folic acid to the active, tetrahydro form. Methotrexate toxicity is treated with folinic acid, which is already fully reduced, and therefore can bypass the inhibited dihydrofolate reductase.

TABLE 8–2	DRUGS THAT CAUSE MEGALOBLASTIC ANEMIA
Agents	Comments
Antifolates	
Methotrexate	Very potent inhibitor of dihydrofolate reductase
Aminopterin	Treat overdose with folinic acid
Pyrimethamine	Much weaker than methotrexate and aminopterin
Trimethoprim	Treat with folinic acid or by withdrawing the drug
Sulfasalazine	Can cause acute megaloblastic anemia in susceptible patients, especially those with low folate stores
Chlorguanide (Proguanil)	
Triamterene	Use of folate and cobalamin during pemetrexed treatment reduces toxicity
Pemetrexed (Alimta)	

Agents	Comments
Purine analogues	
6-Mercaptopurine	Megaloblastosis precedes hypoplasia, usually mild
6-Thioguanine	Responds to folinic acid but not folate
Azathioprine	
Acyclovir	Megaloblastosis at high doses
Pyrimidine analogues	
5-Fluorouracil	Mild megaloblastosis
Floxuridine (5-fluorodeoxyuridine)	
6-Azauridine	Blocks uridine monophosphate production by inhibiting orotidyl decarboxylase; occasional megaloblastosis with orotic acid and orotidine in urine
Zidovudine (AZT)	Severe megaloblastic anemia is the major side effect
Ribonucleotide reductase inhibitors	
Hydroxyurea	Marked megaloblastosis within 1–2 days of starting therapy; quickly reversed by withdrawing drug
Cytarabine (cytosine arabinoside)	Early megaloblastosis is routine
Anticonvulsants	
Phenytoin (diphenylhydantoin)	Occasional megaloblastosis, associated with low folate levels; responds to high-dose folate (1–5 mg/day); how anticonvulsants cause low folate is not understood, but may be related to a drug-induced rise in cytochrome P450
Phenobarbital	
Primidone	
Carbamazepine	
Other drugs that depress folates	
Oral contraceptives	Occasional megaloblastosis; sometimes dysplasia of uterine cervix, corrected with folate
Glutethimide	
Cycloserine	
H+/K+-ATPase inhibitors	
Omeprazole	Long-term use causes decreased serum cobalamin levels
Lansoprazole	
Miscellaneous	
N_2O	See "Acute Megaloblastic Anemia"
p-Aminosalicylic acid	Causes cobalamin malabsorption with occasional mild megaloblastic anemia
Metformin	
Phenformin	Causes cobalamin malabsorption but not anemia
Colchicine	
Neomycin	
Arsenic	Causes myelodysplastic hematopoiesis, sometimes with megaloblastic changes

Source: *Williams Hematology,* 8th ed, Chap. 41, Table 41–7, p. 554.

Megaloblastic Anemia in Childhood

- Cobalamin malabsorption occurs in the presence of normal intrinsic factor in an inherited disorder of childhood (*selective malabsorption of cobalamin, or Imerslund-Graesbeck disease*). There is associated albuminuria. Anemia usually develops before age 2 years. Treatment is with parenteral cobalamin.
- *Congenital intrinsic factor deficiency* is an autosomal recessive disorder in which parietal cells fail to produce intrinsic factor. The disease presents at 6 to 24 months of age. Treatment is with parenteral cobalamin.
- *Transcobalamin II deficiency* is an autosomal recessive disorder that leads to megaloblastic anemia in early infancy. Serum cobalamin levels are normal, but there is severe tissue cobalamin deficiency because transcobalamin II mediates transport of cobalamins into the tissues. The diagnosis is made by measuring serum transcobalamin II concentration. Treatment is with sufficiently large doses of cobalamin to override the deficient transport.
- *True juvenile pernicious anemia* is an extremely rare disorder that usually presents in adolescence. The diagnosis and treatment are the same as for the adult disease.

Other Megaloblastic Anemias and Changes

- Megaloblastic anemia may occur in some patients with inborn errors of cobalamin metabolism, inborn errors of folate metabolism, hereditary orotic aciduria, and the Lesch-Nyhan syndrome. A thiamine responsive megaloblastic anemia has also been reported.
- Anemia with megaloblastic-like red cell morphology ("megaloblastoid") may occur in some patients with congenital dyserythropoietic anemias, myelodysplastic syndromes, and erythroleukemia.

LABORATORY DIAGNOSIS OF TISSUE COBALAMIN DEFICIENCY

- Measurement of serum cobalamin level (a low level alone is insufficient for diagnosis).
- Transcobalamin-bound cobalamin represents about 25 percent of the total plasma cobalamin and is the functionally important fraction. Assays permit measurement of this more relevant cobalamin level.
- Serum cobalamin levels may be low with normal tissue levels in vegetarians, older persons, the chronically ill, people taking megadoses of vitamin C, pregnancy (25%), transcobalamin I deficiency, or folate deficiency (30%).
- Serum cobalamin levels are low in most affected patients, but may be normal in cobalamin deficiency because of nitrous oxide inhalation and in some of the inherited abnormalities of cobalamin metabolism (see below).
- Methylmalonic aciduria and elevated serum levels of methylmalonic acid are reliable indicators of tissue cobalamin deficiency (except in the presence of severe renal insufficiency). They are the earliest changes and precede anemia or morphologic blood cell changes. If normal, they argue strongly against tissue deficiency even if serum levels of the vitamin are low.
- Elevated serum homocysteine can indicate cobalamin deficiency but, unlike abnormalities in methylmalonic acid noted above, it can also be elevated in folic acid deficiency, pyridoxine deficiency, and hypothyroidism.
- Some individuals are able to absorb free cobalamin but cannot release it from food and therefore may become cobalamin deficient.

Folic Acid Deficiency

- Table 8–1 summarizes the causes of folic acid deficiency.
- Because of the possible development of neurologic complications in untreated patients with cobalamin deficiency, it is important to evaluate all patients with macrocytic anemia for both cobalamin and folic acid deficiency.

- Folic acid deficiency responds to physiologic doses of folic acid (200 μg/day), but cobalamin deficiency responds only to folic acid doses of 5 mg/day. Because neurologic complications may develop in patients with cobalamin deficiency treated with folic acid, a trial with folic acid is not recommended as a diagnostic test.
- An inadequate diet is the principal cause of folic acid deficiency. Folic acid reserves are small, and deficiency can develop rapidly.
- Alcohol use can depress absorption and serum folate levels and can accelerate the appearance of megaloblastic anemia in people with early folate deficiency.
- In megaloblastic anemia with laboratory evidence of folic acid deficiency, a full response to physiologic doses of folic acid should occur. If a question of absorptive limitations is present, the folate should be administered intramuscularly.
- Serum folate levels are reduced, but a low level may merely reflect reduced oral intake in the few days preceding the test.
- The red cell folic acid level is a more accurate reflection of tissue folate because it is not affected by recent dietary intake or drugs. Both red cell and serum folate are decreased in folic acid deficiency. In cobalamin deficiency, red cell folate may be low but serum folate is normal or elevated. Thus, both measurements are required to assess tissue folate levels.

THERAPY, COURSE, AND PROGNOSIS

Cobalamin Deficiency

- Treatment consists of parenteral administration of cyanocobalamin (vitamin B_{12}) or hydroxycobalamin in doses sufficient to replete tissue stores and provide daily requirements.
- Vitamin B_{12} has no toxicity per se, but parenteral cobalamin doses larger than 100 μg saturate the transport proteins and much is lost in the urine.
- A typical treatment schedule consists of 1000 μg of vitamin B_{12} intramuscularly daily for 2 weeks, then weekly until the hemoglobin level is normal, and then monthly for life.
- It has been recommended that after initial therapy, to return the hematocrit to normal, patients with neurologic abnormalities should receive 1000 μg every 2 weeks for 6 months.
- Infection can interfere with the response to vitamin B_{12} therapy.
- Transfusion may be required if the clinical picture requires prompt alleviation of anemia. Most patients, however, have adapted to severe anemia and can be treated with vitamin replacement therapy.
- Following initiation of cobalamin therapy, there is often a prompt improvement in the sense of well being.
- Marrow erythropoiesis converts from megaloblastic to normoblastic beginning about 12 hours after treatment is started.
- Reticulocytosis appears on days 3 to 5, and reaches a peak on days 4 to 10. The hemoglobin concentration should become normal within 1 to 2 months.
- Leukocyte and platelet counts normalize promptly, although neutrophil hypersegmentation persists for 10 to 14 days.
- Elevated serum bilirubin, serum iron, and lactic dehydrogenase levels fall to normal rapidly.
- Severe hypokalemia may develop after cobalamin therapy, and death from hypokalemia has occurred. Potassium levels must be monitored and appropriate replacement given.
- Cobalamin therapy should be administered to all patients after total gastrectomy or resection of the terminal ileum. After partial gastrectomy, patients should be monitored carefully for the development of anemia.
- The anemia of the blind loop syndrome will respond to parenteral cobalamin therapy, but it also responds to oral antibiotic therapy or successful correction of an anatomic abnormality.

- About 1 percent of an oral dose of vitamin B_{12} is absorbed even in the absence of intrinsic factor. Therefore, patients with pernicious anemia can be successfully treated with oral vitamin B_{12} in doses of 1000 μg/day. Patients receiving such therapy should be carefully monitored to ensure compliance and a response.

Folic Acid Deficiency

- Folic acid is administered orally at a dose of 1 to 5 mg daily. At this dosage, patients with malabsorption usually respond.
- Pregnant women should receive 1 mg of folic acid daily. Women at risk for cobalamin deficiency, such as strict vegetarians, may also be given vitamin B_{12}, 1 mg parenterally every 3 months, during the pregnancy.

For a more detailed discussion, see Ralph Green: Folate, Cobalamin, and Megaloblastic Anemias. Chapter 41, p. 533 in *Williams Hematology*, 8th ed.

CHAPTER 9
Iron-Deficiency Anemia and Iron Overload

- Iron deficiency is one of the most common chronic maladies in humans. One-third to one-half of healthy females of reproductive age in the United States have absent iron stores, and 10 percent have iron deficiency anemia, also common in infants and adolescents.
- Iron overload denotes an excess of iron in the body.

DEVELOPMENTAL STAGES OF IRON DEFICIENCY

- *Iron depletion:* storage iron decreased or absent.
- *Iron deficiency:* storage iron decreased or absent with low serum iron concentration and transferrin saturation.
- *Iron-deficiency anemia:* storage iron decreased or absent, low serum iron concentration and transferrin saturation, and low hemoglobin level.

CAUSES OF IRON DEFICIENCY

- Chronic blood loss.
- Diversion of maternal iron to fetus/infant during pregnancy/lactation.
- Inadequate dietary intake of iron, primarily in infants and children.
- Malabsorption of iron.
- Intravascular hemolysis with hemoglobinuria.
- Combinations of the above.

Dietary Causes

- Infants most often develop iron deficiency because milk is a poor source of dietary iron and the requirements for iron imposed by rapid growth are not satisfied.
- In children, poor dietary intake plus intestinal parasites and/or bleeding gastrointestinal lesions are the usual causes.
- In the United States, average iron intake is 5 to 7 mg/day. Children and menstruating women are in precarious iron balance and at risk for iron deficiency.

Malabsorption

- Iron absorption is decreased in the malabsorption syndromes.
- After subtotal gastrectomy, malabsorption of dietary iron occurs in 50 percent of patients because of rapid gastrointestinal transit and because food bypasses the site of maximal absorption due to location of anastomosis. In contrast, medicinal iron is well absorbed after partial gastrectomy.
- In postgastrectomy anemia, there may be bleeding from anastomotic ulcer(s).

Chronic Blood Loss

- Menorrhagia is the most common cause of iron deficiency in women.
- Chronic blood loss may occur from the respiratory, gastrointestinal, or genitourinary tracts, or from phlebotomy for blood donation or laboratory testing, or it may be self-induced.
- The most common cause of iron deficiency in men and postmenopausal women is gastrointestinal bleeding.

Pregnancy and Lactation

- The average iron loss from transfer to the fetus and blood in the placenta is 900 mg. Lactation losses of iron average 30 mg/mo.

PATHOGENESIS

- Lack of iron interferes with heme synthesis, which leads to reduced hemoglobin synthesis and defective erythropoiesis.
- There is decreased activity of iron-containing enzymes, such as the cytochromes and succinic dehydrogenase.
- Neurologic dysfunction may occur, with impaired intellectual performance, paresthesias, etc.
- Impaired performance during physical exertion is often present, especially in children and young adults.
- Atrophy of oral and gastrointestinal mucosa may occur, although this is unusual except in severe prolonged deficiency.
- Gastric acid secretion may be reduced, often irreversibly.

CLINICAL FEATURES

- Patients develop the general symptoms of anemia, e.g., easy fatiguability, dyspnea on exertion, loss of sense of well-being.
- There is poor correlation between hemoglobin levels and severity of symptoms. Some patients with marked iron deficiency may deny the common symptoms of fatigue, weakness, or palpitations, while patients with mild iron deficiency may be symptomatic.
- Irritability and headache can occur.
- Children may have poor attention span, poor response to sensory stimuli, retarded developmental and behavioral achievement, and retarded longitudinal growth.
- Paresthesias and burning of the tongue may occur, possibly because of tissue iron deficiency.
- Pica, a craving to eat unusual substances such as clay or ice, is a classic manifestation.

PHYSICAL EXAMINATION

- Pallor.
- Smooth red tongue, stomatitis.
- Angular cheilitis.
- Koilonychia (rare and limited to severe chronic deficiency).
- Retinal hemorrhages/exudates (rare and limited to severe chronic deficiency).
- Splenomegaly (rare and limited to severe chronic deficiency).

LABORATORY CHANGES

Red Blood Cells

- Earliest change is anisocytosis and increased red cell distribution width (RDW) (Fig. 9–1), although at early stages in patients with minimal and even moderate anemia, these abnormalities can be absent.
- Mild ovalocytosis, target cells.
- Progressive hypochromia (low MCHC) and microcytosis (low MCV).
- Reticulocytes normal or reduced.
- Measurement of the reticulocyte hemoglobin content in a flow cytometer is a sensitive index of early iron deficiency. A value of less than 26 pg/cell is indicative, on average, of iron deficiency.

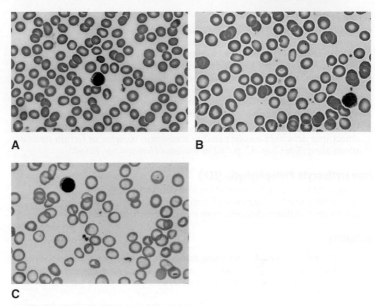

FIGURE 9–1 The characteristic hypochromia and microcytosis of moderately severe iron deficiency anemia. (Reproduced with permission from *Lichtman's Atlas of Hematology,* www.accessmedicine. com.) **A.** Normal blood film. **B.** Mild iron deficiency anemia. **C.** Severe iron deficiency anemia. Note advancing hypochromia and anisocytosis from A through C.
(Source: *Williams Hematology,* 8th ed, Chap. 42, Fig. 42–10, p. 580.)

Leukocytes
- Leukopenia (3 to 4.4 × 10⁹/L) is found in a small number of patients. Differential white count is normal.

Platelets
- Thrombocytopenia develops in approximately one-quarter of iron deficient children but is very uncommon in adults.
- Thrombocytosis is found in approximately one-third of iron deficient children but is very common among adults, usually secondary to chronic active blood loss.

Marrow
- Marrow cellularity and M/E ratio variable.
- Absent sideroblasts.
- Markedly decreased to absent macrophage hemosiderin by Prussian blue staining.
- Erythroblasts may be small, with narrow rim of ragged cytoplasm and poor hemoglobin formation (micronormoblasts with defective hemoglobinization).

Serum Iron Concentration and Total Iron-Binding Capacity (TIBC)
- Serum iron concentration may be in the low-normal range in mild deficiency
- TIBC usually increased but may be in the high-normal range in mild deficiency.
- Saturation (iron/TIBC) is often 15 percent or less, but this is not specific for iron deficiency. Occurs also in chronic inflammation and severe inflammatory states (e.g., arthritis, pericarditis, and others).
- Serum transferrin receptor level may be of utility when ferritin levels are borderline low. Its elevation provides further evidence for the diagnosis of an early stage of iron deficiency (for *soluble transferrin receptor index* see next paragraph).

Serum Ferritin

- Levels of less than 10 μg/L are characteristic of iron-deficiency anemia.
- Levels of 10 to 20 μg/L are presumptive, but not diagnostic.
- May be elevated with concomitant inflammatory diseases (e.g., rheumatoid arthritis), Gaucher disease, chronic renal disease, malignancy, hepatitis, or iron administration.
- Iron deficiency can be suspected in rheumatoid arthritis or other severe inflammatory states if the ferritin level is less than 60 μg/L.
- The ratio of soluble transferrin receptor to the log of the serum ferritin concentration expressed as *soluble transferrin receptor index* (calculated as a ratio of the sTfR/log ferritin; i.e., TfR-F Index) has been proposed as a superior way to detect iron deficiency as compared to transferrin receptor or ferritin measurements alone. See Chap. 42, p. 582 in *Williams Hematology,* 8th ed.

Free Erythrocyte Protoporphyrin (FEP)

- Concentration is usually increased in iron deficiency.
- A sensitive test for diagnosis of iron deficiency and suitable for large-scale screening of children, detecting both iron deficiency and lead poisoning.

DIAGNOSIS

- The physician who establishes a diagnosis of iron deficiency should assiduously search for a source of blood loss if unapparent or if another, much less common, reason for the deficiency is not evident. Determination of the site and cause of the blood loss is essential.
- As in all deficiency states leading to anemia, the diagnostic findings depend on the severity of the deficiency. If early and mild, the expected changes (e.g., decreased serum iron and percent saturation of transferrin) may be mild or within the normal range.

Special Studies

- Gastrointestinal loss is the most prevalent site of blood loss in men and uterine menstrual) loss in women. Multiple stools should be tested for occult blood in every patient with iron deficiency.
  - Bleeding may be intermittent.
  - Common screening tests are insensitive to < 5 to 10 mL blood loss per day.
  - Angiography may be helpful if active bleeding is 0.5 mL/min or greater.
  - Pertechnetate uptake studies may detect a Meckel diverticulum.
  - Radiographic/endoscopic studies, including capsule endoscopy, may detect the source of gastrointestinal bleeding.
- Hemosiderin-laden macrophages in sputum if intrapulmonary bleeding is present.
- Urinary hemosiderin detection (iron laden urine epithelial cells) is a definitive way of confirming iron deficiency due to intravascular hemolysis. The first morning urine is the most sensitive sample collection time for finding iron in the urine. Urinary iron loss can also be measured quantitatively by atomic absorption spectroscopy.

DIFFERENTIAL DIAGNOSIS

- Iron deficiency vs. thalassemia vs. anemia of chronic disease (see Table 9–1).

TREATMENT

Therapeutic Trial

- Should initially be via oral route, if possible.
- Response to expect:
  - Peak reticulocytosis at approximately 10 days, although reticulocyte response is a function of severity of anemia and may be modest.

TABLE 9–1	MICROCYTIC DISORDERS THAT MAY BE CONFUSED WITH IRON DEFICIENCY

Thalassemias and hemoglobinopathies (see Chap. 16)
β-Thalassemia major
β-Thalassemia minor
δβ-Thalassemia minor
α-Thalassemia-minor
Hemoglobin Lepore trait
Hemoglobin E trait
Homozygous hemoglobin E disease
Hemoglobin H disease
Combination of above (compound heterozygotes)

Blockade of heme synthesis caused by chemicals (see Chaps. 11 and 22)
Lead
Pyrazinamide
Isoniazid

Other disorders
Sideroblastic anemias (see Chap. 11)
    Hereditary sex-linked
    Idiopathic acquired
Anemia of chronic inflammation (see Chap. 13)
DMT-1 human mutations

Source: *Williams Hematology,* 8th ed, Chap. 42, Table 42–9, p. 583.

— Significant increase in hemoglobin concentration at 3 to 4 weeks; one-half of hemoglobin deficit corrected at 4 to 5 weeks.
— Hemoglobin level normal at 2 to 4 months.
— Unless there is continued bleeding or evidence for iron malabsorption, absence of a response indicates that iron deficiency is not the cause of anemia. Iron treatment should be stopped and another mechanism of anemia sought. (See also "Failure to Respond to Therapy," below.)

Oral Iron Therapy
• Dietary sources are insufficient for treatment.
• Safest, least expensive are oral ferrous salts (e.g., ferrous sulfate or ferrous gluconate).
• Nonenteric-coated forms should be used.
• Avoid multiple hematinics.
• Do not give with meals or antacids or with inhibitors of acid production.
• Daily total of 150 to 200 mg elemental iron in 3 to 4 doses, each 1 hour before meals (65 mg of elemental iron is contained in 325 mg of ferrous sulfate USP, or in 200 mg dried ferrous sulfate).
• A few patients may complain of gastrointestinal intolerance to pills, pyrosis, constipation, diarrhea, and/or metallic taste and require:
    — Reduction of daily dose.
    — Change of oral iron preparation.

Length of Treatment
• In order to replenish iron stores, continue oral therapy for 12 months after hemoglobin level is normal.
• Therapy may be needed indefinitely if bleeding continues (e.g., menstruating women).

Parenteral Iron Therapy

- Routine use usually not justified, unless used in renal failure patients on dialysis.
- Indications are:
  — Malabsorption.
  — Intolerance to oral iron preparations (colitis, enteritis).
  — Need in excess of amount that can be given orally.
  — Patient uncooperative or unavailable for follow-up.
  — Renal failure patients on dialysis.
- Iron dextran
  — First product available in United States.
  — 50 mg elemental iron per milliliter.
  — Approximately 70 percent readily available for hemoglobin synthesis.
  — May be given intramuscularly or intravenously.
  — Be aware of danger of anaphylaxis or other systemic side effects.
  — Severe reactions are more common than with other parenteral preparations listed below.
  — See *Williams Hematology*, 8th ed, Chap. 42 or product information sheet for dosage calculations.
- Iron sucrose
  — A complex of polynuclear iron ferric hydroxide in sucrose.
  — Recommended by the manufacturer is 5 mL (100 mg of elemental iron).
  — Adverse events reported by more than 5 percent of treated patients: hypotension most common.
- Ferric gluconate complex in sucrose (Ferrlecit)
  — Macromolecular complex of innate and ferric iron.
  — The manufacturer recommends administration of doses of 125 mg of elemental iron with the preparation diluted in 100 mL of 0.9 percent sodium chloride and given intravenously over 1 hour.
  — Adverse events reported by more than 5 percent of treated patients: hypotension most common.
- Ferumoxytol
  — An intravenous iron preparation approved for treatment of the anemia of chronic kidney disease.
  — A carbohydrate-coated, superparamagnetic iron oxide nanoparticle.
  — Limited clinical experience; approved in 2010.

Failure to Respond to Therapy

- Wrong oral preparation (enteric-coated, insoluble iron, too little iron in each dose).
- Bleeding not controlled.
- Therapy not long enough to show response.
- Patient not taking medication.
- Concomitant deficiencies (vitamin B_{12}, folate, thyroid hormone).
- Concomitant illness limiting erythropoietic response:
  — Inflammation, infection, malignancy, hepatic disease, renal disease.
- Diagnosis incorrect:
  — Thalassemia, lead poisoning, etc.

HEREDITARY HEMOCHROMATOSIS

Etiology and Pathogenesis (see Table 9-2)

Classic Hemochromatosis (HFE hemochromatosis) (type 1)

- This diagnosis is applied to persons who have increased body iron as suggested by increased serum ferritin levels, and even to those who merely have the hemochromatosis *HFE* genotype, regardless of the level of their iron stores.
- Autosomal recessive disorder. Heterozygotes do not develop the disease.

TABLE 9–2 **CAUSES OF IRON OVERLOAD**	
Genetic	Acquired
Hereditary hemochromatosis (*HFE* mutation)	Chronic ingestion of medicinal iron
Juvenile hemochromatosis (*HAMP* or *HJV* mutations)	Transfusion iron overload
Hemochromatosis due to transferrin receptor 2 mutations	Acquired sideroblastic anemia
Ferroportin disease (*SLC40A1* mutations)	Siderosis associated with splenorenal or portocaval shunts
Neonatal hemochromatosis	
African hemochromatosis	
Thalassemia major (see Chap. 16)	
Hereditary sideroblastic anemia (see Chap. 11)	
Hereditary hemolytic anemias	
Enzyme deficiencies (see Chap. 15)	
Erythrocyte membrane disorders (see Chap. 14)	
Congenital dyserythropoietic anemias (see Chap. 7)	
Porphyria cutanea tarda (see Chap. 30)	
Hereditary atransferrinemia	
Hereditary aceruloplasminemia	

Source: *Williams Hematology,* 8th ed, Chap. 42, p. 589.

- The identification of the *HFE* gene made it possible to assess accurately the gene frequency and penetrance of the *HFE* mutations.
- The penetrance of the homozygous state is so low that it could be considered a risk factor, rather than the major cause of the disease.
- The major *HFE* mutation is cDNA nt 845 C → G (C282Y).
- The gene frequency is 0.06 to 0.08 in northern European populations so that about 15 percent of people are heterozygous and 0.5 percent are homozygous.
- It is rare in non-Europeans.
- About one-half of homozygotes have increased serum transferrin saturation and/or ferritin levels, but only about 1 percent of homozygotes are clinically affected, and there is no demonstrated effect of the mutation, even in its homozygous form, on life expectancy.
- A common minor mutation of *HFE* is cDNA nt 187 C → G (H63D).
- This gene's frequency is about 0.16 in the European population and is panethnic in its worldwide distribution.
- In the homozygous state (H63D/H63D), or in the compound heterozygous state (C282Y/H63D), this mutation may be also (but far less likely) associated with hemochromatosis.
- A number of "private" *HFE* mutations have been found in individual families.
- Excessive iron absorption through the gastrointestinal mucosa leads to accumulation of ferritin and hemosiderin in most cells in the body, especially in hepatocytes, bile duct epithelium, and macrophages.

Juvenile Hemochromatosis (type 2)
- The penetrance of the rare juvenile form of the disease seems to be high and cardiomyopathies and endocrine deficiencies are the major clinical features.
- For list of mutations refer to Table 9–2.

African Iron Overload

- African hemochromatosis is not caused by *HFE* or other known mutations.
- Not clear to what extent African iron overload is a symptomatic condition.
- Many complicating factors, including malnutrition and high alcohol intake generally present.

Clinical Features

- Hereditary hemochromatosis (symptomatic HFE hemochromatosis) usually presents in the fifth decade or later and is rare in children and young adults. The male:female ratio is 5:1, and the disease is uncommon in premenopausal women.
- Most common symptoms are weakness, lethargy, loss of libido, joint symptoms, and weight loss.
- Arthralgia typically involves second and third metacarpophalangeal joints with swelling and tenderness. Hips and knees may also be involved, but because hemochromatosis is a disease of later life, a cause-and-effect relationship between joint symptoms and hemochromatosis is not established.
- Chondrocalcinosis or calcification of periarticular ligaments is a frequent late manifestation. Synovial fluid may contain calcium pyrophosphate and apatite crystals.
- Skin becomes hyperpigmented primarily from deposition of melanin.
- Cardiac effects are common.
  - Arrhythmias.
  - Cardiomegaly (may be a result of restrictive or dilated cardiomyopathy).
  - Congestive failure.
- Endocrinopathies are common.
  - Pancreas (may show diffuse fibrosis and loss of islets). Diabetes mellitus occurs in some patients.
  - Hypothyroidism (10% of male patients).
  - Hypothalamic pituitary insufficiency, usually involving gonadotropins (about half of patients).
  - Testicular atrophy, azoospermia, reduced libido, and impotence.
  - Premature menopause.
- Hepatomegaly and liver injury are common.
  - Jaundice is uncommon.
  - Liver function tests may be abnormal.
  - Esophageal varices develop late in the disease.
  - Hepatocellular carcinoma occurs in one-third of patients who have fully developed disease.
  - Patients who have hemochromatosis and also consume significant quantities of alcohol are more likely to develop hepatic fibrosis than are patients who abstain from alcohol.
  - Cirrhosis found only in patients who have serum ferritin levels of > 1000 ng/mL and who have abnormal liver function tests.
- Splenomegaly is frequently present.

Laboratory Features

- The transferrin saturation exceeds 50 percent in one-half of homozygotes for the C282Y mutation. The serum ferritin is > 200 ng/mL in one-half of homozygous women and > 250 ng/mL in one-half of homozygous men.
- Patients with fully developed disease may have hyperglycemia and an abnormal glucose tolerance test.
- Serum aminotransferase activities are increased in about 5 to 10 percent of homozygotes and in all of those with cirrhosis.
- Serum concentrations of pituitary gonadotropins and androgens are often low.
- Serum thyroxine levels may be low and TSH concentrations increased.

Diagnosis

- Early diagnosis of clinically affected patients is imperative because body iron reduction therapy is relatively simple and prevents tissue injury and complications may be irreversible and lead to death, for example from hepatocellular carcinoma.
- Serum ferritin levels are useful in screening but may be less sensitive than the serum iron level and transferrin saturation for screening but helpful to discriminate affected (ferritin > 1000 ng/mL) from asymptomatic patients.
- Estimates of the amount of marrow iron have little or no diagnostic value.
- CT scan and MRI can demonstrate increased iron content of the liver, but high cost makes these tests inappropriate for screening.
- Liver biopsy is occasionally useful but is not required for diagnosis in most cases.
- In normal liver, iron content is less than 2.8 mg/g dry weight (50 μmol/g).
- In alcoholic liver disease, iron content is less than 5.6 mg/g (100 μmol/g).
- In hemochromatosis, iron content exceeds 5.6 mg/g (100 μmol/g), and in hemochromatosis with cirrhosis, iron content is usually greater than 11 mg/g (200 μmol/g).
- Genetic analysis for *HFE* mutations is important in family studies in order to detect other affected individuals.

Treatment

- Phlebotomy
  - Removal of 500 mL blood by venesection once or twice a week depletes the body iron burden. Each 500 mL removes about 200 mg iron.
  - The patient with severe disease usually has accumulated 30 to 40 g excess iron.
  - Adequacy of treatment may be gauged by progressive fall in hemoglobin level and the MCV, indicating a decrease of body iron below normal.
  - For maintenance, removal of 500 mL blood every few months is usually sufficient. Serial measurements of serum ferritin levels are more useful than estimates of transferrin saturation in monitoring the effects of phlebotomy and should be used to monitor the patient indefinitely.
  - Alcohol and other hepatotoxins should be avoided.
- Oral chelating agents
  - More expensive and more side effects compared to phlebotomies.
  - May be useful when phlebotomies cannot be used.
  - For details, refer to Chap. 42, p. 565, *Williams Hematology,* 8th ed.

Prognosis

- Life span is normal in patients without cirrhosis.
- Incidence of hepatocellular carcinoma is not diminished by treatment once there is hepatic fibrosis.
- Treatment may improve diabetes, cardiac function, and gonadal insufficiency.

SECONDARY HEMOCHROMATOSIS

Etiology and Pathogenesis

- Hyperabsorption of iron occurs in many hemolytic anemias, particularly in those accompanied by ineffective erythropoiesis.
- Blood transfusion adds to the iron burden.
- The administration of medicinal iron in the mistaken belief that iron will help the anemia is sometimes an aggravating factor.

Clinical Features

- Same as hereditary hemochromatosis.

Laboratory Features
- Those of the underlying disease.
- Elevated serum ferritin and often serum iron.

Diagnosis
- The minimum iron burden can be calculated from the number of transfusions received (1 U contains ~200 mg iron), because daily iron loss is very small (~0.5 to 1.0 mg/dL).
- Elevation of ferritin levels reflects iron burden.

Treatment
- Twenty-four-hour iron excretion in the urine after a subcutaneous or intravenous infusion of 2 g desferrioxamine predicts response to this drug.
- If excretion is > 20 mg, then treatment may be useful: give overnight subcutaneous infusions of 2 to 4 g desferrioxamine or give drug intravenously over as long a period as possible if the patient has an indwelling venous catheter.

For a more detailed discussion, see Ernest Beutler: Disorders of Iron Metabolism. Chap. 42, p. 565 in *Williams Hematology*, 8th ed.

CHAPTER 10
Anemia Resulting from Other Nutritional Deficiencies

VITAMIN A DEFICIENCY

- Prevalent in school children in several underdeveloped African countries (e.g., Malawi).
- Anemia is characterized by reduced MCV, MCHC, and anisocytosis and poikilocytosis.
- Similar to the anemia of chronic disease with reduced serum iron concentration, normal or low serum total iron-binding capacity and increased liver and marrow iron stores (increased serum ferritin), and failure to respond to treatment with medicinal iron.
- Responds to vitamin A repletion.

VITAMIN B₆ DEFICIENCY

- Vitamin B_6 includes pyridoxal, pyridoxine, and pyridoxamine.
- May lead to hypochromic microcytic anemia.
- Microcytic anemia may occur in patients taking isoniazid, which interferes with B_6 metabolism. Such anemias may be corrected with large doses of pyridoxine.
- Some patients who are not vitamin B_6 deficient may have sideroblastic anemia that will partially respond to high doses of pyridoxine (see Chap. 14).

RIBOFLAVIN DEFICIENCY

- Volunteers receiving a riboflavin-deficient diet plus a riboflavin antagonist (galactoflavin) developed vacuolated erythroid precursors, followed by pure red cell aplasia—all reversed by administration of riboflavin.
- Reduced erythrocyte glutathione reductase activity occurs in riboflavin deficiency but is not associated with hemolysis or oxidant-induced injury.

VITAMIN C (ASCORBIC ACID) DEFICIENCY

- Anemia in humans with scurvy may be macrocytic, normocytic, or microcytic, and the marrow may be hypocellular, normocellular, or hypercellular. In 10 percent of patients, the marrow is megaloblastic.
- Macrocytic anemia may develop with vitamin C deficiency because vitamin C interacts with folic acid in the generation of tetrahydrofolic acid.
- Microcytic anemia may develop because vitamin C facilitates the absorption of iron and because of the bleeding manifestation of scurvy.
- Iron deficiency in children is often associated with dietary vitamin C deficiency.
- Normocytic normochromic anemia with a reticulocytosis of 5 to 10 percent also develops in scurvy, perhaps from compromised cellular antioxidant defense mechanisms.
- The anemia of vitamin C deficiency responds promptly to administration of vitamin C. Sufficient folic acid and iron is required for the response to occur.

VITAMIN E (α-TOCOPHEROL) DEFICIENCY

- The vitamin E requirement varies with polyunsaturated fatty acid content of diet and the content of lipids that can peroxidize in tissues.
- Perinatal period: Low-birth-weight infants have low serum and tissue concentrations of vitamin E.
- A diet rich in polyunsaturated fatty acids and adequate in iron but inadequate in vitamin E may lead to hemolytic anemia by 4 to 6 weeks of age.
- Anemia is often associated with altered red cell morphology, thrombocytosis, and edema of the dorsum of the feet and pretibial area.
- These abnormalities are reversed promptly by treatment with vitamin E.
- Chronic fat malabsorption, such as is common in cystic fibrosis, can lead to vitamin E deficiency, if daily supplements of the water-soluble form of this vitamin are not given. In such patients, the red cell life span is mildly reduced and anemia may develop.
- Patients with sickle cell disease often have low serum tocopherol concentrations. Vitamin E deficiency has been associated with an increase in irreversibly sickled cells in the blood. Vitamin E (450 units/day) has been associated with a decrease in irreversibly sickled cells.

COPPER DEFICIENCY

- Copper is required for absorption and utilization of iron, perhaps functioning by maintaining iron in the ferric state for transferrin transport.
- Copper deficiency occurs in malnourished children and in infants and adults receiving parenteral alimentation, and can also be caused by chronic ingestion of massive quantities of zinc, which impairs copper absorption.
- Young children with copper deficiency may have osteoporosis, flaring of ribs, and other bony abnormalities.
- Copper deficiency causes a microcytic anemia with hypoferremia, neutropenia, and vacuolated erythroid precursors in marrow that does not respond to iron therapy.
- Copper deficiency can occur after gastric resection or after bariatric gastric reduction surgery. The macrocytic anemia, neutropenia, and ringed sideroblasts in the marrow can mimic closely the clonal anemia seen in the myelodysplastic syndrome.
- Copper deficiency can be associated with secondary neurologic abnormalities, especially myeloneuropathy. Anemia in this situation can mimic cobalamin deficiency and should be considered in the differential diagnosis of the latter, especially in individuals post-gastrectomy.
- Diagnosis is established by demonstration of low serum ceruloplasmin or copper levels, or by a therapeutic trial with copper at a dose of 0.2 mg/kg day. Copper levels are the more reliable because ceruloplasmin is an acute phase reactant. A 10 percent solution of copper sulfate contains 25 mg of copper per milliliter.
- Low serum copper values may also be seen in hypoproteinemic states (exudative enteropathies, nephrosis) and Wilson disease (see Chap. 22).

ZINC DEFICIENCY

- May accompany thalassemia or sickle cell disease.
- Isolated zinc deficiency does not produce anemia.
- Zinc deficiency can result in growth retardation in children, impaired wound healing, impaired taste perception, and immunologic inadequacies.
- Table 10–1 contains the normal levels in blood for the vitamins and minerals discussed above.

TABLE 10–1	BLOOD VITAMIN AND MINERAL LEVELS (ADULT VALUES)			
Vitamin or Mineral	Serum Level	Plasma Level	Red Cell Level	White Cell Level
Copper	11–24 μmol/L		14–24 μmol/L	
Folate	7–45 nmol/L		>320 nmol/L	
Riboflavin (B₂)	110–640 nmol/L		265–1350 nmol/L	
Vitamin A	1–3 μmol/L			
Vitamin B₆		20–122 nmol/L		
Vitamin C		25–85 μmol/L		11–30 attomol/cell
Vitamin E	12–40 μmol/L			
Selenium	1200–2000 nmol/L			
Zinc	11–18 μmol/L			

Source: *Williams Hematology*, 8th ed, Chap. 43, Table 43–1, p. 608.

ANEMIA OF STARVATION

• Semistarvation causes mild to moderate normocytic normochromic anemia with reduced marrow erythroid precursors. The anemia is principally dilutional.
• Complete starvation for 9 to 12 weeks leads to anemia and marrow hypocellularity, which responds to resumption of a normal diet. The decreased hemoglobin may be a response to a hypometabolic state with consequent decrease in oxygen requirements. Reticulocytosis and correction of the hemoglobin deficit follows refeeding.

ANEMIA OF PROTEIN DEFICIENCY (KWASHIORKOR)

• In protein-calorie malnutrition, the hemoglobin level may fall to 8 g/dL, but some children may not be anemic because the reduced red cell mass is masked by a reduced plasma volume.
• Anemia is normocytic, normochromic, with significant anisocytosis and poikilocytosis.
• Leukocyte and platelet counts are usually normal.
• The marrow is usually normocellular or hypocellular with reduced erythroid precursors.
• Patients respond slowly to high-protein diets (powdered milk or essential amino acids).
• After 3 or 4 weeks of treatment, there may be an episode of erythroid aplasia that responds to riboflavin or prednisone.
• Occult deficiencies may become manifest during the repletion period; e.g., iron, folic acid, vitamin E, and vitamin B₁₂.

ALCOHOLISM

• Chronic alcohol ingestion is often associated with anemia, which may be a result of multiple causes:
  — Nutritional deficiencies.
  — Chronic gastrointestinal bleeding.
  — Hepatic dysfunction.
  — Hemolytic anemia.
  — Hypersplenism from portal hypertension.
  — Direct toxic effects of ethanol on erythropoiesis and on folate metabolism.

- Macrocytic anemia occurs commonly in hospitalized alcoholic patients and is often associated with megaloblastic changes and sometimes with ringed sidero-blasts.
- Megaloblastic anemia in alcoholism is almost always caused by folic acid deficiency.
- Megaloblastic anemia is more common in drinkers of wine or whiskey, which have low folate content, than in drinkers of beer, which is a rich source of folate.
- Alcoholics may have associated iron deficiency, producing a "dimorphic" blood picture (macrocytes, hypersegmented neutrophils, and hypochromic micro-cytes).
- Iron deficiency may be unmasked after treatment with folic acid alone by demonstration of an emerging population of microcytic red cells. Treatment with iron alone may unmask folate deficiency, by demonstration of an emerging population of macrocytes.
- Mild macrocytosis (MCV 100 to 110 fL) is found in 82 to 96 percent of chronic alcoholics. Anemia is usually absent, macrocytes are typically round as opposed to oval and neutrophil hypersegmentation is not present. These patients are not folate deficient, and the macrocytosis persists until the patient abstains from alcohol.

For a more detailed discussion, see Ralph Green: Anemia Resulting From Other Nutritional Deficiencies. Chap. 43, p. 607 in *Williams Hematology*, 8th ed.

CHAPTER 11
Hereditary and Acquired Sideroblastic Anemias

- Sideroblastic anemias may be acquired or hereditary (see Table 11–1) and are characterized by:
  - Ringed (pathologic) sideroblasts and increased storage iron in the marrow are the hallmarks of this group of disorders.
  - Increased red cell precursors in the marrow in the face of anemia and a low reticulocyte count (ineffective erythropoiesis). The anemia is the result of increased apoptosis of late erythroid precursors.
  - A population of hypochromic erythrocytes in the blood film is a common finding.
- All normal red cell precursors have siderosomes, iron-containing cytoplasmic aggregates in the cytoplasm, a normal part of intraerythrocytic iron metabolism and hemoglobin synthesis. They can be seen by transmission electron microscopy. These aggregates are often below the resolution of the light microscope. Thus, in Prussian blue-stained marrow specimens, about 20 to 50 percent of normal red cell precursors can be found to have one to three very small, pinhead sized blue granules in the cytoplasm under oil immersion optics, depending on the quality of the preparation.
- Pathologic sideroblasts are of two types. The classical type is a ringed sideroblast with relatively large, Prussian blue-stained granules in an approximate circumferential position around the nucleus of the erythroblast. This location reflects their intramitochondrial location; mitochondria in erythroblasts being

TABLE 11–1	CLASSIFICATION OF SIDEROBLASTIC ANEMIAS

I. Acquired
  A. Primary sideroblastic anemia (myelodysplastic syndromes) (see Chap. 42)
  B. Sideroblastic anemia secondary to:
    1. Isoniazid
    2. Pyrazinamide
    3. Cycloserine
    4. Chloramphenicol
    5. Ethanol
    6. Lead
    7. Chronic neoplastic and inflammatory disease
    8. Zinc
II. Hereditary
  A. X chromosome–linked
    1. *ALAS2* deficiency
    2. Hereditary sideroblastic anemia with ataxia: *ABCB7* mutations
  B. Autosomal: mitochondrial myopathy and sideroblastic anemia (*PSU1* mutations)
  C. Mitochondrial: Pearson marrow-pancreas syndrome

Source: *Williams Hematology*, 8th ed, Chap. 58, Table 58–1, p. 866.

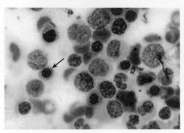 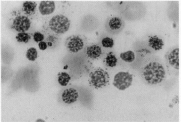

A　　　　　　　　　　**B**

FIGURE 11-1 Marrow films. **A.** Normal marrow stained with Prussian blue. Note several erythroblasts without apparent siderotic (blue-stained) granules. The *arrow* indicates erythroblast with several very small cytoplasmic blue-stained granules. It is very difficult to see siderosomes in most erythroblasts in normal marrow because they are often below the resolution of the light microscope. **B.** Sideroblastic anemia. Note the florid increase in Prussian blue staining granules in the erythroblasts, most with circumnuclear locations. These are classic examples of ringed sideroblast, which are by definition pathologic changes in the red cell precursors. In some cases, cytoplasmic iron granules are also increased in size and number, also a pathologic change. (Reproduced with permission from *Lichtman's Atlas of Hematology,* www.accessmedicine.com.) (Source: *Williams Hematology,* 8th ed, Chap. 58, Fig. 58–1, p. 866.)

positioned closely surrounding the nucleus. The other type of pathologic sideroblast has large and multiple cytoplasmic granules (see Fig. 11–1).

* Drugs that reduce the formation of pyridoxal 5′-phosphate from pyridoxine decrease heme synthesis and cause sideroblastic anemia.
* The main factor responsible for the anemia is ineffective erythropoiesis, with increased plasma iron turnover, normal to decreased red cell survival, and increased excretion of fecal stercobilin.

ACQUIRED SIDEROBLASTIC ANEMIA

Primary

* A clonal (neoplastic) anemia with varying frequencies of neutropenia and thrombocytopenia or occasionally thrombocytosis. This feature of the myelodysplastic syndromes is discussed in Chap. 42.

Secondary

* Most commonly associated with use of isonicotinic acid hydrazide (INH), pyrazinamide, or cycloserine.
* Common in the marrow of abusers of alcohol and a diagnostic feature of the anemia of alcohol abuse.
    — In the anemia of chronic alcoholism, folate deficiency may coexist as a result of inadequate diet. Thus, the anemia may have megaloblastic features and ringed siderblasts. On removal of alcohol and replacement of folate, the megaloblastic features disappear first and the sideroblastic features disappear at a later time as long as abstinence from alcohol is in place.
* May occur in patients with neoplastic or chronic inflammatory diseases.
* Anemia may be severe and is characterized by dimorphic red cells on the blood film, hypochromic and normochromic.
* If drugs are responsible, the anemia responds promptly to withdrawal of the offending agent.
* In cases related to an underlying disease, improvement is associated with successful treatment of the primary disease.

HEREDITARY SIDEROBLASTIC ANEMIA

Inheritance
- The X-linked form is a result of mutations of erythroid-specific ALA synthase *(ALAS2)*.
- Some autosomal forms have also been described.
- A mitochondrial deletion causes *Pearson marrow-pancreas syndrome.*

Clinical and Laboratory Manifestations
- Anemia appears in the first few weeks or months of life.
- Characteristically microcytic and hypochromic.
- Prominent red cell dimorphism, with striking anisocytosis and poikilocytosis.
- Splenomegaly is usually present.
- Hemochromatosis develops frequently in these patients.

Treatment
- Patients with hereditary sideroblastic anemia may respond to pyridoxine in oral doses of 50 to 200 mg daily.
- Folic acid administered concomitantly may increase the response.
- Full normalization of the hemoglobin level is usually not achieved, and relapse occurs if pyridoxine therapy is stopped.
- Efforts should be made to reduce iron overloading by phlebotomy, if possible, or by use of desferrioxamine.

For a more detailed discussion, see Prem Ponka and Josef T. Prchal: Hereditary and Acquired Sideroblastic Anemias. *Williams Hematology,* 8th ed, Chap. 58, p. 865.

CHAPTER 12
Anemia Resulting from Marrow Infiltration

DEFINITIONS

- Anemia or pancytopenia associated with extensive marrow infiltration is called *myelophthisic anemia*
- *Leukoerythroblastosis* refers to anemia with schistocytes, teardrop-shaped red cells, nucleated red cells, megakaryocytic fragments, and immature myeloid cells (e.g., neutrophilic myelocytes) in the blood.

ETIOLOGY AND PATHOGENESIS

- Table 12–1 lists the conditions that cause marrow infiltration.
- Invasion is the essential component of cancer cell metastasis and often involves the loss of E-cadherin.
- In most cases, the infiltration is focal, with surrounding areas of normal or hyperactive marrow.
- Disruption of the microenvironment by infiltration with foreign cells leads to premature release of immature blood cells from the marrow.
- Myelophthisic anemia is most often caused by humoral factors (e.g., cytokines) or injury to the marrow microenvironment.

CLINICAL FEATURES

- The clinical features of marrow infiltrative disorders are usually those of the underlying disease but the marrow replacement may also accentuate associated cytopenias.

LABORATORY FEATURES

- Anemia is mild to moderate.
- Leukocyte and platelet counts may be high or low depending on the nature and extent of marrow replacement.
- Blood film may show anisocytosis and poikilocytosis, with schistocytes, teardrop cells, nucleated red cells, immature granulocytic cells, and megakaryocytic fragments.
- Leukocyte alkaline phosphatase activity is normal or increased.
- Clusters of cancer cells may rarely be found on the blood film (carcinocythemia).
- Marrow biopsy is the most reliable diagnostic procedure. Marrow aspiration may also be of value. Aspiration or biopsy is more likely to be positive if taken from a tender area of bone.
- Sites of marrow infiltration may be detected by technetium-99m sestamibi uptake, magnetic resonance imaging or fluorine-18 fluorodeoxyglucose with positron emission tomography.

DIFFERENTIAL DIAGNOSIS

- Nucleated red cells and leukocytosis can be seen in overwhelming sepsis, primary myelofibrosis acute severe hypoxia (e.g., acute congestive heart failure), thalassemia major, and severe hemolytic anemia.

TABLE 12–1	**CAUSES OF MARROW INFILTRATION**

I. Fibroblasts and Collagen
   A. Primary myelofibrosis (see Chap. 48)
   B. Fibrosis of other myeloproliferative disorders (see Chaps. 43 and 44)
   C. Fibrosis of hairy cell leukemia (see Chap. 57)
   D. Metastatic malignancies
   E. Sarcoidosis
   F. Secondary myelofibrosis with pulmonary hypertension

II. Other Noncellular Material
   A. Oxalosis

III. Tumor Cells
   A. Carcinoma (e.g., lung, breast, prostate, kidney)
   B. Sarcoma

IV. Granulomas (inflammatory cells)
   A. Miliary tuberculosis
   B. Fungal infections
   C. Sarcoidosis

V. Macrophages
   A. Gaucher disease (see Chap. 38)
   B. Niemann-Pick disease (see Chap. 38)

VI. Marrow Necrosis
   A. Sickle cell anemia (see Chap. 17)
   B. Septicemia
   C. Tumors
   D. Arsenic therapy

VII. Failure of Osteoclast Development
   A. Osteopetrosis

Source: *Williams Hematology,* 8th ed, Chap. 44, Table 44–1, p. 614.

- Primary myelofibrosis (see Chap. 48) may be confused with metastatic disease with focal fibrosis.
- In the absence of a known primary site of cancer, it is important to rule out sarcoma of bone.

TREATMENT AND PROGNOSIS

- The goal of treatment is to manage the underlying disease.
- Marrow infiltration may not always adversely affect the response to treatment of malignant disease.
- However, usually short-term survival is seen in patients with cancer metastatic to marrow. Patients with breast and prostate cancer metastatic to marrow have longer survival on average than those with lung cancer.

For a more detailed discussion, see Archana Agarwal and Josef T. Prchal: Anemia Associated with Marrow Infiltration. Chap. 44, p. 613 in *Williams Hematology,* 8th ed.

CHAPTER 13
Anemia of Chronic Inflammation

DEFINITION

- Anemia associated with chronic infection, inflammatory or neoplastic disease.
- Also referred to as anemia of chronic disease.
- One to 2 months of sustained disease is required for anemia to develop.
- Anemia is moderate, with a hemoglobin level between 7 and 11 g/dL, and is rarely symptomatic.
- The characteristic features of anemia of inflammation (AI) are listed in Table 13–1.

PATHOGENESIS

- Inflammation leads to interleukin (IL)-6 production, which induces hepatocyte hepcidin production, which blocks intestinal iron absorption and iron release from macrophages and hepatocytes. Hepcidin binds to and leads to feroportin degradation, the primary cell surface iron exporter.
- Impaired intestinal iron uptake and impaired release of iron from macrophages leads to a low level of serum iron and consequent low saturation of transferrin.
- Enhanced activity of macrophages increases erythrocyte destruction.
- Production of erythropoietin (EPO) is decreased in response to anemia, and the ability of erythroid precursors to respond to EPO is impaired, both also related to inflammatory cytokine production (IL-1, tumor necrosis factor, interferons).

CLINICAL AND LABORATORY FEATURES

- Anemia is usually overshadowed by symptoms of the primary disease.
- Common conditions leading to AI are shown in Table 13–2.

TABLE 13–1 LABORATORY STUDIES OF IRON METABOLISM IN IRON-DEFICIENCY ANEMIA (IDA), ANEMIA OF INFLAMMATION (AI), AND A COMBINATION OF THE TWO.

	IDA (n = 48)	AI (n = 58)	Combination (n = 17)
Hemoglobin, g/L	93 ± 16 (96)	102 ± 12 (103)	88 ± 20 (90)
MCV, fL	75 ± 9 (75)	90 ± 7 (91)	78 ± 9 (79)
Iron, μmol/L (10–40)	8 ± 11 (4)	10 ± 6 (9)	6 ± 3 (6)
Transferrin, g/L (2.1–3.4m, 2.0–3.1f)	3.3 ± 0.4 (3.3)	1.9 ± 0.5 (1.8)	2.6 ± 0.6 (2.4)
Transferrin saturation, %	12 ± 17 (5.7)	23 ± 13 (21)	12 ± 7 (8)
Ferritin, μg/L (15–306m, 5–103f)	21 ± 55 (11)	342 ± 385 (195)	87 ± 167 (23)
TfR, mg/L (0.85–3.05)	6.2 ± 3.5 (5.0)	1.8 ± 0.6 (1.8)	5.1 ± 2.0 (4.7)
TfR/log ferritin	6.8 ± 6.5 (5.4)	0.8 ± 0.3 (0.8)	3.8 ± 1.9 (3.2)

Reproduced with permission from Punnonen K, Irjala K, Rajamaki A: *Blood* 89:1052, 1997.
Source: *Williams Hematology*, 8th ed, Chap. 37, Table 37–2, p. 506.

TABLE 13–2	COMMON CONDITIONS ASSOCIATED WITH AI
Category	Diseases Associated with AI
Infection	AIDS/HIV, tuberculosis, malaria (contributory), osteomyelitis, chronic abscesses, sepsis
Inflammation	Rheumatoid arthritis, other rheumatologic disorders, inflammatory bowel diseases, systemic inflammatory response syndrome
Malignancy	Carcinomas, myeloma, lymphomas
Cytokine dysregulation	Anemia of aging

Source: *Williams Hematology*, 8th ed, Chap. 37, Table 37–1, p. 504.

- Low reticulocyte index for the degree of anemia.
- Diagnosis, especially differentiation from iron-deficiency anemia (IDA), depends on laboratory findings (see Table 13–1):
  — Initially normochromic, normocytic anemia; hypochromic, microcytic features develop as anemia progresses.
  — Low serum iron level and somewhat decreased serum transferrin concentration; decreased percent saturation of transferrin.
  — Level of serum ferritin, an acute phase protein, is inappropriately elevated (approximately threefold) with respect to storage iron.
  — Marrow contains increased storage iron. The M/E ratio is normal, and the percentage of sideroblasts is decreased.

DIFFERENTIAL DIAGNOSIS

- Drug-induced marrow suppression or drug-induced hemolysis.
- Iron-deficiency anemia is characterized by low serum iron, increased transferrin, decreased storage iron, decreased serum ferritin.
- Anemia of chronic renal failure.
- Myelophthisic anemia caused by carcinoma or lymphoma replacing marrow.

THERAPY

- No treatment may be necessary, other than for the underlying disease.
- Iron (by mouth or parenterally) is contraindicated.
- Androgenic steroids may be of benefit but have unacceptable side effects.
- Packed red cell transfusions may be given, if the anemia is symptomatic.
- Recombinant human erythropoietin (rh-EPO) therapy is effective if serum EPO is not elevated.
  — Starting dose: 10,000 U of rh-EPO three times weekly or darbepoetin alfa 200 mcg every 2 weeks, subcutaneously or intravenously.
  — The target hemoglobin should not exceed 12 g/dL after which EPO dose should be lowered to maintain a level between 11 and 12g/dL.
  — If no response in 3 weeks, double dose.
  — If no response to higher dose in 3 more weeks, discontinue.
  — Hypertension and a risk of thrombotic complications with use of EPO preparations.

For a more detailed discussion, see Tomas Ganz: Anemia of Chronic Disease. Chap. 37, p. 503 in *Williams Hematology*, 8th ed.

CHAPTER 14
Hereditary Spherocytosis, Elliptocytosis, and Related Disorders

THE RED CELL MEMBRANE

- The erythrocyte membrane accounts for 1 percent of total weight of the red cell.
- It plays an integral role in the maintenance of erythrocyte integrity.
- The lipid bilayer of the membrane and its associated skeletal proteins provide the flexibility, durability, and tensile strength for the erythrocyte to undergo large deformations during repeated passages through narrow microcirculatory channels.

HEREDITARY SPHEROCYTOSIS

- Hereditary spherocytosis (HS) is the most common inherited anemia of persons of northern European descent. It is characterized by hemolysis of variable intensity, spherocytosis, and increased osmotic fragility of red blood cells. There is a favorable response to splenectomy.

Etiology

- Accelerated red cell destruction results from deficiency or abnormality of one or more of the red cell membrane proteins, resulting in release of membrane lipids, decreased surface area, and formation of poorly deformable spherocytes.
- The underlying molecular defects are heterogeneous and defects affecting the same protein may produce different phenotypes, such as spherocytosis and elliptocytosis or ovalocytosis.
- Table 14–1 summarizes the relationship between red cell membrane proteins and disease phenotype.

Pathophysiology

- With spectrin deficiency, larger areas of lipid bilayer are unsupported by the submembranous skeleton, causing loss of lipid in submicroscopic vesicles.
- The red cell membrane is more permeable to sodium, which activates the Na^+, K^+-ATPase pump and leads to K^+ loss and dehydration.
- A decrease in the surface area-to-volume ratio and an increase in internal viscosity make spherocytes less deformable and unable to penetrate the slits between splenic cords and sinuses.
- While retained in the spleen, the red cells undergo a "conditioning effect," which renders the cells more spherical (loss of membrane surface area) and more osmotically fragile (lower surface area to volume ratio).
- Ultimately, the cells are engulfed by splenic macrophages and destroyed.
- In most cases, the clinical findings are limited to the red cell. However, some genetic defects causing HS have nonerythroid phenotype and may occur in association with a degenerative spinal cord disorder, cardiomyopathy, or mental retardation.

Prevalence/Inheritance

- In persons of northern European ancestry, the prevalence of HS is believed to be 1 in 5000 population or greater. The prevalence in other ethnic groups is unknown.

TABLE 14–1	RED CELL MEMBRANE PROTEIN DEFECTS IN INHERITED DISORDERS OF RED CELL SHAPE	
Protein	Disorder	Comment
Ankyrin	HS	Most common cause of typical dominant HS
Band 3	HS, SAO, NIHF, HAc	"Pincered" HS spherocytes seen on blood film presplenectomy; SAO results from 9 amino acid deletion
β-Spectrin	HS, HE, HPP, NIHF	"Acanthocytic" spherocytes seen on blood film presplenectomy; location of mutation in β-spectrin determines clinical phenotype
α-Spectrin	HS, HE, HPP, NIHF	Location of mutation in α-spectrin determines clinical phenotype; α-spectrin mutations most common cause of typical HE
Protein 4.2	HS	Primarily found in Japanese patients
Protein 4.1	HE	Found in certain European and Arab populations
GPC	HE	Concomitant protein 4.1 deficiency is basis of HE in GPC defects

GPC, glycophorin C; HAc, hereditary acanthocytosis; HE, hereditary elliptocytosis; HPP, hereditary pyropoikilocytosis; HS, hereditary spherocytosis; NIHF, nonimmune hydrops fetalis; SAO, Southeast Asian ovalocytosis.
Source: *Williams Hematology,* 8th ed, Chap. 45, Table 45–2, p. 626.

- The severity of the condition varies greatly among kindreds, but the typical autosomal dominant form is uniform within a family caused predominantly by heterogeneous mutations of ankyrin and band 3 genes.
- In about 75 percent of cases the family history indicates autosomal dominant transmission. The other cases are either caused by new mutations or by autosomal recessive inheritance.
- Several cases of recessively inherited HS have been reported caused by α spectrin and by band 4.2 defects.

Clinical Features

- The condition is highly variable in severity. More severe cases may be diagnosed in infancy or childhood, but mild cases may escape detection until adulthood or may not be uncovered (see Table 14–2).
- An asymptomatic carrier state has been suggested by reports of asymptomatic parents whose children presented with typical HS.
- In some cases, anemia may be absent as increased red cell production in the marrow compensates for the red cell destruction. Changes in red cell morphology may be subtle, and the bilirubin level and reticulocyte count may be normal to slightly elevated.
- Anemia can be accentuated and become more apparent when splenomegaly from other causes, especially infectious mononucleosis, or marrow suppression from any infections, but especially parvovirus in young patients, are superimposed on mild HS.

TABLE 14–2 CLASSIFICATION OF HEREDITARY SPHEROCYTOSIS

Laboratory Findings	HS Trait or Carrier	Mild Spherocytosis	Moderate Spherocytosis	Moderately Severe Spherocytosis*	Severe Spherocytosis†
Hemoglobin (g/dL)	Normal	11–15	8–12	6–8	<6
Reticulocytes (%)	1–2	3–8	± 8	≥10	≥10
Bilirubin (mg/dL)	0–1	1–2	± 2	2–3	≥3
Spectrin content (% of normal)‡	100	80–100	50–80	40–80§	20–50
Blood film	Normal	Mild spherocytosis	Spherocytosis	Spherocytosis	Spherocytosis and poikilocytosis
Osmotic fragility					
Fresh blood	Normal	Normal or slightly increased	Distinctly increased	Distinctly increased	Distinctly increased
Incubated blood	Slightly increased	Distinctly increased	Distinctly increased	Distinctly increased	Markedly increased

*Values in untransfused patients.
†By definition, patients with severe spherocytosis are transfusion dependent. Values were obtained immediately prior to transfusion.
‡Normal, 245 ± 27 × 10³ spectrin dimers per erythrocyte.
§Spectrin content is variable in this group of patients, presumably reflecting heterogeneity of the underlying pathophysiology.
Reproduced with permission from Eber SW, Armbrust R, and Schroter W. *J Pediatr* 117:409, 1990.
Source: *Williams Hematology,* 8th ed. Chap. 45, Table 45–3, p. 629.

- Typically, HS presents as a mild anemia first noted in the neonate; splenomegaly and mild jaundice are characteristic features; occasionally, the spleen becomes very large. The anemia may be mild and escape detection in childhood. Thus, it is not uncommon to have the diagnosis made in mid or late adulthood because of the finding of an enlarged spleen or bilirubin gallbladder stones.
- Severe transfusion-dependent anemia may be seen, improved modestly by splenectomy. Most such affected individuals appear to be homozygous for an autosomal recessive HS gene.

Complications

- Aplastic crises caused by parvovirus infection result in temporary reticulocytopenia and falling hematocrit.
- Acute megaloblastic changes may result from folate deficiency, particularly in the setting of pregnancy.
- Bilirubin gallstones develop in approximately 50 percent of patients, including those with mild disease, and occasionally in older children.
- Recurrent lower leg ulcerations or dermatitis develop in some patients; these heal quickly after splenectomy.
- Rarely, extramedullary hematopoiesis may present as a mass impinging any organ including spinal cord. Masses may also appear in the chest film simulating mediastinal adenopathy.
- Because of frequent transfusions, iron overload may occur in severely affected individuals.

Laboratory Features

- The degree of anemia varies with severity of the disease.
- Spherocytes on the blood film are the hallmark of the disease. They are smaller in diameter and have a deep red stain (hyperchromatic) because of their increased mean cell hemoglobin concentration (MCHC). They also have decreased or absent central pallor. These three features distinguish them from normal red cells (Fig. 14–1). The MCHC is increased in approximately 50 percent of cases and can reach levels as high as 40 g/dL. Spherocytes are less prominent after splenectomy.
- White blood cell and platelet counts are normal.
- Polychromatophilic macrocytes (reticulocytes) are usually increased in the blood film. Nucleated red cells may be found occasionally.
- Reticulocytosis is found in nearly all patients and is greater than usually associated with the degree of anemia present: mild anemia may be associated with high reticulocyte counts.
- Indicators of red cell destruction include increased serum LDH (may be normal in some cases) and unconjugated bilirubin, decreased haptoglobin concentration, and increased urobilinogen in the urine.
- "Pincered" red cells are seen in band 3–deficient individuals.
- HS cells usually hemolyze in hypotonic salt solutions at a molarity of sodium chloride that is higher than the concentration that initiates lysis of normal cells. This difference, which is based on the lower surface-area-to-volume ratio of HS cells, is accentuated after red cells are incubated for 24 hours. Although normal red cells lose surface area during incubation, the loss in HS cells is exaggerated, making the postincubation osmotic fragility a more sensitive measure, especially in cases with a mild defect (Fig. 14–2).
- The value of incubated osmotic fragility tests has been questioned. Occasionally, the only abnormality on testing may be a "tail" of the post-incubation osmotic fragility curve, reflecting the most fragile cells. These HS cells hemolyze in hypotonic salt solutions of a molarity that will not lyse normal cells. The abnormality is more prominent in individuals with intact spleens.

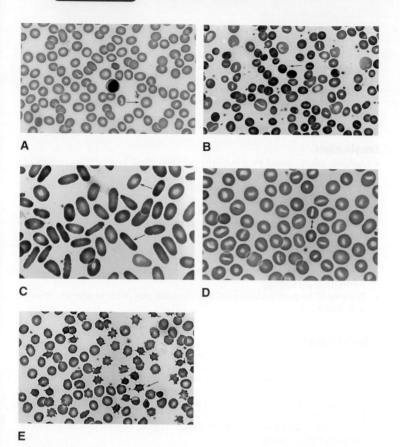

FIGURE 14-1 Red cell shapes in hereditary hemolytic anemia. **A.** Normal blood film. Arrow points to normocytic-normochromic red cell. **B.** Hereditary spherocytosis. Note numerous cells (typified by cell highlighted by arrow) that are hyperchromic with absent or small pale centers, circular-shape, and often with shorter diameters than normal red cells. Larger, paler cells are reticulocytes. **C.** Hereditary elliptocytosis. Numerous elliptocytes with greater length (L) to width (W) ratio (cigar-shaped) (lower arrow) and ovalocytes with lower L/W ratio (American football-shaped) (upper arrow). Because they are such closely related abnormalities, it has been proposed that each should be called elliptocytes and Roman numeral I to III be used to determine the frequency of cells with lower to greater L/W ratio. Thus, elliptocytosis I would be largely ovalocytes, II would be a mixture, and III would be largely elliptocytes. **D.** Hereditary stomatocytosis. Note high prevalence of red cells with either a small central pallor or with a longitudinal slit-like central pallor. An example of each is shown by the double arrow. **E.** Acanthocytosis. Small hyperchromatic red cells with spike like irregularly positioned projections, sometimes turning back on themselves. See arrow for example. (Reproduced with permission from *Lichtman's Atlas of Hematology*, www.accessmedicine.com)

- Other tests for detection of HS have been described but are probably no better than the incubated osmotic fragility test.
- A diligent family study that includes measurement of hemoglobin, reticulocyte count, and examination of the blood film is important because the discovery of family members with a spherocytic hemolytic anemia may secure the diagnosis, affected family members can be evaluated to determine if they need therapy, and diagnosis of the anemia may prevent confusion in their health care at a later date.

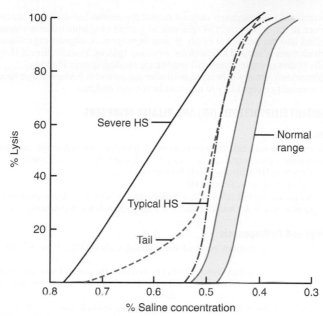

FIGURE 14-2 Osmotic fragility testing. The *shaded area* is the normal range. Results representative of both typical and severe spherocytosis are shown. A "tail," representing very fragile erythrocytes that have been conditioned by the spleen, is common in many HS patients prior to splenectomy. (Reproduced with permission from Gallagher PG, Forget BG, Lux SE: *Hematology of Infancy and Childhood*, p. 544. WB Saunders, Philadelphia, 1998.)
(Source: *Williams Hematology*, 8th ed, Chap. 45, Fig. 45–8B, p. 632.)

Differential Diagnosis
- HS should be considered in patients with incidentally noted splenomegaly, gall-stones at a young age, anemia developing during pregnancy, parvovirus infections, or infectious mononucleosis. Since autoimmune hemolytic disease and HS are the two most common causes of spherocytic anemia, a direct antiglobulin test should be done to eliminate the former as a consideration.
- Immune-mediated hemolysis and unstable hemoglobins may lead to formation of spherocytes. Other rare causes are clostridium sepsis and recluse spider bites. Spherocytes also occasionally occur in patients with an enlarged spleen or with microangiopathic hemolytic anemia. The spherocytes in HS are relatively uniform in shape and are the dominant and sole red cell abnormality.
- Diagnosis can be obscured in obstructive jaundice because red cells may normalize in appearance and increase in survival from accumulation of cholesterol and phospholipid.

Therapy, Course, and Prognosis
- Because of increased red cell turnover, folic acid supplementation is often given.
- Patients with aplastic crises or severe hemolysis may require transfusion.
- If the diagnosis is correct, splenectomy, allows a nearly normal red cell survival, corrects the anemia, and decreases the risk of biliary tract stones. Spherocytosis is much less prominent and osmotic fragility is corrected to nearly normal in most cases. Very uncommonly, in atypical cases, splenectomy may not eliminate the hemolysis completely.

- Occasionally, splenectomy may not correct the anemia because of an accessory spleen or the development of splenosis as a result of splenic tissue accidentally spilled into the peritoneal cavity at time of surgery. A surgeon experienced in splenectomy is advised to search for accessory spleens. Visualization of Howell-Jolly bodies in erythrocytes will confirm the residual splenic function.
- Splenectomy usually is delayed until after the patient is 6 years of age because of increased susceptibility to infection in younger children.

HEREDITARY ELLIPTOCYTOSIS (HE) AND RELATED DISORDERS

Definition

- HE encompasses a heterogeneous group of disorders in which elliptical red cells are common feature and can be divided usually into three major groups:
  — Common HE with discoidal elliptocytes.
  — Spherocytic or ovalocytic HE.
  — Stomatocytic HE (also called Melanesian or Southeast Asian ovalocytosis) in which cells are rounder but have a longitudinal or transverse slit.

Etiology and Pathogenesis

- Table 14–1 summarizes some of the molecular abnormalities associated with HE.
- Most of the defects that cause elliptocytosis render the red cell membrane skeleton unstable. In severely affected individuals, red cell fragmentation may occur under conditions of normal shear stress.
- Red cell precursors in common HE are round, but red cells become more elliptical as they age *in vivo*.
- HE cells appear to be stabilized in their abnormal shape by reorganization of the skeleton with new protein contacts that prevent recovery of normal shape.
- The main features that affect severity of hemolysis are the spectrin content and the percentage of dimeric spectrin.

Prevalence/Inheritance

- In the United States, the prevalence of HE is approximately 3 to 5 per 10,000 population; it is more common in African-Americans, but prevalence data are not available. The prevalence is higher in areas where malaria is endemic (0.6% or more in equatorial Africa).
- In both common HE and stomatocytic HE, the inheritance pattern is autosomal dominant; occasionally, HE can be inherited from an asymptomatic carrier.

Clinical Features

- Most persons with elliptocytosis do not have hemolysis and are asymptomatic.
- Transient hemolysis may be noted in individuals with mild HE if they develop viral, bacterial, or protozoal infections; renal transplant rejection; or vitamin B_{12} deficiency; or if they become pregnant.
- HE may result in significant hemolysis requiring splenectomy. Such patients may be heterozygotes carrying a severely dysfunctional α-spectrin mutant or homozygotes for 4.1 deficiency or β-spectrin mutations. These individuals may have all the clinical features seen in HS: gallstones, leg ulcers, frontal bossing. In addition to elliptocytes, patients with severe disease also have large numbers of poikilocytes and small red cell fragments.

Laboratory Features

- The definition of elliptocytosis is based on red cell shape (see Fig. 14–1).
- Axial ratios of the red cell may vary considerably, as do the number of elliptocytes seen even in patients with a clearly defined biochemical defect.
- The percentage of elliptocytes in normal subjects is less than 1 percent.

- Osmotic fragility is normal in mild HE but increased in severe HE and spherocytic HE.

Differential Diagnosis

- Elliptocytes and poikilocytes are commonly found in many conditions, including megaloblastic anemia, myelophthisic anemias, myelodysplastic syndromes, and pyruvate kinase deficiency. Although they may be numerous, the elliptocytes rarely exceed 60 percent in these conditions and various other red cell shape changes are present.
- Differentiation from HE rests on the negative family history and presence of other clinical features associated with the above diseases.
- Biochemical analysis of the membrane skeletal proteins will establish the diagnosis.

Therapy

- Mild forms need no intervention at all. In the more severely affected, splenectomy will lessen or prevent the need for transfusions.

SPHEROCYTIC HEREDITARY ELLIPTOCYTOSIS

- Shows features of both HE and HS. Also called HE with spherocytosis or hereditary hemolytic ovalocytosis.
- Blood films contain elliptical red cells and spherocytes or round spheroovalocytes are seen. Hemolysis and increased osmotic fragility occur despite mild abnormalities in red cell morphology. The molecular basis is unknown.

SOUTHEAST ASIAN OVALOCYTOSIS

- Dominantly inherited condition that is widespread in certain groups in Southeast Asia and characterized by oval red cells with one or two transverse ridges or a longitudinal slit.
- Other features include increased red cell rigidity, decreased osmotic fragility, increased thermal stability, reduced expression of certain red cell antigens.
- Resistance *in vitro* to invasion by several malaria parasites has been described. The mechanism of this resistance is unknown.
- Caused by an abnormality of band 3 protein.

HEREDITARY PYROPOIKILOCYTOSIS

- Hereditary pyropoikilocytosis (HPP) is a severe hemolytic anemia with marked microspherocytes and micropoikilocytes (MCV as low as 50 fL) and thermal instability of red cells.
- In normal individuals, spectrin denatures and red cells fragment at temperatures of 49 to 50 °C. Generally in HPP, this occurs at temperatures of 45 to 46 °C, although cases of otherwise typical HPP may have normal thermal stability. Thermal instability has also been detected in HE individuals with α-spectrin mutations.
- It is an autosomal recessive disorder.
- The patients are heterozygous for an α-spectrin mutation and a defect in spectrin synthesis. The same phenotype occurs in homozygotes or compound heterozygotes for one or two α-spectrin mutations, respectively.
- Chiefly seen in persons of African ancestry.
- HPP represents a subset of HE; identical spectrin mutations have been noted, but the defect is more severe in HPP where a partial spectrin deficiency is also seen. HPP is clinically indistinguishable from severe homozygous HE.

ACANTHOCYTOSIS

- Spur cells or acanthocytes are red cells with multiple, irregular projections. They have been noted in several conditions.

Severe Liver Disease

- Shape change is a result of accumulation of nonesterified cholesterol in the red cell membrane, but the exact mechanism is unknown. Normal red cells will acquire the defect after transfusion into an affected patient.
- Rapidly progressive hemolytic anemia is noted in some individuals, usually with advanced alcoholic cirrhosis.
- Splenectomy is usually not advised because of severe liver disease. Treatment of the underlying disease, alcohol addiction should be tried.

Abetalipoproteinemia

- A rare autosomal recessive disease with slight increase in membrane cholesterol/phospholipid ratio and definite increase in membrane sphingomyelin. Shape change appears as red cells age.
- Anemia is mild. Acanthocytes constitute 50 to 90 percent of cells (Fig. 14–1).
- Steatorrhea develops early in life; retinitis pigmentosa and other progressive neurologic abnormalities lead to death in the second or third decade.
- Treat with dietary restriction of triglycerides and supplementation of fat-soluble vitamins.

Chorea-Acanthocytosis Syndrome

- A rare inherited, presumably autosomal recessive, choreiform syndrome. The clinical features develop in adults with variable progressive neurologic abnormalities, and acanthocytosis with normal plasma lipids.
- Patients are not anemic.

McLeod Phenotype

- An X-linked disorder that can coexist with chronic granulomatous disease, Duchenne muscular dystrophy, or retinitis pigmentosa.
- Red cells in these individuals lack the 37,000-Da Kx antigen.
- Mild hemolytic anemia with a high percentage of acanthocytes.
- Areflexia, dystonia, and choreiform movements develop after the fifth decade.

Other Conditions

- Acanthocytes may occur in patients with anorexia nervosa, hypothyroidism, and myelodysplasia, and in the postsplenectomy state.

STOMATOCYTOSIS AND RELATED DISORDERS

- In a three-dimensional view, stomatocytes have the shape of a cup or a bowl. The slit-like appearance seen on slides is an artifact caused by folding of the cells (Fig. 14–1).
- Red cell cationic permeability is often disordered, but the red cell volume is variable.
- The cells are seen in a variety of disorders.

Acquired Stomatocytosis

- Stomatocytes make up less than 1 percent of the red cells of normal subjects. About 1 in 40 hospitalized patients have more than this number in association with a variety of medical conditions.

Hereditary Stomatocytosis

- An autosomal dominant disease with moderate to severe hemolytic anemia. From 10 to 30 percent stomatocytes are present and the osmotic fragility is markedly increased. These cells have a major inward sodium leak.

Hereditary Xerocytosis (Desiccocytosis)
- A rare autosomal dominant disease with moderately severe hemolytic anemia characterized by red cell dehydration and decreased osmotic fragility.

Intermediate Syndromes
- Sporadic cases share features of the above disorders with stomatocytes and/or target cells and normal-to-increased osmotic fragility.
- Results of splenectomy in stomatocytosis and xerocytosis are varied.

Rh Deficiency Syndrome
- Rare individuals with absent (Rh null) or markedly reduced (Rh mod) Rh antigen have hemolytic anemia with stomatocytes, occasional spherocytes, and increased osmotic fragility. Splenectomy markedly improves the anemia.

Familial Lecithin–Cholesterol Acyltransferase (LCAT) Deficiency
- A rare autosomal recessive condition with corneal opacities, premature atherosclerosis, proteinuria, and mild hemolytic anemia. Marrow shows sea blue histiocytosis.
- Target cells are numerous and have a marked increase in cholesterol and phosphatidylcholine in the red cell membrane.

Familial Deficiency of High-Density Lipoproteins
- Severe deficiency or absence of HDL results in a moderately severe hemolytic anemia with stomatocytosis and cholesterol ester accumulation in many tissues.

For a more detailed discussion, see Patrick G. Gallagher: The Red Blood Cell Membrane and Its Disorders: Hereditary Spherocytosis, Elliptocytosis, and Related Disorders. Chap. 45, p. 617 in *Williams Hematology*, 8th ed.

CHAPTER 15
Hemolytic Anemia Related to Red Cell Enzyme Defects

- Clinical manifestations of inherited red cell enzyme deficiencies are diverse and may be:
  - — Episodic hemolysis after exposure to oxidants or infection.
  - — Chronic hemolytic anemia (hereditary nonspherocytic anemia).
  - — Acute hemolysis after eating fava beans (favism).
  - — Methemoglobinemia.
  - — Polycythemia.
  - — Icterus neonatorum.
  - — No hematologic manifestations.
- However, only hemolytic complications will be reviewed here. Methemoglobinemia is reviewed in Chap. 19 and polycythemia in Chap. 29.

MECHANISM OF HEMOLYSIS IN PATIENTS WITH RED CELL ENZYME ABNORMALITIES

- In glucose-6-phosphate dehydrogenase (G-6-PD) deficiency, oxidant challenge leads to the formation of denatured hemoglobin and Heinz bodies, which make the red cells less deformable and liable to splenic destruction.
- Metabolic aberrations in most red cell enzymopathies cause hemolysis by undefined mechanism(s).

GLUCOSE-6-PHOSPHATE DEHYDROGENASE DEFICIENCY

- X-linked disorder.
- The normal enzyme is designated G-6-PD B.
- A mutant enzyme with normal activity [G-6-PD A(+)] is found in 16 percent of American men of African descent. It has a single mutation at nt c.376 (c. 376 A>G, amino acid substitution: p.Asn126Asp).
- G-6-PD A− is the principal deficient variant found among people of African ancestry. It has the nt c.376 mutation and an additional mutation, almost always at nt c.202 (c. 202 G>A, p.Val68Met). G-6-PD A− has decreased stability *in vivo*, and the affected hemizygotes have 5 to 15 percent of normal activity. Prevalence of G-6-PD A− in American men of African descent is 11 percent.
- G-6-PD deficiency in Europe is most common in the southern part of the continent and is most often a result of a Mediterranean variant that has a single base substitution at nt c.563 (c. 563 C>T, p.Ser188Phe). Although, there is scarcely any detectable enzymatic activity in the erythrocytes, there are no clinical manifestations unless the patient is exposed to oxidative drugs, infection, or fava beans. Other variants, such as G-6-PD Seattle (p.Asp282His) and G-6-PD A−, are also encountered in Europe.
- Many different G-6-PD mutations, including G-6-PD Mediterranean, are encountered in Asia. Most of these are severe variants. Examples include G-6-PD Canton, Jammu, Bangkok, and Kaiping.

Drugs that Can Incite Hemolysis (see Table 15-1)
- Individual differences in the metabolism of certain drugs as well as the specific G-6-PD mutation influence the extent of RBC destruction.

TABLE 15–1	DRUGS AND CHEMICALS THAT SHOULD BE AVOIDED BY PERSONS WITH G-6-PD DEFICIENCY
Acetanilid	
Dapsone	
Dimercaptosuccinic acid	
Fava beans	
Furazolidone (Furoxone)	
Glibenclamide	
Isobutyl nitrite	
Methylene blue	
Nalidixic acid (NegGram)	
Naphthalene	
Niridazole (Ambilhar)	
Nitrofurantoin (Furadantin)	
Phenazopyridine (Pyridium)	
Phenylhydrazine	
Primaquine	
Sulfacetamide	
Sulfanilamide	
Sulfapyridine	
Thiazolesulfone	
Toluidine blue	
Trinitrotoluene (TNT)	
Urate oxidase	

Source: *Williams Hematology*, 8th ed, Chap. 46, Table 46–5, p. 661.

- Typically, drug-induced hemolysis begins 1 to 3 days after drug exposure. When severe, it may be associated with abdominal or back pain. The urine may become dark, even black.
- Heinz bodies appear in circulating red cells and then disappear as they are removed by the spleen. The hemoglobin concentration then decreases rapidly.
- Hemolysis is self-limited in the G-6-PD A– type but is the more severe and more prolonged in Mediterranean type.

Febrile Illnesses that Can Incite Hemolysis
- Hemolysis may occur within 1 to 2 days of onset of a febrile illness, usually resulting in mild anemia.
- Hemolysis occurs especially in patients with pneumonia or typhoid fever.
- Jaundice may be particularly severe in association with infectious hepatitis.
- Reticulocytosis is usually suppressed, and recovery from anemia is delayed until after the active infection is over.

Favism
- Potentially one of the most severe hematologic consequences of G-6-PD deficiency.
- Hemolysis occurs within hours to days after ingestion of the beans.
- Urine becomes red or dark, and shock, sometimes fatal, may develop rapidly.
- Not all G-6-PD–deficient subjects develop hemolysis when they ingest fava beans. The enzyme deficiency is a necessary but not sufficient factor. The other factors required are not known, but believed to be, in part, genetic.
- More common in children than in adults, and occurs usually with variants that cause severe deficiency.

Icterus Neonatorum

- May occur in some newborns with G-6-PD deficiency and, if not treated, may lead to kernicterus and mental retardation.
- Rare in neonates with the A− variant, but more common in Mediterranean and various Asian variants.
- Is not caused by hemolysis, but rather by impaired conjugation in the liver.
- Occurs particularly in infants who are G-6-PD–deficient who have also inherited a mutation of the UDP-glucuronosyltransferase-1 gene promoter (Gilbert syndrome).

HEREDITARY NONSPHEROCYTIC HEMOLYTIC ANEMIA (HNSHA)

- May occur with severely deficient variants of G-6-PD deficiency (however, these are very rare; referred to as class 1 G-6-PD deficiency) and with deficiency of a variety of other red cell metabolic enzymes.
- Anemia may range from severe (hemoglobin level 5 g/dL) to a fully compensated state with near normal hemoglobin concentration.
- Chronic jaundice, splenomegaly, and gallstones are common, and some patients develop ankle ulcers.
- Nonhematologic manifestations may occur, such as cataracts in some patients with G-6-PD deficiency, muscle glycogen storage deficiency in phosphofructokinase deficiency, or severe neuromuscular disease in triosephosphate isomerase deficiency.
- Pyruvate kinase (PK) deficiency:
  — The most common cause of HNSHA.
  — Estimated to occur at the rate of approximately 50 per 1,000,000 in the white population.
  — Can be so severe that chronic transfusion therapy is required.
  — A partial response to splenectomy is usually observed. As young PK-deficient red cells are selectively sequestered by the spleen in PK deficiency, the postsplenectomy response is accompanied by a paradoxical increase in the number of reticulocytes.
- Glucose phosphate isomerase deficiency:
  — Second most common cause of HNSHA.
  — Anemia is usually relatively mild, but fetal hydrops has been observed several times with this enzyme deficiency.
  — Response to splenectomy is usually very good.
- Triosephosphate isomerase deficiency:
  — The most devastating of the red cell enzyme defects.
  — Adults with the disease are rare because most patients die of neuromuscular complications before the age of 5 years.
- Pyrimidine 5′ nucleotidase deficiency:
  — Characterized by stippled red cells and is, therefore, the only cause of HNSHA in which a provisional morphologic diagnosis is possible.
  — Because of the age-related decay of the normal enzyme, a partial deficiency occurs in patients with decreased erythropoiesis, particularly children with transient erythroblastopenia of childhood.

Laboratory Features

- Erythrocytes with enzyme deficiencies have normal morphology in the absence of hemolysis, except as noted above, or have mild changes that are not distinctive.
- Increased serum bilirubin concentration, decreased haptoglobin levels, and increased serum lactic dehydrogenase activity all may be present when hemolysis occurs.
- Leukopenia may occur in patients with splenomegaly.

Differential Diagnosis

- Depends on demonstration of the enzyme deficiency.
- Start with screening tests for G-6-PD and PK activity.
- Assays or screening tests for G-6-PD deficiency are most reliable in healthy affected (hemizygous) males.
- Diagnosis may be difficult during a hemolytic episode in G-6-PD A– patients because residual young red cells have normal levels of G-6-PD.
- Dense red cells (reticulocyte-depleted) can be tested following differential centrifugation.
- Family studies can be very helpful.
- May have to retest 1 month after patient is fully recovered from hemolytic episode.
- Presence of basophilic stippling suggests lead poisoning or pyrimidine 5′-nucleotidase deficiency.
- When the nucleotide substitution is known, heterozygotes are easily detected by PCR-based analysis, which is also useful for prenatal diagnosis.

Treatment

- G-6-PD–deficient individuals should avoid "oxidant" drugs (see Table 15–1).
- Transfusions should be given only in the most severe cases of G-6-PD deficiency, such as favism, but may be commonly required in PK or other enzyme deficiencies accompanied by severe anemia.
- Exchange transfusion may be necessary in infants with neonatal icterus.
- Splenectomy is sometimes considered in certain patients with HNSHA.
  — Severity of disease and functional impairment are important considerations.
  — Benefit of splenectomy differs according to family defect, and family history of response to splenectomy, if available, is the most useful guide.
  — If cholecystectomy is required, splenectomy may be done at the same time.
- If concomitant iron overload is present, iron chelation is indicated.
- Glucocorticoids are of no known value.
- Folic acid therapy is often given, but is without proven hematologic benefit unless a deficiency is found in the red cells.
- Iron therapy is probably contraindicated unless unrelated causes of iron deficiency are operative.

For a more detailed discussion, see Wouter W. van Solinge and Richard van Wijk: Disorders Of Red Cells Resulting From Enzyme Abnormalities. Chap. 46, p. 613 in *Williams Hematology,* 8th ed.

CHAPTER 16
The Thalassemias

DEFINITION

- A group of disorders, each resulting from an inherited defect in the rate of synthesis of one or more globin chains.
- Resultant imbalance of globin chain production may cause ineffective erythropoiesis, defective hemoglobin production, red cell hemoglobin precipitates, hemolysis, and anemia of variable degree.

ETIOLOGY AND PATHOGENESIS

Genetic Control and Synthesis of Hemoglobin

- Each hemoglobin (Hb) molecule consists of two separate pairs of identical globin chains.
- All normal human hemoglobins found in an adult have one pair of α-chains. The α-chains can combine with β-chains ($\alpha_2\beta_2$), δ-chains ($\alpha_2\delta_2$) and γ-chains ($\alpha_2\gamma_2$).
- Adult Hb is ~97 percent Hb A ($\alpha_2\beta_2$), ~0.5 percent Hb F, and ~2.5 percent Hb A_2 ($\alpha_2\delta_2$).
- Fetal life: Hb F ($\alpha_2\gamma_2$) predominates. Position 136 of some γ-chains is occupied by glycine and in others by alanine. These are designated $^G\gamma$ and $^A\gamma$, respectively: At birth Hb F is a mixture of $\alpha_2{}^G\gamma_2$ and $\alpha_2{}^A\gamma_2$ in a ratio of 3:1.
- Embryonic Hb: Hb Gower 1 ($\zeta_2\epsilon_2$), Hb Gower 2 ($\alpha_2\epsilon_2$), and Hb Portland ($\zeta_2\gamma_2$), before 8th week of intrauterine life.
- During fetal life, globin gene expression switches occur from ζ- to α- and from ϵ- to γ-chain production, followed by β- and δ-chain production after birth.

Globin Gene Clusters

- α-Gene cluster (chromosome 16) consists of one functional ζ gene and two α genes (α_2 and α_1).
- Exons of the two α-globin genes have identical sequences, however, they differ in second intron.
- Production of α_2 mRNA exceeds that of α_1, by factor of 1.5 to 3.
- β-Gene cluster (chromosome 11) consists of one functional ϵ gene, a $^G\gamma$ gene, an $^A\gamma$ gene, a pseudo β gene, a δ gene, and a β gene.
- Flanking regions contain conserved sequences essential for gene expression.

Regulation of Globin Gene Clusters

- Primary transcript is a large mRNA precursor, with both intron and exon sequences, which is extensively processed in the nucleus to yield the final mRNA.
- Expression of the globin genes is regulated by complex control mechanisms.

Developmental Changes in Globin Gene Expression

- β-Globin produced at low levels beginning at 8 to 10 weeks of fetal life, increases considerably at about 36 weeks gestation.
- γ-Globin produced at high levels early, starts to decline at ~36 weeks.
- At birth, β-globin and γ-globin production are approximately equal.
- By age 1 year, γ-globin production is less than 1 percent of total non–α-globin production.

- Mechanism of switches is not clear, but probably involves a "time clock" in the hematopoietic stem cell.
- Fetal hemoglobin synthesis may be reactivated in adults in states of hematopoietic stress.

MOLECULAR BASIS OF THE THALASSEMIAS

- A large number of mutations cause thalassemia (e.g., more than 200 for β-thalassemia).
- The molecular basis of the thalassemias is discussed in detail in Chap. 47, p. 675 in *Williams Hematology,* 8th ed.

DIFFERENT FORMS OF THALASSEMIA

- β-Thalassemias are of two main varieties:
  — β^0-Thalassemia, with total absence of β-chain production.
  — β^+-Thalassemia, with partial deficiency of β-chain production.
  — Hallmark of the common forms of β-thalassemias is elevation of Hb A_2 in heterozygotes.
- δβ-Thalassemias are heterogeneous:
  — In some cases, no δ or β-chains are produced.
  — In others cases, the non-α chains are fusion δβ-chains: N-terminal residue of δ-chain fused to C-terminal residues of the β-chain. Fusion variants are called *Lepore hemoglobins.*
  — Levels of Hb F but not HbA_2 are elevated in heterozygotes.
- Hereditary persistence of fetal hemoglobin (HPFH):
  — Heterogeneous genetically (deletion and nondeletion forms).
  — Characterized by persistence of Hb F in adult life.
  — No clinical significance, but may have mild thalassemic changes.
- α-Thalassemias are usually caused by deletion of one or more of the four α genes (two globin genes per haploid chromosome):
  — If one of the two α-globin loci on chromosome 16 is deleted, the designation α− is used. If both are deleted the designation − − is used. Thus, a patient with two α locus deletions would be designated α−/α− or αα/− − depending on the arrangement of the deletions on the chromosomes.
  — α-Thalassemias also arise from a variety of other mechanisms, such as an elongated α-chain because of a mutated stop codon (Hb Constant Spring) or missense or nonsense mutations.

PATHOPHYSIOLOGY

Imbalanced Globin Chain Synthesis (The Major Problem)

- Homozygous β-thalassemia:
  — β-Globin synthesis absent or greatly reduced, resulting in hypochromic microcytic red cells.
  — As excess α-chains are incapable of forming viable hemoglobin tetramers, they precipitate in red cell precursors, resulting in intramedullary destruction of the abnormal erythroid cells (ineffective erythropoiesis) and hemolysis.
  — Clinical manifestations appear after neonatal switch from γ-chain to β chain production.
- Heterozygous β-thalassemia:
  — Usually only mild hypochromic microcytic anemia with elevated Hb A_2.
  — Some are more severe because of poor heme-binding properties and instability, with red cell inclusions containing precipitated β-chains as well as excess α-chains. These are sometimes designated as *hyperunstable hemoglobins.*

- α-Thalassemias:
  — Defective α-chain production: manifestations in both fetal and adult life as α-chains are present in both fetal and adult hemoglobins.
  — In the newborn, excess γ-chains become soluble γ_4 homotetramers designated Hb Bart's.
  — After infancy, as the switch from γ- to β-chains takes place, excess β-chains if sufficiently large become β_4 (Hb H).
  — As both γ_4 and β_4 homotetramers are soluble, they do not precipitate to any significant degree; explaining the less severe degree of ineffective erythropoiesis in α-thalassemias compared to β-thalassemias.
  — However, Hb H is unstable and precipitates readily, forming inclusion bodies.
  — Both Hb Bart's and Hb H have high oxygen affinity.
  — Defect in hemoglobin synthesis leads to hypochromic, microcytic cells.

Persistent Fetal Hemoglobin Production and Cellular Heterogeneity

- In β^0-thalassemias, Hb F is the only hemoglobin produced except for small amounts of Hb A_2.
- In thalassemias, as in normal individuals, Hb F is heterogeneously distributed among the red cells.
- Because of elevated Hb F levels in β-thalassemias, red cells have high oxygen affinity.
- The mechanism of persistent γ-chain synthesis in thalassemias is incompletely understood.

Consequence of Compensatory Mechanisms for the Anemia of Thalassemia

- Severe anemia and the high oxygen affinity of Hb F in homozygous β-thalassemia produce severe tissue hypoxia.
- High oxygen affinity of Hb Bart's and Hb H accentuates hypoxia in severe forms of α-thalassemia.
- Erythropoietin production and consequent expansion of marrow lead to deformities of skull with frequent sinus and ear infections, porous long bones, and pathologic fractures.
- Massive erythropoiesis diverts calories and also leads to hyperuricemia, gout, and folate deficiency.

Splenomegaly; Dilutional Anemia

- Constant exposure of the spleen to red cells of precipitated globin chains leads to "work hypertrophy" of spleen, ultimately leading to splenomegaly.
- The enlarged spleen may sequester red cells and expand plasma volume, exacerbating anemia.

Abnormal Iron Metabolism

- β^0-Thalassemia homozygotes accumulate large amounts of iron because of increased absorption and red cell transfusions.
- Iron accumulates in endocrine glands, liver and, most importantly, myocardium.
- Consequences: diabetes, hypoparathyroidism, hypogonadism, and death from heart failure.
- The role of hepcidin in the abnormal regulation of iron absorption in thalassemias is discussed in Chap. 9 of this Manual and Chap. 42 of *Williams Hematology*, 8th ed.

Infection

- All forms of severe thalassemia appear to be associated with an increased susceptibility to bacterial infection.

Coagulation Defects

- Patients with thrombocytosis after splenectomy may develop progressive pulmonary hypertension as a result of platelet aggregation in the pulmonary circulation.

Clinical Heterogeneity

- Most manifestations of β-thalassemia are related to excess α-chains.
- Degree of globin-chain imbalance determines severity.
- Coinheritance of α-thalassemia or of genes for enhanced γ-chain production may reduce the severity of β-thalassemias.

POPULATION GENETICS

- β-Thalassemias: Mediterranean populations, Middle East, India and Pakistan, Southeast Asia, southern Russia, China.
  - Rare in Africa, except Liberia and parts of North Africa.
  - Occurs sporadically in all races.
- α-Thalassemias: Widespread in Africa, Mediterranean populations, Middle East, Southeast Asia.
  - Loss of both functional α-globin loci on the same chromosome occurs in Mediterranean and Asian populations and is extremely rare in Africa and the Middle East. Thus, Hb Bart's hydrops syndrome and Hb H disease are largely restricted to Southeast Asia and Mediterranean populations.
- Thalassemic red cells are less likely to be infected with the plasmodial organisms of malaria.

CLINICAL FEATURES

β-Thalassemias

- β-Thalassemia major: clinically severe, requiring transfusions.
- β-Thalassemia intermedia: milder, later onset, requiring either few or no transfusions.
- β-Thalassemia minor: heterozygous carrier, clinically asymptomatic.

β-Thalassemia Major

- Homozygous or compound heterozygous state.
- Infants well at birth; anemia develops in first few months of life and becomes progressively more severe and coincide with switch from γ to β-chains. Failure to thrive.
- Onset of symptoms after first year of life more typical of β-thalassemia intermedia.
- Inadequately transfused child
  - Stunted growth. Expanded marrow leads to bossing of skull, expanded maxilla, widened diploë, gross skeletal deformities.
  - Grossly enlarged liver and spleen. Secondary thrombocytopenia and leukopenia.
  - Skin pigmentation. Chronic leg ulceration.
  - Hypermetabolic state: fever, wasting, hyperuricemia.
  - Frequent infections, folate deficiency, spontaneous fractures, dental problems.
  - Symptoms of iron loading by time of puberty; poor growth; endocrine problems (diabetes mellitus, adrenal insufficiency); cardiac problems, death by the third decade as a result of cardiac siderosis.
- Adequately transfused child
  - Grows and develops normally until effects of iron loading appear by end of first decade.

β-Thalassemia Intermedia
- Wide spectrum of disability:
  — Severe forms: later appearing anemia than β-thalassemia major; usually requires transfusion. Retarded growth and development, skeletal deformities, splenomegaly.
  — Milder forms: asymptomatic, transfusion-independent, Hb levels 10 to 12 g/dL.

β-Thalassemia Minor
- Often slight anemia without functional impairment. Discovered by blood cell examination.

α-Thalassemias
- Interactions of α-thalassemia haplotypes result in four broad phenotypic categories:
  — Normal (αα/αα).
  — Silent carrier (α–/αα).
  — α-Thalassemia trait (α–/α–) or (– –/αα). Mild hematologic changes, but no clinical abnormality. Low MCV, low MCH, varying levels of Hb Bart's (γ_4) at birth.
  — Hb H disease (– –/α–). Hypochromic, severe to moderately severe hemolytic anemia often with marked splenomegaly. Red cells contain precipitates of Hb H(β_4), which is an unstable hemoglobin.
- Hb Bart's *hydrops fetalis* syndrome (– –/– –). Incompatible with extrauterine life.
  — Frequent cause of stillbirth in Southeast Asia. If alive at birth, infant dies within hours.
  — Pallor, massive edema, hepatosplenomegaly. Hydrops resembles that of Rh incompatibility.
  — High incidence of maternal toxemia of pregnancy. Enlarged placenta.
  — At autopsy: massive extramedullary hematopoiesis.

LABORATORY FEATURES

β-Thalassemias
β-Thalassemia Major
- Severe anemia: Hb 2 to 3 g/dL. Blood film: marked anisopoikilocytosis, hypochromia, target cells, basophilic stippling, large poikilocytes. Nucleated red cells numerous. Reticulocytes moderately increased. Inclusions of Hb in hypochromic red cells (these can be supravitally stained by methyl violet). After splenectomy: more inclusions; large, flat macrocytes; small, deformed microcytes.
- Leukocyte and platelet counts normal or slightly elevated.
- Marrow: marked erythroid hyperplasia; abnormal erythroblasts with stippling, increased sideroblasts. Markedly increased storage iron.
- Markedly ineffective erythropoiesis. Shortened red cell survival.
- Hemoglobin: fetal hemoglobin increased, from less than 10 percent to greater than 90 percent. Hb A is absent in β^0-thalassemia. Hb A_2 levels are low, normal, or high; always invariably elevated, however, if expressed as a proportion of Hb A.

β-Thalassemia Minor
- Mild anemia: hemoglobin 9 to 11 g/dL.
- Microcytic hypochromic red cells: MCV 50 to 70 fL, MCH 20 to 22 pg. MCV is a valuable screen for thalassemia trait.
- Hemoglobin A_2 level is increased to 3.5 to 7 percent.

α-Thalassemias

Hemoglobin Bart's Hydrops Fetalis Syndrome

- Blood film: severe thalassemic changes; many nucleated red blood cells.
- Hemoglobin: Hb Bart's predominates; Hb Portland ($\zeta_2\gamma_2$) 10 to 20 percent.

Hemoglobin H Disease

- Blood film: hypochromic microcytic red blood cells, increased polychromasia.
- Mild reticulocytosis (~5%).
- Hb H inclusions demonstrable in almost all red blood cells in blood incubated with brilliant cresyl blue.

α⁰-Thalassemia Trait (αα/– – or α-/α-)

- Similar appearance of blood film and cell counts as in β-thalassemia trait.
- Five to 15 percent Hb Bart's at birth, disappears during maturation.
- Rare cells with Hb H inclusions can be demonstrated in some cases.

Silent Carrier or α⁺-Thalassemia Trait (αα/α-)

- One to 2 percent Hb Bart's at birth in some but not all cases.
- Gene mapping analysis is only certain method of diagnosing α-thalassemia carrier states.

DIFFERENTIAL DIAGNOSIS

- For an approach to the diagnosis of thalassemia syndromes see Fig. 16–1.
- In childhood, hereditary sideroblastic anemias may resemble thalassemia, but marrow examination should permit differentiation (see Chap. 11).
- High fetal hemoglobin levels found in juvenile chronic myelomonocytic leukemia rarely can cause confusion, but examination of the marrow should be definitive (see Chap. 47).
- Diagnosis of the rarer forms of thalassemia is discussed in Chap. 47, of *Williams Hematology,* 8th ed.

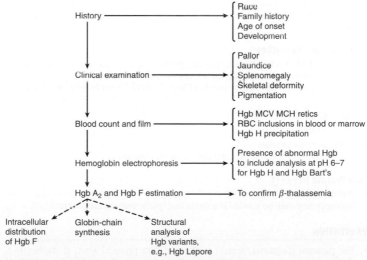

FIGURE 16-1 A flowchart showing an approach to the diagnosis of the thalassemia syndromes. MCH, mean cell hemoglobin; MCV, mean corpuscular volume; RBC, red blood cell count. (Source: *Williams Hematology,* 8th ed, Chap. 47, Fig. 47–20, p. 675.)

THERAPY, COURSE, AND PROGNOSIS

β-Thalassemia Major

General Considerations

- High standard of pediatric care required.
- Early treatment of infections.
- Folate supplements.
- Careful attention to respiratory infections and dental care because of bony deformities of skull.
- When iron-loading is present, endocrine replacement therapy may be needed.

Allogeneic Hematopoietic Stem Cell Transplantation

- Very good results with HLA-identical sibling donors if performed early.
- In the absence of risk factors (irregular chelation, hepatomegaly, portal fibrosis), approximately 90 percent of children have 5-year, event-free survival with a mortality risk of 4 percent.
- For patients with one or two risk factors, the disease-free survival rate is 82 percent; with all three risk factors, the disease-free survival rate is 51 percent.
- No case of hematologic malignancies has been observed after transplantation.

Transfusion

- In children, maintain Hb at 9.5 to 14 g/dL by transfusing red cells every 4 weeks to ensure normal growth and development. Use washed, filtered, or frozen cells to avoid transfusion reactions. Children maintained at high Hb level do not develop hypersplenism.

Iron Chelation

- Rationale: Every child on high-transfusion regimen will develop and die of myocardial siderosis.
- Subcutaneous infusion of deferoxamine, 12 hours, overnight: determine dose to achieve adequate urinary iron excretion.
- Continue nightly infusions of deferoxamine on outpatient basis, monitor by measurements of urinary iron excretion. Ascorbic acid, 50 to 100 mg/d, increases iron excretion but should be given only after deferoxamine infusion has been started.

Experimental Approaches

- Increase γ-globin synthesis in patients with β-thalassemia or sickle cell anemia using demethylating or cytotoxic agents, or arginine butyrate.
- Somatic gene therapy is discussed in Chap. 27 in *Williams Hematology,* 8th ed.

α-Thalassemia

Hydrops Fetalis (--/--)

- There is no treatment.
- Genetic counseling and prenatal diagnosis are options.

Hb H Disease (α -/--)

- Avoid "oxidant" drugs.
- Splenectomy may be needed if anemia and splenomegaly are severe.

PREVENTION

- For prenatal diagnosis, screen mothers at first prenatal visit; if mother is a thalassemia carrier, screen father; if both are carriers of gene for severe form of thalassemia, offer prenatal diagnostic testing and termination of pregnancy.
- Chorionic villus sampling at 9 to 10 weeks and fetal DNA analysis.

PROGNOSIS

β-Thalassemia
Thalassemia Major
- Cardiac complications have decreased dramatically in patients who are adequately treated by transfusion and iron chelation.
- Hematopoietic stem cell transplantation done early in life with HLA-identical sibling donors can lead to cure.

Thalassemia Intermedia
- May develop iron loading and severe bone disease in 3 to 4 decades.
- High incidence of diabetes mellitus, due to iron loading of pancreas.

For a more detailed discussion, see Januario E. Castro and Thomas J. Kipps: Principles of Gene Transfer Therapy. Chap. 27, p. 391; Ernest Beutler: Disorders of Iron Metabolism. Chap. 42, p. 565; Sir David Weatherall: The Thalassemias. Chap. 47, p. 675 in *Williams Hematology,* 8th ed.

CHAPTER 17
The Sickle Cell Diseases and Related Disorders

DEFINITIONS

- The molecular biology of these hemoglobinopathies is well understood, but clinical progress in treatment has been limited.
- Hemoglobin variants were initially designated by letter, but after the letters of the alphabet were exhausted, newly identified variants were named according to the place in which they were first found. If they had a particular feature previously described by a letter, the location was added as a subscript (e.g., Hb $M_{Saskatoon}$).
- In a fully characterized hemoglobin variant, the amino acid position and change is described in a superscript to the appropriate globin chain (e.g., Hb S, $\alpha_2 \beta_2^{6Glu-Val}$).
- The term *sickle cell disorder* describes states in which sickling of red cells occurs on deoxygenation.
- Sickle cell anemia (Hb SS), hemoglobin SC, sickle cell–β thalassemia, and hemoglobin SD produce significant morbidity and are therefore designated *sickle cell diseases*. These diseases are marked by periods of relative well-being interspersed with episodes of illness, but the severity of clinical manifestations varies widely among patients. Generally, sickle cell anemia is the most severe, but there is considerable overlap in clinical behavior among these diseases.
- Hb E might be the most prevalent abnormal hemoglobin and is found principally in Burma, Thailand, Laos, Cambodia, Malaysia, and Indonesia.

ETIOLOGY AND PATHOGENESIS

Hemoglobin Polymerization

- The hemoglobin S mutation is the result of the substitution of valine for glutamic acid at position 6 in the β chain.
- Molecules of deoxyhemoglobin S have a strong tendency to aggregate and form polymers. Polymer formation alters the biophysical properties of the red cells, making them much less deformable and adherent to endothelium.
- The sickling process is initially reversible, but repeated sickling and unsickling leads to irreversibly sickled cells due to membrane damage.
- Sickle cells lead to vascular stasis, tissue damage, and increase in microvascular blood viscosity.
- Susceptibility to sickling is dependent on several factors including intracellular hemoglobin concentration, presence of hemoglobins other than hemoglobin S (e.g., Hg F), blood oxygen tension, pH, temperature, and 2,3-BPG levels.
- Cellular dehydration (such as in the hyperosmolar milieu in renal papillae) increases sickling by increasing the concentration of intracellular hemoglobin, and some of the clinical findings of sickle trait individuals, such as inability to concentrate urine and rarely hematuria, are to the result of this phenomenon.
- Some protection against sickling is conferred by elevated hemoglobin F levels; apparently a threshold phenomenon exists, so that there is no effect beneath a certain level of hemoglobin F.
- In the microvasculature, flow is affected by the rigidity of the sickled cells and adherence to the endothelium. Shear stresses in higher flow areas can break down the gel structure of hemoglobin S. Because the duration of hypoxia is also

important, areas of vascular stasis (such as the spleen) with lower oxygen tension are particularly prone to vascular occlusion and infarction. Most patients with sickle cell anemia have splenic atrophy from multiple infarctions by early adulthood.

Nitric Oxide Scavenging and Other Factors Involved in Pathophysiology of Sickle Cell Disease

- NO (nitric oxide) has vasodilatory, antiinflammatory, and platelet aggregation effects.
- Chronic hemolysis with release of free hemoglobin into the circulation leads to scavenging of NO with endothelial dysfunction and increased sickle cell adherence.
- Several adhesion molecules and pro-inflammatory mediators (e.g., TNF-α) are up-regulated.
- Inflammatory stimuli lead to neutrophil, monocyte and endothelial activation with increased white cell-red cell adhesion resulting in increased vaso-occlusion.
- Coagulation system is also activated.

Inheritance

- Patients with sickle cell anemia are homozygous for the sickle hemoglobin gene and have inherited one gene from each parent. Because 8 percent of Americans of African ancestry have sickle trait, about 1 in 500 Americans of African descent are born with the sickle cell anemia genotype.
- Occurrence of sickle disease can theoretically be prevented by detection of carriers and counseling regarding birth control or elective interruption of pregnancies with fetuses that are homozygous from hemoglobin S.
- Although the sickle cell gene is found in a variety of areas (Middle East, Greece, India), its greatest prevalence is in tropical Africa, with heterozygote frequency as high as 40 percent. A geographic association with areas of high malaria prevalence suggests an advantage to individuals with sickle cell trait, and it appears that this advantage is enhanced resistance to falciparum malaria.

CLINICAL MANIFESTATIONS

- The manifestations of all sickle cell diseases are sufficiently similar that they are discussed together here.
- High levels of fetal hemoglobin protect against sickling for the first 8 to 10 weeks of life; thereafter, the manifestations of sickle cell disease may become apparent.
- There is great variability between affected individuals, but many patients are in good health most of the time.
- In children, most problems are related to pain, infection, or inflammation. In adults, clinical manifestations are likely to be more chronic, related to organ damage.

Crises

- *Vaso-occlusive or painful crises* are the most common manifestation, occurring with a frequency from almost daily to yearly while some affected individuals never have a painful crisis. Tissue hypoxia and infarction can occur anywhere in the body. It is important to carefully evaluate the patient to distinguish between painful crises and pain caused by another process.
- *Aplastic crises* occur when erythropoiesis is suppressed. As red blood cell survival is greatly shortened in sickle cell disease, even temporary reduction in erythropoiesis is rapidly manifested by a dramatic fall in blood hemoglobin concentration. Infection (most notably parvovirus B19) usually causes this type of

crisis, but it may also result from folic acid deficiency, which is of particular concern during pregnancy.

- *Sequestration crises* occur in infants or rarely in older children, and in the occasional adult with an enlarged spleen. There is a sudden massive pooling of red blood cells in the spleen; this can cause hypotension and even death.
- *Hyperhemolytic episodes* occur uncommonly as a result of enhanced hemolysis in certain conditions, such as resolution phase of vaso-occlusive crisis where irreversibly sickled red cells are rapidly destroyed.

Other Clinical Manifestations
Cardiopulmonary System

- The "acute chest syndrome" consists of fever, leukocytosis, and a new pulmonary infiltrate. Infections or pulmonary fat microembolization are the two common causes of the acute chest syndrome.
- Chronic pulmonary hypertension is another common manifestation in adult sickle cell disease patients. The likely reasons are NO scavenging, increased reactive oxygen species, increased arginase activity, and increased platelet activation.
- Asthma, abnormal pulmonary function tests, and airway hyperreactivity are other pulmonary presentations.
- In vaso-occlusive crisis, tachycardia and high-output cardiac (flow) murmurs are commonly seen.

Central Nervous System

- Strokes occur more commonly in children, usually without warning. Risk is highest during first decade of life. Recurrence is common (in at least two-thirds), usually within 3 years.
- The best predictor for stroke risk is an increased blood flow velocity in major intracranial arteries on transcranial Doppler (TCD) ultrasound.
- Patients with two abnormal readings defined as TCD velocities > 200 cm/sec should be offered a chronic red cell transfusion program for primary stroke prevention.

Genitourinary System

- The environment of the renal medulla (hyperosmolar, hypoxic) predisposes to sickling. Hyposthenuria, papillary necrosis, and hematuria are commonly present.
- Priapism is most commonly seen in hemoglobin SS disease, while nocturnal enuresis is prevalent in approximately 30 percent of the adolescent sickle cell population.
- The prevalence of microalbuminuria and proteinuria increases with age. Infants with sickle cell disease have glomerular hyperfiltration. This may evolve into microalbuminuria, proteinuria, and to chronic kidney disease/end-stage renal disease in some.

Musculoskeletal System

- Young children with hemoglobin SS tend to be short. Puberty is delayed, but growth occurs in late adolescence and adults are of normal size.
- Erythroid hyperplasia in the marrow results in widening of the medullary spaces and thinning of the cortex. The vertebral bodies may show biconcavities on the upper and lower surface (codfish spine).
- Bone infarctions can be followed by periosteal reaction and areas of osteosclerosis. Dactylitis occurs in children, usually up to 4 years of age, probably related to avascular necrosis. In adults, avascular necrosis occurs chiefly in the femoral and humeral heads; joint replacement is occasionally required.

Spleen

- In hemoglobin SS disease, splenomegaly (but poor splenic function) in childhood is followed by repeated infarction, leaving a small fibrotic spleen in the adult (auto-splenectomy). However, splenomegaly usually persists in patients with hemoglobin SC, SE, or sickle β-thalassemia.

Hepatobiliary System

- About one-third of sickle cell disease patients will manifest hepatic dysfunction of multifactorial origin.
- Sickle cell–induced cholestasis can be very serious and even fatal, although exchange transfusion has been reported as an effective treatment.
- Hepatitis may develop from transfusions, usually in regions in which testing for hepatitis B and C virus in blood is not performed fastidiously.
- The liver, sometimes chronically enlarged, can also enlarge transiently during a painful crisis.
- Gallstones are seen in 50 to 75 percent of adults; they have been seen in children as young as 6 years of age. Although there is some debate, patients with asymptomatic cholelithiasis probably should not be subjected to surgery.

Iron Overload

- Organ effects from iron overload is being recognized increasingly in adults with sickle cell disease; it develops in patients who have been transfused repeatedly.

Eye

- Neovascularization occurs after obstruction of retinal vessels, resulting in a proliferative retinopathy; however, spontaneous regression can occur in up to 60 percent of cases. Laser coagulation can prevent this complication. This is more common in hemoglobin SC disease than in hemoglobin SS disease.

Leg Ulcers

- Leg ulcers occur with varying frequency in adults and are related to multiple factors (low blood hemoglobin concentration, brisk hemolysis, stasis). They typically occur on lower extremity with the medial malleolus area being more likely affected than the lateral malleolus.

Infection

- Children less than 5 years of age are susceptible to infection by encapsulated organisms due to functional asplenia.

Pregnancy

- Complications to mother include increased frequency sickle cell painful crises, preeclampsia, and infections.
- Complications to fetus include miscarriage, intrauterine growth restriction, preterm birth, low birth weight, and stillbirth and newborn death.
- Oral contraceptives may slightly increase the risk of thromboembolism, but this is less of a risk than pregnancy.

Laboratory Features

- The hemoglobin level is usually between 5 and 11 g/dL. Anemia is normochromic and normocytic, but considerable variation in red cell size and shape is noted. Sickled cells and target cells are seen on the blood film; reticulocytosis is almost always present (see Fig. 17–1).
- Leukocytosis and thrombocytosis are common, even in patients without acute problems; these may be caused by a reactive marrow along with demargination of peripheral leukocytes, and possibly contributed by functional asplenia.
- Modest elevations in whole body iron burden are common; however, hemochromatosis is rare.

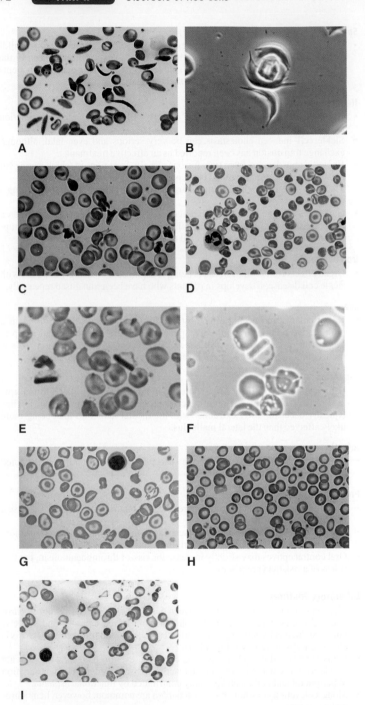

- Hemoglobin electrophoresis is utilized to detect hemoglobin S. Hemoglobins A_2 and often F are particularly increased in patients with sickle cell–β thalassemia; however, many laboratories cannot accurately measure hemoglobins A_2 in the presence of hemoglobin S. Despite high levels of hemoglobin F at birth, electrophoresis can detect hemoglobin S in the newborn.
- Prenatal diagnosis is performed by examining DNA from a chorionic villus biopsy or from cells obtained at amniocentesis.

TREATMENT

Nonspecific Measures

- The administration of folic acid may be useful. Pneumococcal vaccine should be given to children and to those adults who have not received it. Penicillin prophylaxis is administered up to the age of 6 years. Infections should be identified and treated early.

Specific Measures

- Hydroxyurea
  - Chronic administration at a starting dose of 15 mg/kg per day has been shown to decrease the incidence of painful crises, and should therefore be considered for patients with frequent and severe crises; therapy may be associated with improved survival, and this agent is underutilized in sickle cell disease. The precise mechanism of the hydroxyurea effect is uncertain. It was used initially to increase red cell hemoglobin F, but this does not occur in most sickle cells in treated patients and is quantitatively modest. The drug decreases the neutrophil concentration in the blood. Neutrophils play a key role in fostering sickle cell crisis. Both effects may play a role. Other agents are being studied that can encourage the switch from beta to gamma hemoglobin chains, resulting in higher hemoglobin F in the cells.
- Allogeneic hematopoietic stem cell transplantation
  - Only curative treatment for sickle cell disease, but because of the attendant risks, including death, it is suitable only for carefully selected patients with an HLA-matched donor.
- Red cell transfusion
  - Used frequently in sickle cell disease to increase hemoglobin concentration and to decrease the proportion of sickle cells in the blood. Chronic red cell transfusion therapy has been conclusively demonstrated to prevent strokes. See Chap. 91 for considerations of chronic red cell transfusion therapy.

FIGURE 17-1 Blood cell morphology in patients with structural hemoglobinopathies. **A.** Blood film. Hb SS disease with characteristic sickle-shaped cells and extreme elliptocytes with dense central hemoglobin staining. Both shapes are characteristic of sickled cells. Occasional target cells. **B.** Phase contrast microscopy of wet preparation. Note the three sickled cells with terminal fine-pointed projections as a result of tactoid formation and occasional target cells. **C.** Hb SC disease. Blood film. Note high frequency of target cells characteristic of Hb C and the small dense, irregular, contracted cells reflective of their content of Hb S. **D.** Hb CC disease. Blood film. Characteristic combination of numerous target cells and a population of dense (hyperchromatic) microspherocytes. Of the nonspherocytic cells, virtually all are target cells. **E.** Hb CC disease postsplenectomy. Blood film. Note the rod-like inclusions in two cells as a result of Hb C paracrystalinization. These cells are virtually all removed in patients with spleens. **F.** Hb CC disease postsplenectomy. Phase contrast microscopy of wet preparation. Note the Hb C crystalline rod in a cell. **G.** Hb DD disease. Blood film. Note frequent target cells admixed with population of small spherocytes, poikilocytes, and tiny red cell fragments. **H.** Hb EE disease. Blood film. Hypochromia, anisocytosis, and target cells. **I.** Hb E thalassemia. Blood film. Marked anisocytosis (primarily microcytes) and poikilocytosis. Hypochromia. (Reproduced with permission from *Lichtman's Atlas of Hematology*, www.accessmedicine.com.)

(Source: *Williams Hematology,* 8th ed, Chap. 48, Fig. 48–7, p. 716.)

Management of Complications

- Patients in vascular crises should be kept warm and given adequate hydration and pain control; oxygen may be beneficial only for hypoxic patients. The period of crisis usually resolves in hours to days. Hydroxyurea therapy (see "Specific Measures," above) may be considered for prevention or decreased frequency of recurrences.
- Patients undergoing anesthesia are at increased risk for a crisis and should be observed closely for development of hypoxia or acidosis, which could precipitate a crisis.
- The acute chest syndrome is a life-threatening complication, and exchange transfusions or red cell transfusions appear beneficial.
- Because strokes in children are a recurring complication, vigorous therapy of children who have had this complication is recommended. A regular transfusion program is instituted to reduce hemoglobin S levels below 30 percent. Hematopoietic stem cell transplantation can be considered for children with an HLA-matched sibling.
- Priapism, if recent, should be treated immediately by rapid hydration, red cell transfusion, and analgesia for a short period of observation, while awaiting an urgent urologic consultation. If unsuccessful, urologic intervention, usually by injection of a dilute solution of epinephrine into the corpus cavernosum, can be performed. This approach has a high frequency of success and preserves penile function. Surgical procedures, such as shunts, should be avoided if at all possible. Maintenance therapy with an oral α-adrenergic blocker, such as phenylephrine, can be used.
- Patients should be closely watched during pregnancy; prophylactic transfusions have been given, but it is doubtful whether they are of benefit. Low birth weight and increased fetal loss are probably related to placental vascular occlusions.
- Bed rest, elevation, and zinc sulfate dressings are used to treat leg ulcers. A transfusion program or skin grafting can enhance healing. Often, they are quite resistant to therapeutic measures and require a long time to heal.

SICKLE CELL TRAIT

- In sickle cell trait, less than half of the hemoglobin in each red blood cell is hemoglobin S (approximately 40%) and the rest is normal hemoglobin, principally A. This effectively protects against sickling except under special circumstances, such as severe hypoxia or the hyperosmolarity encountered in the renal circulation.
- Numerous anecdotal reports suggest that sickle cell trait may be injurious, but the morbidity and mortality are extremely low and difficult to quantitate.
- A slightly higher incidence of concentrating defect, hyposthenuria, hematuria, and pulmonary embolus has been documented in persons with sickle cell trait.

HEMOGLOBIN C DISEASE

- Glutamic acid in the sixth position of the β chain is replaced by lysine in hemoglobin C.
- In the homozygous state, most of the hemoglobin in the cell is hemoglobin C, the red blood cells are more rigid than normal, and intracellular crystals of hemoglobin C are found; target cells are numerous. In addition, a population of spherocytes is a characteristic finding.
- In Americans of African descent, the prevalence of the heterozygous state (hemoglobin C trait), which is asymptomatic, is approximately 2 percent.
- Splenomegaly and mild hemolytic anemia are almost always present in the homozygous state. Some patients develop bilirubin gallstones.
- No treatment is required and the prognosis is excellent.

HEMOGLOBIN D DISEASE

- These hemoglobin variants have normal solubility but migrate like hemoglobin S on electrophoresis.
- The highest prevalence is in northwest India (2 to 3%).
- The heterozygous state as well as the homozygotes are asymptomatic with normal red cell indices.
- Hemoglobin SD occurs rarely and presents as severe sickle cell disease. Hemoglobin D-β thalassemia is also rare.

HEMOGLOBIN E DISEASE

- A β-chain mutation ($\beta^{26Glu-Lys}$) results in hemoglobin designated hemoglobin E. Some of the hemoglobin E mRNA undergoes alternative splicing, giving rise to a thalassemia-like picture.
- This is a relatively common abnormal hemoglobin in Southeast Asia.
- Hemoglobin E trait is asymptomatic, but mild microcytosis occurs.
- In association with β thalassemia, a moderate anemia and splenomegaly are present; splenectomy may be considered in this setting.
- Homozygous patients have been described; they have microcytosis and mild anemia.

OTHER HEMOGLOBINOPATHIES

- Many other abnormal hemoglobins have been described; most are uncommon and of no clinical significance. Others can produce cyanosis because of a low oxygen affinity, erythrocytosis because of a high oxygen affinity, or a hemolytic anemia because of instability. These are described in Chaps. 18, 19, and 29.

For a more detailed discussion, see Kavita Natarajan, Tim M. Townes, and Abdullah Kutlar: Disorders of Hemoglobin Structure: Sickle Cell Anemia and Related Abnormalities. Chap. 48, p. 709 in *Williams Hematology,* 8th ed.

CHAPTER 18
Hemoglobinopathies Associated with Unstable Hemoglobin

DEFINITION

- The unstable hemoglobins discussed here result from a mutation that changes the amino acid sequence of one of the globin chains, leading to instability and precipitation of the hemoglobin molecule.
- Homotetramers of normal β chains (hemoglobin H) or γ chains (hemoglobin Bart's) are also unstable. These hemoglobins are found in α-thalassemia (see Chap. 16).

ETIOLOGY AND PATHOGENESIS

- The tetrameric hemoglobin molecule has numerous noncovalent forces that maintain the structure of each subunit and bind the subunits to each other.
- Amino acid substitutions or deletions that weaken noncovalent forces, allow hemoglobin to denature and precipitate as insoluble globins, which may attach to the cell membrane, forming Heinz bodies.
- Heinz bodies impair erythrocyte deformability, impeding the ability to negotiate the splenic sinuses; "pitting" of Heinz bodies causes loss of membrane and ultimately destruction of red cells, and a hemolytic anemia.

INHERITANCE

- An autosomal dominant disorder. The patients are heterozygotes and have a combination of hemoglobin A and unstable hemoglobin in their red cells. Homozygous and compound heterozygotes are not observed because they are thought to be lethal.
- Sometimes patients develop an unstable hemoglobin as a *de novo* mutation. More than 80 percent of patients have a defect in the β globin chain; α-globin defects are less likely to cause a clinical disorder because there are four α-globin genes normally and a mutation in one gene results in a minor proportion of abnormal globin in the cell.

CLINICAL FEATURES

- Hemolysis is usually compensated. Also, a patient with an unstable hemoglobin with high oxygen affinity may have a hemoglobin level in the upper normal range.
- Infection or treatment with oxidant drugs may precipitate hemolytic episodes, making the diagnosis apparent.
- In β-chain mutations, chronic hemolytic anemia becomes evident after neonatal period but during the first year of life as γ chains (fetal hemoglobin) are replaced by mutant β chains.
- Physical findings may include pallor, jaundice, splenomegaly.
- Some patients have dark urine probably from the catabolism of free heme groups or Heinz bodies.

LABORATORY FEATURES

- Hemoglobin concentration may be normal or decreased. The MCV may be decreased because of loss of hemoglobin from denaturation and pitting.

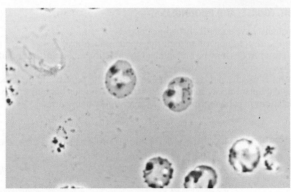

FIGURE 18-1 Wet preparation stained with crystal violet. Inclusions in red cells (Heinz bodies) usually attached to membrane. (Used with permission from *Lichtman's Atlas of Hematology,* www.accessmedicine.com.)
(Source: *Williams Hematology,* 8th ed, Chap. 47, Fig. 47–18 Panel B, p. 696.)

- Blood film may show hypochromia, poikilocytosis, polychromasia, anisocytosis, and basophilic stippling.
- Heinz bodies are commonly found in circulating red cells; after splenectomy they become more abundant.
- Reticulocytosis is often disproportionate to the severity of the anemia, particularly when the abnormal hemoglobin has a high oxygen affinity.
- Diagnosis is confirmed by demonstration of an unstable hemoglobin. This may be done by:
  — Isopropanol precipitation test: a simple screening test that involves the incubation of the hemolysate with a 17 percent of isopropanol; hemolysates containing unstable hemoglobin variants form a precipitate, whereas a normal hemolysate remains clear.
  — Heat denaturation test: cumbersome and usually not used.
  — Heinz body detection: requires the incubation of erythrocytes with a supravital stain (see Fig. 18–1).
  — Hemoglobin electrophoresis: may be useful, but a normal pattern does not rule out an unstable hemoglobin and thus electrophoresis is not a screening or reliable test for unstable hemoglobins. Some unstable globin variants can be identified by reverse phase high performance liquid chromatography (HPLC), due to changes in their hydrophobicity.
- Determination of the $P_{50}O_2$, a measure of hemoglobin oxygen affinity, may be helpful to detect unstable hemoglobins with altered oxygen-hemoglobin affinity.
- Unstable hemoglobins can be detected and identified by DNA analysis.

DIFFERENTIAL DIAGNOSIS

- Consider the possibility of an unstable hemoglobin in all patients with a hereditary nonspherocytic hemolytic anemia (see Chap. 15), especially with hypochromic red cells and reticulocytosis out of proportion to the degree of anemia.
- Not all patients with a positive test for unstable hemoglobin have this disorder; a false-positive isopropanol stability test may be seen in patients with sickle hemoglobin, elevated levels of methemoglobin, or hemoglobin F.
- Hemoglobin H and hemoglobin Bart's are also unstable. These can be detected by electrophoresis and are found in patients with α-thalassemia.

TREATMENT, COURSE, AND PROGNOSIS

- Most patients have a relatively benign course.
- Gallstones are common, often requiring cholecystectomy.
- Hemolytic episodes may be precipitated by infection or administration of oxidative drugs.
- Treatment is usually not required. Folic acid is often given, although benefit is not proven. Splenectomy may be useful in some patients but may cause serious complications in patients with high oxygen-affinity hemoglobins.

For a more detailed discussion, see Kavita Natarajan, Tim M. Townes, Abdullah Kutlar: Disorders of Hemoglobin Structure: Sickle Cell Anemia and Related Abnormalities. Chap. 48, p. 709 in *Williams Hematology,* 8th ed.

CHAPTER 19
Methemoglobinemia and Other Dyshemoglobinemias

DEFINITION

- Cyanosis is most frequently caused by low arterial oxygen saturation because of cardiac or pulmonary disease, but rarely, it may be caused by increased concentrations of methemoglobin or sulfhemoglobin, or by abnormal hemoglobins with low oxygen affinity.

METHEMOGLOBINEMIA

Toxic Methemoglobinemia

- Drugs or chemicals may cause methemoglobinemia either by oxidizing hemoglobin directly or by enhancing its oxidization by molecular oxygen.
- Table 19–1 lists common agents that cause methemoglobinemia.
- Infants are more susceptible because of low levels of NADH diaphorase (cytochrome b5 reductase) in the newborn period. A syndrome of diarrhea, acidosis, and methemoglobinuria of yet unexplained etiology occurs in infancy.
- Severe acute methemoglobinemia impairs oxygen delivery, and levels exceeding 50 percent can be fatal.
- Chronic methemoglobinemia is usually asymptomatic, but at levels greater than 20 percent, mild erythrocytosis is often present.
- Treatment with intravenous methylene blue (given at 1 to 2 mg/kg over 5 minutes) is rapidly effective. Excessive amounts of methylene blue, or its use in G-6-PD–deficient patients, can cause acute hemolysis.

Cytochrome b₅ Reductase Deficiency

- Cytochrome b₅ reductase deficiency (also known as NADH diaphorase) catalyzes the reduction of cytochrome b₅, which, in turn, reduces methemoglobin to hemoglobin.

TABLE 19–1	**SOME DRUGS THAT CAUSE METHEMOGLOBINEMIA**
Phenazopyridine (Pyridium)	
Sulfamethoxazole	
Dapsone	
Aniline	
Paraquat/monolinuron	
Nitrate	
Nitroglycerin	
Amyl nitrite	
Isobutyl nitrite	
Sodium nitrite	
Benzocaine	
Prilocaine	
Methylene blue	
Chloramine	

Source: *Williams Hematology*, 8th ed, Chap. 49, Table 49–1, p. 744.

- Hereditary cytochrome b_5 reductase deficiency results in an accumulation of methemoglobin and is inherited as a recessive disorder.
- If restricted to erythrocytes, cyanosis is the only phenotype (type I cytochrome b_5 reductase deficiency). This is seen sporadically in all racial groups but is reported to be endemic in certain native Siberian ethnic groups, Navajo Indians, and Athabascan natives of Alaska.
- In some patients, cells other than erythrocytes may be involved, and a less common hereditary syndrome of cyanosis with mental retardation and other neurologic defects may occur (type II cytochrome b_5 reductase deficiency).
- Methemoglobin levels vary between 8 and 40 percent, and the cytochrome b_5 reductase level is less than 20 percent of normal.
- Treatment with ascorbic acid (200 to 600 mg/d orally, divided into four doses) lowers the methemoglobin level.
- Infants have transiently low levels of cytochrome b_5 reductase and are more likely to develop acute toxic methemoglobinemia.

Cytochrome b_5 Deficiency
- Rarely, cytochrome b_5 itself is deficient, causing the same clinical picture as type II cytochrome b_5 reductase deficiency.

Hemoglobins M
- Some amino acid substitutions in hemoglobin lead to enhanced formation and inability to reduce methemoglobin. These abnormal proteins are termed *hemoglobins M* and the resultant cyanosis from methemoglobinemia is inherited as a recessive disorder.
- Cyanosis may be evident at birth in hemoglobin M disease with the α-chain mutant; in the β-chain variant, this will evolve over 6 to 9 weeks as γ-globin chains are replaced by β-chains.
- No effective treatment for methemoglobinemia due to hemoglobin M is known.
- The characteristics of M hemoglobins are shown in Table 19–2.

LOW OXYGEN AFFINITY HEMOGLOBINS
- Some hemoglobin variants have a decreased oxygen affinity, and therefore, an abnormal proportion of the hemoglobin is not oxygenated.
- The result may be cyanosis and mild anemia, the latter resulting from the fact that the body perceives adequate oxygen delivery and erythropoietin levels are therefore decreased.
- Table 19–3 gives features and effects of low oxygen affinity hemoglobins.

SULFHEMOGLOBIN
- In vitro sulfhemoglobin can be produced by addition of hydrogen sulfide to hemoglobin.
- *In vivo* sulfhemoglobin can be induced in some individuals by ingestion of drugs or may occur without apparent cause.
- Cyanosis is present and occasionally mild hemolysis occurs. Sulfhemoglobinemia is usually well tolerated and does not affect overall health. Sulfhemoglobin cannot be changed back to normal hemoglobin.

CARBOXYHEMOGLOBIN
- Carbon monoxide (CO) is an odorless, colorless, and tasteless gas. It can be unknowingly inhaled to dangerous levels when present in high concentration in the atmosphere.
- Acute CO intoxication is one of the most common causes of morbidity as a result of poisoning in the United States.

TABLE 19-2   **PROPERTIES OF M HEMOGLOBINS**

Hemoglobin	Amino Acid Substitution	Oxygen Dissociation and Other Properties	Clinical Effect
Hgb M$_{Boston}$	α58 (E7)His $\rightarrow$ Tyr	Very low oxygen affinity, almost nonexistent heme–heme interaction, no Bohr effect	Cyanosis resulting from formation of methemoglobin
Hgb M$_{Saskatoon}$	β63 (E7)His $\rightarrow$ Tyr	Increased oxygen affinity, reduced heme–heme interaction, normal Bohr effect, slightly unstable	Cyanosis resulting from methemoglobin formation, mild hemolytic anemia exacerbated by ingestion of sulfonamides
Hgb M$_{Iwate}$	α87 (F8)His $\rightarrow$ Tyr	Low oxygen affinity, negligible heme–heme interaction, no Bohr effect	Cyanosis resulting from formation of methemoglobin
Hgb M$_{Kankakee}$			
Hgb M$_{Oldenburg}$			
Hgb M$_{Sendai}$			
Hgb M$_{HydePark}$	β92 (F8)His $\rightarrow$ Tyr	Increased oxygen affinity, reduced heme interaction, normal Bohr effect, slightly unstable	Cyanosis resulting from formation of methemoglobin, mild hemolytic anemia
Hgb Milwaukee 2			
Hgb M$_{Akita}$			
Hgb M$_{Milwaukee}$	β67 (E11)Val $\rightarrow$ Glu	Low oxygen affinity, reduced heme–heme interaction, normal Bohr effect, slightly unstable	Cyanosis resulting from methemoglobin formation
Hgb FM$_{Osaka}$	$^G\gamma$63His $\rightarrow$ Tyr	Low oxygen affinity, increased Bohr effect. Methemoglobinemia	Cyanosis at birth
Hgb FM$_{FortRipley}$	$^G\gamma$92His $\rightarrow$ Tyr	Slightly increased oxygen affinity	Cyanosis at birth

Source: *Williams Hematology*, 8th ed, Chap. 49, Table 49–2, p. 745.

- Sign and symptoms of CO poisoning are nonspecific. A high index of suspicion should attend the simultaneous presentation of multiple patients from the same housing complex. Common symptoms of mild to moderate CO poisoning are irritability, headache, nausea, lethargy, and sometimes a flu-like condition. Acute and severe poisoning can result in cerebral edema, pulmonary edema,

TABLE 19–3	LOW-AFFINITY HEMOGLOBINS		
Hemoglobin	Amino Acid Substitution	Oxygen Dissociation and Other Properties	Clinical Effect
Hgb$_{Seattle}$	β70 (E14)Ala → Asp	Decreased oxygen affinity normal heme-heme interaction	Mild chronic anemia associated with reduced urinary erythropoietin; physiologic adaptation to more efficient oxygen release to tissues
Hgb$_{Kansas}$	β102 (G4)Asn → Thr	Very low oxygen affinity, low heme-heme interaction, dissociates into dimers in ligand form	Cyanosis resulting from deoxyhemoglobin, mild anemia

Source: *Williams Hematology*, 8th ed, Chap. 49, Table 49–3, p. 748.

cardiac arrhythmias that may be deadly and significant residual neurologic deficits may remain in survivors.

- The most important step in the treatment for CO poisoning is prompt removal of patients from the source of CO (for mild to moderate cases of CO poisoning) followed by administering 100 percent supplemental oxygen via a tight-fitting mask (in severe cases of CO poisoning).

NITRIC OXIDE-HEMOGLOBIN

- Nitric oxide (NO), a soluble gas, is continuously synthesized in endothelial cells by isoforms of the NO synthase (NOS) enzyme. Vasodilation is caused by diffusion of NO into the smooth muscle cells.
- According to the S-nitroso hemoglobin (SNO-Hb) hypothesis, this vasodilator function is carried by a population of hemoglobin that have undergone the addition of NO to a critical cysteine (cysβ93) via S-nitrosylation, forming SNO-Hb. The allosterically controlled equilibrium of NO groups between hemes and cysteine thiols enables erythrocytes to convey a graded signal for vasodilatation, thereby enhancing perfusion.
- Another mechanism by which Hb may be converted to SNO-Hb is by Hb function as nitrite reductase. Deoxygenated Hb reacts with nitrite to form NO and methemoglobin. Products of the nitrite-hemoglobin reaction generate NO, promote vasodilation, and form SNO-Hb.

 For a more detailed discussion, see Neeraj Agarwal and Josef T. Prchal: Methemoglobinemia and Other Dyshemoglobinemias. Chap. 49, p. 743 in *Williams Hematology*, 8th ed.

CHAPTER 20
Traumatic Hemolytic Anemia, March and Sports-Related Hemoglobinuria, Traumatic Cardiac Hemolytic Anemia

Definition
- Also referred to as macroangiopathic hemolytic anemia, a type of fragmentation hemolytic anemia.
- Complications of prosthetic heart valves (or less commonly cardiac valve disorders, especially severe aortic or subaortic stenosis) or other mechanical cardiac devices, such as left ventricular assistance devices.
- Turbulence and high shear stresses within a space enclosed by a foreign surface result in red cell fragmentation and hemolysis.

Clinical Features
- Patients with ball-and-cage valves, bilcaflet valves (as compared to tilting disc valves), mechanical valve prostheses versus xenograft tissue prostheses, and double-valve as compared to single-valve replacement are more likely to experience clinically significant hemolysis.
- Hemolytic anemia is usually mild and compensated but may be severe.
- Coexistent other causes of anemia (iron or folate deficiencies, see Chaps. 8 and 9), and increased cardiac output as a consequence of strenuous physical exertion, can convert mild hemolysis without anemia to moderate or severe hemolysis and a more severe anemia resulting from increased shear stress.
- More important clinically is the thrombogenicity of nonendothelialized surfaces, as well as the loss of nitric oxide-mediated reduction in platelet reactivity and vasodilation, which promote platelet thrombosis and embolization (see Chapter 19).

Laboratory Features (see Table 20–1)
- Blood film: moderate poikilocytosis, schistocytosis, and polychromasia may be present.
- Serum levels of total and indirect bilirubin, and LDH can be elevated, whereas the serum haptoglobin is depressed.
- Urine hemosiderin present as a result of intravascular hemolysis.
- Iron deficiency may result from chronic hemoglobinuria and hemoglobinuria.
- Decreased platelet count may indicate platelet thrombi on valve surfaces.

Diagnosis
- Based on the presence of schistocytes on the blood film and evidence of chronic intravascular hemolysis in a patient with a cardiac valve disorder or an artificial heart valve or cardiac device.

Treatment
- Appropriate therapy is to replace iron and folate (if deficient).
- Surgical repair or replacement of the malfunctioning prosthesis (if indicated).
- Transfusion may be necessary preoperatively and may diminish the rate of hemolysis by decreasing the heart rate and flow velocity.
- For severe anemia ineligible for reoperation, recombinant human erythropoietin treatment may diminish or eliminate transfusion requirements.

TABLE 20-1	SEVERITY OF PROSTHETIC VALVE HEMOLYSIS		
	Mild	Moderate	Severe
Hemosiderinuria	Present	Present	Marked
Hemoglobinuria	Absent	Absent	Absent
Schistocytosis	< 1%	> 1%	> 1%
Reticulocytosis	< 5%	> 5%	> 5%
Haptoglobin	Decreased	Absent	Absent
LDH	< 500 Units/L	> 500 Units/L	> 500 Units/L

LDH, lactic acid dehydrogenase.
Source: *Williams Hematology*, 8th ed, Chap. 50, Table 50–2, p. 759.

MARCH HEMOGLOBINURIA AND SPORTS ANEMIA

Definition

- First described in a German soldier in whom hemoglobinuria was brought on by marching.
- Also seen in young athletes with frequent participation in severe and prolonged exertion.
- Hemoglobinuria has also been seen following other types of trauma in activities as diverse as repetitive slapping of the forehead, karate exercises, congo drum playing.

Clinical and Laboratory Features

- Because the estimated quantity of blood hemolyzed in an average paroxysm is only 6 to 40 mL, anemia is uncommon; however, repeated episodes may eventually lead to iron deficiency (see Chap. 9).
- Reticulocyte count may be mildly increased, especially in active runners.
- Serum iron, ferritin, and haptoglobin concentrations are usually decreased.
- Hemoglobinuria may be noted for 6 to 12 hours in runners after a race and hemosiderinuria for several weeks after an acute episode.

Diagnosis

- Hemoglobinuria follows exercise or physical insult.
- The Donath-Landsteiner test for paroxysmal cold hemoglobinuria and a test for paroxysmal nocturia hemoglobinuria may be performed to rule out these causes of hemoglobinuria.
- Myoglobinuria can be distinguished from hemoglobinuria by chemical tests of urine.
- Athletes with occult blood in stools should be tested for an underlying gastrointestinal tract abnormality, despite the frequency of subclinical gastrointestinal bleeding after strenuous exercise.
- Anemia also occurs in astronauts but it is not related to shear stress in erythrocytes (see Chap. 2).

Therapy

- For march hemoglobinuria, reassure the patient, add cushioned insoles to the shoes, and suggest that changing the gait may ameliorate the condition.
- Correct iron or folate deficiency, if present.

 For a more detailed discussion, see Kelty R. Baker and Joel Moake: Hemolytic Anemia Resulting from Physical Injury to Red Cells. Chap. 50, p. 755 in *Williams Hematology*, 8th ed.

CHAPTER 21
Microangiopathic Hemolytic Anemia

DEFINITION

- Intravascular hemolysis caused by fragmentation of normal red cells passing through abnormal arterioles and other small vessels.
- The hemolytic anemia generated by red cell damage in small vessels is referred to as microangiopathic hemolytic anemia, a type of fragmentation hemolytic anemia.
- "Split" red cells of varying shapes, referred to as schistocytes, are prominent on blood films.
- Less-extensive red cell fragmentation, development of schistocytes, and hemolysis may also occur under conditions of more moderate vascular occlusion or endothelial surface abnormalities, sometimes under conditions of lower shear stress.
- Excessive platelet aggregation, fibrin polymer formation, and secondary fibrinolysis in the arterial or venous microcirculation are seen in disseminated intravascular coagulation (see Chap. 86), preeclampsia, giant cavernous hemangiomas (the Kasabach-Merritt phenomenon), or in the HELLP (*h*emolysis *e*levated *l*iver enzyme and *l*ow *p*latelets) syndrome.

ETIOLOGY AND PATHOGENESIS

- Intravascular coagulation, with deposition of platelets and fibrin in small arterioles, is the common antecedent.
- Red cells stick to fibrin and are fragmented by force of blood flow, resulting in both intravascular and extravascular hemolysis.
- Underlying disorders include:
  — Invasive carcinoma, especially mucin-producing adenocarcinomas (see Table 21–1).
  — Abruptio placentae.
  — Malignant hypertension.
  — Thrombotic thrombocytopenic purpura (TTP); hemolytic uremic syndrome (HUS), (see Chap. 91).
- The effect of certain drugs:
  — Antineoplastic agents are most often the offender (e.g., mitomycin, bleomycin, daunorubicin in combination with cytosine arabinoside, cisplatin (see Chap. 91, Table 91–2 for more comprehensive list).
  — A TTP-like syndrome may occur weeks or months after discontinuing mitomycin therapy.
- Posttransplantation of kidney or liver. Rejection of kidney graft associated with a vasculitis that can be accompanied by red cell fragmentation.
- Postallogeneic or autologous marrow transplantation as a result of high-dose chemotherapy or radiation, immunosuppressive drugs, graft-versus-host disease, or infections.
- Generalized vasculitis associated with immune disorders; e.g., systemic lupus erythematosus, polyarteritis nodosa, Wegener granulomatosis, scleroderma.
- Kasabach-Merritt syndrome
  — Usually develops in early childhood.
  — Characterized by thrombocytopenia, microangiopathic hemolytic anemia, consumptive coagulopathy, and hypofibrinogenemia.

TABLE 21–1	CANCERS ASSOCIATED WITH MICROANGIOPATHIC HEMOLYTIC ANEMIA
I. Gastric (55%)	
II. Breast (13%)	
III. Lung (10%)	

IV. Other Adenocarcinomas
  A. Prostate
  B. Colon
  C. Gallbladder
  D. Pancreas
  E. Ovary
  F. Unknown primary	

V. Other Malignancies
  A. Hemangiopericytoma
  B. Hepatoma
  C. Melanoma
  D. Small cell cancer of the lung
  E. Testicular cancer
  F. Squamous cell cancer of the oropharynx
  G. Thymoma
  H. Erythroleukemia	

Source: *Williams Hematology,* 8th ed, Chap. 50, Table 50–1, p.757.

- — Caused by an enlarging kaposiform hemangioendothelioma or tufted angioma.
- Localized vascular abnormalities: cutaneous cavernous hemangiomas, hemangioendothelioma of the liver.
- Preeclampsia and HELLP syndrome:
  - — During normal pregnancy, specialized placental epithelial cells replace the endothelium of the uterine spiral arteries and intercalate within the muscular tunica, increasing the vessels' diameters and decreasing their resistance. As a result, the vasculature is converted into a high flow system much less responsive to vasoconstrictors circulating in the maternal blood.
  - — In a preeclamptic pregnancy, this process fails and the spiral arteries do not adequately penetrate the uterus. This results in platelet-fibrin deposition in the capillaries and may progress to multiorgan microvascular injury, microangiopathic hemolytic anemia, elevated liver enzymes because of hepatic necrosis, and thrombocytopenia because of peripheral consumption, i.e., the HELLP syndrome.

CLINICAL FEATURES

- Symptoms and signs are related to the primary process and to the organs affected by the intravascular deposition of platelets and fibrin.
- Fever, hemolytic anemia, thrombocytopenia, kidney failure, and neurologic symptoms that may progress to coma are often combined and are referred to as the pentad of the microangiopathic hemolytic anemia associated with TTP (see Chap. 91).
- Kasabach-Merritt hemangioendotheliomas are locally invasive, but never metastasize and show little tendency to resolve spontaneously.

LABORATORY FEATURES

- Blood film: schistocytes prominent, including helmet cells, arrowhead cells, and other odd shapes.

- Elevation of reticulocyte count, decreased serum haptoglobin level, increased concentrations of plasma hemoglobin and urine hemoglobin, and hemosiderinuria, the latter three signs of intravascular hemolysis.
- An increased concentration of serum lactic acid dehydrogenase (LDH) activity correlates with disease activity.
- Coagulation abnormalities due to consumption coagulopathy include low fibrinogen and platelets.
- In HELLP: The high LDH seen in HELLP is most likely the result of liver damage rather than hemolysis. Serum levels of aspartic acid transaminase (AST) and alanine transaminase (ALT) can be more than 100 times normal, whereas alkaline phosphatase values are typically only about twice normal. Liver enzymes usually return to baseline within 3 to 5 days postpartum.
- Elevated levels of the extracellular domain (soluble) form of FMS-like tyrosine kinase 1 (sFLT-1), also known as soluble vascular endothelial growth factor receptor-1 (sVEGF receptor-1), functions as an antiangiogenic protein because it binds to vascular endothelial growth factor (VEGF) and placental growth factor (PGF).

DIFFERENTIAL DIAGNOSIS

- Other types of intravascular hemolysis: paroxysmal nocturnal hemoglobinuria (see Chap. 45), disseminated intravascular coagulation (see Chap. 86), vasculitis, heart-associated traumatic hemolysis (see Chap 20).
- Distinguishing features: schistocytes on the blood film, thrombocytopenia, negative direct antiglobulin test, evidence of intravascular coagulation, identification of the primary process (see Table 21–1).

TREATMENT, COURSE, AND PROGNOSIS

- Directed toward management of primary process underlying the microangiopathy.
- Red cell transfusions to maintain adequate level of hemoglobin.
- Platelet transfusions for bleeding caused by thrombocytopenia.
- Heparin use is controversial.
- Kasabach-Merritt phenomenon
  — Resection of hemangioma is always followed by normalization of hematologic parameters; for large or recurrent lesions, numerous systemic therapies have been attempted.
  — The mortality rate of Kasabach-Merritt phenomenon can be as high as 30 percent because of complications from aggressive, often extensive local lesions, and complications arising from disseminated vascular coagulation (see Chap. 86).

For a more detailed discussion, see Kelty R. Baker and Joel Moake: Hemolytic Anemia Resulting from Physical Injury to Red Cells. Chap. 50, p. 755 in *Williams Hematology,* 8th ed.

CHAPTER 22
Hemolytic Anemia Resulting from a Chemical or Physical Agent

- Hemolysis can be mainly intravascular (i.e., hypotonic lysis or heat damage) or predominantly extravascular (i.e., arsine gas and oxygen).
- Certain drugs can induce hemolysis in individuals with abnormalities of erythrocytic enzymes, such as glucose-6-phosphate dehydrogenase, or with an unstable hemoglobin (see Chaps. 15 and 18). Such drugs can also cause hemolysis in normal individuals if given in sufficiently large doses.
- Other drugs induce hemolytic anemia through an immunologic mechanism (see Chap. 26).
- The drugs and chemicals discussed here cause hemolysis by other mechanisms.

ARSENIC HYDRIDE (ARSINE, AsH$_3$)

- Arsine gas is formed in many industrial processes.
- Inhalation of arsine gas can lead to severe anemia and jaundice.

LEAD

- Lead poisoning in children usually is a result of ingestion of lead paint flakes or chewing lead-painted objects. In adults, it usually is the result of industrial exposure.
- Lead intoxication leads to anemia largely caused by inhibition of heme synthesis. There is also a modest decrease in red cell life span.
- Lead also inhibits pyrimidine 5'-nucleotidase (see Chap. 15), which may be responsible for the basophilic stippling of red cells found in lead poisoning. Basophilic stippling may be fine or coarse and is most likely found in polychromatophilic cells.
- The anemia is usually mild in adults but may be severe in children. Red cells are normocytic and slightly hypochromic.
- Ringed sideroblasts are frequently found in the marrow.

COPPER

- Hemolytic anemia may be induced by high levels of copper in patients hemodialyzed with fluid contaminated by copper tubing, or in patients with Wilson disease.
- Wilson disease may present or be called to medical attention by a hemolytic anemia, often having spherocytes and Heinz bodies as a result of copper injury to red cells. The presence of liver disease with a hemolytic anemia should raise the question of Wilson disease. (See Table 22–1 for laboratory findings in Wilson disease.)
- The hemolysis is probably caused by inhibition of several erythrocyte enzymes.

CHLORATES

- Ingestion of sodium or potassium chlorate, or contamination of dialysis fluid with chloramines, can cause oxidative damage with formation of Heinz bodies and methemoglobin and with development of hemolytic anemia.

TABLE 22–1	LABORATORY FINDINGS IN WILSON DISEASE	
Variable	Normal Value	Wilson Disease
Serum ceruloplasmin (mg/L)	200–400	< 200
Serum copper (μM)	11–24	< 11
Urinary copper (μg/24 h)	≤ 40	> 100
Liver copper (μg/g dry weight)	20–50	> 200

MISCELLANEOUS DRUGS AND CHEMICALS

- Other drugs and chemicals that can cause hemolytic anemia are listed in Table 22–2.

WATER

- Water administered intravenously, inhaled in near-drowning, or gaining access to the circulation during irrigation procedures can cause hemolysis.

OXYGEN

- Hemolytic anemia has developed in patients receiving hyperbaric oxygenation and in astronauts exposed to 100 percent oxygen.

INSECT AND ARACHNID VENOMS

- Severe hemolysis may occur in some patients following bites by bees, wasps, spiders, or scorpions.
- Snake bites are only rarely a cause of hemolysis.

HEAT

- Patients with extensive burns may develop severe hemolytic anemia, apparently as a result of direct damage to the red cells by heat.
- Blood films of many burned patients show spherocytes and fragmentation, and the osmotic fragility may be increased.

TABLE 22–2	DRUGS AND CHEMICALS THAT HAVE BEEN REPORTED TO CAUSE HEMOLYTIC ANEMIA
Chemicals	Drugs
Aniline	Amyl nitrite
Apiol	Mephenesin
Dichlorprop (herbicide)	Methylene blue
Formaldehyde	Omeprazole
Hydroxylamines	Pentachlorophenol
Lysol	Phenazopyridine (Pyridium)
Mineral spirits	Salicylazosulfapyridine (Azulfidine)
Nitrobenzene	Tacrolimus
Resorcin	

Source: *Williams Hematology*, 8th ed, Chap. 51, Table 51–1, p. 764.

NEOCYTOLYSIS

- Neocytolysis, the selective destruction of young red cells is a phenomenon unique to microgravity and is associated with a rapid decrease in erythropoietin levels.
- Experienced by astronauts after space flight even in the presence of normal ambient oxygen concentration or in people rapidly descending from high altitude to sea level.
- Radiolabeling studies of erythrocytes indicated that the anemia was caused by selective hemolysis of young erythrocytes less than 12 days old.

 For a more detailed discussion, see Brian S. Bull and Paul C. Herrmann: Hemolytic Anemia Resulting from Chemical and Physical Agents. Chap. 51, p. 763 in *Williams Hematology,* 8th ed.

CHAPTER 23
Hemolytic Anemia Resulting from Infectious Agents

- Hemolysis represents a prominent part of the overall clinical picture in many infections. Table 23–1 lists the microorganisms associated with the induction of hemolytic anemia.

MECHANISMS

- Hemolysis may be caused by:
  — Direct invasion by infecting organisms (malaria).
  — Elaboration of hemolytic toxins (*Clostridium perfringens*).
  — Development of autoantibodies against red blood cell antigens (*Mycoplasma pneumoniae*).

MALARIA

Etiology and Pathogenesis
- The world's most common cause of hemolytic anemia.
- Transmitted by bite of an infected female *Anopheles* mosquito.
- Parasites grow intracellularly and parasitized cells are destroyed in the spleen.
- Uninvaded cells are also destroyed (estimated at 10 × the number of infected cells).
- Erythropoietin low for degree of anemia secondary to release of inhibitory cytokines, especially in *Plasmodium falciparum* infection.
- Certain heterozygous mutations that interfere with invasion of red blood cells by parasites have developed in endemic areas (G-6-PD deficiency, thalassemia, other hemoglobinopathies, and hereditary elliptocytosis).

Clinical Features
- Febrile paroxysms are characteristically cyclic: *Plasmodium vivax* every 48 hours, *Plasmodium malariae* every 72 hours, and *P. falciparum* daily.
- Rigors, headache, abdominal pain, nausea and vomiting, and extreme fatigue accompany the fever.
- Splenomegaly typically is present in chronic infection.
- Falciparum malaria is occasionally associated with very severe hemolysis and dark, almost black urine (blackwater fever).
- Cerebral malaria may result in delirium, other neurologic manifestations.
- Organ dysfunction (respiratory insufficiency and renal failure) may be present.

Laboratory Features
- Signs of hemolytic anemia.
- Thrombocytopenia nearly always present.
- Diagnosis depends on demonstration of the parasites on the blood film (Fig. 23–1) or the appropriate DNA sequences in the blood.
- If greater than 5 percent of red cells parasitized or if two ring forms in a red cell, *P. falciparum* infection usually present.

Treatment and Prognosis
- The blood form of malaria should be treated as soon as possible. Artemisinins are effective against *P. falciparum*, but numerous studies are in progress to determine efficacy of individual drugs and drug combinations.

TABLE 23–1	ORGANISMS THAT CAUSE HEMOLYTIC ANEMIA

Aspergillus
Babesia microti and *Babesia divergens*
Bartonella bacilliformis
Campylobacter jejuni
Clostridium welchii
Coxsackie virus
Cytomegalovirus
Diplococcus pneumoniae
Epstein-Barr virus
Escherichia coli
Haemophilus influenzae
Hepatitis A
Hepatitis B
Herpes simplex virus
Human immunodeficiency virus
Influenza A virus
Leishmania donovani
Leptospira ballum and/or butembo
Mumps virus
Mycobacterium tuberculosis
Mycoplasma pneumoniae
Neisseria intracellularis (meningococci)
Parvovirus B19
Plasmodium falciparum
Plasmodium malariae
Plasmodium vivax
Rubella virus
Rubeola virus
Salmonella
Shigella
Streptococcus
Toxoplasma
Trypanosoma brucei
Varicella virus
Vibrio cholerae
Yersinia enterocolitica

Source: *Williams Hematology,* 8th ed, Chap. 52, Table 52–1, p. 770.

- Tissue stages of vivax malaria have been treated with primaquine. Primaquine, as well as certain sulfones, may produce severe hemolysis in patients with G-6-PD deficiency.
- Transfusions may be necessary in treatment of severe blackwater fever, and if renal failure occurs, dialysis may be required.
- In patients with severe malaria, cerebral malaria, or high levels of parasitemia, erythrocytapheresis or erythrocyte exchange may be beneficial.
- With early treatment, prognosis is excellent. When therapy is delayed or the strain is resistant, malaria (particularly falciparum) may be fatal.

BARTONELLOSIS (OROYA FEVER)

- *Bartonella bacilliformis* is transmitted by the sand fly.
- The organism adheres to the exterior surface of red blood cells, which are rapidly removed from the circulation by the spleen and liver.

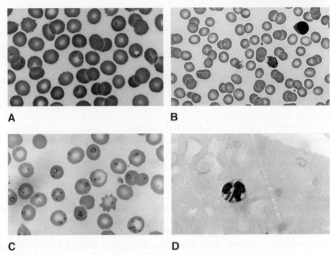

FIGURE 23-1 A. Blood film from a patient with malaria caused by *Plasmodium falciparum*. Several red cells contain ring forms. Note red cell with double ring form in center of the field, characteristic of *P. falciparum* infection. Note the ring form with double dots at the left edge of figure, suggestive of *P. falciparum* infection. Note also high rate of parasitemia (~10% of red cells in this field) characteristic of *P. falciparum* infection. **B.** Blood film from a patient with malaria caused by *Plasmodium vivax*. Note mature schizont. **C.** Blood film from a patient with *Babesia microti* infection. The heavy parasitemia is characteristic of babesiosis (about two-thirds of red cells infected). **D.** Blood film from a patient with *Clostridium perfringens* septicemia. Few red cells evident as a result of intense erythrolysis. Neutrophil with two bacilli (*C. perfringens*). *(Reproduced with permission from* Lichtman's Atlas of Hematology *www.accessmedicine.com.)*
(Source: *Williams Hematology*, 8th ed, Chap. 52, Fig. 52–1, p. 771.)

Clinical Features
- Disease develops in two stages:
  — Acute hemolytic anemia (Oroya fever).
  — Chronic granulomatous disorder (verruca peruviana).
- Most patients manifest no other clinical symptoms during the Oroya fever phase, but some may develop severe hemolytic anemia accompanied by anorexia, thirst, sweating, and generalized lymphadenopathy. Severe thrombocytopenia may occur.
- Verruca peruviana is a nonhematologic disorder characterized by bleeding warty reddish-purple nodules over the face and extremities.

Laboratory Features
- Severe anemia develops rapidly.
- Large numbers of nucleated red cells appear in the blood and the reticulocyte count is elevated.
- Diagnosis is established by demonstrating the organisms on the surface of red cells on a Giemsa-stained smear (red-violet rods 1 to 3 μm in length).

Treatment and Prognosis
- Mortality in untreated patients is very high. Those who survive experience sudden clinical improvement with increase in red cell count and change of the organisms from an elongated to a coccoid form.
- The acute phase usually responds to treatment with ciprofloxacin, chloramphenicol, and β-lactam antibiotics or combinations of the aforementioned, especially in children.

BABESIOSIS

- Intraerythrocytic protozoa transmitted by ticks infect many species of wild and domestic animals (rodents and cattle).
- Humans are rarely infected, usually via ticks, but transmission by transfusion has been reported.
- Most common in the U.S. northeastern coastal region, but also encountered in the midwest.
- Gradual onset with malaise, anorexia, fatigue, followed by fever, sweats, myalgias, and arthralgias.
- May be more severe in splenectomized patients.
- Parasites seen in the red blood cells on Giemsa-stained blood films (Fig. 23–1).
- Treatment with clindamycin and quinine.
- Whole-blood exchange has been used with marked improvement.

CLOSTRIDIUM PERFRINGENS (welchii)

- Most common in patients with septic abortion and occasionally seen following acute cholecystitis.
- In *C. perfringens* septicemia, the toxin (a lecithinase) reacts with red blood cell lipids, leading to severe, often fatal hemolysis with striking hemoglobinemia and hemoglobinuria; serum may be a brilliant red and the urine a dark-brown mahogany color.
- Acute renal and hepatic failure usually develops.
- The blood film shows microspherocytosis, leukocytosis with a left shift, and thrombocytopenia and occasionally intracellular gram-positive rods. (Fig. 23–1).
- The hematocrit may approach zero, but the blood (plasma) hemoglobin may be about 60 to 100 g/L at the time of acute massive intravascular hemolysis.
- Treatment is with intravenous fluid support, high-dose penicillin or a similar antibiotic (e.g., ampicillin) and surgical debridement.
- Mortality is greater than 50 percent, even with appropriate therapy.

OTHER INFECTIONS

- Viral agents may be associated with autoimmune hemolysis (see Chap. 24). The mechanisms include absorption of immune complexes, crossreacting antibodies, and loss of tolerance.
- Evidence for CMV infection is found in a high percentage of children with lymphadenopathy and hemolytic anemia.
- High cold agglutinin titer may develop with *M. pneumoniae* infection and occasionally results in hemolytic anemia or compensated hemolysis (see Chap. 25).
- *Microangiopathic hemolytic anemia* (see Chap. 21) may be triggered by a variety of infections, including *Shigella*, *Campylobacter*, and *Aspergillus*.
- Thrombotic microangiopathy with fragmentation hemolytic anemia (hemolytic uremic syndrome), especially in children, can be caused by enterotoxigenic gram-negative microorganisms, notably *Escherichia coli* serotype O157:H7 (see Chap. 21).

For a more detailed discussion, see Marshall A. Lichtman: Hemolytic Anemia Resulting from Infections with Microorganisms. Chap. 52, p. 769 in *Williams Hematology*, 8th ed.

CHAPTER 24
Hemolytic Anemia Resulting from Warm-Reacting Antibodies

- In autoimmune hemolytic anemia (AHA), shortened red blood cell (RBC) survival is the result of host antibodies that react with autologous RBC.
- AHA may be classified by whether an underlying disease is present (secondary) or not (primary or idiopathic) (Table 24–1).
- AHA may also be classified by the nature of the antibody (Table 24–2).
- "Warm-reacting" antibodies are usually of the IgG type, have optimal activity at 37 °C, and bind complement.
- "Cold-reacting" antibodies show affinity at lower temperatures (see Chap. 25).
- Occasionally, mixed disorders occur with both warm and cold antibodies.
- Warm antibody AHA is the most common type.

ETIOLOGY AND PATHOGENESIS

- AHA occurs in all age groups, but the incidence rises with age, probably because the frequency of lymphoproliferative malignancies increases with age.
- In primary AHA, the autoantibody often is specific for a single RBC membrane protein, suggesting that an aberrant immune response has occurred to an autoantigen or a similar immunogen; a generalized defect in immune regulation is not seen.
- In secondary AHA, the autoantibody most likely develops from an immunoregulatory defect.
- Certain drugs (e.g., α-methyldopa) can induce specific antibodies in otherwise normal individuals by some unknown mechanism. These subside spontaneously when the drug is stopped.
- The red cells of some apparently normal individuals may be found coated with warm-reacting autoantibodies similar to those of patients with AHA. Such antibodies are noted in otherwise normal blood donors at a frequency of 1 in 10,000. A few develop AHA.
- RBC autoantibodies in AHA are pathogenic.
- RBCs that lack the targeted antigen have a normal survival.
- Transplacental passage of autoantibodies to a fetus can cause hemolytic anemia.
- Antibody-coated RBCs are trapped by macrophages primarily in the spleen, where they are ingested and destroyed or partially phagocytosed and a spherocyte with a lower surface area:volume ratio is released.
- Macrophages have cell surface receptors for the Fc portion of IgG and for fragments of C3 and C4b. These immunoglobulin and complement proteins on the RBC surface can act cooperatively as opsonins and enhance trapping of RBC.
- Large quantities of IgG, or the addition of C3b, will increase trapping of RBC by macrophages in the liver and spleen.
- Direct RBC lysis by complement is unusual in warm antibody AHA, probably as a result of interference with complement activity by several mechanisms. Lysis by complement is seen in cold antibody type AHA and paroxysmal cold hemoglobinuria (see Chap. 25).
- RBC may be destroyed by monocytes or lymphocytes by direct cytotoxic activity, without phagocytosis. The proportion of hemolysis caused by this mechanism is unknown. Antibodies may also attach to late erythroid precursors and suppress erythropoiesis.

TABLE 24–1	CLASSIFICATION OF WARM-ANTIBODY–MEDIATED AUTOIMMUNE HEMOLYTIC ANEMIA (AHA)

I. On basis of presence or absence of underlying or significantly associated disorder
   A. Primary or idiopathic AHA (no apparent underlying disease)
   B. Secondary AHA
      1. Associated with lymphoproliferative disorders (e.g., Hodgkin or non-Hodgkin lymphoma)
      2. Associated with the rheumatic disorders, particularly systemic lupus erythematosus
      3. Associated with certain infections (e.g., *Mycoplasma pneumoniae*)
      4. Associated with certain non-lymphoid neoplasms (e.g., ovarian tumors)
      5. Associated with certain chronic inflammatory diseases (e.g., ulcerative colitis)
      6. Associated with ingestion of certain drugs (e.g., α-methyldopa)

CLINICAL FEATURES

- Generally, symptoms of anemia draw attention to the disease, although jaundice may also be a presenting complaint.
- Symptoms are usually slow in onset, but rapidly developing anemia can occur.
- Uncommonly severe anemia may require urgent care. The patient may display air-hunger, profound pallor, and weakness. This syndrome can be seen in patients with AHA in the setting of chronic lymphocytic leukemia.
- Physical examination may be normal if the anemia is mild. Splenomegaly is common but not always observed. Jaundice and physical findings related to more pronounced anemia may be noticed.
- AHA may be aggravated or first noticed during pregnancy. Both mother and fetus generally fare well if the condition is treated early.

LABORATORY FEATURES

General

- Anemia can range from mild to life-threatening.
- Blood film reveals polychromasia (indicating reticulocytosis) and spherocytes (see Fig. 24–1).
- With severe cases, nucleated RBC, RBC fragments, and, occasionally, erythrophagocytosis by monocytes may be seen (see Fig. 24–1).
- Reticulocytosis is usually present if the marrow has not been injured by some other condition; initially, a short period of relative reticulocytopenia occurs in one-third of the cases.
- Most patients have mild neutrophilia and normal platelet count, but occasionally immune neutropenia and thrombocytopenia occur concomitantly.
- Evans syndrome is a rare condition in which both autoimmune-mediated RBC and platelet destruction occur. A low neutrophil count may also be present.
- Marrow examination usually reveals erythroid hyperplasia; occasionally an underlying lymphoproliferative disease may be uncovered.
- Unconjugated hyperbilirubinemia is often present, but usually the total bilirubin level does not exceed 5 mg/dL, with less than 15 percent conjugated.
- Haptoglobin levels are usually low, and serum lactic acid dehydrogenase (LDH) activity is elevated.
- Urinary urobilinogen is routinely increased, but hemoglobinuria is uncommon.

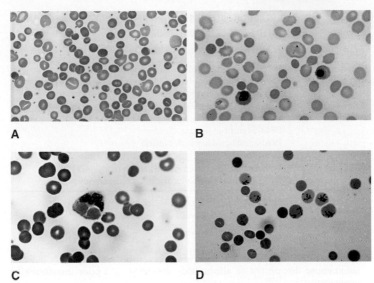

FIGURE 24-1 A. Blood film. Autoimmune hemolytic anemia. Moderately severe. Note high frequency of microspherocytes (small hyperchromatic RBCs) and the high frequency of macrocytes (putative reticulocytes). **B.** Blood film. Autoimmune hemolytic anemia. Severe. Note the low density of red cells on the film (profound anemia), high frequency of microspherocytes (hyperchromatic), and the large red cells (putative reticulocytes). Note the two nucleated RBCs and the Howell-Jolly body (nuclear remnant) in the macrocyte. Nucleated RBCs and Howell-Jolly bodies may be seen in autoimmune hemolytic anemia with severe hemolysis or after splenectomy. **C.** Blood film. Autoimmune hemolytic anemia. Severe. Monocyte engulfing two red cells (erythrophagocytosis). Note frequent microspherocytes and scant red cell density. **D.** Reticulocyte preparation. Autoimmune hemolytic anemia. Note high frequency of reticulocytes, the large cells with precipitated ribosomes. Remaining cells are microspherocytes. (*Reproduced with permission from* Lichtman's Atlas of Hematology, *www.accessmedicine.com.*)
(Source: *Williams Hematology,* 8th ed, Chap. 53, Fig. 53–2, p. 786.)

Serologic Features (Table 24-2)

- The diagnosis of AHA requires demonstration of immunoglobulin and/or complement bound to the RBC.
- This is achieved by the direct antiglobulin test (DAT) in which rabbit antiserum to human IgG or complement is added to suspensions of washed patient's RBC. Agglutination of the RBC signifies the presence of surface IgG or complement.
- The DAT is first performed with broad-spectrum reagents, including antibodies against both complement and immunoglobulin. If this is positive, further testing is done to define the offending antibody or complement component.
- RBC may be coated with:
  — IgG alone.
  — IgG and complement.
  — Complement only.
- Rarely, anti-IgA and anti-IgM reactions are encountered.
- Autoantibody exists in a dynamic equilibrium between RBC and plasma.
- Free autoantibody may be detected by the indirect antiglobulin test (IAT) in which the patient's serum is incubated with normal donor RBC, which are then tested for agglutination by the addition of antiglobulin serum.
- Binding affinity for antibodies varies, but in general, serum autoantibody is detectable in those with heavily coated RBC.

TABLE 24–2	MAJOR REACTION PATTERNS OF THE DIRECT ANTIGLOBULIN TEST AND ASSOCIATED TYPES OF IMMUNE INJURY
Reaction Pattern	Type of Immune Injury
IgG alone	Warm-antibody autoimmune hemolytic anemia Drug-immune hemolytic anemia: hapten drug adsorption type or autoantibody type
Complement alone	Warm-antibody autoimmune hemolytic anemia with subthreshold IgG deposition Cold-agglutinin disease Paroxysmal cold hemoglobinuria Drug-immune hemolytic anemia: ternary complex type
IgG plus complement	Warm-antibody autoimmune hemolytic anemia Drug-immune hemolytic anemia: autoantibody type (rare)

Source: *Williams Hematology,* 8th ed, Chap. 53, Table 53–4, p. 787.

- A positive indirect test with a negative direct test probably does not indicate autoimmune disease but an alloantibody generated by a prior transfusion or pregnancy.
- Occasional patients exhibit all the features of AHA but have a negative DAT. The amount of their RBC-bound autoantibody is too low for detection by DAT but can often be demonstrated by more sensitive methods, such as enzyme-linked immunoassay or radioimmunoassay.
- The relationship between the amount of bound antibody and degree of hemolysis is variable.
- Subclasses IgG_1 and IgG_3 are generally more effective in causing hemolysis than IgG_2 and IgG_4, apparently because of greater affinity of macrophage Fc receptors for these subclasses as well as increased complement fixation abilities.
- Autoantibodies from AHA patients usually bind to all the types of RBC used for laboratory screening and therefore appear to be "nonspecific."
- However, the autoantibodies from individual patients usually react with antigens that are present on nearly all RBC types, the so-called "public" antigens, and only appear to lack specificity.
- Nearly half of the antibodies have specificity for epitopes on Rh proteins (Rh related) and hence will not react with cells of the rare Rh-null type.
- The remaining autoantibodies have a variety of specificities, but many are not defined.

DIFFERENTIAL DIAGNOSIS

- Other conditions may have spherocytosis, including hereditary spherocytosis, Zieve syndrome, Wilson disease, and clostridial sepsis. DAT is negative in these conditions.
- AHA and autoimmune thrombocytopenia may also occur as a manifestation of systemic lupus erythematosus (secondary AHA).
- Paroxysmal nocturnal hemoglobinuria and microangiopathic hemolytic anemia should also be considered, but minimal or no spherocytosis is seen and the DAT is negative.
- If the DAT is positive for complement alone, further serologic characterizations are warranted to distinguish cold-reacting from warm-reacting autoantibodies.
- In recently transfused patients, alloantibody against donor RBC may be detected by a positive DAT.

- Organ transplant recipients may develop a picture of AHA usually when an organ from a blood group O donor is transplanted into a group A recipient, probably because B lymphocytes persist in the transplanted organ and form alloantibodies against host RBC.
- Marrow transplant patients of blood group O who receive blood group A or B marrow may develop a briefly positive DAT, and RBC synthesized by the engrafted marrow may be hemolyzed until previously made recipient anti-A or anti-B disappears.
- Mixed chimera also occurs so that the immunocompetent host B lymphocyte continues to generate alloantibodies.

THERAPY

- Occasional patients have a positive DAT but minimal hemolysis and stable hematocrit. These patients need no treatment but should be observed for possible progression of the disease.

Transfusion

- Generally, anemia develops slowly so that RBC transfusion is not required; however, for rapid hemolysis or patients otherwise compromised (i.e., cardiac disease), transfusion may be lifesaving.
- Virtually all units are incompatible on cross-match unless one has an autoantibody that is specific for a single RBC antigen and RBC units lacking that antigen can be obtained.
- Transfused RBCs are destroyed as fast as or faster than host RBC but may tide the patient through a dangerous time.
- The blood bank should try to ascertain the ABO type of patient's RBC to avoid alloantibody-mediated hemolysis of donor cells.

Glucocorticoids

- Glucocorticoids slow or stop hemolysis in two-thirds of the patients.
- Twenty percent of patients will achieve a complete remission.
- Ten percent will show little or no response.
- Best results are seen in patients with primary AHA or AHA secondary to lupus erythematosus.
- Initial treatment should be with oral prednisone at 60 to 100 mg/d, orally.
- For the gravely ill, intravenous methylprednisolone at 100 to 200 mg in divided doses over the first 24 hours can be given.
- When the hematocrit stabilizes, prednisone may be slowly tapered to 15 to 20 mg/d at a rate of about 5 mg per week and continued for 2 to 3 months before slowly tapering off the drug entirely. In some cases in which tapering cannot be completed, alternative day therapy may be tried, 20 to 30 mg every other day by mouth.
- Relapses are common, and the patient should be closely monitored.
- The mechanism(s) of action of glucocorticoids in AHA has not been fully established but presumably they impair macrophage ingestion of antibody-coated RBC, early after treatment is started and suppress autoantibody production.

Splenectomy

- In patients who cannot be tapered off prednisone (approximately one-third), splenectomy is the next modality of therapy to use. If response is slow and the anemia is severe, splenectomy should be considered.
- Splenectomy removes the main site of RBC destruction. Hemolysis can continue, but much higher levels of RBC-bound antibody are necessary to cause the same rate of destruction. Sometimes the amount of cell-bound antibody will decrease after splenectomy, but often no change is noted.

- Approximately two-thirds of patients have complete or partial remission after splenectomy, but relapses frequently occur. If glucocorticoids are still necessary, it is often possible to use a lower dosage.
- Splenectomy slightly increases the risk of pneumococcal sepsis (children more than adults), and pneumococcal vaccine should be given several weeks before surgery, if feasible. In addition, prophylactic oral penicillin is often given to children after splenectomy.

Rituximab

- A monoclonal antibody directed against CD20 may be used to treat AHA based on its ability to eliminate B lymphocytes producing autoantibodies to RBCs. The rapid response in many patients in whom autoantibody is still circulating makes that an unlikely initial mechanism.
- Opsonized B lymphocytes may decoy macrophages and monocytes from autoantibody complexes and normalize autoreactive T lymphocyte responses.
- The response rate has averaged about 60 percent of patients treated with anti-CD20.

Immunosuppressive Drugs

- Either cyclophosphamide (60 mg/m^2) or azathioprine (80 mg/m^2) given daily can be used. Close attention to blood counts is crucial because erythropoiesis can be suppressed, temporarily worsening the anemia. Treatment can be continued for up to 6 months awaiting a response, and then tapered if and when the desired response is attained.

Other Treatments

- Plasmapheresis has been used with occasional success reported, but its efficacy is unpredictable.
- Variable success has been achieved with high-dose intravenous immunoglobulin (400 mg/kg daily for 5 days), danazol, 2-chlorodeoxyadenosine, thymectomy in children, and administration of vinblastine-loaded RBC.

COURSE AND PROGNOSIS

- Idiopathic warm-antibody AHA runs an unpredictable course characterized by remissions and relapses.
- Survival at 10 years is approximately 70 percent.
- In addition to anemia, deep venous thrombosis, pulmonary emboli, splenic infarcts, and other cardiovascular events occur during active disease.
- In secondary warm-antibody AHA, prognosis is related to the underlying disease.
- Overall mortality rate in children is lower than in adults, ranging from 10 to 30 percent.
- AHA related to infection is self-limited and responds well to glucocorticoids.
- Children who develop chronic AHA tend to be older.

 For a more detailed discussion, see Charles H. Packman: Hemolytic Anemia Resulting from Immune Injury. Chap. 53, p. 777 in *Williams Hematology*, 8th ed.

CHAPTER 25
Cryopathic Hemolytic Anemia

- Caused by autoantibodies that bind red cells best at temperatures below 37 °C, usually below 31°C.
- Mediated through two major types of "cold antibody": cold agglutinins and Donath-Landsteiner antibodies.
- Clinical features vary considerably, but in both types, the complement system plays a major role in red cell destruction.

COLD AGGLUTININ-MEDIATED AUTOIMMUNE HEMOLYTIC ANEMIA

- Cold agglutinins are IgM autoantibodies that agglutinate red cells optimally between 0 °C and 5 °C. Complement fixation occurs at higher temperatures.
- Classified as either primary (chronic cold agglutinin disease) or secondary (generally as a result of *Mycoplasma pneumoniae* infection or Epstein-Barr virus (EBV)–related infectious mononucleosis) (see Table 25–1).
- Peak incidence for the primary (chronic) syndrome is in persons older than 50 years.
- This disorder characteristically has monoclonal IgM cold agglutinins and may be considered a symptomatic monoclonal gammopathy.
- Some patients develop a B-cell lymphoproliferative disorder (e.g. Waldenström macroglobulinemia).

Pathogenesis

- The specificity of cold agglutinins is usually against I/i antigens. I is expressed heavily in adult red cells, weakly on neonatal red cells. The reverse is true of the i antigen, which also may still be expressed on reticulocytes.
- High proportions of IgM cold agglutinins with either anti-I or anti-i specificity have heavy-chain variable regions encoded by V_H4–34, a conserved immunoglobulin variable region gene.
- Naturally occurring cold agglutinins are present in low titer (less than 1:32) in normal persons. Transient hyperproduction of less clonally restricted antibodies occurs in the recovery phase of infections, such as EBV, mycoplasma, or cytomegalovirus.
- I/i antigens serve as mycoplasma receptors, which may lead to altered antigen presentation and to subsequent autoantibody production.
- In B-cell lymphomas, cold agglutinins may be produced by the malignant cells.
- The highest temperature at which antibodies can cause red cell agglutination is termed the thermal amplitude. The higher the thermal amplitude, the greater the risk for clinically significant hemolysis, depending on the ambient temperature.
- Cold agglutinins bind red cells in the superficial vessels impeding capillary flow, producing acrocyanosis.
- Hemolysis is dependent on the antibody's ability to bind complement to the red cell membrane; concurrent agglutination is not required for this process. This is termed complement fixation.
- Red cell injury then occurs either by direct lysis or enhanced phagocytosis by macrophages.
- Direct lysis results from propagation of the full complement sequence, but severe intravascular hemolysis from this cause is rare.
- Commonly, fragments C3b and C4b are deposited on the red cell surface, providing a stimulus for phagocytosis. The affected red cell may be engulfed and

TABLE 25–1	**AUTOIMMUNE HEMOLYTIC ANEMIA: COLD ANTIBODY TYPE***

  I. Mediated by cold agglutinins
      A. Idiopathic (primary) chronic cold-agglutinin disease (usually associated with clonal
          B-lymphocyte disease)
      B. Secondary cold-agglutinin hemolytic anemia
          1. Postinfectious (e.g., *Mycoplasma pneumoniae* or infectious mononucleosis)
          2. Associated with preexisting malignant B-cell lymphoproliferative disorder
 II. Mediated by cold hemolysins
      A. Idiopathic (primary) paroxysmal cold hemoglobinuria—very rare
      B. Secondary
          1. Donath-Landsteiner hemolytic anemia, usually associated with an acute viral
             syndrome in children—relatively common
          2. Congenital or tertiary syphilis in adults—very rare

*Uncommonly, cases may have mixed cold and warm autoantibodies (e.g., primary or idiopathic mixed autoimmune hemolytic anemia) or secondary mixed autoimmune hemolytic anemia associated with the rheumatic disorders, particularly systemic lupus erythematosus.
Source: *Williams Hematology,* 8th ed, Chap. 53, Table 53-1, p. 778.

destroyed or released back into circulation as a spherocyte because of loss of some plasma membrane.
- Red cells are released with a coating of C3dg, an inactive fragment that protects the red cells from further complement fixation and agglutination but causes a positive direct antiglobulin test.

Clinical Features
- Cold-agglutinin–mediated hemolysis accounts for 10 to 20 percent of all cases of autoimmune hemolytic anemia.
- Women are affected more commonly than men.
- Hemolysis is generally chronic, although episodes of acute hemolysis can occur upon chilling.
- Acrocyanosis is frequently observed, but skin ulceration and necrosis are uncommon.
- Splenomegaly may occasionally be seen in the idiopathic form.
- The hemolysis caused by mycoplasma infection develops as the patient recovers from the infection and is self-limited, lasting 1 to 3 weeks.
- In patients with mycoplasma infections, clinically significant hemolysis is uncommon.

Laboratory Features
- Anemia is usually mild to moderate. On the blood film the red cells show autoagglutination (Fig. 25–1), polychromasia, and spherocytosis.
- In the chronic syndrome, serum titers of cold agglutinins (generally IgM) can be greater than 1:100,000. The direct antiglobulin test is positive with anticomplement reagents. The cold agglutinin itself (IgM) is not detectable as it readily dissociates from the red cell at 37 °C.
- As a rule, the higher the cold agglutinin titer the higher the thermal amplitude, although there are exceptions to this rule (lower titer and high thermal amplitude).
- Testing for cold agglutinin titer and thermal amplitude requires blood collection and serum separation at 37 °C.
- Anti-I specificity is seen with idiopathic disease, *M. pneumoniae*, and some lymphoma cases. Anti-i occurs with infectious mononucleosis and lymphomas. Rarely, the antibodies have other specificities, including Pr, M, or P antigens.

Differential Diagnosis

- When peripheral vaso-occlusive symptoms occur, especially if related to cold temperatures (Raynaud phenomenon), cryoglobulinemia should also be considered.
- In drug-induced immune hemolytic anemia, the direct antiglobulin test also may be positive only for complement.
- Mixed type autoimmune hemolysis can occur with a direct antiglobulin test positive for both IgG and complement, along with elevated cold agglutinin titers.
- Episodic hemolysis can result from paroxysmal cold hemoglobinuria (see below), paroxysmal nocturnal hemoglobinuria (see Chap. 45), and march hemoglobinuria (see Chap. 20).

Therapy, Course, and Prognosis

- Keeping the patient warm is important and may be the only treatment needed for mild conditions.
- Rituximab is useful in symptomatic cases.
- Chlorambucil and cyclophosphamide are useful for more severe chronic cases; interferon-α can be useful.
- Splenectomy and glucocorticoids generally are not helpful (they may have some efficacy in low titer, high thermal amplitude cases), although very high dose glucocorticoids may be useful in the severely ill patient.
- In critically ill patients, plasmapheresis may provide temporary relief.
- Generally, patients with the chronic syndrome have a stable condition and long-term survival.
- Postinfectious syndromes are self-limited, resolving in a few weeks.

PAROXYSMAL COLD HEMOGLOBINURIA

- A very rare form of hemolytic anemia characterized by recurrent massive hemolysis following exposure to cold. Formerly, this condition was more common, because of its association with syphilis. A self-limited form occurs in children following several types of viral infections.

Pathogenesis

- In the extremities, the cold reactive autoantibody (Donath-Landsteiner antibody), which is an IgG antibody, and early complement proteins bind to the red cells at low temperatures. Upon return to the 37 °C environment, lysis occurs as a consequence of propagation of the classic complement sequence.

Clinical Features

- Two to 5 percent of all patients have autoimmune hemolytic anemia; the incidence of hemolytic anemia may exceed 30 percent in the pediatric population.
- Paroxysms of hemolysis occur with associated systemic symptoms—rigors, fever, diffuse myalgias, headache. These symptoms and hemoglobinuria usually last several hours. Cold-induced urticaria may also occur.

Laboratory Features

- Hemoglobinuria with a rapid fall in hemoglobin level is usual and is associated with depressed complement levels. Spherocytes and erythrophagocytosis may be seen on the blood film.
- The direct antiglobulin test is positive for complement RBC coating during and immediately after an attack; the Donath-Landsteiner antibody itself is not detected by the test because it readily dissociates from the red cells.
- Antibody is detected by the biphasic Donath-Landsteiner test. Red cells are incubated with the patient's serum at 4 °C, then warmed to 37 °C, at which point intense hemolysis occurs.

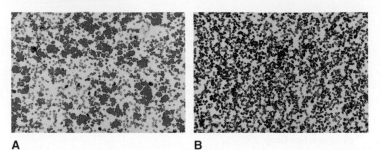

A   **B**

FIGURE 25-1 Blood films. **A.** Cold-reactive (IgM) antibody. Red cell agglutination at room temperature. **B.** Same blood examined at 37°C. Note marked reduction in agglutination. *(Reproduced with permission from* Lichtman's Atlas of Hematology, *www.accessmedicine.com.)* (Source: *Williams Hematology,* 8th ed, Chap. 53, Fig. 53–3. p.787.)

- Classically, the antibody (IgG type) has specificity for P blood group antigens, although other specificities have been noted.
- The Donath-Landsteiner antibody is a far more potent hemolysin than most cold agglutinins.

Differential Diagnosis
- Patients with paroxysmal cold hemoglobinuria lack elevated titers of cold agglutinins, distinguishing it from cold agglutinin disease.

Therapy, Course, and Prognosis
- Attacks can be prevented by avoiding cold exposure.
- Splenectomy and glucocorticoids are not of value.
- Urticaria may be treated with antihistamines.
- If related to syphilis, the hemolysis will resolve with antibiotic treatment of the infection.
- Postinfectious paroxysmal cold hemoglobinuria may resolve spontaneously in days to weeks, although the antibody may be detectable for years.
- In the idiopathic chronic form, long-term survival is common.
- Children may have a high mortality rate.

For a more detailed discussion, see Charles H. Packman: Hemolytic Anemia Resulting from Immune Injury. Chap. 53, p. 777 in *Williams Hematology,* 8th ed.

CHAPTER 26
Drug-Induced Hemolytic Anemia

ETIOLOGY AND PATHOGENESIS

- Table 26–1 lists the drugs implicated in the production of a positive direct antiglobulin test and accelerated red cell destruction.
- Three mechanisms of drug-related immunologic injury to red cells are defined:
  — Hapten/drug adsorption involving drug-dependent antibodies.
  — Ternary complex formation involving drug-dependent antibodies.
  — Induction of autoantibodies that react with red cells in the absence of the inciting drug.
- Drug-related nonimmunologic protein adsorption may also result in a positive direct antiglobulin test without red cell injury.

HAPTEN OR DRUG ADSORPTION MECHANISM

- Occurs with drugs that bind firmly to red cell membrane proteins. Penicillin is the classic example.
- In patients receiving high-dose penicillin, red cells have a substantial coating of the drug. In a small proportion of patients, an antipenicillin antibody (usually IgG) develops and binds to the penicillin on the red cell. The direct antiglobulin test then becomes positive and hemolytic anemia may ensue.
- Hemolytic anemia caused by penicillin typically occurs after 7 to 10 days of treatment and ceases a few days to 2 weeks once the drug is stopped.
- Other manifestations of penicillin allergy are usually not present.
- Antibody-coated ("opsonized") red cells are destroyed mainly in the spleen.
- Antibodies eluted from red cells, or present in sera, react only against penicillin-coated red cells. This specificity distinguishes drug-dependent antibodies from true autoantibodies.
- Hemolytic anemia similar to that seen with penicillin has also been ascribed to other drugs (see Table 26–1).

TERNARY COMPLEX MECHANISM: DRUG-ANTIBODY TARGET-CELL COMPLEX

- The mechanism of red cell injury is not clearly defined, but it appears to be mediated by a cooperative interaction to generate a *ternary complex* involving the drug or drug-metabolite, a drug-binding membrane site on the target cell, and antibody, with consequent activation of complement (see Fig. 26–1B).
- The antibody attaches to a neoantigen consisting of loosely bound drug and red cell antigen; binding of drug to the target cell is weak until stabilized by the attachment of the antibody to both drug and cell membrane.
- Some of these antibodies have specificity for blood group antigens, such as Rh, Kell, or Kidd, and are nonreactive with red cells lacking the alloantigen even in the presence of drug.
- The direct antiglobulin test is usually positive with anticomplement reagents.
- Intravascular hemolysis may occur after activation of complement, with hemoglobinemia and hemoglobinuria, and C3b-coated red cells may be destroyed by the spleen and liver.

| TABLE 26–1 | ASSOCIATION BETWEEN DRUGS AND POSITIVE DIRECT ANTIGLOBULIN TESTS* |

Drugs

Hapten or Drug Adsorption Mechanism

Penicillins	Carbromal
Cephalosporins	Tolbutamide
Tetracycline	Cianidanol
6-Mercaptopurine	Hydrocortisone
	Oxaliplatin

Ternary Complex Mechanism

Stibophen	Probenecid
Quinine	Nomifensine
Quinidine	Cephalosporins
Chlorpropamide	Diethylstilbestrol
Rifampicin	Amphotericin B
Antazoline	Doxepin
Thiopental	Diclofenac
Tolmetin	Etodolac
Metformin	Hydrocortisone
	Oxaliplatin
	Pemetrexed

Autoantibody Mechanism

Cephalosporins	Cianidanol
Tolmetin	Latamoxef
Nomifensine	Glafenine
α-Methyldopa	Procainamide
l-Dopa	Diclofenac
Mefenamic acid	Pentostatin
Teniposide	Fludarabine
Oxaliplatin	Cladribine
Efalizumab	Lenalidomide

Nonimmunologic Protein Adsorption

Cephalosporins	Cisplatin
Oxaliplatin	Carboplatin

Uncertain Mechanism of Immune Injury

Mesantoin	Streptomycin
Phenacetin	Ibuprofen
Insecticides	Triamterene
Chlorpromazine	Erythromycin
Melphalan	5-Fluorouracil
Isoniazid	Nalidixic acid
p-Aminosalicylic acid	Sulindac
Acetaminophen	Omeprazol
Thiazides	Temafloxacin
Efavirenz	Carboplatin

*It is not always possible to infer the mechanism of immune injury induced by a drug. Moreover, some drugs can act by more than one mechanism. In cases of uncertain mechanism, the cited drug use is coincident with the hemolytic anemia, and causality is inferred, not established experimentally. These cases are included so that the reader may be aware of these potential associations.

Source: *Williams Hematology*, 8th ed, Chap. 53, Table 53–2, p. 780.

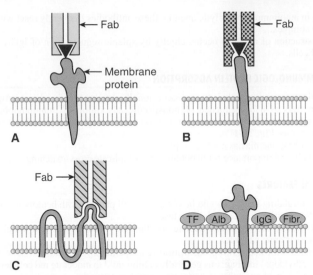

FIGURE 26-1 Effector mechanisms by which drugs mediate a positive direct antiglobulin test. Relationships of drug, antibody-combining site, and red blood cell membrane protein are shown. Panels A, B, and C show only a single immunoglobulin Fab region (bearing one combining site). **A.** Drug adsorption/hapten mechanism. The drug (▼) binds avidly to an unknown red blood cell membrane protein *in vivo.* Antidrug antibody (usually IgG) binds to the protein-bound drug. The direct antiglobulin test (with anti-IgG) detects IgG antidrug antibody on the patient's circulating (drug-coated) red blood cells. **B.** Ternary complex mechanism. Drug binds loosely or in undetectable amounts to red blood cell membrane. However, in the presence of appropriate antidrug antibody, a stable trimolecular (ternary) complex is formed by drug, red blood cell membrane protein, and antibody. In this mechanism, the direct antiglobulin test typically detects only red blood cell–bound complement components (e.g., C3 fragments) that are bound covalently and in large number to the patient's red blood cells *in vivo.* The antibody itself escapes detection. **C.** Autoantibody induction. Some drug-induced antibodies can bind avidly to red blood cell membrane proteins (usually Rh proteins) in the absence of the inducing drug and are indistinguishable from the autoantibodies of patients with autoimmune hemolytic anemia. The direct antiglobulin test detects the IgG antibody on the patient's red blood cells. **D.** Drug-induced non-immunologic protein adsorption. Certain drugs cause plasma proteins to attach nonspecifically to the red blood cell membrane. The direct antiglobulin test detects nonspecifically bound IgG and complement components. In contrast to the other mechanisms of drug-induced red blood cell injury, this mechanism does not shorten red blood cell survival *in vivo.*
(Source: *Williams Hematology,* 8th ed, Chapter 53, Fig. 53–1, p. 779.)

AUTOANTIBODY MECHANISM

- Many drugs induce the formation of autoantibodies to autologous (or homologous) red cells, most importantly α-methyldopa (see Table 26–1). The mechanism by which a drug can induce formation of an autoantibody is unknown.
- Positive direct antiglobulin tests are seen in 8 to 36 percent of those taking α-methyldopa. The positive test develops 3 to 6 months after the start of therapy. In contrast, less than 1 percent of those taking α-methyldopa develop hemolytic anemia.
- Infrequently, patients with chronic lymphocytic leukemia treated with purine analogues (e.g., fludarabine) develop autoimmune hemolytic anemia.
- Antibodies in the serum or eluted from red cells react optimally at 37 °C with autologous or homologous red cells in the absence of drug.

- As in autoimmune hemolytic anemia, these antibodies frequently react with the Rh complex.
- Destruction of red cells occurs chiefly by splenic sequestration of IgG-coated red cells.

NONIMMUNOLOGIC PROTEIN ADSORPTION

- Patients receiving cephalosporins occasionally develop positive direct antiglobulin tests as a consequence of nonspecific adsorption of immunoglobulins, complement, albumin, fibrinogen, and other plasma proteins to red cell membranes (see **Fig. 26–1D**).
- Hemolytic anemia has not been reported.
- The clinical importance is the potential to complicate cross-matching.

CLINICAL FEATURES

- A careful drug history should be obtained in all patients with hemolytic anemia and/or positive direct antiglobulin test.
- The severity of symptoms depends on the rate of hemolysis, and the clinical picture is quite variable.
- Patients with hapten/drug adsorption (e.g., penicillin) and autoimmune (e.g., α-methyldopa) mechanisms generally exhibit mild to moderate red cell destruction with insidious onset of symptoms over days to weeks.
- If the ternary complex mechanism is operative (e.g., cephalosporins or quinidine), there may be sudden onset of severe hemolysis with hemoglobinuria and acute renal failure.
- Hemolysis can occur after only one dose of the drug if the patient has been previously exposed.

LABORATORY FEATURES

- Findings are similar to those of autoimmune hemolytic anemia, with anemia, reticulocytosis, and high MCV.
- Leukopenia, thrombocytopenia, hemoglobinemia, or hemoglobinuria may be observed in cases of ternary complex-mediated hemolysis.
- The serologic features are included under "Differential Diagnosis," below.

DIFFERENTIAL DIAGNOSIS

- Immune hemolysis caused by drugs should be distinguished from autoimmune hemolytic anemia (warm or cold antibodies), congenital hemolytic anemias (e.g., hereditary spherocytosis), and drug-mediated hemolysis caused by disorders of red cell metabolism (e.g., G-6-PD deficiency).
- In drug-related hemolytic anemia, the direct antiglobulin test is positive.
- In the hapten/drug mechanism, the key difference from autoimmune hemolytic anemia is that serum antibodies react only with drug-coated red cells. This serologic distinction plus a history of the specific drug exposure should be decisive.
- In the ternary complex mechanism, the direct antiglobulin test is positive with anticomplement serum, similar to cold autoimmune hemolytic anemia. However, the cold agglutinin titer and Donath-Landsteiner test are normal and the indirect antiglobulin test is positive only in the presence of drug. The direct antiglobulin test becomes negative shortly after stopping the drug.
- In hemolytic anemia caused by α-methyldopa, the direct antiglobulin reaction is strongly positive for IgG (rarely for complement) and the indirect antiglobulin reaction is positive with unmodified red cells, often showing Rh specificity. There is no specific serologic test to differentiate this disorder from warm-autoimmune hemolytic anemia with Rh complex specificities. The diagnosis is

supported by recovery from anemia and disappearance of antibodies upon discontinuing the drug.

- With a clinical picture of drug-induced immune hemolysis, it is reasonable to stop any drug while serologic studies are performed and to monitor for increase in hematocrit, decrease in reticulocytosis, and disappearance of positive antiglobulin test.
- Rechallenge with the suspected drug may confirm the diagnosis but should be tried only for compelling reasons.

THERAPY, COURSE, AND PROGNOSIS

- Discontinuation of the offending drug is often the only treatment needed, and may be lifesaving in severe hemolysis mediated by the ternary complex mechanism.
- Transfuse only for severe, life-threatening anemia.
- Glucocorticoids are generally unnecessary and are of questionable efficacy.
- If high-dose penicillin is the treatment of choice in life-threatening infection, therapy need not be changed as a result of a positive direct antiglobulin test, unless there is overt hemolytic anemia.
- A positive direct antiglobulin test alone is not necessarily an indication for stopping α-methyldopa, although it may be prudent to consider alternative antihypertensive therapy.
- Hemolysis associated with α-methyldopa ceases promptly after stopping the drug. The positive direct antiglobulin test gradually diminishes over weeks or months.
- Problems with cross-matching may occur in patients with a strongly positive indirect antiglobulin test.
- Immune hemolysis caused by drugs is usually mild, but occasional episodes of severe hemolysis with renal failure or death have been seen, usually as a consequence of the ternary complex mechanism.

For a more detailed discussion, see Charles H. Packman: Hemolytic Anemia Resulting from Immune Injury. Chapter 53, p. 777 in *Williams Hematology*, 8th ed.

CHAPTER 27
Alloimmune Hemolytic Disease of the Newborn

DEFINITION

- A disease in which there is fetal to maternal transfer of red cells that results in immunization of the mother. Then, transplacental transfer of maternal anti–red cell antibodies to the fetus shortens the life span of fetal or newborn red cells.
- Manifestations include fetal anemia, jaundice, and hepatosplenomegaly; in more severe cases, anasarca and kernicterus also occur.

PATHOGENESIS

- Asymptomatic transplacental passage of fetal red cells occurs in 75 percent of pregnancies.
- If there is blood group incompatibility between mother and fetus, the chance of maternal immunization increases with the volume of any transplacental hemorrhage.
- Approximately 95 percent of pregnant women have fetomaternal hemorrhage of less than 1.0 mL at delivery.
- Intrapartum fetomaternal hemorrhage of more than 30 mL occurs in approximately 1.0 percent of deliveries.
- Larger volume transplacental hemorrhages are more likely to occur at delivery or during invasive obstetric procedures.
- The risk of sensitization increases with each trimester of pregnancy and is greatest (65%) at delivery.
- Fetomaternal transfusion can occur at the time of chorionic villous sampling, amniocentesis, therapeutic abortion, cesarean section, abdominal trauma, and other situations.
- Prior blood transfusions or abortions also can immunize the mother.
- Maternal red cell antibodies fall into three classes: antibodies directed against the D antigen in the Rh blood group, antibodies directed against the A or B antigens, and antibodies directed against the remaining red cell antigens.
- The D antigen of the Rh blood group system is involved in most serious cases.
- Without prophylaxis, immunization occurs in approximately 12 percent of those at risk with an RhD-positive, ABO-compatible fetus and 2 percent of these with an RhD-positive, ABO-incompatible fetus.
- Anti-D IgG crosses the placenta and leads to a positive antiglobulin test and hemolysis in the infant.
- In ABO hemolytic disease, the mother is usually type O and the fetus is type A or B.
- Anti-A and anti-B antibodies ordinarily cause mild and rarely severe hemolysis. Numerous other causative antibodies have been described but are less common (see Epidemiology).

EPIDEMIOLOGY

- The distribution of blood group antigens among different ethnic groups determines their risk of alloimmune hemolytic disease.
- Approximately 16 percent of Americans of European descent are RhD-negative, compared to 8 percent of Americans of African ancestry, 5 percent of persons of Asian Indian ancestry, and 0.3 percent of those of Chinese ancestry.

- More than 50 different red cell antigens have been associated with maternal alloimmunization and with alloimmune hemolytic disease with varying degrees of severity.
- Women can have naturally occurring antigens to blood group A or B (e.g., Mother type O) or may develop other antibodies not screened for prior to blood transfusion.
- Antenatal screening programs detect antibodies in approximately 0.2 percent of pregnant women.
- After anti-RhD, the following antigens may be involved in alloimmunization: Rhc, C, e, cc, Ce, Kell, Duffy, Kidd, and the MNS antigen system.
- The presence of maternal antibodies is not predictive of alloimmune hemolytic disease because of the following: (a) they may be IgM antibodies and not traverse the placenta, (b) the antigens may not be present on fetal red cells or their density very low, (c) the concentration of antibody in maternal blood may be very low, (d) the antibody Ig subclass may not interact with fetal red cells, and other mitigating factors.

CLINICAL FEATURES

Distinctions between ABO and RhD Alloimmunization

- RhD and ABO hemolytic disease differ in several respects (see Table 27–1):
  — ABO hemolytic disease can occur in (a) mothers with O red cells and fetuses with blood group A or B red cells, (b) mothers of type B and fetuses of type A, (c) mothers of type A and fetuses of type B.
  — ABO incompatibility is present in 15 percent of O group pregnancies, but hemolytic disease of the fetus or newborn occurs in about 2 percent of births.

TABLE 27–1	COMPARISON OF RH AND ABO HEMOLYTIC DISEASE OF THE NEWBORN	
	Rh	ABO
Blood groups		
Mother	Negative	O
Infant	Positive	A or B
Type of antibody	IgG$_1$ and /or IgG$_3$	IgG$_2$
Clinical aspects		
Occurrence in first-born	5%	40–50%
Predictable severity in subsequent pregnancies	Usually	No
Stillbirth and/or hydrops	Frequent	Rare
Severe anemia	Frequent	Rare
Degree of jaundice	+++	+ to ++
Hepatosplenomegaly	+++	+
Laboratory findings		
Maternal antibodies	Always present	Not clear-cut
Direct antiglobulin test (infant)	+	+ or −
Microspherocytes	0	+
Treatment		
Antenatal measures	Yes	No
Exchange transfusion frequency	Approx. 2/3	Occasional
Donor blood type	Rh-negative, group specific when possible	Group O only
Incidence of late anemia	Common	Rare

Source: *Williams Hematology,* 8th ed, Chap. 54, Table 54–2, p. 802.

— The low frequency of ABO hemolytic disease is the result of most anti-A and anti-B being IgM antibodies, which do not easily traverse the placenta.

— Prenatal testing for maternal anti-A or anti-B antibodies is not predictive of occurrence of alloimmune hemolytic disease because of the unpredictable time of expression of A or B on fetal red cells and the sink for maternal antibodies provided by other fetal tissues that express A or B antigen.

— ABO incompatibility may be observed during the first pregnancy because of preexisting anti-A and anti-B in the mother. Not so in RhD alloimmunization, unless the mother was previously immunized by transfusion or, rarely, by sharing needles with an RhD-positive intravenous drug abuser.

— ABO alloimmune hemolytic disease usually results in early neonatal jaundice requiring phototherapy, but only rarely requires exchange transfusion. Moderate anemia and mild hepatosplenomegaly may also be evident.

— ABO fetomaternal incompatibility rarely leads to severe disease (hydrops fetalis).

— A somewhat higher degree of jaundice is seen in some ethnic groups (e.g., Americans of African, Southeast Asian, or Hispanic descent). This finding may have to do with variant glucuronyltransferase gene expression.

Hemolytic Disease

• Anemia, jaundice, and hepatosplenomegaly in the newborn are the major findings in alloimmune hemolytic disease.

• The spectrum of severity is wide. In RhD alloimmunization, half the newborn have mild disease and do not need intervention, one-quarter are born at term with moderate anemia and severe jaundice, and one-quarter of fetuses developed hydrops fetalis *in utero* prior to the availability of intrauterine intervention.

• With severe hemolysis, usually in RhD-sensitized mothers, profound anemia can lead to hydrops fetalis (anasarca caused by hypoproteinemia, cardiac failure), and such fetuses can die *in utero*.

• Hydrops fetalis is associated with marked extramedullary hematopoiesis in the liver, spleen, kidneys, and adrenal glands. Portal and umbilical vein hypertension, hypoproteinemia (liver dysfunction), and pleural effusions and ascites.

• With milder cases, hemolysis persists until incompatible red cells or the offending IgG is cleared (half-life of IgG is 3 weeks).

• If severe anemia is present, infant displays pallor, tachypnea, tachycardia; cardiovascular collapse and tissue hypoxia can occur if hemoglobin is less than 40 g/L.

• Most affected infants are not jaundiced at birth because of transplacental transport of bilirubin. Jaundice appears during the first postpartum day or in hours after birth if severe hemolysis is present.

• Generally, with mild disease, the bilirubin peaks at day 4 or 5 postpartum and declines slowly thereafter.

• Premature infants may have higher levels of bilirubin of longer duration because of decreased hepatic glucuronyltransferase activity.

• With marked elevation of the serum bilirubin level, kernicterus may develop from deposition of unconjugated bilirubin in the basal ganglia and brainstem nuclei.

• Acute bilirubin encephalopathy is marked initially by lethargy, poor feeding, and hypotonia. If unaddressed, may progress to high-pitched cries, fever, hypertonia, opisthotonus, and irregular respiration.

• Severe involvement can be fatal or lead to long-lasting severe neurologic defects (e.g., choreoathetoid cerebral palsy, sensorineural hearing loss, gaze abnormalities, cognitive abnormalities).

• Occasionally, severe thrombocytopenia or hypoglycemia also occurs and is a poor prognostic sign.

LABORATORY EVALUATION

Historical Guideposts

- Obstetric history often guides the laboratory approach. Prior history of transfusions, alloimmunization, severity of prior alloimmune hemolytic disease, prior hydrops fetalis (recurs in 90% of immunized mothers), neonatal death, determining paternity in subsequent pregnancies since the fetus is at risk only if the father is positive for the antigen in question, and related factors may guide the timing and extent of fetal surveillance.

Maternal Red Cell Antigen Typing and Titering

- All pregnant patients should have ABO and RhD typing and testing for unusual red cell alloantibodies early in the pregnancy (10th to 16th week) (see **Fig. 27–1**).
- Whether RhD-positive or -negative, the mother should be tested again at 28 weeks gestation.

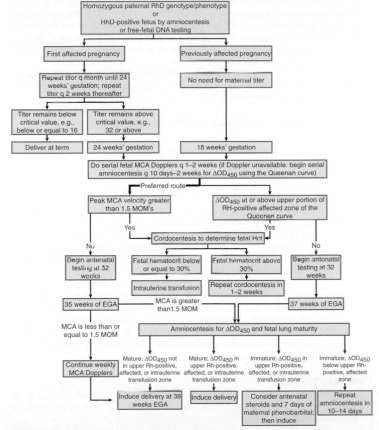

FIGURE 27-1 Algorithm for clinical management of Rh alloimmunized pregnancy. ΔOD, deviation in amniotic fluid optical density; EGA, estimated gestational age; Hct, hematocrit; MCA, middle cerebral artery; MOM, multiples of the median for gestational age; Rh, rhesus. (Reproduced with permission from Moise KJ: *Obstet Gynecol* 112:164, 2008.)

- If alloimmunized, the mother's titer should be determined at 4-week intervals from 20 to 28 weeks and every 2 weeks thereafter.
- Antibody titers are reported as the reciprocal of the highest dilution at which agglutination is observed. A difference of two dilutions is considered significant. If the titer becomes greater than 16 (varies from 8 to 32 in different laboratories), ultrasonography and amniocentesis can be performed to test for the bilirubin level, which predicts disease severity.
- In the United States and the United Kingdom, the anti-D level is compared to an international standard and reported in international units per milliliter (IU/mL). Levels above 4 IU/mL require prompt referral to fetomaternal specialist for monitoring and risk assessment. IU of 4 to 15/mL indicates moderate alloimmune hemolytic disease is likely and over 15 IU/mL implies a severe risk of alloimmune hemolytic disease is likely.
- The significance for antibody titer levels, if anti-D is not involved (e.g., anti-Kell antibodies), has not been determined.

Paternal Zygosity Testing
- In pregnancies in which maternal sensitization occurs or there is a past history of alloimmunization, determining paternal zygosity for all common antigens involved in alloimmune hemolytic disease may determine the risk to the fetus. If the father is homozygous for the antigen in question, one can assume the fetal red cells will carry that antigen. If the father is heterozygous, the fetus will have a 50 percent chance of carrying the antigen.
- If paternal zygosity is unknown, testing fetal red cell blood type early in pregnancy permits appropriate monitoring of the fetus or determines that invasive fetal monitoring is unnecessary.

Fetal DNA, Amniotic Fluid Bilirubin, and Middle Cerebral Artery Doppler Measurements
- Fetal DNA can be obtained from maternal plasma in the first trimester of pregnancy (as early as 5 weeks). Real-time quantitative polymerase chain reaction methods can distinguish maternal from fetal DNA and then amplify fetal exons that include RhD. Accuracy of RhD phenotyping using fetal DNA is 95 percent.
- Amniotic fluid spectrophotometry for bilirubin is an indirect measure of degree of hemolysis. Bilirubin is measured at an optical density (OD) of 450 nm and the elevation in OD_{450} reflects the concentration of bilirubin derived from the fetus. A special nomogram is used to determine the bilirubin for gestational age and four zones in which the bilirubin may fall, providing the probability ranging from no risk of hemolysis to severe hemolytic anemia.
- Because of the risk of amniocentesis, this approach has been replaced by serial noninvasive middle cerebral artery Doppler ultrasound measurements for measuring fetal anemia. Measuring peak blood flow, usually at 1 to 2 week intervals after week 18 until week 35 is a more accurate assessment of anemia than amniotic fluid bilirubin levels. After week 38 of gestation, because of a high false-positive rate with Doppler measurements, amniocentesis and measurement of amniotic fluid OD_{450} is required.

Ultrasonography
- Ultrasonography allows noninvasive description of the fetal condition, an estimate of the need for aggressive management, and a biophysical profile to determine fetal well-being.
- Ultrasonography can be done serially and can detect signs of hydrops such as polyhydramnios, placental enlargement, hepatomegaly, pericardial effusion, ascites, scalp edema, and pleural effusion in roughly that sequence of appearance.

Percutaneous Umbilical Blood Sampling

- More specific information can be obtained by percutaneous umbilical blood sampling (PUBS) (mortality less than 1%) or chorionic villus sampling.
- PUBS (syn. cordocentesis) allows direct measurement of fetal red cell antigens, blood hemoglobin, reticulocyte count, direct antiglobulin test, bilirubin level, blood gases, and lactate levels and can be done at 18 weeks gestation, if severe fetal anemia is indicated by amniotic fluid bilirubin levels or by middle cerebral artery Doppler peak flow measurements.
- PUBS can be done through a 22 gauge spinal needle inserted into the umbilical vein at the site of the cords insertion into the placenta under ultrasonic guidance. If necessary, red cell transfusion can be given by this route.
- Complications of PUBS include umbilical cord bleeding, chorioamnionitis, fetomaternal hemorrhage and maternal red cell sensitization, and fetal death. The latter reported as approximately 3 percent.

Neonatal Assessment

- After delivery, cord blood of the neonate should be sampled for hemoglobin and bilirubin concentrations, the ABO and Rh type, and the direct antiglobulin test. The blood film may show nucleated red blood cells, microspherocytes, and polychromatophilia, if alloimmune hemolytic anemia has occurred. Such testing with a blood group O RhD-positive mother is useful to detect ABO alloimmunization before the newborn is discharged.
- One hour after delivery, blood should be drawn from the mother to evaluate the degree of fetomaternal hemorrhage, so that an appropriate dose of anti-Rh IgG can be given (see "Therapy, Course, and Prognosis" section below).
- Hematopoiesis may be suppressed in the newborn, but marrow recovery is usually complete by 2 months.
- Other diseases can cause hydrops but are distinguished from alloimmune hemolysis by the absence of maternal antibodies.

THERAPY, COURSE, AND PROGNOSIS

Fetus

- PUBS (see "Laboratory Evaluation" section above) can be used to deliver a red cell transfusion to a severely affected fetus, based on level of anemia, development of ascites, or a rising bilirubin concentration. This approach has replaced exchange transfusion in some centers because it is a more rapid procedure.
- Packed red cells are transfused to the fetus to achieve a hematocrit of 40 to 45 percent. The red cells are packed to about 75 percent and a calculation made as to what volume of red cells should be necessary to achieve the desired hematocrit in the fetus.
- Intraperitoneal fetal transfusions may be necessary if (a) intravascular access is not possible because the umbilical vessels are too narrow in early pregnancy or (b) fetal size blocks access to the cord later in pregnancy.
- For a woman alloimmunized in a previous pregnancy, fetal transfusions should begin 10 weeks before the time of the earliest prior fetal death or transfusion, but not before 18 weeks gestation unless hydrops is present. Transfusions are given to keep the hematocrit of the fetus in the 20 to 25 percent range and to prevent hydrops.
- O-negative, antigen-negative for any other identified antibody, CMV-negative, irradiated packed red cells are used, cross-matched against the mother's blood.
- The decision about when to deliver the fetus is complex; if possible, transfusions are given up to 34 weeks with delivery at 36 weeks gestation.
- Other treatments to desensitize the mother (maternal immunomodulation) have included intravenous immunoglobulin with or without plasmapheresis, glucocorticoids, or administration of recombinant D-specific antibodies that do not

destroy RhD-positive red cells. The nonhemolytic anti-D enters the fetal circulation and competes with natural, hemolytic anti-D for red cell sites, ameliorating the hemolysis.

Neonatal

- The aim of treatment is to prevent bilirubin neurotoxicity.
- Indications for immediate exchange transfusion:
  — The cord blood hemoglobin level is significantly less than normal (perhaps a threshold of ≤110 g/L).
  — The bilirubin level is greater than 4.5 mg/dL.
  — Cord blood bilirubin is rising rapidly (> 0.5 mg/dL per hour).
- If the infant is premature or has unstable vital signs, less stringent criteria are used to give an exchange transfusion. After the first exchange, the rate of rise of bilirubin is used to guide to subsequent transfusions.
- Double volume exchanges will remove, perhaps, 85 percent of sensitized red cells and greater than 50 percent of intravascular bilirubin, and also some maternal anti-D antibody.
- In some centers, prior to exchange, intravenous albumin is given to mobilize extravascular, interstitial bilirubin. Removal of sensitized red cells and prevention of bilirubin formation is the most efficient approach.
- ABO-compatible, RhD-negative, irradiated blood is used, cross-matched against the mother.
- Potential newborn complications of exchange transfusion include hypocalcemia, hypoglycemia, thrombocytopenia, dilutional coagulopathy, neutropenia, disseminated intravascular coagulation, umbilical venous or arterial thrombosis, enterocolitis, and infection. Permanent serious sequelae or neonatal death has been reported in a rate as high as 12 percent in sick infants compared to <1 percent in healthy infants over a period of observation from 1981 to 1995.
- Recombinant human erythropoietin, 200 U/kg, subcutaneously, three times per week for 6 weeks, has been used to enhance recovery of the hemoglobin concentration and decrease the need for postnatal exchange transfusions. It is also useful in Kell antigen-mediated alloimmune disease, since in that case, erythroid hypoplasia is an important factor.
- Phototherapy is used prophylactically in any patient with moderate or severe hemolysis or in infants with bilirubin levels rising at >0.5 mg/dL per hour and is the mainstay of treatment for unconjugated hyperbilirubinemia. The object is to prevent bilirubin neurotoxicity.
- Intensive phototherapy (≥30 microWatts/cm^2) in the 430–490 nm band delivered to as much of the infants surface area as possible.
- In full-term infants (at least 38 weeks gestation) with alloimmune hemolytic disease, intensive phototherapy should be instituted if total serum bilirubin is ≥5.0 mg/dL at birth, ≥10 mg/dL at 24 hours after birth, or ≥13 mg/dL 48 to 72 hours after birth.
- Phototherapy is recommended at lower bilirubin levels for preterm or ill infants or infants with a positive direct antiglobulin test, often at serum bilirubin less than 5.0 mg/dL to lessen the need for exchange transfusions.
- Other treatments have been applied. For example, administration of high-dose intravenous immunoglobulin as soon as possible after diagnosis of alloimmune hemolysis is made, decreases the need for phototherapy or exchange transfusion by nonspecific blockade of macrophage Fc receptors and, thereby, a decrease in hemolysis.
- Perinatal survival is greater than 90 percent with intrauterine transfusions in nonhydropic fetuses with severe alloimmune hemolytic disease. The overall survival for hydropic fetuses is approximately 85 percent despite intrauterine transfusion.
- A first trimester screening program increased survival in Kell antigen induced alloimmune hemolytic disease from 61 to 100 percent in the Netherlands.

PREVENTION

- Transfusion of red cells matched for RhD, other Rh antigens, and for Kell antigens should be used in premenopausal women.
- RhIg immunoprophylaxis is standard practice for an RhD-negative mother (Table 27–2).
- Intramuscular doses of 100 to 300 µg of Rh immune globulin to nonsensitized RhD-negative mothers within 72 hours of delivery have decreased Rh immunization by greater than 90 percent.
- If the mother is Rh-D-negative with an RhD-positive newborn, administration of antepartum Rh immunoglobulin at 28 weeks has decreased immunization to about 0.1 percent. Rarely, sensitization may occur before the 28th. This approach is standard practice in the United States.
- The standard dose of 300 µg of RhIg (1500 IU) affords protection for a fetomaternal transfusion of 15 mL of RhD-positive red cells or 30 mL or RhD-positive whole blood.
- Larger fetomaternal transfusions can occur in certain circumstances. The blood of RhD-negative women should be tested 1 hour after delivery of an RhD-positive infant. If abruptio placenta or abdominal trauma occurred, the testing can be done after 20 weeks gestation. Testing uses a rosette test requiring very small amounts of maternal blood, followed by a Kleihauer-Betke test for fetal red cells in the maternal blood. Flow cytometric methods are particular useful for quantification of fetal red cells in the maternal blood.

TABLE 27–2	DOSAGE OF RH IMMUNOGLOBULIN	
Indication	Route of Administration	Dose
Pregnancy termination < 12 weeks' gestation	IM	50 µg
Abortion, miscarriage, ectopic pregnancy, or other pregnancy complications > 12 weeks' gestation	IM, IV	300 µg
Amniocentesis or chorionic villus sampling < 34 weeks' gestation	IM	300 µg[1]
	IV	300 µg
Amniocentesis, chorionic villus sampling, or other manipulation during pregnancy > 34 weeks' gestation	IM	300 µg[2]
Obstetric complication (e.g., abruptio placentae or placenta previa)	IM, IV 300 µg	
Antepartum, 28 weeks' gestation	IM, IV	300 µg
Postpartum[3]	IM	300 µg[4]
	IV	120 µg[4]
Transfusion of Rh-positive blood	IM	20 µg/mL RBCs

[1]To be repeated at 12-week intervals until delivery.
[2]Same dose should be administered if procedure is repeated 21 days after first dose.
[3]Infant should be RhD-positive
[4]Dose should be adjusted for fetal-maternal hemorrhage >15 mL.
Abbreviations: RBC, red blood cell; IM, intramuscular; IV, intravenous.
Reproduced with permission from Hartwell EA: *Am J Clin Pathol* 110:281, 1998.

- In patients found to have large fetomaternal transfusions, larger doses of RhIg can be calculated to try to prevent maternal immunization.
- Although immunoprophylaxis has greatly reduced the incidence of alloimmune hemolytic disease, alloimmune sensitization still occurs in 10.6 per 10,000 births in the United States.
- Because the only adequate prophylaxis is for the D-antigen, other less common antibodies will continue to cause hemolytic disease.

For a more detailed discussion, see Jayashree Ramasethu and Naomi L. C. Luban: Alloimmune Hemolytic Disease of the Fetus and Newborn. Chapter 54, p. 799 in *Williams Hematology*, 8th ed.

CHAPTER 28
Hypersplenism and Hyposplenism

THE SPLEEN

- The white pulp (lymphoid tissue) functions in antigen processing and antibody production.
- The red pulp (monocyte-macrophage system) serves as a filter, retaining defective or effete blood cells and foreign particles.

HYPERSPLENISM (INCREASED SPLENIC FUNCTION)

- Hypersplenism is considered "appropriate" if it is an exaggeration of normal function, as in hereditary spherocytosis or idiopathic thrombocytopenic purpura, or "inappropriate" if the hyperfunction is a result of vascular congestion or infiltrative disease.
- Usually associated with splenomegaly.
- Causes cytopenias with associated compensatory bone marrow hyperplasia.
- Usually corrected by splenectomy, if indicated.
- Table 28–1 lists the causes of hypersplenism; Table 28–2 lists the causes of massive splenomegaly.

Pathophysiology

- The normal spleen carries out filtration and elimination of aged and defective blood cells.
- This same process also removes red cells with hereditary abnormalities of red blood cell membrane and antibody-coated blood cells.
- An enlarged spleen may sequester and destroy normal blood cells, leading to symptomatic cytopenias.
- An expanded splenic (systemic) plasma pool may cause further anemia by dilution.
- Massively increased splenic blood flow, especially if there is decreased hepatic compliance, may cause portal hypertension, further splenomegaly, and associated gastroesophageal varices.

Effect on Platelets

- Normally about one-third of the platelet mass is sequestered in the spleen.
- Up to 90 percent of platelets may be sequestered temporarily by a very enlarged spleen.
- Platelets survive almost normally in the spleen and are available, albeit slowly, when needed.

Effect on Neutrophils

- Large fraction of circulating neutrophil pool may be marginated in an enlarged spleen.
- Neutrophils survive almost normally in the spleen and, like platelets, slowly become available on demand.

Effect on Red Blood Cells

- Red blood cells are metabolically more vulnerable than leukocytes or platelets and may be destroyed prematurely in red pulp.
- Spherocytes may be formed during repeated or prolonged metabolic conditioning in the red pulp.

TABLE 28–1	CLASSIFICATION AND THE MOST COMMON CAUSES OF SPLENOMEGALY AND HYPERSPLENISM

I. Congestive
  A. Right-sided congestive heart failure
  B. Budd-Chiari syndrome (inferior vena cava and hepatic vein thrombosis)
  C. Cirrhosis with portal hypertension
  D. Portal or splenic vein thrombosis
II. Immunologic
  A. Viral infection
    1. Acute HIV infection/chronic infection
    2. Acute mononucleosis
    3. Dengue fever
    4. Rubella (rare except newborns)
    5. Cytomegalovirus infection (rare except newborns)
    6. Herpes simplex (rare except newborns)
  B. Bacterial infection
    1. Subacute bacterial endocarditis
    2. Brucellosis
    3. Tularemia
    4. Melioidosis
    5. Listeriosis
    6. Plague
    7. Secondary syphilis
    8. Relapsing fever
    9. Psittacosis
    10. Ehrlichiosis
    11. Rickettsial diseases (scrub typhus, Rocky Mountain spotted fever, Q fever)
    12. Tuberculosis
    13. Splenic abscess (most common organisms are *Enterobacteriaceae*, *Staphylococcus aureus*, streptococcus group D, and anaerobic organisms as part of mixed flora infections)
  C. Fungal Infection
    1. Blastomycosis
    2. Histoplasmosis
    3. Systemic candidiasis and hepatosplenic candidiasis
  D. Parasitic infection
    1. Malaria
    2. Kala-azar
    3. Leishmaniasis
    4. Schistosomiasis
    5. Babesiosis
    6. Coccidioidomycosis
    7. Paracoccidioidomycosis
    8. Trypanosomiasis (cruzi, brucei)
    9. Toxoplasmosis (rare except newborns)
    10. Echinococcosis
    11. Cysticercosis
    12. Visceral larva migrans (*Toxocara* infection)
  E. Inflammatory/autoimmune
    1. Systemic lupus erythematosus (SLE)
    2. Felty syndrome
    3. Juvenile rheumatoid arthritis
    4. Autoimmune lymphoproliferative syndrome (ALP syndrome)
    5. Hemophagocytic syndrome
    6. Common variable immunodeficiency
    7. Anti-D immunoglobulin administration

III. Associated with hemolysis
   A. Thalassemia major and intermedia
   B. Pyruvate kinase deficiency
   C. Hereditary spherocytosis
   D. Autoimmune hemolytic anemia (rare)
   E. Sickle cell disease, more common in early childhood (splenic sequestration), hemoglobin C disease, and some other hemoglobinopathies

IV. Infiltrative

   A. Nonmalignant
      1. Splenic hematoma (splenic cysts are usually a late complication of a hematoma)
      2. Littoral cell angioma
      3. Disorders of sphingolipid metabolism
         a. Gaucher disease
         b. Niemann-Pick disease
      4. Cystinosis
      5. Amyloidosis (light-chain amyloid and amyloid A protein)
      6. Multicentric Castleman disease
      7. Mastocytosis
      8. Hypereosinophilic syndrome
      9. Sarcoidosis
   B. Extramedullary hematopoiesis
      1. Primary myelofibrosis
      2. Osteopetrosis (childhood)
      3. Thalassemia major
   C. Malignant
      1. Hematologic
         a. Chronic lymphocytic leukemia (especially prolymphocytic variant)
         b. Chronic myeloid leukemia
         c. Polycythemia vera
         d. Hairy cell leukemia
         e. Heavy chain disease
         f. Hepatosplenic lymphoma
         g. Acute leukemia (acute lymphoblastic leukemia/acute myeloid leukemia)
         h. Hodgkin and other lymphomas
      2. Nonhematologic
         a. Metastatic carcinoma (rare)
         b. Neuroblastoma
         c. Wilms tumor
         d. Leiomyosarcoma
         e. Fibrosarcoma
         f. Malignant fibrous histiocytoma
         g. Kaposi sarcoma
         h. Hemangiosarcoma
         i. Lymphangiosarcoma
         j. Hemangioendothelial sarcoma

V. Iatrogenic

   A. Granulocyte colony-stimulating factor administration
   B. Erythropoietin administration

Source: *Williams Hematology*, 8th ed, Chap. 55, Table 55–1, p. 817.

TABLE 28–2	CAUSES OF MASSIVE SPLENOMEGALY

I. Myeloproliferative disorders
   A. Primary myelofibrosis
   B. Chronic myeloid leukemia
II. Lymphomas
   A. Hairy cell leukemia
   B. Chronic lymphocytic leukemia (especially prolymphocytic variant)
III. Infectious
   A. Malaria
   B. Leishmaniasis (kala azar)
IV. Extramedullary hematopoiesis
   A. Thalassemia major
V. Infiltrative
   A. Gaucher disease

Source: *Williams Hematology*, 8th ed, Chap. 55, Table 55–2, p. 818.

Symptoms of Splenomegaly

- Splenomegaly may be asymptomatic.
- Very rapid enlargement of the spleen may cause some pain due to strain on the splenic capsule.
- Greatly enlarged spleens may cause abdominal discomfort, trouble sleeping on the left side, and early satiety.
- Splenic infarction may cause pleuritic-like left upper quadrant or shoulder pain, with or without a friction rub.
- In young patients with sickle cell anemia, the spleen may become acutely enlarged and painful due to obstruction of the splenic outflow, with sudden aggravation of anemia (sequestration crisis).

Estimation of Splenic Size

- A normal size spleen may be palpable in young and thin patients with low diaphragms. Otherwise, a palpable spleen should be considered to be enlarged.
- Splenic size can be assessed with abdominal ultrasound (Fig. 28–1) or CT examination (Fig. 28–2).
- Cysts, tumors, or infarcts of the spleen may be identified by radionuclide colloid scanning, abdominal computed tomography, or magnetic resonance imaging.

Hematologic Features of Splenomegaly

- The blood concentration of erythrocytes, leukocytes, or platelets is reduced in the blood, with corresponding hyperplasia in the marrow.
- Cellular morphology is usually normal, but spherocytes may be present.

Splenectomy

- May be required for severe, dangerous cytopenias and can lead to dramatic improvement of blood counts, sometimes to normal, in patients with hypersplenism.
- May alleviate portal hypertension but is not the preferred primary treatment.
- Will alleviate painful splenic infarcts.
- After splenectomy there may be a rapid, but temporary, increase in the platelet count, which can lead to thromboembolic complications especially in the elderly or bedridden patients.

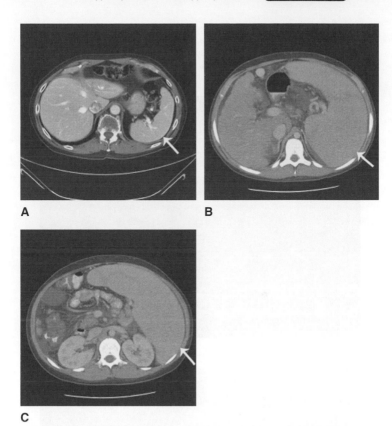

FIGURE 28-1 A three-way composite of abdominal computed tomography. **A.** Normal spleen size. **B.** Enlarged spleen. **C.** Massively enlarged spleen at the level of mid-kidney. Normally the spleen would either not be visualized or only a small lower pole would be evident at the latter level. (*White arrow* in the three images mark edge of splenic silhouette.) (Reproduced with permission from Deborah Rubens, MD, The University of Rochester Medical Center.)

- Chronic changes in the blood after splenectomy are listed below under "Hyposplenism, Laboratory Findings."
- Removes a protective filter bed and renders the patient vulnerable to bacteremia, especially due to encapsulated gram-positive organisms. Therefore, vaccination against such organisms (e.g., *Streptococcus pneumoniae*, *Haemophilus influenzae*) should precede elective splenectomy by 2 to 3 weeks.
- Diminishes resistance to preexisting parasitic disease (malaria, bartonellosis, babesiosis) and transforms dormant infestation into active disease.
- Partial splenectomy has been used in special circumstances to decrease hypersplenism and prevent hyposplenism.
- The frequency of splenectomy for some disorders has decreased in recent years because of improved alternative therapies or a higher threshold for recommending the procedure.
- Splenectomy is still recommended under specific conditions for some disorders, as discussed in specific chapters (e.g., Chap. 14, Hereditary Spherocytosis,

Elliptocytosis, and Related Disorders; Chap. 24, Hemolytic Anemia Resulting from Warm-Reacting Antibodies; Chap. 48, Primary Myelofibrosis, and Chap. 74, Thrombocytopenia). However, as a result of higher risks of overwhelming infection, splenectomy should be postponed, if at all possible, until after age 5.

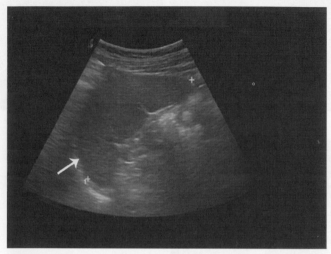

A

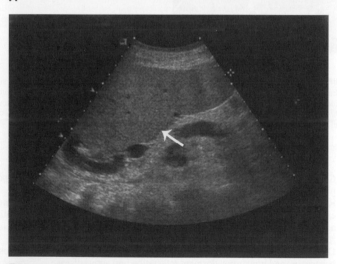

B

FIGURE 28–2 A two-way composite of ultrasonographic examination for spleen size. Patient's head is to the left side of the longitudinal image. **A.** Image of echo indicating normal spleen size with cranial to caudal longitudinal dimension of 10.3 cm. **B.** Image of echo indicating enlarged spleen with cranial to caudal longitudinal dimension of 16.2 cm. (*White arrows* mark edge of splenic silhouette.) The normal spleen is usually less than 13 cm in length, but the examiner has to consider other dimensions in assessing spleen size (volume). (Reproduced with permission from Deborah Rubens, MD, The University of Rochester Medical Center.)

HYPOSPLENISM (DECREASED SPLENIC FUNCTION)

- Splenic function may be reduced by disease or surgical removal.
- Hyposplenism may or may not be associated with reduced splenic size.
- Impaired filtering causes mild thrombocytosis and increased risk of severe bloodstream infections.
- Causes of hyposplenism are listed in Table 28–3.

Infectious Complications

- Overwhelming sepsis is often fatal.
- Usually caused by encapsulated bacteria, such as pneumococcus or *H. influenzae*.
- Risk greatest in very young and splenectomy usually contraindicated before age 4 years.
- Healthy adults with splenectomy because of accidental rupture of normal spleen are still at some increased risk.

Laboratory Findings

- Slight to moderate increase in leukocyte and platelet counts.
- Target cells, acanthocytes, other misshapen erythrocytes.
- Howell-Jolly bodies (nuclear fragment remnants) in 1 red cell per 100 to 1000.

TABLE 28–3	CONDITIONS ASSOCIATED WITH HYPOSPLENISM

Miscellaneous
  Surgical splenectomy
  Splenic irradiation
  Sickle hemoglobinopathies
  Congenital asplenia
  Thrombosis of splenic artery or vein
  Normal infants

Gastrointestinal and hepatic diseases
  Celiac disease
  Dermatitis herpetiformis
  Inflammatory bowel disease
  Cirrhosis

Autoimmune disorders
  Systemic lupus erythematosus
  Rheumatoid arthritis
  Vasculitis
  Glomerulonephritis
  Hashimoto thyroiditis
  Sarcoidosis

Hematologic and neoplastic disorders
  Graft-versus-host disease
  Chronic lymphocytic leukemia
  Non-Hodgkin lymphoma
  Hodgkin lymphoma
  Amyloidosis
  Advanced breast cancer
  Hemangiosarcoma

Sepsis/infectious diseases
  Malaria
  Disseminated meningococcemia

Source: *Williams Hematology*, 8th ed, Chap. 55, Table 55–3, p. 819.

- Pitted erythrocytes (wet preparation, using direct interference-contrast microscopy).
- Increased numbers of Heinz bodies on supravital examination.
- Increased numbers of nucleated red cells in patients splenectomized for various hemolytic disorders.
- ^{99m}Tc sulfur colloid uptake is a reliable measure of the capacity of the spleen to clear particulates from the blood.

Treatment of Hyposplenic or Post-splenectomy Patient

- Immunize with polyvalent pneumococcal vaccine before splenectomy.
- Vaccinate children against *H. influenzae*.
- Prophylactic penicillin is usually given to asplenic children.
- All febrile infections should be considered serious. Administer an appropriate antibiotic regimen immediately upon onset of symptoms.
- Treat with broad-spectrum antibiotics at the time of all dental work (especially extractions).

For a more detailed discussion, see Jaime Caro and Ubaldo Martinez Outschoorn: Hypersplenism and Hyposplenism. Chap. 55, p. 815 in *Williams Hematology*, 8th ed.

CHAPTER 29
Polyclonal Polycythemias (Primary and Secondary)

- Polycythemia (also known as erythrocytosis) is characterized by an increased red cell blood volume. Polycythemias can be primary or secondary and either inherited or acquired.
- Classification of polycythemic disorders appears in Table 2–2 in Chap. 2.
- Primary polycythemias are caused by somatic or germline mutations causing changes within hematopoietic stem cells or erythroid progenitors causing an augmented response to erythropoietin.
- Secondary polycythemias are caused by either an appropriate or inappropriate increase in the red cell mass as a result of augmented levels of erythropoietin.

PRIMARY POLYCYTHEMIA

- The most common primary polycythemia, polycythemia vera, is a clonal acquired multipotential hematopoietic progenitor cell disorder discussed in Chap. 43.

Primary Familial and Congenital Polycythemia
- Autosomal dominant disorder, with normal leukocytes and platelets.
- Many affected persons are misdiagnosed as having polycythemia vera.
- Always low erythropoietin level (see Fig. 29–1).
- Erythroid progenitors in *in vitro* cultures are hypersensitive to erythropoietin but do not grow independent of erythropoietin.
- Caused by a truncation of erythropoietin receptor and deletion of negative regulatory cytoplasmic domain.
- Affected individuals may have an increased risk of cardiovascular complications regardless of control of elevated hematocrit by phlebotomies.

SECONDARY POLYCYTHEMIA (ERYTHROCYTOSIS)

- A group of disorders with increased red cell mass (absolute polycythemia) because of stimulation of red cell production by increased erythropoietin production. The polycythemia is considered:
  — *Appropriate* if there is tissue hypoxia and the increased red cell mass minimizes the hypoxia.
  — *Inappropriate* if tissue hypoxia is absent and the polycythemia serves no useful purpose.

Appropriate Secondary Polycythemias
High-Altitude Acclimatization
- There is a great variability in an individuals' susceptibility to acute and chronic mountain sickness complications. Some populations such as Tibetans, Aymaras and Quechua natives of High Andes, and Ethiopian dwellers of high mountains have a genetically determined resistance to these complications.
- Acute mountain sickness:
  — Caused by cerebral hypoxia and may be life-threatening. Polycythemia does not occur.

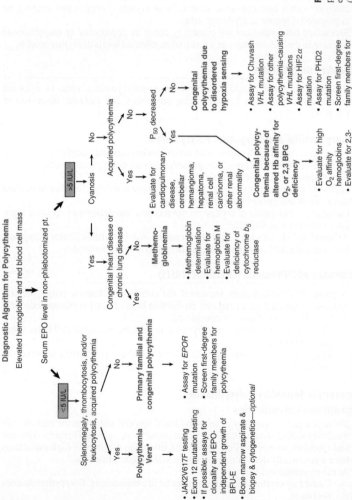

FIGURE 29-1 Diagnostic algorithm for polycythemia based on erythropoietin level. BFU–E, burst-forming unit–erythroid. (Source: *Williams Hematology*; 8th ed, Fig. 56–6, p. 832.)

Diagnostic Algorithm for Polycythemia

Elevated hemoglobin and red blood cell mass

Serum EPO level in non-phlebotomized pt.

<5 IU/L

Splenomegaly, thrombocytosis, and/or leukocytosis, acquired polycythemia

Yes → **Polycythemia Vera***
- JAK2V617F testing
- Exon 12 mutation testing
- If possible: assays for clonality and EPO-independent growth of BFU-E
- Bone marrow aspirate & biopsy & cytogenetics—*optional*

No → **Primary familial and congenital polycythemia**
- Assay for *EPOR* mutation
- Screen first-degree family members for polycythemia

>5 IU/L

Cyanosis

Yes → Congenital heart disease or chronic lung disease

  Yes

  No → **Methemoglobinemia**
- Methemoglobin determination
- Evaluate for hemoglobin M
- Evaluate for deficiency of cytochrome b_5 reductase

No → Acquired polycythemia

Yes → Evaluate for cardiopulmonary disease, cerebellar hemangioma, hepatoma, renal cell carcinoma, or other renal abnormality

No → P_{50} decreased

Yes → **Congenital polycythemia because of altered Hb affinity for O_2 or 2,3 BPG deficiency**
- Evaluate for high O_2 affinity hemoglobins
- Evaluate for 2,3-BPG deficiency

No → **Congenital polycythemia due to disordered hypoxia sensing**
- Assay for Chuvash *VHL* mutation
- Assay for other polycythemia-causing *VHL* mutations
- Assay for HIF2α mutation
- Assay for PHD2 mutation
- Screen first-degree family members for polycythemia

*Some patients may have a normal EPO level.

- Persons may have headaches, insomnia, palpitations, weakness, nausea, vomiting, and mental dullness, and may develop pulmonary and cerebral edema.
- Treatment is with oxygen, dexamethasone, and acetazolamide and/or rapid return to lower altitude.
- Chronic mountain sickness:
  - Occurs after prolonged exposure to high altitudes; there appears to be a genetic predisposition.
  - Characterized by marked polycythemia, cyanosis, plethora, pulmonary hypertension, clubbing of the fingers, and signs of right heart failure.
  - Treatment with the angiotensin-converting enzyme inhibitor enalapril has been reported to be effective.
  - A return to a normal state develops slowly.

Pulmonary Disease
- Associated with cyanosis, clubbing, and arterial oxygen desaturation.
- In chronic obstructive pulmonary disease, chronic infection and inflammation may blunt erythropoietin expression and red cell production.
- Venesection is controversial; many consider it ill-advised, but some recommend it to maintain the hematocrit at no more than 55 percent, presumably to optimize oxygen carrying capacity and blood flow characteristics.

Alveolar Hypoventilation
- Central: May be a result of cerebral vascular accident, parkinsonism, encephalitis, or barbiturate intoxication.
- Peripheral: May be a result of myotonic dystrophy, poliomyelitis, spondylitis, or extreme obesity.

Cardiovascular (Eisenmenger syndrome)
- In patients with congenital right-to-left intracardiac shunts, arterial Po_2 decreases significantly, erythropoietin secretion increases, and the hematocrit may reach 75 to 85 percent.
- Reduction of the hematocrit by phlebotomy may not be beneficial, and such therapy is controversial.
- Treatment with phlebotomy is indicated for cerebral symptoms (headaches, difficulty to concentrate); however if prompt improvement after phlebotomies does not ensue, phlebotomies are probably of no benefit.
- Dehydration should be avoided to prevent further increase in hematocrit.
- Other right-to-left shunts can result in secondary polycythemia in hepatic cirrhosis (pulmonary arteriovenous or portopulmonary venous shunts), hereditary hemorrhagic telangiectasia, and idiopathic pulmonary arteriovenous aneurysms.

Acquired High-Affinity Hemoglobinopathy
- May be a result of elevated blood carboxyhemoglobin (smoking).

Tissue Hypoxia (Histotoxic Anoxia)
- Cobalt chloride treatment inhibits oxidative metabolism and leads to an increased hematocrit. Particularly high hematocrits are recorded in cobalt miners in high Andes Peruvian mines (as high as 90).

Inappropriate Secondary Acquired Polycythemias
Post-Renal Transplantation Erythrocytosis
- Defined as a persistent elevation of the hematocrit over 51 percent.
- Found in approximately 5 to 10 percent of renal allograft recipients; incidence may be decreasing because of widespread use of angiotensin-converting enzyme inhibitors.

- Develops within 8 to 24 months after transplantation, despite good function of the allograft.
- Therapy with either angiotensin-converting enzyme inhibitor enalapril or with angiotensin II receptor type 1 blocker, losartan.

Renal Cysts and Hydronephrosis

- Erythropoietin can be demonstrated in cyst fluid or is due to cyst-induced mechanical renal ischemia downstream of the cyst.

Renal Tumors

- One to 3 percent of patients with hypernephroma have erythrocytosis, probably as a consequence of excess erythropoietin formed by the tumor.
- Remission of polycythemia occurs after tumor removal.
- Reappearance of polycythemia heralds recurrence.
- May be associated with von Hippel-Lindau (*VHL*) gene mutation.

Cerebellar Hemangiomas

- About 15 percent of patients have erythrocytosis, and erythropoietin can be demonstrated in cyst fluid and stromal cells.
- May be associated with *VHL* gene mutations.

Other Tumors

- Uterine myoma, usually huge. Removal of the myoma routinely followed by return to normal hemoglobin concentration.
- Hepatoma can cause erythrocytosis, probably because of erythropoietin production by the neoplastic cells.

Endocrine Disorders

- Pheochromocytoma, aldosterone-producing adenomas, Bartter syndrome, or dermoid cyst of ovary may be associated with increased erythropoietin levels and erythrocytosis, which respond to removal of the tumor.
- Pheochromocytoma may be associated with *VHL* gene mutations.
- Cushing syndrome: Hydrocortisone and other glucocorticoids may cause general marrow stimulation and mild polycythemia.

Androgen Usage

- Androgens of the 5α-H configuration stimulate erythropoietin production and result in erythrocytosis.
- Androgens of the 5α-H configuration also enhance differentiation of stem cells.

Neonatal Erythrocytosis

- Normal physiologic response to intrauterine hypoxia and high oxygen-affinity fetal hemoglobin.
- May be excessive in infants of diabetic mothers.
- Late cord clamping may be contributory.
- Partial exchange transfusion sometimes performed if the hematocrit is above 65 percent at birth.

Autotransfusion (Blood Doping)

- Autotransfusion of stored red cells prior to competition improves performance in cross-country skiers and long-distance runners but at the risk of life-threatening hyperviscosity when associated with fluid losses from strenuous activity.
- Should be suspected when an elevated hematocrit is associated with very low level of erythropoietin in an athlete.

- Injection of commercial erythropoietin preparations will achieve the same effect as autotransfusion. This approach, in addition to being unethical to improve athletic performance, bears the risk of overdose and life-threatening hyperviscosity under periods of athletic stress and dehydration.

Congenital Secondary Polycythemias

Hereditary High-Affinity Hemoglobins

- Autosomal dominant inheritance.
- Only about fifty percent of the abnormal hemoglobins are demonstrable by hemoglobin electrophoresis.
- The initial and sensitive test is determination of hemoglobin-oxygen affinity (estimated by measuring the p50).
- Increased hemoglobin-oxygen affinity (decreased p50) results in tissue hypoxia, erythropoietin may be high or normal.
- Phlebotomies are generally ill advised unless severe symptoms of hyperviscosity.
- For more details, see Chap. 19.

2,3-Biphosphoglycerate Deficiency

- Results in an increased oxygen affinity of hemoglobin (decreased p50).
- Caused by bisphosphoglyceromutase deficiency (see Chaps. 15 and 19).

Congenital Methemobinemias

- Mild polycythemia occurs in patients with methemoglobinemia caused by recessively inherited cytochrome b_5 reductase deficiency (see Chap. 15) or globin mutations causing dominantly inherited methemoglobinemia (see Chap. 19).

Congenital Disorders of Hypoxia Sensing

Chuvash Polycythemia

- Only known endemic congenital polycythemia, endemic in Chuvash autonomous region of Russia, Italian island of Ischia; sporadic worldwide.
- Autosomal recessive disorder.
- Caused by mutation in the von Hippel-Lindau (*VHL*) gene (*VHL* C598T) that upregulates HIF transcription factors that increase transcription of many genes including erythropoietin (see *Williams Hematology,* 8th ed, Chap. 56, p. 823.)
- Erythropoietin levels are normal or increased.
- Erythroid progenitors in *in vitro* cultures are hypersensitive to erythropoietin, thus shares features of both primary and secondary polycythemia.
- Strokes and other thrombotic vascular complications and pulmonary hypertension lead to early mortality are not affected by phlebotomies.

Congenital Polycythemia from Other VHL Gene Mutations

- Most patients are compound heterozygotes for Chuvash *VHL* C598T and other VHL gene mutations.
- Rare patients have only a single VHL mutation.

Proline Hydroxylase Deficiency

- Rare disorder causing mild or borderline polycythemia associated with upregulated HIF transcription factors.
- Because of its rarity, little is known about its clinical manifestations.

HIF-2α Gain-of-Function Mutations

- Rare disorder due to increased activity of HIF-2 that increases transcription of many genes including erythropoietin.
- Because of its rarity, little is known about its clinical manifestations.

Apparent Polycythemia (Relative or Spurious Polycythemia)

- Characterized by an increased hematocrit, normal red cell mass, and low plasma volume.
- In the past, referred to as Gaisbock syndrome; pseudo-polycythemia; or stress, spurious, and smokers' polycythemia.
- Associated with obesity, hypertension, use of diuretics, and smoking.
- Differential diagnosis includes severe dehydration.
- Treatment should be directed toward any underlying condition, if present, such as obesity (weight reduction) or cigarette smoking (cessation of smoking).

For a more detailed discussion, see Josef T. Prchal: Primary and Secondary Polycythemias (Erythrocytosis). Chap. 56, p. 823 in *Williams Hematology*, 8th ed.

CHAPTER 30
The Porphyrias

- The porphyrias are inherited or acquired disorders in which the activity of an enzyme in the heme biosynthetic pathway is altered. Metabolic intermediates are produced in excess, initially either in the marrow or the liver, and result in neurologic or photocutaneous symptoms and signs.

CLASSIFICATION

- See Table 30–1.
- The two organs most active in heme biosynthesis are the marrow and the liver. Photosensitivity (indicated below with the following symbols as either **blistering*** or **nonblistering**†) and/or (indicated below with the following symbol as) **neurovisceral symptoms**‡ may be part of the porphyria phenotype. Therefore, porphyrias are classified as erythropoietic or hepatic and as cutaneous or acute.

Erythropoietic Porphyrias

- Principal site of initial accumulation of pathway intermediates is the erythroblast.
- Congenital erythropoietic porphyria (CEP).*
- Erythropoietic protoporphyria (EPP).†

Hepatic Porphyrias

- Principal site of initial accumulation of pathway intermediates is the liver.
- δ-Aminolevulinic acid dehydratase porphyria (ADP).‡
- Acute intermittent porphyria (AIP).‡
- Hereditary coproporphyria (HCP).*‡
- Variegate porphyria (VP).*‡
- Porphyria cutanea tarda (PCT).*
- Hepatoerythropoietic porphyria (HEP).*

SPECIFIC DISORDERS

General Considerations

- Synthesis of heme is catalyzed by a series of eight enzymes. Altered activity of each of these enzymes is associated with a specific form of porphyria (see Fig. 30–1).
- Diagnostic biochemical findings in the individual porphyrias are summarized in Table 30–2.

ERYTHROPOIETIC PORPHYRIAS

Congenital Erythropoietic Porphyria
Pathogenesis

- Rare (~200 cases reported), autosomal recessive disorder, caused by an almost complete (<5 percent of normal) deficiency of uroporphyrinogen III synthase activity.

Clinical Findings

- Cutaneous photosensitivity appears early in life. Subepidermal bullous lesions develop and progress to crusted erosions that heal with scarring, pigmentary changes, hypertrichosis, and alopecia. Bacterial infections contribute to mutilation of facial features and fingers.

TABLE 30–1 HUMAN PORPHYRIAS: SPECIFIC ENZYMES AFFECTED BY MUTATIONS, MODES OF INHERITANCE, CLASSIFICATION, AND MAJOR CLINICAL FEATURES OF EACH OF THE HUMAN PORPHYRIAS

Porphyria[a]	Affected Enzyme	Known Mutations	Inheritance	Classification	Principal Clinical Features
Erythropoietic protoporphyria (EPP)—X-linked form	δ-Aminolevulinic acid (ALA) synthase erythroid-specific form (ALAS2)	2 (gain of function)	Sex-linked recessive	Erythropoietic	Nonblistering photosensitivity
δ-Aminolevulinic acid dehydratase porphyria (ADP)	ALA dehydratase (ALAD)	11	Autosomal recessive	Hepatic[b]	Neurovisceral
Acute intermittent porphyria (AIP)	PBG deaminase (PBGD)	273	Autosomal dominant	Hepatic	Neurovisceral
Congenital erythropoietic porphyria (CEP)	Uroporphyrinogen III synthase (UROS)	36	Autosomal recessive	Erythropoietic	Neurovisceral
Porphyria cutanea tarda (PCT)	Uroporphyrinogen decarboxylase (UROD)	70 (includes HEP)	Autosomal dominant[c]	Hepatic	Blistering photosensitivity
Hepatoerythropoietic porphyria (HEP)	UROD	—	Autosomal recessive	Hepatic[b]	Blistering photosensitivity
Hereditary coproporphyria (HCP)	Coproporphyrinogen oxidase (CPO)	42	Autosomal dominant	Hepatic	Neurovisceral; blistering photosensitivity (uncommon)
Variegate porphyria (VP)	Protoporphyrinogen oxidase (PPO)	130	Autosomal dominant	Hepatic	Neurovisceral; blistering photosensitivity (common)
EPP—classic form	Ferrochelatase (FECH)	90	Autosomal dominant[d]	Erythropoietic	Nonblistering photosensitivity

[a]Porphyrias are listed in the order of the affected enzyme in the heme biosynthetic pathway.

[b]These porphyrias also have erythropoietic features, including increases in erythrocyte zinc protoporphyrin.

[c]Heterozygous UROD mutations are present in "familial" (type 2) but not in the more common "sporadic" (type 1) PCT. In all cases, an acquired inhibition of hepatic UROD reduces the enzyme activity to less than ~20% of normal.

[d]Because both alleles are abnormal in affected individuals (in most cases with a severe FECH mutation trans to a hypomorphic FECH allele), EPP is now regarded as recessive at the molecular level.

Source: *Williams Hematology*, 8th ed, Chap. 57, Table 57–1, p. 840.

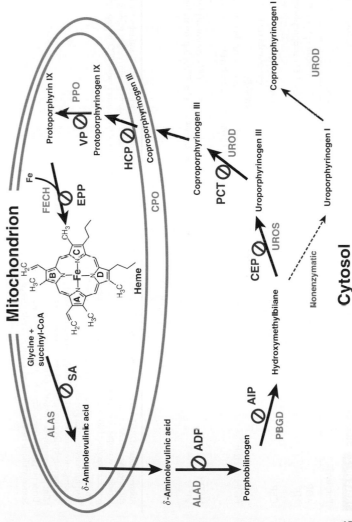

FIGURE 30-1 Enzymes and intermediates in the heme biosynthetic pathway and the type of porphyria associated with a deficiency of each enzyme (indicated by ⊘). Gain of function mutation of the erythroid form of ALA synthase is not shown. Abbreviations: ADP, ALA dehydratase porphyria; AIP, acute intermittent porphyria; ALA, δ-aminolevulinic acid; ALAD, δ-aminolevulinic acid dehydratase; ALAS, δ-aminolevulinic acid synthase; CEP, congenital erythropoietic porphyria; CPO, coproporphyrinogen oxidase; EPP, erythropoietic protoporphyria; FECH, -ferochelatase HCP, hereditary coproporphyria; PBG, porphobilinogen; PBGD, porphobilinogen deaminase; PCT, porphyria cutanea tarda; PPO, protoporphyrinogen oxidase; SA, sideroblastic anemia; UROD, uroporphyrinogen decarboxylase; UROS, uroporphyrinogen III synthase; VP, variegate porphyria. (Source: *Williams Hematology*, 8th ed, Chap. 57, Fig. 57–1, p. 841.)

TABLE 30–2   BIOCHEMICAL FINDINGS INCLUDING MAJOR INCREASES IN PORPHYRINS AND PORPHYRIN PRECURSORS IN THE HUMAN PORPHYRIAS[a]

Porphyria	Erythrocytes	Plasma	Urine	Stool
ADP	Zinc protoporphyrin	ALA[b]	ALA, coproporphyrin III	[b]
AIP	Decreased PBGD activity (most cases)[b]	ALA, PBG[b] (~620 nm)[c]	ALA, PBG, uroporphyrin	[b]
CEP	Uroporphyrin I; coproporphyrin I	Uroporphyrin I, coproporphyrin I (~620 nm)[c]	Uroporphyrin I; coproporphyrin I	Coproporphyrin I
PCT and HEP	Zinc protoporphyrin (in HEP)	Uroporphyrin, heptacarboxyl porphyrin (~620 nm)[c]	Uroporphyrin, heptacarboxyl porphyrin	Heptacarboxyl porphyrin, isocoproporphyrins
HCP	[b]	[d] (~620 nm)[c]	ALA, PBG, coproporphyrin III	Coproporphyrin III
VP	[b]	Protoporphyrin (~628 nm)[c]	ALA, PBG, coproporphyrin III	Coproporphyrin III, protoporphyrin
EPP	Free protoporphyrin	Protoporphyrin[e] (~634 nm)[c]	[f]	Protoporphyrin[b]

Abbreviations: ADP, ALA dehydratase porphyria; AIP, acute intermittent porphyria; ALA, δ-aminolevulinic acid; ALAD, δ-aminolevulinic acid dehydratase; HEP, Hepatoerythropoietic porphyria. ALAS, δ-aminolevulinic acid synthase; CEP, congenital erythropoietic porphyria; CPO, coproporphyrinogen oxidase; EPP, erythropoietic protoporphyria; HCP, hereditary coproporphyria; PBG, porphobilinogen; PBGD, porphobilinogen deaminase; PCT, porphyria cutanea tarda; PPO, protoporphyrinogen oxidase; UROD, uroporphyrinogen decarboxylase; UROS, uroporphyrinogen III synthase; VP, variegate porphyria.

[a]Porphyrias are listed in the order of the affected enzyme in the heme biosynthetic pathway.

[b]Porphyrin levels normal or slightly increased.

[c]Fluorescence emission peak of diluted plasma at neutral pH.

[d]Plasma porphyrins usually normal, but increased when blistering skin lesions develop.

[e]Zinc protoporphyrin ≤5% of total in classic EPP, but 15–50% in variant form.

[f]Urine porphyrins (especially coproporphyrin) increase only with hepatopathy.

Source: *Williams Hematology*, 8th ed, Chap. 57, Table 57–2, p. 841.

- Red teeth with red fluorescence under UV light is characteristic.
- Hemolytic anemia is common, with splenomegaly and compensatory marrow expansion.
- Late onset cases may be associated with myeloproliferative or myelodysplastic disorders.

Diagnosis and Laboratory Findings
- *In utero*, dark brown porphyrin-rich amniotic fluid is characteristic.
- In newborns, pink or dark brown staining of diapers may suggest the diagnosis.
- Erythrocyte and urinary porphyrins (predominantly uroporphyrin and coproporphyrin, isomer I), and fecal porphyrins (predominantly coproporphyrin I) are markedly increased.
- Mutations should be confirmed by DNA studies in all cases.

Treatment
- Avoid sunlight and skin trauma and treat infections promptly. Topical sunscreens that block UVA and visible light of some value.
- Hematopoietic stem cell transplantation in early childhood is most effective.
- Suppression of marrow with hypertransfusion or hydroxyurea, splenectomy and oral charcoal have been of limited value.

Erythropoietic Protoporphyria
Pathogenesis
- The third most common porphyria and the most common in children, caused either by loss of function mutations of ferrochelatase (FECH) or gain of function mutations of the erythroid form of ALAS (ALAS2). At the molecular level, EPP is an autosomal recessive disorder (with both FECH alleles affected by loss-of-function mutations) or sex-linked (gain of function mutation of one ALAS2 allele).
- In the classic form, functional deficiency in the enzyme to less than ~20 percent of normal results from a severe FECH mutation trans to a common hypomorphic FECH allele.
- In the X-linked form, a truncated ALAS2 allele leads to gain of function, resulting in significantly increased production of δ-ALA, which accumulates as protoporphyrin IX in erythroblasts.

Clinical Features
- Childhood onset of nonblistering cutaneous photosensitivity is characteristic.
- Symptoms include burning pain, itching, redness and swelling of the skin soon after light exposure (Table 30–3).
- Gallstones containing protoporphyrin and presenting at an early age are common.
- No neurovisceral symptoms.

TABLE 30–3	COMMON CLINICAL FEATURES OF ERYTHROPOIETIC PROTOPORPHYRIA
Symptoms and Signs	Incidence (% of Total)
Burning	97
Edema	94
Itching	88
Erythema	69
Scarring	19
Vesicles	3
Anemia	27
Cholelithiasis	12
Abnormal liver function results	4

Source: *Williams Hematology,* 8th ed, Chap. 57, Table 57–3, p. 848.

- May have impaired iron absorption and mild microcytic anemia.
- Less than 5 percent of cases may develop cholestatic liver disease (protoporphyric hepatopathy) which may present with abdominal pain and jaundice and progress rapidly.
- Late onset cases may be associated with myeloproliferative or myelodysplastic disorders.

Diagnosis and Laboratory Findings

- Diagnosis is more delayed than in any other type of porphyria in part because symptoms out of proportion to physical findings, and urine porphyrins are normal.
- Excess concentrations of protoporphyrin in red cells, plasma, bile, and feces.
- Diagnosis established by finding marked increase in total erythrocyte protoporphyrin with a predominance for metal-free protoporphyrin rather than zinc protoporphyrin.

Treatment

- Avoidance of sun exposure, use of topical sunscreens that block UVA and visible light, and oral β-carotene (120 to 180 mg/d).
- Protoporphyric hepatopathy is treated with erythrocyte transfusions, plasmapheresis, hemin, cholestyramine, ursodeoxycholic acid and vitamin E, and liver transplantation is often necessary.

HEPATIC PORPHYRIAS

ALA Dehydratase Porphyria

Pathogenesis

- Autosomal recessive disorder due to a severe deficiency of ALA dehydratase.

Clinical Findings

- The rarest form of porphyria (6 documented cases).
- Patients have neurovisceral symptoms similar to those of AIP (see below).

Laboratory Findings

- Urine ALA and coproporphyrin III excretion is markedly increased; porphobilinogen (PBG) excretion is normal or only slightly increased. Erythrocyte zinc protoporphyrin is markedly increased.
- Red cell ALA dehydratase activity of less than 5 percent of normal.
- Must distinguish from other causes of ALA dehydratase deficiency, such as lead poisoning (measure blood lead) and hereditary tyrosinemia I (measure succinylacetone in urine), and identify the causative ALAD mutations.

Treatment

- The same approach as for AIP; hemin appears to be most effective.

Acute Intermittent Porphyria

Pathogenesis

- Autosomal dominant disorder caused by partial deficiency of porphobilinogen deaminase.

Clinical Findings

- Symptoms usually occur as neuropathic acute attacks lasting for days or if not treated, for weeks.
- Abdominal pain is the most common and often the initial symptom.
- Extremity pain, nausea, vomiting, constipation or diarrhea, abdominal distention, ileus, urinary retention are frequently present.
- Abdominal tenderness, fever and leukocytosis are usually not prominent.

- Neuropathy, predominantly motor may lead to quadraparesis, respiratory impairment, and bulbar paralysis.
- Seizures (sometimes associated with hyponatremia and inappropriate antidiuretic hormone secretion) and mental symptoms indicate central nervous system involvement.
- Tachycardia, hypertension, sweating and tremors indicate sympathetic overactivity.
- Pain and depression may become chronic.
- **Up to 90 percent of individuals with decreased PBG deaminase activity remain asymptomatic.**
- Attacks may be precipitated by:
  — Drugs and hormones (especially progesterone) that induce hepatic ALAS1 and cytochrome P450 enzymes.
  — Reduced caloric or carbohydrate intake.
  — Intercurrent illnesses, infection, surgery.
- Increased risk of hepatocellular carcinoma.
- Some drugs that precipitate acute attacks are listed in Table 30–4.

TABLE 30–4 SOME DRUGS CONSIDERED UNSAFE IN ACUTE PORPHYRIAS[a]

Alcohol
Barbiturates[a]
Carbamazepine[a]
Carisoprodol[a]
Clonazepam (high doses)
Danazol[a]
Diclofenac[a] and possibly other NSAIDs
Ergots
Estrogens[a,b]
Ethchlorvynol[a]
Glutethimide[a]
Griseofulvin[a]
Mephenytoin
Meprobamate[a] (also mebutamate[a], tybamate[a])
Methyprylon
Metoclopramide[a]
Phenytoin[a]
Primidone[a]
Progesterone and synthetic progestins[a]
Pyrazinamide[a]
Pyrazolones (aminopyrine, antipyrine)
Rifampin[a]
Succinimides (ethosuximide, methsuximide)
Sulfonamide antibiotics[a]
Valproic acid[a]

NSAIDs, nonsteroidal antiinflammatory drugs.
[a]Porphyria is listed as a contraindication, warning, precaution, or adverse effect in U.S. labeling for these drugs.
[b]Estrogens are unsafe for porphyria cutanea tarda, but can be used with caution in the acute porphyrias.
NOTE: More complete sources, such as the websites of the American Porphyria Foundation (www.porphyriafoundation.com) and the European Porphyria Initiative (www.porphyria-europe.com), should be consulted before using drugs not listed here.
Adapted with permission from Anderson KE, Bloomer JR, Bonkovsky HL: *Ann Intern Med* 142:439, 2005.
Source: *Williams Hematology,* 8th ed, Chap. 57, Table 57–4, p. 851.

Diagnosis and Laboratory Findings

- Urine may be dark (porphobilin) or red (porphyrins).
- A kit for screening for a substantial increase in urinary PBG is recommended.
- Measurement of ALA and PBG concentration in urine (typically ALA 25 to 100 mg/d; PBG 50 to 200 mg/d during attacks) (see Fig. 30–2).
- Decreased PBG deaminase activity (~50 percent of normal) in ~90 percent of cases.
- Diagnosis should be confirmed by finding the disease-causing mutation, which is often family-specific.

Treatment

- Ensure adequate caloric intake.
- Avoid precipitating drugs (an up-to-date list is available at http://www.porphyriafoundation.com/testing-and-treatment/drug-safety-in-acute-porphyria).
- Initiate prompt treatment of fasting, intercurrent disease, or infection.
- Acute attacks usually require admission to hospital:
  — Mild attacks may be treated by glucose loading (at least 300 g/d intravenously).
  — Intravenous hemin (3 to 4 mg/kg once daily for 4 days) is the treatment of choice for all but mild attacks. Reconstitution with human albumin rather than sterile water is recommended to prevent infusion site phlebitis.
- Long-acting agonists of gonadotrophic hormone releasing hormone can be effective in preventing frequent premenstrual attacks in women.
- Liver transplantation can be curative in patients who become refractory to other therapies.

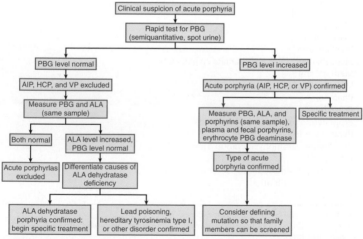

FIGURE 30–2 Recommended laboratory evaluation of patients with concurrent symptoms suggesting an acute porphyria, indicating how the diagnosis is established or excluded by biochemical testing and when specific therapy should be initiated. This schema is not applicable to patients who have been recently treated with hemin or who have recovered from past symptoms suggestive of porphyria. Levels of δ-aminolevulinic acid (*ALA*) and porphobilinogen (*PBG*) may be less increased in hereditary coproporphyria (*HCP*) and variegate porphyria (*VP*) and decrease more quickly with recovery than in acute intermittent porphyria (*AIP*). Mutation detection provides confirmation and greatly facilitates detection of relatives with latent porphyria. (Source: *Williams Hematology,* 8th ed, Chap. 57, Fig. 57–6, p.853.)

Hereditary Coproporphyria
Pathogenesis
- Autosomal dominant disorder caused by partial deficiency of coproporphyrinogen oxidase.

Clinical Findings
- Neurovisceral manifestations are the same as in AIP.
- Attacks are precipitated by the same factors as in AIP.
- Blistering skin lesions resembling PCT may occur but much less commonly than in VP.
- Increased risk of hepatocellular carcinoma.

Diagnosis and Laboratory Findings
- Excessive urinary ALA, PBG, and uroporphyrin in the urine during attacks, as in AIP. Urine coproporphyrin III also increased.
- Distinguished from AIP by marked increase in fecal porphyrins with a predominance of coproporphyrin III.
- DNA studies can identify the causative CPO mutation in almost all cases.

Treatment
- Same as in AIP.

Variegate Porphyria
Pathogenesis
- Autosomal dominant disorder caused by partial deficiency of protoporphyrinogen oxidase.

Clinical Findings
- Neurovisceral manifestations are the same as in AIP and HCP.
- Attacks are precipitated by the same factors as in AIP and HCP.
- Blistering skin lesions resembling PCT are common and may occur apart from the neurovisceral symptoms.
- Increased risk of hepatocellular carcinoma.

Laboratory Findings
- Excessive urinary ALA, PBG, and uroporphyrin in the urine during attacks, as in AIP. Urine coproporphyrin III also increased.
- Distinguished from AIP and HCP by marked increase in fecal porphyrins with a predominance of both coproporphyrin III and protoporphyrin IX.
- Increased plasma porphyrins with a fluorescence emission peak at ~628 nm is diagnostic.
- DNA studies can identify the causative PPO mutation in almost all cases.

Treatment
- Neurovisceral attacks treated as in AIP.
- Protective clothing and avoidance of sunlight is important in patients with blistering photosensitivity. Treatments for PCT are not effective in VP.

Porphyria Cutanea Tarda
Pathogenesis
- The most common human porphyria.
- Results from a substantial deficiency of hepatic uroporphyrinogen (URO) decarboxylase activity, which is due to generation of an inhibitor (uroporphomethene).
- An iron-related disorder, with hepatic siderosis in almost all cases.
- In each patient, at least several of the following susceptibility factors are found: ethanol use, smoking, estrogen use (in females), hepatitis C, HFE mutations, HIV infection, and UROD mutations.

- Most patients do not have UROD mutations and are referred to as type 1 (or type 3 if additional family members have PCT).
- Type 2 patients are heterozygous for UROD mutations, sometimes have affected relatives or earlier onset of disease, but are otherwise indistinguishable from type 1.

Clinical Findings

- Patients have increased skin fragility and blistering of sun exposed areas, especially the backs of the hands.
- Other findings may include hyperpigmentation, hypertrichosis, alopecia, and scarring.
- Cirrhosis and increased risk of hepatocellular carcinoma may result from one or more susceptibility factors or PCT itself.
- Outbreaks due to environmental or occupational exposure to halogenated cyclic aromatic hydrocarbons, such as hexachlorobenzene, have been reported.

Diagnosis and Laboratory Findings

- Levels of highly carboxylated porphyrins, especially uroporphyrin and hepta-carboxyl porphyrin are markedly increased in urine and plasma.

Treatment

- Susceptibility factors should be identified, and exposures to alcohol and estrogens discontinued. Hepatitis C should be treated later.
- Repeated phlebotomy to reduce the serum ferritin to ~20 ng/mL is the preferred treatment and is highly effective.
- A low-dose regimen of hydroxychloroquine (100 mg twice weekly) is also effective when phlebotomies are contraindicated or poorly tolerated.

Hepatoerythropoietic Porphyria

Pathogenesis

- HEP is a rare disorder caused by homozygous or compound heterozygosity for mutations in the URO decarboxylase gene. This is the homozygous form of familial (type 2) PCT, but at least one allele must express some enzyme activity.

Clinical Findings

- HEP is characterized by childhood onset and is clinically similar to CEP.
- Anemia and hepatosplenomegaly may be present.

Diagnosis and Laboratory Findings

- Porphyrin elevations in urine, serum and feces resemble PCT, but in addition there is marked elevation of erythrocyte zinc protoporphyrin.
- Erythrocyte URO decarboxylase activity is reduced to 2 to 10 percent of normal.

Treatment

- Avoidance of sun exposure is most important; topical sunscreens that block UVA and visible light may be of some benefit.
- Treatments used in PCT are generally not effective.

For a more detailed discussion, see John D. Phillips and Karl Anderson: The Porphyrias. Chap. 57, p. 839 in *Williams Hematology*, 8th ed.

PART III

DISORDERS OF GRANULOCYTES

CHAPTER 31
Classification and Clinical Manifestations of Neutrophil Disorders

GENERAL CONSIDERATIONS

- Initially, one should use appropriate normal neutrophil concentration values for certain ethnic groups in which neutrophil counts are significantly lower than persons of European ancestry (e.g., African ancestry, Yemeni Jewish ancestry).
- In this classification, diseases resulting from neutrophil abnormalities in which the neutrophil is either the only cell type affected or is the dominant cell type affected are considered (Table 31–1).
- Neutropenia or neutrophilia occurs as part of disorders that affect multiple blood cell lineages, (e.g., aplastic anemia [see Chap. 3], myelodysplastic syndrome [see Chap. 42], acute and chronic myelogenous leukemias [see Chaps. 46 and 47], chronic myeloproliferative diseases [see Chaps. 43, 44, and 48]).
- A pathophysiologic classification of neutrophil disorders has proved elusive because:
  - The low concentration of blood neutrophils in neutropenic states makes measuring the circulatory kinetics of autologous cells technically difficult.
  - The two compartments of neutrophils in the blood, the random disappearance of neutrophils from the circulation, the extremely short circulation time of neutrophils ($t_{1/2}$ = ~6 hours), the absence of techniques to measure the size of the tissue neutrophil compartment, and the disappearance of neutrophils by apoptosis or excretion from the tissue compartment make multicompartment kinetic analysis difficult.
- Thus, the classification of neutrophil disorders is partly pathophysiologic and partly descriptive (see Table 31–1).

NEUTROPENIA

- Certain childhood syndromes have been listed under decreased neutrophilic granulopoiesis. They could have been listed under chronic hypoplastic or

TABLE 31-1 **CLASSIFICATION OF NEUTROPHIL DISORDERS**

I. Quantitative disorders of neutrophils
  A. Neutropenia
    1. Decreased neutrophilic granulopoiesis
      a. Congenital severe neutropenias (Kostmann syndrome and related disorders)
      b. Reticular dysgenesis (congenital aleukocytosis)
      c. Neutropenia and exocrine pancreas dysfunction (Shwachman-Diamond syndrome)
      d. Neutropenia and immunoglobulin abnormality (e.g., hyper-IgM syndrome)
      e. Neutropenia and disordered cellular immunity (cartilage hair hypoplasia)
      f. Mental retardation, anomalies, and neutropenia (Cohen syndrome)
      g. X-linked cardioskeletal myopathy and neutropenia (Barth syndrome)
      h. Myelokathexis
      i. Warts, hypogammaglobulinemia, infection, myelokathexis (WHIM) syndrome
      j. Neonatal neutropenia and maternal hypertension
      k. Griscelli syndrome
      l. Glycogen storage disease 1b
      m. Hermansky-Pudlak syndrome
      n. Wiskott-Aldrich syndrome
      o. Chronic hypoplastic neutropenia
        (1) Drug-induced
        (2) Cyclic
        (3) Branched-chain aminoacidemia
      p. Acute hypoplastic neutropenia
        (1) Drug-induced
        (2) Infectious
      q. Chronic idiopathic neutropenia
        (1) Benign
          (a) Familial
          (b) Sporadic
        (2) Symptomatic
    2. Accelerated neutrophil destruction
      a. Alloimmune neonatal neutropenia
      b. Autoimmune neutropenia
        (1) Idiopathic
        (2) Drug-induced
        (3) Felty syndrome
        (4) Systemic lupus erythematosus
        (5) Other autoimmune diseases
        (6) Complement activation-induced neutropenia
        (7) Pure white cell aplasia
    3. Maldistribution of neutrophils
      a. Pseudoneutropenia
  B. Neutrophilia
    1. Increased neutrophilic granulopoiesis
      a. Hereditary neutrophilia
      b. Trisomy 13 or 18
      c. Chronic idiopathic neutrophilia
        (1) Asplenia
      d. Neutrophilia or neutrophilic leukemoid reactions
        (1) Inflammation
        (2) Infection

        (3) Acute hemolysis or acute hemorrhage
        (4) Cancer, including granulocyte colony-stimulating factor (G-CSF)-secreting tumors
        (5) Drugs (e.g., glucocorticoids, lithium, granulocyte- or granulocyte-monocyte colony-stimulating factor, tumor necrosis factor-α)
        (6) Ethylene glycol exposure
        (7) Exercise
    e. Sweet syndrome
    f. Cigarette smoking
    g. Cardiopulmonary bypass
  2. Decreased neutrophil circulatory egress
    a. Drugs (e.g., glucocorticoids)
  3. Maldistribution of neutrophils
    a. Pseudoneutrophilia

II. Qualitative disorders of neutrophils
  A. Defective adhesion of neutrophils
    1. Leukocyte adhesion deficiency
    2. Drug-induced
  B. Defective locomotion and chemotaxis
    1. Actin polymerization abnormalities
    2. Neonatal neutrophils
    3. Interleukin-2 administration
    4. Cardiopulmonary bypass
  C. Defective microbial killing
    1. Chronic granulomatous disease
    2. RAC-2 deficiency
    3. Myeloperoxidase deficiency
    4. Hyperimmunoglobulin E (Job) syndrome
    5. Glucose-6-phosphate dehydrogenase deficiency
    6. Extensive burns
    7. Glycogen storage disease 1b
    8. Ethanol toxicity
    9. End-stage renal disease
    10. Diabetes mellitus
  D. Abnormal structure of the nucleus or of an organelle
    1. Hereditary macropolycytes
    2. Hereditary hypersegmentation
    3. Specific granule deficiency
    4. Pelger-Huët anomaly
    5. Alder Reilly anomaly
    6. May-Hegglin anomaly
    7. Chédiak-Higashi disease

III. Neutrophil-induced vascular or tissue damage
  A. Pulmonary disease
  B. Transfusion-related lung injury
  C. Renal disease
  D. Arterial occlusion
  E. Venous occlusion
  F. Myocardial infarction
  G. Impaired ventricular function
  H. Stroke
  I. Neoplasia

Source: *Williams Hematology*, 8th ed, Chap. 64, Table 64–1, p. 934.

chronic idiopathic neutropenia; however, they seem to hold a special interest as pediatric conditions and the causative gene mutations are known in many cases.

- Three childhood syndromes, although associated with neutropenia, are omitted because the neutropenia is part of a more global suppression of hematopoiesis: Pearson syndrome, Fanconi syndrome, and dyskeratosis congenita (see Chap. 3).
- Chronic idiopathic neutropenias include:
  — Cases with normocellular marrows but an inadequate compensatory increase in granulopoiesis for the degree of neutropenia.
  — Cases with hyperplastic granulopoiesis that is apparently ineffective.
- The clinical manifestations of decreased concentrations or abnormal function of neutrophils are the result of infection.
  — The relationship of frequency or type of infection to neutrophil concentration is an imperfect one.
  — The cause of the neutropenia, the coincidence of monocytopenia or lymphopenia, concurrent use of alcohol or glucocorticoids, and other factors can influence the likelihood of infection.
  — Infections in neutropenic persons not otherwise compromised are most likely to result, initially, from gram-positive cocci and usually are superficial, involving skin, oropharynx, bronchi, anal canal, or vagina. However, any site may become infected, and gram-negative organisms, viruses, or opportunistic organisms may be involved.
  — There is a decrease in the formation of pus in patients with severe neutropenia. This failure to suppurate can mislead the clinician and delay identification of the site of infection because minimal physical or radiographic findings develop.
  — Exudate, swelling, and regional adenopathy are much less prevalent in severely neutropenic patients. Fever is common, and local pain, tenderness, and erythema are nearly always present despite a marked reduction in neutrophils.
- Some individuals may have apparent neutropenia because a larger proportion of their blood neutrophils is in the marginal rather than the circulating blood pool. In this type of neutropenia, the total blood neutrophil pool is normal, neutrophil ability to enter tissues is normal, and infections do not result from this atypical circulatory distribution of neutrophils. This type of alteration has been called *pseudoneutropenia*.

QUALITATIVE (FUNCTIONAL) NEUTROPHIL ABNORMALITIES

- Neutrophil function depends on the ability of neutrophils to adhere to vascular endothelium, penetrate endothelium, migrate along chemotactic gradients, and ingest and kill microorganisms. Loss of any of these functions can predispose to infection (see Chap. 33).
- Defects in cytoplasmic contractile proteins, granule synthesis or contents, or intracellular enzymes may underlie a movement, ingestion, or killing defect.
- These defects may be inherited or acquired.
- Chronic granulomatous disease and Chédiak-Higashi disease are two examples of the former (see Chap. 33).
- Among the acquired disorders are those extrinsic to the cell, such as in the movement, chemotactic, or phagocytic defects of diabetes mellitus, alcohol abuse, and glucocorticoid excess.
- Acquired intrinsic disorders are usually manifestations of clonal myeloid diseases (e.g., deficient granules in leukemic neutrophils) (see Chap. 41).
- Severe functional abnormalities in neutrophils can result in *Staphylococcus aureus, Klebsiella aerobacter, Escherichia coli,* and other catalase-positive microorganism infections (see Chap. 33).

NEUTROPHILIA

- An overabundance of neutrophils has not been shown to result in specific clinical manifestations.
- Impairment of post-ischemic reperfusion of the coronary microcirculation has been thought to be dependent, in part, on neutrophil plugging of myocardial capillaries.

NEUTROPHIL-INDUCED VASCULAR OR TISSUE DAMAGE

- Neutrophil products may contribute to the pathogenesis of inflammatory skin, bowel, synovial, glomerular, bronchial, retinal, and interstitial pulmonary diseases.
- Highly reactive oxygen products of neutrophils may be mutagens that increase the risk of neoplasia.
  - Development of carcinoma of the bowel in patients with chronic ulcerative colitis.
  - Relationship between chronically elevated leukocyte count and the occurrence of lung cancer, independent of the effect of cigarette usage.
- The oxidants, especially hypochlorous acid and chloramines, released by the neutrophils are extremely short-lived but may inactivate protease inhibitors in tissue fluids, permitting elastase, collagenase, gelatinase, and other proteases or cationic proteins to cause tissue injury.
- Expression of neutrophil selectins and integrin molecules (e.g., intracellular adhesion molecule-1, endothelial-leukocyte adhesion molecule-1) contribute to neutrophils as pathogens. They contribute to microvascular damage by adherent neutrophils (e.g., diabetic retinopathy; sickle cell vasculopathy (see Chap. 17); transfusion-related acute lung injury (see Chap. 92); specific types of renal, cerebral, retinal, and coronary vasculopathies; and other situations).
- Thrombogenesis has also been ascribed to leukocyte products, especially tissue factor.

 For a more detailed discussion, see Marshall A. Lichtman: Classification and Clinical Manifestations of Neutrophil Disorders. Chap. 64, p. 933 in *Williams Hematology*, 8th ed.

CHAPTER 32
Neutropenia and Neutrophilia

NEUTROPENIA

- *Leukopenia* refers to a reduced total leukocyte count.
- *Granulocytopenia* refers to a reduced granulocyte (neutrophils, eosinophils, and basophils) count.
- *Neutropenia* refers to a reduced neutrophil count: less than 1.5×10^9/L in patients from age 1 month to 10 years, and less than 1.8×10^9/L in patients older than age 10 years. Table 31–1 outlines the classification of neutrophil disorders.
- Agranulocytosis literally means a complete absence of blood granulocytes but is used to indicate very severe neutropenia, usually a neutrophil count $< 0.5 \times 10^9$/L.
- Americans of African descent (as do some other ethnic groups) have lower mean neutrophil counts than do Americans of European descent.
- The risk of infections is inversely related to the severity of the neutropenia: patients with qualitatively normal neutrophils and neutrophil counts of 1.0 to 1.8×10^9/L are at little risk; patients with counts of 0.5 to 1.0×10^9/L are at low or slight risk; and patients with counts less than 0.5×10^9/L are at higher risk.
- Patients with severe, prolonged neutropenia are at particular risk for bacterial and fungal infections.
- The risk is calculated not only by the neutrophil count but by complicating factors as follows:
  — The longer the duration of severe neutropenia, the greater the risk of infection.
  — The risk of infection is greater when the count is falling rapidly or when there is associated monocytopenia, lymphocytopenia, or hypogammaglobulinemia.
  — Neutropenia caused by disorders of hematopoietic progenitor cells (e.g., chemotherapy-induced marrow suppression, severe inherited neutropenia) generally results in a greater susceptibility to infections compared with neutropenia resulting from accelerated turnover (e.g., immune neutropenia).
  — Integrity of the skin and mucous membranes, blood supply to tissues, presence of an indwelling catheter, and nutritional status are also important in considering infection risk.
- Neutropenia can be classified as: (1) disorders of production; (2) disorders of distribution and turnover; (3) drug-induced neutropenia; and (4) neutropenia with infectious diseases.

DISORDERS OF PRODUCTION

Inherited Neutropenia Syndromes
Kostmann Syndrome

- Can be an autosomal dominant (mutation in gene for neutrophil elastase, *ELA-2*), recessive (mutation in gene encoding mitochondrial protein, *HAX-1*)), or a sporadic (mutation in *ELA-2*) disease. Mutation in the gene for the glucose-6-phosphate catalytic subunit (*G6PC3*) also can cause severe neutropenia.
- Mutations in the receptor for granulocyte colony-stimulating factor (G-CSF) and in *RAS* may be present but are not the cause of the neutropenia but may predispose to evolution to acute myelogenous leukemia.

- Otitis, gingivitis, pneumonia, enteritis, peritonitis, and bacteremia usually occur in the first month of life.
- Neutrophil count is often less than 0.2×10^9/L. Eosinophilia, monocytosis, and mild splenomegaly may be present.
- Marrow usually shows some early neutrophil precursors but few myelocytes or mature neutrophils.
- Immunoglobulin levels are usually normal or increased and chromosome analyses are normal.
- Treatment with G-CSF is usually effective in all types of hereditary neutropenia. It decreases recurrent fevers and infections. About 5 percent of patients do not respond.
- Risk of development of acute myelogenous leukemia.
- Allogeneic hematopoietic stem cell transplantation may be curative.

Neutropenia Associated with Congenital Immunodeficiency Diseases

- X-linked agammaglobulinemia, common variable immunodeficiency, and X-linked hyper-IgM syndrome are each accompanied by neutropenia in a proportion of patients.
- G-CSF may correct the neutropenia.
- Allogeneic hematopoietic stem cell transplantation may correct the primary immune disorder.
- Neutropenia is usually a production disorder based on marrow examinations showing decreased granulopoiesis.
- In X-linked agammaglobulinemia of Bruton (mutation in *BTK* gene), severe neutropenia is present in about 25 percent of patients.
- Children with common variable immunodeficiency commonly have neutropenia (and thrombocytopenia and hemolytic anemia).
- In X-linked hyperimmunoglobulin-M syndrome (mutation in gene encoding CD40 ligand), neutropenia is present in approximately 50 percent of patients.
- In severe combined immunodeficiency, neutropenia is a constant feature.
- Reticular dysgenesis results from thymic aplasia and inability to produce neutrophils or thymus- or marrow-derived lymphocytes. Neutropenia is severe, and patients have extreme susceptibility to bacterial and viral infections and often die at an early age.
- Allogeneic hematopoietic stem cell transplantation should be considered.

Cartilage-Hair Hypoplasia Syndrome

- Rare autosomal recessive disorder.
- Short-limbed dwarfism with hyperextensible digits, fine hair.
- Neutropenia, lymphopenia, and frequent infections.
- The marrow shows granulocytic hypoplasia.
- A defect in cellular immunity is present, also.
- Allogeneic hematopoietic stem cell transplantation can correct the hematopoietic and immune abnormality.

Shwachman-Diamond Syndrome

- Autosomal recessive inheritance. Mutation in *SBDS* gene results in proliferative defect in and exaggerated apoptosis of hematopoietic precursors.
- Characterized by short stature, pancreatic exocrine deficiency, steatorrhea, skeletal abnormalities, developmental retardation.
- Neutropenia beginning in the neonatal period. May be intermittent or cyclic and may be as low as 0.2×10^9/L. Anemia and thrombocytopenia occur in about one-third of patients.
- May develop aplastic anemia, oligoblastic or acute myelogenous leukemia (> 20 percent of patients who do not have successful allogeneic hematopoietic stem cell transplantation).
- Some patients may have an increase in neutrophil count with G-CSF.

- Allogeneic hematopoietic stem cell transplantation can correct the hematopoietic abnormality and markedly decrease the risk of transformation to acute myelogenous leukemia.

Chédiak-Higashi Syndrome

- Autosomal recessive disorder with oculocutaneous albinism. Mutation in *LYST* gene regulating lysosomal trafficking.
- Neutropenia is usually mild.
- Giant granules in granulocytes, monocytes, and lymphocytes.
- Recurrent infections result from moderate neutropenia and ineffective killing of microorganisms.

Failure of Neutrophil Marrow Egress

- Myelokathexis is a rare disorder associated with neutrophil counts of less than 0.5×10^9/L.
  — Marrow contains abundant myeloid precursors and mature neutrophils.
  — Marrow neutrophils show hypersegmentation, cytoplasmic vacuoles, and abnormal nuclei.
  — Neutrophil count does not rise with infection, suggesting that the primary disorder is neutrophil release from the marrow.
- Warts, hypogammaglobulinemia, infections, and myelokathexis (WHIM syndrome).
  — Caused by mutation in *CXCR-4* gene (encodes the receptor for the stromal cell-derived factor 1) resulting in abnormal trafficking of cells out of marrow.
  — May improve after G-CSF administration.
  — Can evolve into myelodysplastic syndrome or acute myelogenous leukemia.
- Lazy leukocyte syndrome
  — Has ample marrow precursors and neutrophils, but few circulating cells. The neutrophils have a defect in intrinsic motility and do not migrate out of the marrow efficiently.

Glycogen Storage Disease Ib

- Characterized by hypoglycemia, hepatosplenomegaly, seizures, and failure to thrive in infants. Attributable to mutation in gene for intracellular transport protein for glucose.
- Severe neutropenia gradually develops despite normal-appearing marrow.
- Neutrophils have reduced oxidative burst and chemotaxis.
- Neutropenia may improve with G-CSF.
- May evolve into acute myelogenous leukemia.

Cyclic Neutropenia

- Onset is usually in childhood.
- One-third of patients have an autosomal dominant pattern of inheritance. Mutations in *ELA-2* gene.
- Recurring episodes of severe neutropenia, every 21 days, lasting 3 to 6 days.
- Malaise, fever, mucous membrane ulcers, and lymphadenopathy.
- The result of a defect in the regulation of hematopoietic stem cells.
- Diagnosis can be made by serial differential counts, at least three times per week for a minimum of 6 weeks.
- Cycling of other white cells, reticulocytes, and platelets may accompany neutrophil cycles.
- Most patients survive to adulthood, and symptoms are often milder after puberty.
- Fatal clostridial bacteremia has been reported.
- Careful observation is warranted with each neutropenic period.
- Treatment with G-CSF is effective. It does not abolish cycling but shortens the neutropenic periods sufficiently to lessen symptoms and infections.

Transcobalamin II Deficiency

- Neutropenia as an early feature of pancytopenia from vitamin B_{12} deficiency and megaloblastic hematopoiesis as a result of a deficiency in the cobalamin carrier. It is corrected by vitamin B_{12} treatment.

Neutropenia with Dysgranulopoiesis

- Notable for ineffective granulopoiesis.
- Neutrophil precursors show abnormal granulation, vacuolization, autophagocytosis, and nuclear abnormalities.

Acquired Neutropenia Syndromes

Neutropenia in Neonates of Hypertensive Mothers

- Low birth weight infants with low neutrophil counts common.
- Neutropenia severe and a high risk of infection in first several weeks postpartum.
- G-CSF may increase neutrophil count. Clinical benefit (decreased incidence of infection) has not been documented.

Chronic Idiopathic Neutropenia

- Includes familial, severe or benign neutropenia, chronic benign neutropenia of childhood, and chronic idiopathic neutropenia in adults.
- Some patients with chronic neutropenia may have large granular lymphocyte leukemia (see Chap. 58).
- Patients have selective neutropenia and normal or near-normal red cell, reticulocyte, lymphocyte, monocyte, and platelet counts and immunoglobulin levels.
- The spleen size is normal or minimally enlarged.
- Marrow examination shows normal cellularity or selective neutrophilic hypoplasia; the ratio of immature to mature cells is increased, suggesting ineffective granulocytopoiesis.
- Clinical course can usually be predicted based on the degree of neutropenia, marrow examination, and prior history of fever and infections.
- Treatment with G-CSF will increase neutrophils in most patients, if symptomatic with recurrent infections.

Cytotoxic Drug Therapy

- Causes neutropenia by decreasing cell production; probably the most frequent cause of neutropenia in the United States.

Neutropenia as a Result of Diseases Causing Impaired Production

- Diseases affecting hematopoietic stem and progenitor cells, such as acute leukemia and aplastic anemia.

Neutropenia as a Consequence of Nutritional Deficiencies

- Neutropenia is an early and consistent feature of megaloblastic anemias due to vitamin B_{12} or folate deficiency.
- Copper deficiency can cause neutropenia in patients receiving total parenteral nutrition with inadequate supplies of trace metals, in patients who have had gastric resection, and in malnourished children.
- Mild neutropenia may occur in patients with anorexia nervosa.

Pure White Cell Aplasia

- Rare disorder exhibiting selective severe neutropenia.
- Marrow devoid of neutrophils and their precursors.
- Counterpart to pure red cell aplasia.
- May be associated with thymoma or agammaglobulinemia.
- Presumptive autoimmune mechanism.
- Treat with antithymocyte globulin, glucocorticoids, and/or cyclosporine.

DISORDERS OF NEUTROPHIL DISTRIBUTION AND TURNOVER

Alloimmune (Isoimmune) Neonatal Neutropenia
- Neutropenia caused by the transplacental passage of maternal IgG antibodies against neutrophil-specific antigens inherited from the father.
- The disorder occurs in about 1 in 2000 neonates and usually lasts 2 to 4 months.
- Often not recognized until bacterial infections occur in an otherwise healthy infant and may be confused with neonatal sepsis.
- Hematologic picture usually consists of isolated severe neutropenia and marrow with normal cellularity but reduced numbers of mature neutrophils.
- Diagnosis is usually made with antineutrophil agglutination or immunofluorescence tests.
- Antibiotic treatment used only when necessary; glucocorticoids should be avoided.
- Exchange transfusions to decrease antibody titers may be useful.

Autoimmune Neutropenia
Idiopathic Immune Neutropenia
- Neutrophil autoantibodies may accelerate neutrophil turnover and impair production.
- Patients usually have selective neutropenia and one or more positive tests for antineutrophil antibodies.
- Difficult to distinguish cases of autoimmune neutropenia from chronic idiopathic neutropenia.
- Spontaneous remissions sometimes occur; intravenous immunoglobulin is effective for some pediatric patients; response to glucocorticoids is unpredictable.

Systemic Lupus Erythematosus
- Neutropenia occurs in 50 percent of patients, anemia in 75 percent (direct antiglobulin test positive in one-third), thrombocytopenia in 20 percent, and splenomegaly in 15 percent.
- Increased IgG on the surface of neutrophils, and marrow cellularity and maturation are normal.
- Neutropenia usually does not increase susceptibility to infections in the absence of treatment with glucocorticoids or cytotoxic drugs.

Rheumatoid Arthritis
- Less than 3 percent of patients with classic rheumatoid arthritis have leukopenia.

Sjögren Syndrome
- About 30 percent of patients have leukocyte counts of 2.0 to 5.0 $\times$ 10^9/L, with a normal differential count. Severe neutropenia with recurrent infections is rare.
- Treatment of the neutropenia should be reserved for patients with recurrent infections.

Felty Syndrome
- Rheumatoid arthritis, splenomegaly, leukopenia represent classic triad.
- Prominent neutropenia is a constant feature.
- Troublesome infections are common in patients with absolute neutrophil counts below 0.2 $\times$ 10^9/L.
- High levels of circulating immune complexes may play a role in neutropenia.
- Lymphopenia and a very high rheumatoid factor titer. A subset of patients has large granular lymphocytic leukemia (see Chap. 58).
- No clear relationship exists between spleen size and neutrophil count.
- Two-thirds of patients respond to splenectomy with an increase in neutrophil count, but two-third of these responders relapse later.

- Splenectomy should be reserved for patients with severe, recurrent, or intractable infections.
- Improvement has been reported with lithium, gold, and methotrexate. Some clinicians favor weekly methotrexate therapy because of ease of administration, effectiveness, and comparatively lower toxicity.
- Rituximab and tocilizumab have been used but response is unpredictable.
- Treatment with G-CSF or GM-CSF may improve neutropenia but may exacerbate arthritic manifestations.
- Treatment of the neutropenia should be reserved for patients with recurrent infections.

Autoimmune Neutropenia

- Sporadically reported in Hodgkin lymphoma, chronic autoimmune hepatitis, and Crohn disease.

Other Neutropenias Associated with Splenomegaly

- A variety of diseases may cause this type of neutropenia including sarcoidosis, lymphoma, tuberculosis, malaria, kala-azar, and Gaucher disease, usually in association with thrombocytopenia and anemia.
- Neutropenia associated with splenomegaly may be due to immune mechanisms or sluggish blood flow through the spleen with trapping of neutrophils.
- The neutropenia is usually not of clinical significance and splenectomy is rarely indicated to correct neutropenia.

DRUG-INDUCED NEUTROPENIA

- Drugs may cause neutropenia because of (1) dose-related toxic effects or (2) by immune mechanisms.
- Table 32–1 lists drugs implicated. Information about new drugs can be obtained from the manufacturer, a drug information center, or a poison control center.
- Dose-related toxicity refers to nonselective interference of the drug with protein synthesis or cell replication.
- Phenothiazines, antithyroid drugs, and chloramphenicol cause neutropenia by this mechanism.
- Dose-related toxicity is more likely to occur with multiple drugs, high plasma concentrations, slow metabolism, or renal impairment.
- Cases not dose-related may be allergic (i.e., the immunologic mechanism is poorly understood but appears to be similar to drug-induced hemolytic anemia). Neutropenia tends to occur relatively early in the course of treatment with drugs to which the patient has been previously exposed.
- Women, older persons, persons with history of allergies are more commonly affected with drug-induced neutropenia.
- Patients usually present with fever, myalgia, sore throat, and severe neutropenia.
- A high level of suspicion and careful clinical history are critical to identifying the offending drug.
- Differential diagnosis includes acute viral infections and acute bacterial sepsis.
- If other hematologic abnormalities are also present, hematologic diseases that cause bi- and tricytopenia should be considered.
- Once the offending drug is stopped, patients with sparse marrow neutrophils but normal-appearing precursor cells will have neutrophil recovery in 4 to 7 days. When early precursor cells are severely depleted, recovery may take considerably longer.
- Marrow biopsy soon after recovery may reveal a very large cohort of normal promyelocytes, simulating promyelocytic leukemia. Observation for 2 or 3 days establishes the normal recovery process.
- If febrile, cultures of throat, nasal cavities, blood and urine should be done and broad-spectrum antibiotics used.

TABLE 32–1 **CLASSIFICATION OF WIDELY USED DRUGS ASSOCIATED WITH IDIOSYNCRATIC NEUTROPENIA**

Analgesics and Antiinflammatory Agents
Indomethacin*
Gold salts
Pentazocine
Para-aminophenol derivatives*
Acetaminophen
Phenacetin
Pyrazolone derivatives*
Aminopyrine
Dipyrone
Oxyphenbutazone
Phenylbutazone

Antibiotics
Cephalosporins
Chloramphenicol*
Clindamycin
Gentamicin
Isoniazid
Para-aminosalicylic acid
Penicillins and semisynthetic penicillins*
Rifampin
Streptomycin
Sulfonamides*
Tetracyclines
Trimethoprim-sulfamethoxazole
Vancomycin

Anticonvulsants
Carbamazepine
Mephenytoin
Phenytoin

Antidepressants
Amitriptyline
Amoxapine
Desipramine
Doxepin
Imipramine

Antihistamines—H₂-Blockers
Cimetidine
Ranitidine

Antimalarials
Amodiaquine
Chloroquine
Dapsone
Pyrimethamine
Quinine

Antithyroid Drugs*
Carbimazole
Methimazole
Propylthiouracil

Cardiovascular Drugs
  Captopril
  Disopyramide
  Hydralazine
  Methyldopa
  Procainamide
  Propranolol
  Quinidine
  Tocainide

Diuretics
  Acetazolamide
  Chlorthalidone
  Chlorothiazide
  Ethacrynic acid
  Hydrochlorothiazide

Hypoglycemic Agents
  Chlorpropamide
  Tolbutamide

Hypnotics and Sedatives
  Chlordiazepoxide and other benzodiazepines
  Meprobamate

Phenothiazines*
  Chlorpromazine
  Phenothiazines

Other Drugs
  Allopurinol
  Clozapine
  Levamisole
  Penicillamine
  Ticlopidine

---

*More frequently reported to cause neutropenia in epidemiologic studies.
NOTE: Documentation of the role of specific drugs in the causation of neutropenia is dependent on (1) the frequency of the occurrence among patients, (2) the timing of the event in relationship to drug use, (3) the absence of alternative explanations, or (4) the inadvertent or intentional reuse of the drug (rechallenges) with a similar response. Readers who require supplementary lists of putative drugs involved in the development of neutropenia or wish to read original references for these interactions are referred to references 111 to 113 in *Williams Hematology*, 8th ed, Chap. 65, p. 939.
Source: *Williams Hematology*, 8th ed, Chap. 65, Table 65–1, p. 945.

NEUTROPENIA WITH INFECTIOUS DISEASES

• Occurs with acute or chronic bacterial, viral, parasitic, or rickettsial diseases.
• Some agents such as those causing infectious hepatitis, Kawasaki disease, and HIV infection may cause neutropenia and pancytopenia by infecting hematopoietic progenitor cells.
• In severe gram-negative bacterial infections, neutropenia is probably a result of increased adherence to the endothelium, as well as increased utilization of neutrophils at the site of infection. This mechanism may also occur in rickettsial infections and some viral infections.
• Chronic infections causing splenomegaly, such as tuberculosis, brucellosis, typhoid fever, and malaria, probably cause neutropenia by splenic sequestration and marrow suppression.

CLINICAL APPROACH TO THE PATIENT PRESENTING WITH NEUTROPENIA

- *Acute onset of severe neutropenia* often presents with fever, sore throat, and inflammation of the skin or mucous membranes. This is an urgent clinical situation requiring prompt cultures, intravenous fluids, and broad-spectrum antibiotics.
- In the absence of recent hospitalization and antibiotic exposure, infections are usually caused by organisms found on the skin, nasopharynx, and intestinal flora, and are sensitive to several antibiotics. Immediate evaluation should include a careful history with particular attention to drug use and physical examination with attention to skin; oronasopharynx; sinuses; lungs; lymph nodes; abdomen, including liver and spleen size or bone tenderness.
- Prompt blood counts, microbial cultures, institution of intravenous fluids, and other supportive measures may be critical in an acute and severe situation. The history and physical examination may point to other needs such as chest or abdominal imaging.
- *Chronic neutropenia* is usually found by chance or during evaluation of recurrent fevers or infections. It is useful to determine whether the neutropenia is chronic or cyclic, and the average neutrophil count when the patient is well.
- The absolute monocyte, lymphocyte, eosinophil, and platelet counts, as well as hemoglobin and immunoglobulin levels, should be determined, and the blood film should be studied carefully for reactive lymphocytes and abnormal cells.
- Marrow examination is useful if multilineage involvement suggests a clonal myeloid disease or another cause of multicytopenia (e.g., aplastic anemia or megaloblastosis).
- It may be useful to measure antinuclear antibodies (ANA) and rheumatoid factor, or to obtain other serologic tests for collagen vascular diseases, especially if skin rashes or articular symptoms or signs are present.
- Examination of the blood and marrow may identify abnormal cells (e.g., Chédiak-Higashi syndrome or large granular lymphocytic leukemia).
- Infectious and nutritional causes for chronic neutropenia are rare and seldom difficult to recognize.
- Measurements of antineutrophil antibodies, *in vitro* marrow colony-forming activity, and studies of drug-induced neutropenia may require laboratory techniques available only in specialized laboratories.

NEUTROPHILIA

- Neutrophilia is an increase in the absolute neutrophil count (bands and mature neutrophils) to greater than 7.5×10^9/L.
- For infants younger than 1 month of age, the normal range is as high as 26×10^9/L.
- Extreme neutrophilia is often referred to as a *leukemoid reaction* because the height of the leukocyte count may simulate leukemia.
- Neutrophilia may occur as a result of:
  - An increase in neutrophil production. Required for sustained neutrophilia.
  - Accelerated release of neutrophil from the marrow "storage pool" into the blood.
  - Shift from the marginal to circulating pool (demargination). (Cannot generate more than a twofold to threefold increase in neutrophil count.)
  - Reduced egress of neutrophils from the blood to tissues.
  - A combination of these mechanisms.
- The time required to develop neutrophilia may be:
  - Minutes (demargination).
  - Hours (accelerated release of neutrophils from marrow).
  - Days (increase in cell production).

ACUTE NEUTROPHILIA

- The causes are listed in Table 32–2.
- Pseudoneutrophilia is caused by a shift from the marginated to circulating pool (demargination) induced by vigorous exercise, by acute physical and emotional stress, or by the infusion of epinephrine.
- Marrow storage pool shifts involve the release of segmented neutrophils and bands from the marrow reserve in response to inflammation, infections, or colony-stimulating factors (CSFs).

TABLE 32–2	**MAJOR CAUSES OF NEUTROPHILIA**
Acute Neutrophilia	**Chronic Neutrophilia**

Physical stimuli
    Cold, heat, exercise, convulsions,
    pain, labor, anesthesia, surgery
	Infections
	    Persistence of infections that cause
	    acute neutrophilia

Emotional stimuli
    Panic, rage, severe stress, depression
	Inflammation
	    Most acute inflammatory reactions,
	    such as colitis, dermatitis,
	    drug-sensitivity reactions, gout,
	    hepatitis, myositis, nephritis,
	    pancreatitis, periodontitis,
	    rheumatic fever, rheumatoid
	    arthritis, vasculitis, thyroiditis,
	    Sweet syndrome

Infections
    Many localized and systemic acute
    bacterial, mycotic, rickettsial,
    spirochetal, and certain viral
    infections
	Tumors
	    Gastric, bronchogenic, breast, renal,
	    hepatic, pancreatic, uterine, and
	    squamous cell cancers; rarely
	    Hodgkin lymphoma, lymphoma,
	    brain tumors, melanoma, and
	    multiple myeloma

Inflammation or tissue necrosis
    Burns, electric shock, trauma,
    infarction, gout, vasculitis,
    antigen-antibody complexes,
    complement activation
	Drugs, hormones, and toxins
	    Continued exposure to many
	    substances that produce acute
	    neutrophilia, lithium; rarely as a
	    reaction to other drugs

Drugs, hormones, and toxins
    Colony-stimulating factors,
    epinephrine, etiocholanolone,
    endotoxin, glucocorticoids,
    smoking tobacco, vaccines,
    venoms
	Metabolic and endocrinologic disorders
	    Eclampsia, thyroid storm, overpro-
	    duction of adrenocorticotropic
	    hormone

	Hematologic disorders
	    Rebound from agranulocytosis or
	    therapy of megaloblastic anemia,
	    chronic hemolysis or hemorrhage,
	    asplenia, myeloproliferative
	    disorders, chronic idiopathic
	    leukocytosis

	Hereditary and congenital disorders Down syndrome, congenital

Source: *Williams Hematology*, 8th ed, Chap. 65, Table 65–2, p. 947.

CHRONIC NEUTROPHILIA

- Table 32–2 lists the causes of chronic neutrophilia.
- The neutrophil production rate increases up to threefold with chronic infections and even more in clonal myeloid disorders and in response to therapeutic administration of G-CSF or GM-CSF. The maximum response requires at least 7 to 10 days to develop.
- Neutrophilia as a result of decreased egress from the vascular compartment occurs with glucocorticoids, leukocyte adhesion deficiency (CD11/CD18 deficiency) (see Chap. 33), and recovery from infection.
- Chronic neutrophilic leukemia is a rare disorder with a very high blood concentration of neutrophils, often with few immature cells (see Chap. 46).

DISORDERS ASSOCIATED WITH NEUTROPHILIA (TABLE 32–2)

- Perhaps the most frequent are conditions with elevations of endogenous epinephrine and cortisol, such as exercise or emotional stress.
- The mean neutrophil count of people who smoke two packs of cigarettes daily is twice normal on average.
- Gram-negative infections, particularly those resulting in bacteremia or septic shock, may cause extreme neutrophilia or neutropenia.
- Some infections characteristically do not cause neutrophilia (e.g., typhoid fever, brucellosis, many viral infections).
- Neutrophilia in association with cancer may be a result of tumor cell secretion of colony-stimulating factors (esp. G-CSF) or because of tumor necrosis and infection.
- In patients with cancer, subarachnoid hemorrhage, or coronary artery disease, neutrophilia may portend a less favorable prognosis.
- In addition to the clonal myeloid diseases, several unusual hematologic conditions may be associated with neutrophilia:
  — Hereditary disorders associated with thrombocytopenia may also be accompanied by leukemoid reactions (e.g., thrombocytopenia with absent radii, see Chap. 74).
  — Benign idiopathic neutrophilic leukocytosis may be acquired or may occur as an autosomal dominant trait.
  — In Down syndrome, neonatal leukemoid reactions may resemble myelogenous leukemia.

Neutrophilia and Drugs

- Catecholamines and glucocorticoids are common causes of neutrophilia.
- Lithium causes neutrophilia, presumably because of G-CSF release.
- Rarely, other drugs will cause neutrophilia (e.g., ranitidine or quinidine).

EVALUATION OF NEUTROPHILIA

- In most instances, the finding of neutrophilia, with an increase in bands and with toxic granules in the mature cells, can be related to an infection or inflammatory condition or, less commonly, the release of G-CSF by a neoplasm such as lung cancer.
- The history should make note of smoking, drug usage, or symptoms of occult malignancy.
- If the neutrophilia is accompanied by myelocytes, promyelocytes, increased basophils, and splenomegaly, a clonal myeloid disorder (e.g., chronic myelogenous leukemia, primary myelofibrosis, chronic myelomonocytic leukemia) should be considered.

THERAPY

- There are no direct adverse effects of an elevated neutrophil count in most situations in which the response is to an infection. Sickle cell crisis has been associated with chronic or recurring neutrophilia, as have some vasculopathies (see Chapter 31, Section on Neutrophil-Induced Vascular or Tissue Damage"). In the clonal myeloid diseases in which there are very elevated blast cell counts, adverse effects may occur (see "Hyperleukocytic Syndromes" in Chap. 41). The retinoic acid syndrome in acute promyelocytic leukemia treated with all-*trans* retinoic acid is a special situation in which morbid effects are often correlated with simultaneous neutrophilia (see Chap. 46).
- In some inflammatory diseases, glucocorticoids and immunosuppressive therapies are used to reduce inflammation in part by reducing production or altering distribution of neutrophils.
- Specific therapy, if indicated, is generally directed at the underlying cause of neutrophilia.

For a more detailed discussion, see Wayne C. Smith: Production, Distribution, and Fate of Neutrophils. Chap. 61, p. 891; Marshall A. Lichtman: Classification and Clinical Manifestations of Neutrophil Disorders. Chap. 64, p. 933; David C. Dale: Neutropenia and Neutrophilia. Chap. 65, p. 939 in *Williams Hematology*, 8th ed.

CHAPTER 33
Disorders of Neutrophil Functions

CATEGORIES OF NEUTROPHIL DYSFUNCTION

- Antibody or complement defects.
- Abnormalities of cytoplasmic movement (chemotaxis and phagocytosis).
- Abnormal microbicidal activity.
- See Table 33–1 for features of major the abnormalities of neutrophil function.

ANTIBODY/COMPLEMENT DEFECTS

- Interactions between antibodies and complement generate opsonins and stimulate chemotactic factor development.
- C3 deficiency (autosomal recessive inheritance) results in the most severe disorder.
- Homozygotes have no detectable C3 and suffer severe recurrent bacterial infections.
- Deficiency of other less centrally active complement proteins results in a milder condition.
- C3b inactivator or properdin deficiency results in deficiency of C3 also.
- Affected individuals usually suffer from infections due to encapsulated organisms.

GRANULE ABNORMALITIES

Chédiak-Higashi Syndrome
Pathogenesis

- A rare autosomal recessive disorder of abnormal, increased granule fusion with generalized cell dysfunction, resulting in defects in chemotaxis, degranulation, and microbicidal activity.
- Caused by mutation in *LYST* gene on chromosome 1q.
- Increased membrane fluidity in Chédiak-Higashi neutrophils, monocytes, and natural killer cells.
- Spontaneous fusion of granules results in huge lysosomes with diluted hydrolytic enzymes.
- Phagocytosis and the respiratory burst are normal, but killing of organisms is slow.
- Neutropenia occurs as a consequence of precursor death (apoptosis) in the marrow.

Clinical Features

- Because of abnormal association of melanosomes, decreased pigment is noted in skin, hair, iris, and ocular fundus. Characteristic light skin, silvery hair, solar sensitivity, and photophobia.
- Total leukocyte counts average about 2×10^9/L and neutrophil counts range from 0.5 to 2.0×10^9/L.
- Neutrophils and monocytes have impaired microbial killing as a result of inconsistent delivery of diluted granule contents into phagosome.
- Natural killer cell dysfunction may contribute to the predisposition to infection.
- Infections are common, primarily involving mucous membranes, skin, and the respiratory tract; a variety of bacteria and fungi are involved, but *Staphylococcus aureus* is the most common.

TABLE 33–1   CLINICAL DISORDERS OF NEUTROPHIL FUNCTION

Disorder	Etiology	Impaired Function	Clinical Consequence
Degranulation abnormalities			
Chédiak-Higashi syndrome	Autosomal recessive; disordered coalescence of lysosomal granules; responsible gene is CHS1/LYST which encodes a protein hypothesized to regulate granule fusion	Decreased neutrophil chemotaxis; degranulation and bactericidal activity; platelet storage pool defect; impaired NK function, failure to disperse melanosomes	Neutropenia; recurrent pyogenic infections, propensity to develop marked hepatosplenomegaly as a manifestation of the hemophagocytic syndrome
Specific granule deficiency	Autosomal recessive; functional loss of myeloid transcription factor arising from a mutation or arising from reduced expression of Gfi-1 or C/EBPε, which regulates specific granule formation	Impaired chemotaxis and bactericidal activity; bilobed nuclei in neutrophils; defensins, gelatinase, collagenase, vitamin B_{12}-binding protein, and lactoferrin	Recurrent deep-seated abscesses
Adhesion abnormalities			
Leukocyte adhesion deficiency I	Autosomal recessive; absence of CD11/CD18 surface adhesive glycoproteins (β_2 integrins) on leukocyte membranes most commonly arising from failure to express CD18 mRNA	Decreased binding of C3bi to neutrophils and impaired adhesion to ICAM-1 and ICAM-2	Neutrophilia; recurrent bacterial infection associated with a lack of pus formation
Leukocyte adhesion deficiency II	Autosomal recessive; loss of fucosylation of ligands for selectins and other glycol conjugates arising from mutations of the GDPfucose transporter	Decreased adhesion to activated endothelium expressing ELAM	Neutrophilia; recurrent bacterial infection without pus
Leukocyte adhesion deficiency III (LAD-1 variant syndrome)	Autosomal recessive; impaired integrin function arising from mutations of FERMT3 which encodes kindlin-3 in hematopoietic cells; kindlin-3 binds to β-integrin and thereby transmits integrin activation	Impaired neutrophil adhesion and platelet activation	Recurrent infections, neutropenia, bleeding tendency

(continued)

TABLE 33–1 (CONTINUED)

Disorder	Etiology	Impaired Function	Clinical Consequence
Disorders of cell motility			
Enhanced motile responses; FMF	Autosomal recessive gene responsible for FMF on chromosome 16, which encodes for a protein called "pyrin"; pyrin regulates caspase–1 and thereby IL-1β secretion; mutated pyrin may lead to heightened sensitivity to endotoxin, excessive IL-1β production, and impaired monocyte apoptosis	Excessive accumulation of neutrophils at inflamed sites which may be the result of excessive IL-1β production	Recurrent fever, peritonitis, pleuritis, arthritis, and amyloidosis
Depressed motile responses			
Defects in the generation of chemotactic signals	IgG deficiencies; C3 and properdin deficiency can arise from genetic or acquired abnormalities; mannose-binding protein deficiency predominantly in neonates	Deficiency of serum chemotaxis and opsonic activities	Recurrent pyogenic infections
Intrinsic defects of the neutrophil, e.g., leukocyte adhesion deficiency, Chédiak-Higashi syndrome, specific granule deficiency, neutrophil actin dysfunction, neonatal neutrophils; direct inhibition of neutrophil motility, e.g., drugs	In the neonatal neutrophil, there is diminished ability to express β2 integrins and there is a qualitative impairment in β2-integrin function; ethanol, glucocorticoids, cyclic AMP	Diminished chemotaxis; impaired locomotion and ingestion; impaired adherence	Propensity to develop pyogenic infections; possible cause for frequent infections; neutrophilia seen with epinephrine arises from cyclic AMP release from endothelium
Immune complexes	Bind to Fc receptors on neutrophils in patients with rheumatoid arthritis, systemic lupus erythematosus, and other inflammatory states	Impaired chemotaxis	Recurrent pyogenic infections
Hyperimmunoglobulin-E syndrome	Autosomal dominant; responsible gene is Stat 3	Impaired chemotaxis at times; impaired regulation of cytokine production	Recurrent skin and sinopulmonary infections, eczema, mucocutaneous candidiasis, eosinophilia, retained primary teeth, minimal trauma fractures, scoliosis, and characteristic facies

Hyperimmunoglobulin-E syndrome	Autosomal recessive; more then one gene likely contributes to its etiology	High IgE levels, impaired lymphocyte activation to staphylococcal antigens	Recurrent pneumonia without pneumatoceles sepsis, enzyme, boils, mucocutaneous candidiasis, neurologic symptoms, eosinophilia
Microbicidal activity			
Chronic granulomatous disease	X-linked and autosomal recessive; failure to express functional gp91 $phox$ in the phagocyte membrane in p22 $phox$ (autosomal recessive); other autosomal recessive forms of CGD arise from failure to express protein p47 $phox$ or p67 $phox$	Failure to activate neutrophil respiratory burst leading to failure to kill catalase-positive microbes	Recurrent pyogenic infections with catalase-positive microorganisms
G-6-PD deficiency	Less than 5% of normal activity of G-6-PD	Failure to activate NADPH-dependent oxidase, and hemolytic anemia	Infections with catalase-positive microorganisms
Myeloperoxidase deficiency	Autosomal recessive; failure to process modified precursor protein arising from missense mutation	H_2O_2-dependent antimicrobial activity not potentiated by myeloperoxidase	None
Rac-2 deficiency	Autosomal dominant; dominant negative inhibition by mutant protein of Rac-2 mediated functions	Failure of membrane receptor-mediated O_2 generation and chemotaxis	Neutrophilia, recurrent bacterial infections
Deficiencies of glutathione reductase and glutathione synthetase	Autosomal recessive; failure to detoxify H_2O_2	Excessive formation of H_2O_2	Minimal problems with recurrent pyogenic infections

AMP, adenosine monophosphate; C, complement; CD, cluster designation; CGD, chronic granulomatous disease; G-6-PD, glucose-6-phosphate dehydrogenase; GDP, glucose diphosphate; ELAM, endothelial-leukocyte adhesion molecule; FMF, familial Mediterranean fever; ICAM, intracellular adhesion molecule; Ig, immunoglobulin; IL, interleukin; LAD, leukocyte adhesion deficiency; NADPH, nicotinamide adenine dinucleotide phosphate; NK, natural killer.
Source: *Williams Hematology*, 8th ed, Chap. 66, Table 66–2, p. 964.

- Peripheral neuropathies (sensory and motor), cranial neuropathies, and autonomic dysfunction occur, as well as ataxia.
- Platelet counts are normal but impaired platelet aggregation, storage pool deficiency, and prolonged closure times are common.
- An accelerated phase may occur at any age, characterized by rapid lymphocytic proliferation (not neoplastic) resulting in a syndrome of hepatosplenomegaly, lymphadenopathy, high fever in the absence of bacterial infection. Subsequently, pancytopenia and a high susceptibility to infection usually lead to death. The syndrome is the result of an inherited predisposition to hemophagocytic lymphohistiocytosis, probably related to the inability to contain Epstein-Barr virus infection.

Laboratory Features

- In addition to the characteristic phenotypic features noted above, the principal confirmatory test is the presence of giant granules in neutrophils on the blood film. Molecular testing is not generally available. Heterozygotes are normal and cannot be detected clinically or biochemically.

Treatment

- High-dose ascorbic acid (200 mg/day in infants, 2 g/day in adults) is usually prescribed in the stable phase and improves the clinical state in occasional patients.
- Infections are treated as they arise. Prophylactic antibiotics are generally not useful.
- The only curative treatment is allogeneic hematopoietic stem cell transplantation from a histocompatible donor. The hematologic, immunologic, and natural killer cell abnormalities are corrected by successful transplantation. Other cell abnormalities are not.
- In the accelerated phase, vincristine and glucocorticoids have been used but are not clearly efficacious.

Specific Granule Deficiency

- Exceedingly rare, autosomal recessive disorder characterized by bilobed neutrophils lacking specific granules on the blood film and "empty" specific granules by transmission electron microscopy.
- Vitamin B_{12}-binding protein, lactoferrin, and collagenase are absent from specific granules. Defensins are absent from primary granules. Gelatinase activity is absent from tertiary granules. Microbicidal activity is moderately impaired because of a lack of defensins and lactoferrin.
- Chemotaxis is abnormal because of a lack of adhesion molecules in tertiary and specific granules.
- Eosinophil granule proteins are also deficient (major basic protein, eosinophilic cationic protein, eosinophil-derived neurotoxin). Thus, this disorder is a global abnormality of phagocyte granules and is not limited to neutrophil specific granules as its name implies.
- The diagnosis can be confirmed by a severe deficiency of lactoferrin or B_{12}-binding protein in the plasma.
- Recurrent skin and pulmonary infections are common, usually from infection with *S. aureus* and *Pseudomonas aeruginosa*. *Candida albicans* infections also may occur.
- Treatment is supportive. Antibiotics for acute infections and surgical drainage of chronic abscesses.

ADHESION ABNORMALITIES

Leukocyte Adhesion Deficiency-I

- A rare, autosomal recessive disease, with delayed detachment of umbilical cord, delayed wound healing, frequent severe periodontal or soft-tissue infection, and markedly decreased pus formation despite blood neutrophilia.

- Underlying defect is decreased or absent expression of the β_2 integrin family of leukocyte adhesion proteins (CD11/CD18 complex). These integral membrane glycoproteins (including LFA-1, Mac-1, and p150,95) have noncovalently bonded α and β subunits. Several mutations in the gene encoding the β subunit have been found; these mutations result in profoundly impaired chemotaxis or phagocytosis; degranulation and the respiratory burst are diminished. As a result, the neutrophils can enter the circulation but cannot egress into the tissues.
- See Table 33–2 for features of leukocyte adhesion deficiency disorders.
- Markedly elevated blood neutrophil concentrations (15 to 60×10^9/L), but cells do not enter tissues. Neutrophil concentrations may increase to as high as 150×10^9/L if patient is infected.
- Typically, there is marrow granulocytic hyperplasia and blood neutrophilia. Diagnosis made by flow cytometric measurement of CD11a, CD11b, CD11c, and CD18 on neutrophils. Decreased expression of these surface molecules are the characteristic finding.
- Severely affected patients have recurrent and chronic soft tissue infections (subcutaneous and mucous membranes). *S. aureus, Pseudomonas* spp., other gram-negative enteric rods, and *Candida* spp. are the usual offenders.
- Prophylactic trimethoprim-sulfamethoxazole lowers the risk of recurrent infection.
- Treatment of choice for the severely affected is allogeneic hematopoietic stem cell transplantation.

MOVEMENT DISORDERS

Neutrophil Actin Dysfunction

- Abnormal chemotaxis and phagocytosis are expressed as neonatal recurrent severe bacterial infections.
- Defective actin polymerization occurs; an intracellular inhibitor of polymerization has been isolated.
- A rare lethal disease requiring allogeneic hematopoietic stem cell transplantation.

Familial Mediterranean Fever

- Autosomal recessive disease that primarily affects populations surrounding the Mediterranean basin. Result of a mutation in the *PYRIN* gene expressed primarily in leukocytes and synovial and peritoneal fibroblasts.
- The gene mutation may be identified by polymerase chain reaction methodology.
- The pathogenesis is a predisposition for neutrophils to migrate to serosal surfaces, accumulate and generate an inflammatory response.
- The disease is characterized by acute limited attacks of fever often accompanied by pleuritis, peritonitis, arthritis, pericarditis, inflammation of the tunica vaginalis of the testes, and erysipelas-like skin disease on the lower leg, ankle, or dorsum of the foot.
- Arthralgia and monarticular arthritis can accompany febrile attacks.
- Approximately 25 percent of affected patients develop renal amyloidosis. This finding can progress to renal failure and may be the cause of death.
- Prophylactic colchicine, 0.6 mg orally, two to three times a day, prevents or substantially reduces the acute attacks in most patients. Some patients, who have prodromes, can abort attacks with doses of colchicine beginning at the onset of attacks (0.6 mg orally every hour for 4 hours, then every 2 hours for four doses, and then every 12 hours for 2 days).

Other Disorders of Neutrophil Motility

- Neonatal neutrophils have impaired β_2 integrin function with abnormal transendothelial movement.
- Direct inhibitors of neutrophil motility include ethanol and glucocorticoids.
- Circulating immune complexes also inhibit motility by binding to neutrophil Fc receptors.

186

TABLE 33–2 BIOGLOGIC AND CLINICAL FEATURES OF LEUKOCYTE ADHESION DEFICIENCIES 1 AND 2

	Genetic Defect	Leukocyte Functional Abnormalities	Clinical Features	Diagnosis
LAD-1	Molecular mutations affecting expression of the β_2-integrin CD18	Neutrophils; adherence spreading, homotypic aggregation, chemotaxis receptor CR3 activities; C3bi binding affecting phagocytosis, respiratory burst, and degranulation in response to C3bi-coated particles* Monocytes; adherence, CR3 activities Lymphocytes; cytotoxic T-lymphocyte activities; NK cytotoxic activities; blastogenesis	Autosomal recessive; delayed umbilical cord separation; neutrophilia; defective neutrophil migration into tissue; recurrent bacterial infections; impaired wound healing	Flow cytometry for expression of CD11b/CD18 (Mac-1)
LAD-2 (CDG-IIc)	Mutations affecting function of GDPfucose transporter 1 resulting in defective glycosylation expression at the α1,3–position of selectin ligands including sLe^x and other fucosylated proteins requiring fucosylation	Neutrophils; rolling mediated by sLe^x to endothelium; neutro-philia†	Autosomal recessive; recurrent bacterial infections, periodontitis; growth retardation; developmental retardation; Bombay red cell phenotype	Flow cytometry for leukocyte sLe^x (CD15)

*These functional abnormalities and clinical features are a consequence of lack of the CD11b/CD18, which includes CD11a, CD11b, CD11c, and CD11d markers of four different á chains and the common B2 chain CD18 of molecular mass 95 kDa.
†These functional abnormalities and clinical features are a consequence of lack of sLex expression on leukocytes.
Source: *Williams Hematology*, 8th ed, Chap. 66, Table 66–3, p. 967.

Hyperimmunoglobulin E Syndrome

- Usually an autosomal dominant disorder as a result of mutations in *STAT3* gene.
- Patients have markedly elevated serum IgE levels, chronic eczematoid dermatitis, and recurrent bacterial infections (skin abscesses, sinusitis, otitis media, pneumonia). They may also have coarse facial features, growth retardation, and osteoporosis.
- Coarse facial features, prominent forehead, broad nasal bridge, wide nasal tip, prognathism, hyperextensible joints, and scoliosis may be present. Delayed shedding of primary dentition.
- Chemotaxis is impaired but the molecular mechanism is unknown.
- Serum IgE levels usually exceed 2000 IU/mL, but, as opposed to atopic patients, most of this antibody is directed against *S. aureus*.
- Marked blood and sputum eosinophilia are constant features. Poor antibody responses to neoantigens is also seen.
- Prophylactic trimethoprim-sulfamethoxazole is used to minimize frequency of *S. aureus* infections.
- Early diagnosis and staphylococcal antibiotic prophylaxis can markedly improve the prognosis.
- Topical glucocorticoids may reduce symptoms of the eczematoid dermatitis.
- Orthopedic care for scoliosis, fractures, degenerative joint disease and dental care for delayed loss of first dentition important.
- Incision and drainage of abscesses and superinfected pneumatoceles.

DEFECTS IN MICROBICIDAL ACTIVITY

Chronic Granulomatous Disease (CGD)

- Neutrophils and monocytes have impaired production of superoxide, with markedly reduced microbicidal activity.
- Caused by mutations in any of the genes encoding the NADPH oxidase, an electron transport chain that catalyzes the formation of superoxide.
- About two-thirds of the patients inherit the neutrophil defect as an X chromosome–linked abnormality. The remaining patients have several types of autosomal inheritance.
- In the resting state, the oxidase components are in two locations. The membrane-bound portion, cytochrome b558, is composed of two subunits: gp91-*phox* and p22-*phox*. The heavy chain has binding sites for heme, FAD, and NADPH. Three other proteins reside in the cytosol, but upon stimulation, move to the membrane and interact with gp91-*phox*. These are p47-*phox*, p67-*phox*, and a GTP-binding protein. Severity of CGD depends upon which of these components is affected. The most frequent form is due to mutation of gp91-*phox* gene on chromosome Xp21.1. Other mutations also cause CGD, but occur less frequently. See Table 33–3 for the genetic and molecular classification of chronic granulomatous disease.

Pathogenesis

- Normally, neutrophils form hydrogen peroxide, which acts as substrate for myeloperoxidase to oxidize chloride to hypochlorous acid and chloramines. These accumulate in the phagosome and kill the microbe.
- Oxidase activation acutely produces an alkaline phase in the phagosome that is important for function of neutral hydrolases. In CGD cells, this alkaline phase does not occur, impairing the enzymes that digest bacteria.

Clinical Features

- The X-linked form can be evident in the first months of life, whereas autosomal forms may not be diagnosed until adulthood.
- Skin abscesses, recurrent lymphadenitis, dermatitis, pneumonias, osteomyelitis in small bones of hands or feet, and bacterial hepatic abscesses are each common and require consideration of chronic granulomatous disease. See Table 33–4.

TABLE 33–3			DIAGNOSTIC CLASSIFICATION OF CHRONIC GRANULOMATOUS DISEASE		
Affected Component	Inheritance	Subtype	Membrane Bound Cytochrome b558*	Cytosol $p47^{phox}$*	Cytosol $p67^{phox}$*
$gp91^{phox}$	X	$X91^0$	Not detectable	Normal	Normal
		$X91^+$	Normal quantity, but nonfunctional	Normal	Normal
		$X91^-$	Defective gp 91 ^{phox}, which is poorly functional or expressed in a small fraction of phagocytes	Normal	Normal
$p22^{pho}$	A	$A22^0$	Not detectable	Normal	Normal
		$A22^+$	Normal quantity, but nonfunctional	Normal	Normal
$p47^{phox}$	A	$A47^0$	Normal quantity	Not detectable	Normal
$p67^{phox}$		$A67^0$	Normal	Normal	Not detectable

*Detected by spectral analysis or immunoblotting. In this nomenclature, the first letter represents the mode of inheritance (X-linked [X] or autosomal recessive [A]). The number indicates the phox component, which is genetically affected. The superscript symbols indicate whether the level of protein of the affected component is undetectable (0), diminished (–), or normal (+) as measured by immunoblot or spectral analysis.
Source: *Williams Hematology*, 8th ed, Chap. 66, Table 66–4, p. 973.

- Organisms commonly involved are *S. aureus, Aspergillus* sp., and *C. albicans* (see Table 33–4).
- Granulomata are common and cause chronic lymphadenopathy.

Laboratory Features

- For diagnosis, neutrophil superoxide or hydrogen peroxide generation is measured in response to soluble and particulate stimuli. Read out can be done using flow cytometry with dihydrorhodamine-123 label. The later compound detects oxidative products because it increases fluorescence upon oxidation.
- In addition, the nitroblue tetrazolium (NBT) test can be used. In normal neutrophils, NBT is reduced to purple formazan, and this assay is read out by microscopic examination of individual neutrophils for purple formazan crystals. With most forms of CGD, no reduction to the purple color occurs.
- The NBT test can also detect the X-linked carrier state, as a varied percentage of cells will be NBT-negative and the remainder of the cells will be NBT-positive (mosaicism).
- More sophisticated procedures can define the molecular defect.
- Rare severe forms of glucose-6-phosphate dehydrogenase deficiency can mimic CGD; NADPH is inadequate for normal superoxide generation.

Therapy and Prognosis

- Treatment consists of long-term trimethoprim-sulfamethoxazole prophylaxis, appropriate antibiotics for particular infections, and surgical management of abscesses.
- Interferon-γ (50 μg/m², 3 times per week) has been found to decrease the number of serious bacterial and fungal infections.
- The only curative therapy is allogeneic hematopoietic stem cell transplantation.

		X-Linked	Autosomal
Infection Type	**Organism**	**Recessive (%)**	**Recessive (%)**
	Aspergillus spp.	41	29
	Staphylococcus spp.	11	13
	Burkholderia cepacia	7	11
	Nocardia spp.	6	13
	Serratia spp.	4	5
Abscess			
Subcutaneous	*Staphylococcus* spp.	28	21
	Serratia spp.	19	9
	Aspergillus spp.	7	0
Liver	*Staphylococcus* spp.	52	52
	Serratia spp.	19	9
	Candida spp.	7	0
Lung	*Aspergillus* spp.	27	18
Perirectal	*Staphylococcus* spp.	9	15
Brain	*Aspergillus* spp.	75	25
Suppurative	*Staphylococcus* spp.	29	12
adenitis	*Serratia* spp.	9	15
	Candida spp.	7	4
Osteomyelitis	*Serratia* spp.	32	12
	Aspergillus spp.	25	18
Bacteremia/	*Salmonella* spp.	20	13
fungemia	*B. cepacia*	13	0
	Candida spp.	9	25
	Staphylococcus spp.	11	0

TABLE 33–4   COMMON INFECTING ORGANISMS ISOLATED FROM CHRONIC GRANULOMATOUS DISEASE PATIENTS

Source: *Williams Hematology,* 8th ed, Chap. 66, Table 66–5, p. 976.

- Some affected persons and carriers who have only a small percent of normal functioning neutrophils have mild disease and a much better prognosis. This finding is most common in X chromosome–linked forms. Gene therapy is being studied, since one could predict that a very small increase in normally functioning neutrophils (e.g., 5%) might significantly ameliorate the disease.

Myeloperoxidase Deficiency (MPO)

- A common autosomal recessive disorder, with a prevalence of 1:2000 in the general population.
- Absence of MPO in primary granules of neutrophils and monocytes (but not eosinophils).
- MPO catalyzes formation of hypochlorous acid; the MPO-deficient neutrophil is slower to kill ingested organisms, but after 1 hour, microbicidal activity is similar to normal as a result of MPO-independent killing systems in the cell.
- The disorder usually does not lead to increased susceptibility to infection.
- In a few patients with diabetes mellitus and MPO deficiency, severe infection with *Candida sp.* has occurred.
- Acquired MPO deficiency can be seen in lead intoxication, myelodysplasia, acute myelogenous leukemia, and ceroid lipofuscinosis.

EVALUATION OF SUSPECTED NEUTROPHIL DYSFUNCTION

- Frequent bacterial infections should alert the clinician to the possibility of a functional neutrophil defect. Many of the tests used to evaluate neutrophils are bioassays, so are subject to great variability; they must be interpreted with caution, always in light of the patient's clinical condition. These tests are reviewed in Fig. 33–1.

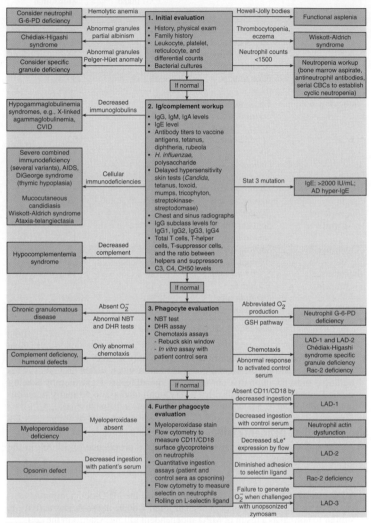

FIGURE 33-1 Algorithm for the evaluation of patients with recurrent infections. (Source: *Williams Hematology*, 8th ed, Chap. 68, Fig. 66–8, p. 979.)

For a more detailed discussion, see Niels Borregaard and Laurence Boxer: Disorders of Neutrophil Function. Chap. 66, p. 951 in *Williams Hematology*, 8th ed.

CHAPTER 34
Eosinophils and Their Diseases

EOSINOPHIL COUNTS

- The normal absolute eosinophil count in adults is less than 0.5×10^9 cells/L.
- The eosinophil count is higher in neonates.
- Eosinophils are primarily tissue dwelling, with 300 cells in the tissues for every blood eosinophil.

CAUSES OF EOSINOPHILIA

- The degree of eosinophilia is described as:
  — Mild (0.5 to 1.5×10^9 eosinophils/L).
  — Moderate (1.5 to 5.0×10^9 eosinophils/L).
  — Marked ($>5.0 \times 10^9$ eosinophils/L).
- The most common causes of eosinophilia include:
  — Worldwide: infections with helminthic parasites.
  — In industrialized countries: asthma and other allergic disorders (drug allergy, allergic rhinitis, atopic dermatitis).
  — Allergic diseases generally result in only mild eosinophilia.
  — The major causes of eosinophilia are listed in Table 34–1.

EOSINOPHILS AND DISEASE

- Eosinophils appear to have a role in both ameliorating inflammatory responses and producing tissue damage.
- They may be important in wound healing and may act as accessory cells in T cell–mediated reactions.
- Because eosinophils can kill parasites, it has been hypothesized that their principal role is to counter parasitic infection.
- Eosinophils can cause airway damage in asthma and severe tissue damage in hypereosinophilic syndromes.

Asthma

- Inhaled antigen produces:
  — An early response, with fall in forced expiratory volume caused by release of mediators from mast cells.
  — A late response with influx of large numbers of eosinophils, activated T cells, and monocytes to the airways.
  — Correlation exists between the numbers of airway eosinophils and the severity of asthma.
  — Basic proteins secreted by eosinophils are toxic for airway epithelium and may be a better guide to the degree of inflammation than eosinophil numbers.

Parasitic Disease

- The mechanism of eosinophilia in parasitic disease is similar to allergic disease.
- The more pronounced eosinophilia in parasitic disease is presumably caused by the systemic nature of the disease compared with the more localized nature of allergic disease.
- Eosinophils can kill a number of opsonized parasite larvae but not adult worms.
- Table 34–2 describes the major parasitic causes of eosinophilia.

TABLE 34–1	CAUSES OF AN EOSINOPHILIA		
Disease	Frequency	Usual Degree of Eosinophilia	Comment
Infections			
Parasitic	Common worldwide	Moderate to high	
Bacterial	Rare		Usually cause eosinopenia, although serum ECP levels may be raised, suggesting eosinophil involvement in tissue.
Mycobacterial	Rare		More often secondary to drug therapy.
Invasive fungal	Rare		Apart from allergic reactions, which are common, and coccidioidomycosis, in which as many as 88% of patients have an eosinophilia.
Rickettsial infections	Rare		
Fungi	Rare		Cryptococcus reported as causing CSF eosinophilia.
Viral infections	Rare		There are occasional case reports of an eosinophilia in a variety of viral infections, including herpes and HIV infection.
Allergic diseases			
Allergic rhinitis	Common worldwide	Mild	
Atopic dermatitis	Common especially children	Mild	
Urticaria/ angioedema	Common	Variable	Eosinophilia seen in skin even with normal blood count.
Asthma	Common	Mild	Syndrome of intrinsic asthma, nasal polyps, and aspirin intolerance are associated with higher-than-usual eosinophil counts.
Drug reactions			
Many drugs	Uncommon	Mild to high	Antibiotics, NSAIDs, and antipsychotics are the most common groups; count usually returns to normal on stopping drug.
Neoplasms			
Acute eosinophilic leukemia	Rare	High	

Disease	Frequency	Usual Degree of Eosinophilia	Comment
Neoplasms (*continued*)			
Acute myelogenous leukemia with marrow eosinophilia	Uncommon	Mild to high in marrow only	Often associated with chromosome 16 abnormalities.
Chronic eosinophilic leukemia	Rare	High	See text on HES.
Chronic myelogenous leukemia	Uncommon	Moderate to high	Raised eosinophil counts can be seen uncommonly in chronic myelogenous leukemia.
Lymphomas	Uncommon	Moderate	Often intense tissue eosinophilia with moderately elevated blood eosinophil count; Hodgkin lymphoma most common type. T-cell lymphomas elaborating IL-5 or other eosinopoietic cytokines.
Langerhans cell histiocytosis	Uncommon	Mild	Intense tissue eosinophilia in granulomata but blood eosinophilia unusual.
Solid tumors	Uncommon	Mild to high	Many different tumors reported.
Musculoskeletal disorders			
Rheumatoid arthritis	Uncommon	Mild to high	Occasional case reports. More usually secondary to therapy.
Eosinophilic fasciitis	Rare	High	
Gastrointestinal disorders			
Eosinophilic gastroenteritis	Rare	Mild to moderate	As with many GI diseases there is often a marked tissue eosinophilia with only a mild or no blood eosinophilia.
Eosinophilic esophagitis	Increasingly recognized	Mild	Marked tissue eosinophilia with mild blood eosinophilia.
Celiac disease	Uncommon	None	Tissue eosinophilia.
Inflammatory bowel disease			Eosinophils seen in biopsies in both Crohn disease and ulcerative colitis, but blood eosinophilia unusual.
Allergic gastroenteritis	Uncommon	Mild to high	Young children.

(*continued*)

TABLE 34–1 **(CONTINUED)**

Disease	Frequency	Usual Degree of Eosinophilia	Comment
Respiratory tract (for asthma, see allergic diseases)			
Churg-Strauss syndrome	Rare	Moderate to high	Syndrome of eosinophilic vasculitis and asthma.
Pulmonary eosinophilia including eosinophilic pneumonia	Uncommon	Mild to high	Syndrome of eosinophilia and pulmonary infiltrates. Apart from ABPA usually of unknown cause.
Bronchiectasis; cystic fibrosis	Common	Mild	Often associated with asthma or ABPA.
Skin diseases (for atopic dermatitis see allergic diseases)			
Bullous pemphigoid	Uncommon	Moderate	
Eosinophilic cellulitis	Uncommon	Moderate to high	High eosinophil count distinguishes from bacterial cause.
Miscellaneous causes			
IL-2 therapy	Rare	Moderate to high	For renal cell carcinoma or melanoma.
Hypereosinophilic syndrome	Uncommon	High	
Endomyocardial fibrosis	Uncommon	High	Secondary to any cause of a high eosinophil count.
Hyper-IgE syndrome	Uncommon	Moderate to high	
Eosinophilia-myalgia syndrome and toxic oil syndrome	Rare	High	Two related conditions, one caused by poisoning with contaminated cooking oil in Spain and the other by a batch of contaminated tryptophan.

ABPA, allergic bronchopulmonary aspergillosis; CSF, cerebrospinal fluid; GI, gastrointestinal; HES, hypereosinophilic syndrome; NSAID, nonsteroidal antiinflammatory drug.
Source: *Williams Hematology*, 8th ed, Chap. 62, Table 62–4, p. 905.

TABLE 34–2 **HELMINTHIC CAUSES OF AN EOSINOPHILIA**

Parasite (Disease)	Comment
Nematodes	
Ascaris (Ascariasis)	Ascariasis results in higher eosinophil counts in children. Larvae migrate from intestine to lungs where they cause Loeffler syndrome, a form of pulmonary eosinophilia.
Toxocara canis (Toxocariasis)	Infective eggs are present in feces of puppies and pregnant bitches. Larvae in hosts such as chicken. Eosinophilia seen mainly in children younger than age 9 years. Can migrate to eye and cause blindness. Serologic evidence suggests infection not uncommon in industrialized countries.

Parasite (Disease)	Comment
Nematodes (*continued*)	
Loa loa (Filariasis, Loiasis); *Wuchereria bancrofti* (Filariasis, Elephantiasis); *Brugia malayi* (Filariasis, Elephantiasis); *Onchocerca volvulus* (Filariasis, River Blindness)	Common. Invariably result in marked eosinophilia, especially *L. loa* filariasis infection. Filariasis is the cause of tropical pulmonary eosinophilia caused by migration of adult worms to lung, elephantiasis caused by involvement of lymphatics (*W. bancrofti* and *B. malayi*) and river blindness (*O. volvulus*). Treatment can result in systemic reaction called Mazzotti reaction, possibly as a result of massive eosinophil degranulation.
Ancylostoma duodenale (Ancylostomiasis, Old World Hookworm) and *Necator americanus* (New World Hookworm)	Hookworm infection. *A. duodenale* and *N. americanus*. One of the main causes of eosinophilia in patients returning from tropical countries. Eosinophil counts in region of $2000 \times 10^6/\mu L$.
Strongyloides stercoralis (Strongyloidiasis)	Subclinical infection can persist for more than 20 years. Stool examinations often negative. Cause of eosinophilia in ex-servicemen who spent time in tropics. If *Strongyloides* infection is not considered and these patients are given glucocorticoids for suspected hypereosinophilic syndrome or as trial of therapy, they can develop disseminated disease.
Trichinella spiralis (Trichinosis)	Trichinosis is caused by ingestion of encysted muscle larvae of *T. spiralis*. Most prominent eosinophilia seen during early stages of infection when larvae migrating into striated muscle via the blood. Fatal cases reported of which only 20% were noted to have an eosinophilia.
Others	Other nematodes that can cause eosinophilia include *Trichuris trichiura* (Trichuriasis), *Capillaria philippinensis* (Capillariasis), and *Gnathostoma spinigerum* (Gnathostomiasis). The thread worm, *Enterobius vermicularis* (Pinworm), occasionally causes an eosinophilia when they invade tissues.
Trematodes	
Schistosoma mansoni, *S. haematobium*, *S. japonicum* (Schistosomiasis, Bilharzia)	Infection with one of the *Schistosoma* (blood flukes), *S. mansoni*, *S. haematobium*, or *S. japonicum*, is perhaps the commonest cause of a moderate to high eosinophilia worldwide with 200 million people infected. Infection is nearly always associated with an eosinophilia.
Fasciola	Adult worms of *Fasciola hepatica* reside in the bile ducts, where they are associated with abnormal liver function tests and an eosinophilia.
Cestodes	
Echinococcus	Eosinophilia occurs in 25–50% of patients with hydatid disease.

Source: *Williams Hematology*, 8th ed, Chap. 62, Table 62–5, p. 907.

Idiopathic Hypereosinophilic Syndrome (Myeloid and Lymphoid Variants)

Definition

- The sporadic occurrence of striking eosinophilia ($>1.5 \times 10^9/L$) in the absence of a disease that is associated with reactive eosinophilia.

Myeloid Type

- Monoclonal eosinophilia, reflecting the expression of chronic eosinophilic leukemia. Marrow contains principally eosinophilic myelocytes and mature eosinophils, some with hypersegmented nuclei (>2 segments).
  - Onset with some or all of the following: anorexia, weight loss, fatigue, nausea, abdominal pain, diarrhea, nonproductive cough, pruritic rash, fever, night sweats, and venous thrombosis.
  - Skin signs: urticaria, papules, pruritus.
  - Cardiac involvement: endocardial fibrosis, restrictive cardiomyopathy, mitral or tricuspid valve incompetence, ventricular failure.
  - Neurologic findings: neuropathies.
  - Organ involvement as a consequence of the noxious effects of eosinophil granule contents is a feature of chronic eosinophilic leukemia.
  - Most patients have cardiac involvement, with congestive heart failure, new murmurs, conduction defects, and arrhythmias.
  - Hepatosplenomegaly, interstitial pulmonary infiltrates, and pleural effusions can occur.
  - Nervous system dysfunction may be profound, including confusion, delirium, dementia, and coma.
  - Anemia occurs in most patients.
  - Thrombocytopenia is seen occasionally.
  - All patients have leukocytosis with a striking eosinophilia, usually eosinophil counts greater than $1.5 \times 10^9/L$, and counts of $50.0 \times 10^9/L$ or more are found in more than half the patients.
  - The eosinophilia may be progressive.
  - Cytogenetic abnormalities may be found in the leukemic eosinophilic cells in a proportion of patients. One of several translocations involving chromosome 5 may occur. Of particular importance is the occurrence of the *FILIPI-PDGFR-α* fusion gene since, if present, the patient will usually respond to tyrosine kinase inhibitor drugs, such as imatinib mesylate.
  - Elevated serum tryptase is common (suggesting unapparent mast cell involvement).
  - The disease is sometimes indolent, but more often progressive and fatal.
  - Signs and symptoms may remit and relapse, but organ damage is usually progressive.
  - Cardiac failure may result from endomyocardial fibrosis.
  - Central nervous system dysfunction may lead to encephalopathy, polyneuropathy, or stroke.
  - Episodes of venous thrombosis may complicate the course.
  - In patients unresponsive to tyrosine kinase inhibitors, hydroxyurea and glucocorticoids may be of benefit in decreasing the eosinophil count and the risk of tissue injury.
  - Other therapies include etoposide, interferon-α, cladribine, and leukapheresis.
  - Surgical replacement of severely damaged heart valves has been successful.
  - Allogeneic hematopoietic stem cell transplantation has been used in some patients.

Lymphoid Type

- A less common cause of hypereosinophilia is a clonal T-lymphocyte disorder (lymphoma) with polyclonal eosinophilia resulting from lymphoma cell elaboration of eosinopoietic cytokines, especially interleukin-5.

— In this lymphoid form of hypereosinophilia, eosinophil-induced tissue damage is not a feature of the disease, suggesting that the tissue damage is a feature of leukemic eosinophils.

— The treatment is directed principally at the underlying lymphoma.

- Table 34–3 contains tests that may be helpful in evaluating patients with the hypereosinophilic syndrome.

Other Types

- The causes of the remaining cases of hypereosinophilia that are neither chronic eosinophilic leukemia nor related to lymphoma are still unclear.

Eosinophilia-Myalgia Syndrome

- First described in 1989, with more than 1500 cases reported and 30 deaths in the next 2 years.
- Caused by the ingestion of L-tryptophan, a nutritional supplement, containing a contaminant.
- Constant features are severe myalgia and eosinophil count greater than 1.0×10^9/L.
- Common findings are arthralgias, cough, dyspnea, edema, hair loss, peripheral neuropathy, and scleroderma-like skin changes.
- Pathologic features mimic eosinophilic fasciitis (see below).
- Glucocorticoids improved symptoms and signs.

Toxic Oil Syndrome

- In 1981, in Spain, more than 20,000 people developed a syndrome of fever, cough, dyspnea, neutrophilia, and eosinophilia. More than 300 deaths occurred.
- Thought to be caused by ingestion of aniline-denatured rapeseed oil.
- Pulmonary infiltrates, pleural effusion, and hypoxemia were common findings.

TABLE 34–3	EVALUATION OF PATIENTS WITH UNEXPLAINED HYPEREOSINOPHILIA

Complete blood counts with examination of blood film
Serum immunoglobulins
Serum vitamin B_{12}
Serum tryptase
Marrow aspirate and biopsy with cytogenetic analysis
Polymerase chain reaction assay or fluorescence in situ hybridization for
    FILIPI-PDGFRa fusion gene
Lymphocyte immunophenotyping
T-cell receptor gene rearrangements
Serum IL-5 measurement
Chest radiograph
Electrocardiogram
Cardiac ultrasound
Complete neurologic examination

Special Tests of Organ Site Damage as Warranted

Nerve conduction studies and electromyography if neuromuscular
    abnormalities
Cardiac magnetic resonance imaging if myocardial or endocardial damage
Chest computed tomography if significant lung or pleural disease
Lung function tests if suspected breathing disorder or decreased arterial blood
    oxygen saturation
Gastrointestinal endoscopy if esophageal or gastric signs or symptoms

- One-half the patients developed a chronic illness that mimicked the eosinophilia–myalgia syndrome (see above), with myalgias, eosinophilia, peripheral neuritis, scleroderma-like skin lesions, hair loss, and sicca syndrome.
- Glucocorticoids may have improved the pulmonary symptoms.

Reactive Hypereosinophilia and Neoplasms

- Marked eosinophilia has been reported in association with a variety of solid tumors and lymphomas (e.g., Hodgkin lymphoma), believed to be caused by IL-5 and other cytokines elaborated by tumor cells.
- Eosinophilia may precede the diagnosis but usually occurs concomitantly.
- Successful treatment of the malignancy may be associated with amelioration of eosinophilia.

Acute Eosinophilic Leukemia

- Rare forms of AML (see Chap. 46).

Eosinophilia, Angiitis, and Asthma

- Polyarteritis nodosa and allergic granulomatosis (Churg-Strauss angiitis) are associated with prominent eosinophilia.
- In patients with asthma and eosinophilia, the development of multiorgan signs (skin, nervous system, kidney, joints, lung, heart, gastrointestinal tract) should lead to consideration of this disorder.

Eosinophilic Fasciitis

- Characterized by stiffness, pain, and swelling of the arms, forearms, thighs, legs, hands, and feet in descending order of frequency.
- Malaise, fever, weakness, and weight loss also occur.
- Absolute eosinophil counts of greater than $1.0 \times 10^9/L$ are found in most patients.
- Biopsy is usually required for diagnosis and shows inflammation, edema, thickening, and fibrosis of the fascia and synovia.
- Aplastic anemia, cytopenias, pernicious anemia, and myelogenous leukemia have been associated.

EOSINOPHILS IN URINE AND CEREBROSPINAL FLUID

- Excretion of eosinophils in the urine is seen most often in urinary tract infection or acute interstitial nephritis.
- Cerebrospinal fluid eosinophilia may occur with infection, shunts, allergic reactions involving the meninges, and Hodgkin lymphoma.

EOSINOPENIA

- The eosinophil count in hospitalized patients is less than $0.01 \times 10^9/L$ in only 0.1 percent of patients.
- Acute infections, glucocorticoids, and epinephrine all decrease the eosinophil count.

For a more detailed discussion, see Andrew J. Wardlaw: Eosinophils and Their Disorders. Chap. 62, p. 897 in *Williams Hematology*, 8th ed.

CHAPTER 35
Basophils and Mast Cells and Their Diseases

BASOPHILIA

- Normal basophil count is 0.015 to 0.08×10^9/L.
- The causes of basophilia are listed in Table 35–1.
- An increase in the absolute basophil count among other blood cell abnormalities may be a useful sign of a chronic clonal myeloid disease (see Table 35–1).
- In chronic myelogenous leukemia (CML), an increased absolute basophil count occurs in virtually all patients.
- *De novo* acute basophilic leukemia is very rare, but marrow basophilia may be associated uncommonly with other subtypes of acute myelogenous or acute promyelocytic leukemia (see Table 35–2).
- Basophils in acute or chronic clonal myeloid diseases are derived from the malignant clone and occasionally may cause symptoms of histamine release (flushing, pruritus, hypotension) or severe peptic ulcer disease reflecting hypersecretion of gastric acid and pepsin.

BASOPHILOPENIA

- The causes of basophilopenia are listed in Table 35–1.

MAST CELLS

- Mast cells are produced in the marrow, transit the blood to the tissues where they reside. They cannot be identified in transit in the blood of healthy individuals by standard techniques.
- Mast cells contain mediators that may be preformed in granules (e.g., histamine, heparin, and chemotactic factors) or newly formed (e.g., arachidonic acid metabolites, such as prostaglandin D_2 and leukotrienes).

REACTIVE MASTOCYTOSIS

- An increased number of mast cells may be seen in any tissue involved in a hypersensitivity reaction.
- An increased number may be seen in the lymph nodes and marrow as a reaction to a variety of benign and malignant tumors.

BENIGN MAST CELL DISEASES

- *Cutaneous mastocytosis* may be expressed as a solitary lesion in infants or as multiple nodules in older children.
- *Urticaria pigmentosa* occurs before age 2 years in 50 percent of cases and is characterized by dermal accumulations of mast cells resulting in brown papules symmetrically distributed, especially over the trunk.
- Intense pruritus and urticaria may occur from mild friction of the skin (Darier sign).
- Demonstration of infiltrates of mast cells on the skin biopsy is diagnostic.

TABLE 35–1	**CONDITIONS ASSOCIATED WITH ALTERATIONS IN NUMBERS OF BLOOD**

Basophils

I. Decreased Numbers (Basopenia)
- A. Hereditary absence of basophils (very rare)
- B. Elevated levels of glucocorticoids
- C. Hyperthyroidism or treatment with thyroid hormones
- D. Ovulation
- E. Hypersensitivity reactions
  1. Urticaria
  2. Anaphylaxis
  3. Drug-induced reactions
- F. Leukocytosis (in association with diverse disorders)

II. Increased Numbers (Basophilia)
- A. Allergy or inflammation
- B. Ulcerative colitis
- C. Drug, food, inhalant hypersensitivity
- D. Erythroderma, urticaria
- E. Juvenile rheumatoid arthritis
- F. Endocrinopathy
  1. Diabetes mellitus
  2. Estrogen administration
  3. Hypothyroidism (myxedema)
- G. Infection
  1. Chicken pox
  2. Influenza
  3. Smallpox
  4. Tuberculosis
- H. Iron deficiency
- I. Exposure to ionizing radiation
- J. Neoplasia
  1. "Basophilic leukemias" (see text)
  2. Myeloproliferative neoplasms (especially chronic myelogenous leukemia; also polycythemia vera, primary myelofibrosis, essential thrombocytemia)
  3. Carcinoma

Source: *Williams Hematology*, 8th ed, Chap. 63, Table 63–2, p. 921.

TABLE 35–2	**LEUKEMIAS ASSOCIATED WITH STRIKING BASOPHILIA**

I. Chronic myelogenous leukemia with exaggerated basophilia

II. Blast transformation of chronic myelogenous leukemia, including acute basophilic transformation, of chronic myelogenous leukemia

III. Acute myeloid leukemia with t(9;22), t(6;9), t(3;6) or 12p abnormalities and marrow basophilia

IV. Acute promyelocytic leukemia with basophilic maturation

V. Acute basophilic leukemia

Source: *Williams Hematology*, 8th ed, Chap. 63, Table 63–3, p. 922.

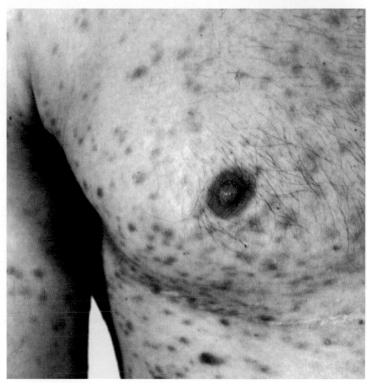

FIGURE 35-1 Urticaria pigmentosa in an adult man with indolent systemic mastocytosis. Multiple pigmented macules are present. If local pressure is applied to the skin, individual lesions show urtication and become raised, pruritic, and erythematous.
(Source: *Williams Hematology*, 8th ed, Chap. 63, Fig. 63–2, p. 924.)

- Urticaria pigmentosa usually subsides at puberty but can continue into adulthood (see **Fig. 35–1**), and later patients may develop systemic mastocytosis.
- A 10-fold increase in mast cells in skin biopsies of chronic inflammatory sites is considered consistent with cutaneous mastocytosis.
- **Table 35–3** lists causes of alterations in mast cell numbers.

SYSTEMIC MASTOCYTOSIS

Clinical Features
- Affects men and women equally.
- Half the patients are older than 60 years of age at the time of diagnosis.
- Malaise, weight loss, and fever are frequent.
- Symptoms of mediator release include urticaria, pruritus, dermatographism, abdominal cramps, diarrhea, nausea, vomiting, musculoskeletal pain, flushing, headaches, dizziness, palpitations, dyspnea, hypotension, syncope, and shock.
- Hyperpigmented skin lesions may be present.
- Lymphadenopathy, hepatomegaly, splenomegaly, and bone pain are frequently present, especially in aggressive disease.
- Osteoporosis complicated by fractures occurs in half the patients.
- **Table 35–4** contains a classification of systemic mast cell disease.

TABLE 35–3	**CONDITIONS ASSOCIATED WITH SECONDARY CHANGES IN MAST CELL NUMBERS**

I. Decreased Numbers
   A. Long-term treatment with glucocorticoids
   B. Primary or acquired immunodeficiency disorders (certain mast cell populations)

II. Increased Numbers
   A. IgE-associated disorders
      1. Allergic rhinitis
      2. Asthma
      3. Urticaria
   B. Connective tissue disorders
      1. Rheumatoid arthritis
      2. Psoriatic arthritis
      3. Scleroderma
      4. Systemic lupus erythematosus
   C. Infectious diseases
      1. Tuberculosis
      2. Syphilis
      3. Parasitic diseases
   D. Neoplastic disorders
      1. Lymphoproliferative diseases* (lymphoplasmacytic lymphoma/ Waldenström macroglobulinemia, other lymphomas, chronic lymphocytic leukemia)
      2. Hematopoietic multipotential progenitor cell diseases* (acute or chronic myelogenous leukemias, myelodysplastic syndromes)
   E. Lymph nodes draining areas of tumor growth
   F. Osteoporosis*
   G. Chronic liver disease*
   H. Chronic renal disease*

* Indicates increase numbers of mast cells may be principally in marrow.
Source: *Williams Hematology*, 8th ed, Chap. 63, Table 63–4, p. 922.

TABLE 35–4	**WORLD HEALTH ORGANIZATION CLASSIFICATION OF SYSTEMIC MASTOCYTOSIS**

  I. Cutaneous mastocytosis (CM)
    A. Urticaria pigmentosa (UP)/Maculopapular cutaneous mastocytosis (MPCM)
    B. Diffuse cutaneous mastocytosis
    C. Solitary mastocytoma of skin

  II. Indolent systemic mastocytosis (ISM)

 III. Systemic mastocytosis with associated clonal, hematologic non–mast-cell lineage disease (SM-AHNMD)

 IV. Aggressive systemic mastocytosis (ASM)

  V. Mast cell leukemia (MCL)

 VI. Mast cell sarcoma (MCS)

VII. Extracutaneous mastocytoma

Modified with permission from Horney HP, Metcalfe DD, Bennett JM, et al: Mastocytosis, in WHO Classification of Tumours of Haematopoietic and Lymphoid Tissues, ed. Swerdlow E, et al. IARC Press, Lyon, 2008:54.
Source: *Williams Hematology*, 8th ed, Chap. 63, Table 63–5, p. 923.

Laboratory Features

- Anemia is present in about half the cases at the time of diagnosis.
- Marrow biopsy shows an increase in mast cells in about 90 percent of patients. Immunohistochemical staining for mast cell tryptase is best for visualizing and quantifying mast cell involvement.
- Mast cells in paraffin tissues are strongly positive for CD117, as are a subset of leukemic myeloblasts. Mast cells, unlike the later, are not positive for peroxidase, however.
- Mast cells in the blood indicate a transformation to leukemia.
- Elevated alkaline phosphatase, aminotransaminases, γ-glutamyltranspeptidase in about 50 percent of patients, reflect liver involvement.
- Skin biopsy shows mast cell accumulations.
- Osteoporosis, osteoblastic, or osteolytic lesions are common on bone imaging studies.
- Aberrant mast cell phenotype by flow cytometry: high side scatter cells (granular) with surface IgE, and CD2+, CD25+, CD35+, CD117+, and CD34− immunophenotype.
- Finding of elevated plasma histamine levels and urinary excretion of the histamine metabolite 1-methyl-4-imidazoleacetic acid are useful diagnostic tests.
- Elevated mast cell tryptase in the serum is an important confirmatory finding.
- Elevated serum or urine histamine or serum tryptase is not pathognomonic of mastocytosis, however, and needs to be integrated with the clinical findings.
- Gain-of-function *KIT* gene mutation, Asp816Val, is a virtually universal finding in adults and many children with mastocytosis.
- Table 35–5 lists the diagnostic criteria for systemic mastocytosis.

Management

- Local lesions may be excised.
- Avoid triggers such as temperature extremes, physical exertion, or in some cases opiate analgesics, nonsteroidal antiinflammatory drugs, ingestion of ethanol containing drinks.
- Anaphylaxis may follow stings by venomous insects. Epinephrine-filled syringes and instructions for self-administration should be carried by patients considered at risk. These patients may also benefit from prophylactic

---

TABLE 35–5 **DIAGNOSTIC CRITERIA FOR SYSTEMIC MASTOCYTOSIS**

I. Major Criteria
   A. Multifocal, dense infiltrates of mast cells ($\geq$15 mast cells in an aggregate) detected in sections of marrow and/or other extracutaneous organ(s)

II. Minor Criteria
   A. In biopsy sections of marrow or other extracutaneous organs, >25% of the mast cells in the infiltrate are spindle shaped or have atypical morphology, or, of all mast cells in marrow aspirate smears, >25% are immature or atypical mast cells
   B. Detection of a point mutation in *KIT* at codon 816 (Asp816V) in marrow, blood, or other extracutaneous organ
   C. Mast cells in marrow, blood, or other extracutaneous organs that co-express CD117 with CD2 and/or CD25
   D. Serum total tryptase persistently >20 μg/L (if there is an associated clonal myeloid disorder, this criterion is not valid)

The diagnosis of systemic mastocytosis can be made if one major and one minor criterion are present or if three minor criteria are met.

Source: *Williams Hematology*, 8th ed, Chap. 63, Table 63–6, p. 925.

antihistamines in settings and during seasons that insect stings are prevalent. Patients with mastocytosis can also have anaphylaxis from iodinated contrast material.

- Mastocytosis currently has no curative therapy and symptomatic therapy, although transiently helpful, does not alter course of the disease.
- Histamine-2 (H_2)-receptor antagonists (e.g., cimetidine, ranitidine, famotidine) can decrease gastric hyperacidity, and can be used to treat gastritis or peptic ulcer. Proton pump inhibitors may also be useful in treating gastric hypersecretion. They may, in combination with histamine-1 (H_1)-receptor antagonists, contribute to ameliorating mast-cell constituent release–related signs and symptoms.
- H_1-receptor antagonists (e.g., diphenhydramine, chlorpheniramine, tricyclic antidepressants) can decrease flushing, vasodilation, and headache. More potent H_1-receptor blockers (hydroxyzine and doxepin) may be useful in more severe cases.
- Oral disodium cromoglycate may alleviate gastrointestinal cramping, diarrhea, and headache. It has also been useful in childhood cutaneous mast cell disease.
- Ketotifen may ameliorate pruritus and wheal formation and may minimize osteoporosis.
- Diphosphonates have also been used to stop or reverse osteopenia.
- Cutaneous glucocorticoids and 8-methoxypsoralen and ultraviolet light (PUVA) have been reported to decrease pruritus or improve the appearance of skin lesions.
- Oral glucocorticoids can be used for malabsorption or ascites. In adults, the doses used to start therapy are approximately 0.75 mg/kg for 2 to 3 weeks and then they are tapered, eventuating in alternate day use, if they are helpful.
- Insufficient data are available to determine the usefulness of cytotoxic agents, such as cladrabine, for progressive mastocytosis. Chemotherapy, generally, has been disappointing in cases of aggressive systemic disease.
- Allogeneic stem cell transplantation has been used very infrequently, especially if an associated clonal myeloid disease coexists, but the mastocytic component of disease seems not to have been benefitted, usually.
- In all the therapy noted above, success is unpredictable, the treatment has its own consequential side effects, and one must exercise judgment continually about whether the treatment is resulting in a net benefit to the patient.
- Avoid mast cell stimulants such as alcohol, anticholinergics, aspirin, other non-steroidal antiinflammatory agents, and morphine derivatives.
- Inhibitors of mutant *KIT*-encoded tyrosine kinase (e.g., imatinib mesylate) have been generally unsuccessful in therapy because the most prevalent *KIT* mutation at codon 816 (Asp816Val) is resistant to these drugs. Rare mutations such as *KIT* (Phe522Cys) are responsive. Some diseases not technically mastocytosis but with elevated mast cells and elevated serum tryptase and with the *FIPIL1-PDGFRA* fusion gene do respond. (e.g., chronic eosinophilic leukemia, see Chaps. 34 and 47). If possible, mutational analysis on the mastocytosis cells should be done to determine if a drug-sensitive mutated kinase is present.

Course and Prognosis

- Symptoms range from absent to progressive and disabling. Patients with urticaria pigmentosa and indolent systemic mast cell disease may live a normal life span with symptomatic treatment. Progression to advanced disease is rare and some improve spontaneously.
- About one-third of patients have systemic mastocytosis with an associated hematologic malignancy. In these cases, the prognosis is related to the ability to manage the hematologic disease. Usually this combination portends a foreshortened life span.
- Elevated serum lactic dehydrogenase and more advanced age tend to be poor prognostic findings.
- Overall 3-year survival is about 50 percent.

MAST CELL LEUKEMIA

- Patients may have fever, constitutional symptoms, and severe clinical manifestations of mediator release (see above).
- Hepatomegaly, splenomegaly, and lymphadenopathy are common.
- Anemia and thrombocytopenia are nearly always present; the white count varies from 10.0 to 150×10^9/L, and mast cells make up 5 to 90 percent of the blood leukocytes.
- Marrow shows a striking increase in mast cells, sometimes up to 90 percent of cells.

MAST CELL SARCOMA

- A rare tumor, characterized by nodules at various cutaneous and mucosal sites; subsequently, almost every organ becomes involved by extensive mast cell infiltration; terminally, the blood cells are nearly all immature mast cells with a monocytoid appearance.

For a more detailed discussion, see Stephen J. Galli, Dean D. Metcalf, Daniel A. Arber, Ann M. Dvorak: Basophils and Mast Cells and Their Diseases. Chap. 63, p. 915 in *Williams Hematology*, 8th ed.

PART IV

DISORDERS OF MONOCYTES AND MACROPHAGES

CHAPTER 36
Monocytosis and Monocytopenia

- Monocytes in the blood are in transit. They function in the tissues, where they mature into macrophages and participate in:
  — Inflammation, including granulomatous reactions, atheroma formation, and tissue repair.
  — Immunologic reactions, including delayed hypersensitivity.
  — Reactions to neoplasia and allografts.
- The need for macrophages in tissues also can be met by local proliferation of macrophages, not requiring increased transit of blood monocytes.
- Ninety percent of blood monocytes intensely express CD14 (lipopolysaccharide receptor) but not CD16 and 10 percent have weak expression of CD14 and strongly express CD16.
- Older persons have a striking decrease in the proportion of CD14+CD16− to CD14+CD16+ monocytes compared with younger persons.
- Disorders rarely produce abnormalities of monocytes alone, in the absence of other blood cell abnormalities.

NORMAL BLOOD MONOCYTE CONCENTRATION

- The monocyte count averages 1.0×10^9/L in neonatal life, gradually decreasing to a mean of 0.4×10^9/L in adult life.
- Monocytosis (in adults): $>0.8 \times 10^9$/L.
- Monocytopenia: $<0.2 \times 10^9$/L.

HEMATOLOGIC DISORDERS ASSOCIATED WITH MONOCYTOSIS

- See Table 36–1.

Neoplastic or Clonal Monocytic Proliferations
- Oligoblastic myelogenous leukemia (refractory leukemia with excess blasts or myelodysplastic syndrome).
- Acute myelogenous leukemia (myelomonocytic or monocytic types).
- Chronic myelomonocytic leukemia.

TABLE 36–1   **DISORDERS ASSOCIATED WITH MONOCYTOSIS**

I. Hematologic disorders
  A. Myeloid neoplasms
    1. Myelodysplastic states
    2. Acute monocytic leukemia
    3. Acute myelomonocytic leukemia
    4. Acute monocytic leukemia with histiocytic features
    5. Acute myeloid dendritic cell leukemia
    6. Chronic myelomonocytic leukemia
    7. Juvenile myelomonocytic leukemia B. Infections
    8. Chronic myelogenous leukemia (m-*BCR*–positive type)
    9. Polycythemia vera
  B. Chronic neutropenias
  C. Drug-induced neutropenia
  D. Postagranulocytic recovery
  E. Lymphocytic neoplasms
    1. B-cell Lymphoma
    2. T-cell Lymphoma
    3. Hodgkin disease
    4. Myeloma
    5. Macroglobulinemia
  F. Drug-induced pseudolymphoma
  G. Immune hemolytic anemia
  H. Idiopathic thrombocytopenic purpura
  I. Postsplenectomy state

II. Inflammatory and Immune Disorders
  A. Connective tissue diseases
    1. Rheumatoid arthritis
    2. Systemic lupus erythematosus
    3. Temporal arteritis
    4. Myositis
    5. Polyarteritis nodosa
    6. Sarcoidosis
  B. Infections
    1. Mycobacterial infections
    2. Subacute bacterial endocarditis
    3. Brucellosis
    4. Dengue hemorrhagic fever
    5. Resolution phase of acute bacterial infections
    6. Syphilis
    7. Cytomegalovirus infection
    8. Varicella-zoster virus

III. Gastrointestinal disorders
  A. Alcoholic liver disease
  B. Inflammatory bowel disease
  C. Sprue

IV. Nonhematopoietic malignancies

V. Exogenous cytokine administration

VI. Myocardial infarction

VII. Cardiac bypass surgery

VIII. Miscellaneous conditions
   A. Tetrachloroethane poisoning
   B. Parturition
   C. Glucocorticoid administration
   D. Depression
   E. Thermal injury
   F. Marathon running
   G. Holoprosencephaly
   H. Kawasaki disease
   I. Wiskott-Aldrich syndrome

Source: *Williams Hematology*, 8th ed, Chap. 71, Table 71–1, p. 1042.

- Juvenile myelomonocytic leukemia
- Unusual type of *BCR-ABL* (p190)-positive chronic myelogenous leukemia with monocytosis.

Reactive (Nonclonal) Monocytic Proliferations

- Neutropenic states: cyclic neutropenia; chronic granulocytopenia of childhood; familial benign neutropenia; infantile genetic agranulocytosis; chronic hypoplastic neutropenia.
- Drug-induced agranulocytosis (transient monocytosis, especially in the recovery phase).
- Chlorpromazine toxicity, monocytosis precedes the agranulocytosis.
- Lymphoma.
- Hodgkin lymphoma.
- Postsplenectomy state.
- Myeloma.

INFLAMMATORY AND IMMUNE DISORDERS ASSOCIATED WITH MONOCYTOSIS

- See Table 36–1.

Collagen Vascular Diseases

- Rheumatoid arthritis.
- Systemic lupus erythematosus.
- Temporal arteritis.
- Myositis.
- Polyarteritis nodosa.

Chronic Infections

- Bacterial infections, e.g., subacute bacterial endocarditis, tonsillitis, dental infections, recurrent liver abscesses (probably *not* in typhoid fever or brucellosis).
- Tuberculosis.
- Syphilis: neonatal, primary, and secondary.
- Viral infections: cytomegalovirus, varicella-zoster virus.

Other Inflammatory Disorders

- Sprue.
- Ulcerative colitis.
- Regional enteritis.
- Sarcoidosis (the degree of monocytosis is inversely related to reduction in number of T lymphocytes).

NONHEMATOPOIETIC MALIGNANCIES

- Found in about 20 percent of patients who have monocytosis; independent of metastatic disease.

MISCELLANEOUS CONDITIONS ASSOCIATED WITH MONOCYTOSIS

- Alcoholic liver disease.
- Tetrachloroethane poisoning.
- Langerhans cell histiocytosis.
- Parturition.
- Severe depression.
- See also Table 36–1.

DISORDERS ASSOCIATED WITH MONOCYTOPENIA

- Aplastic anemia.
- Hairy cell leukemia:
  — May be a helpful diagnostic clue.
  — Contributes to the frequent infections.
- Chronic lymphocytic leukemia.
- Cyclic neutropenia.
- Severe thermal injury.
- Rheumatoid arthritis.
- Systemic lupus erythematosus.
- HIV infections.
- Postradiation therapy.
- Following the administration of:
  — Glucocorticoids.
  — α-Interferon.
  — Tumor necrosis factor-α.

Blood Dendritic Cells

- Blood dendritic cells are composed of two phenotypic subtypes: myeloid-derived (HLA-Dr+CD11c+CD123+) and lymphoid-plasmacytoid-derived (HLA-Dr+CD11c–CD123+).
- The total blood dendritic cell count can be measured by flow cytometry.
- Dendritic cells make up approximately 0.6 percent of blood cells (range: 0.15 to 1.30%) and represent 14×10^6 cells/L (range: 3 to 30×10^6 cells/L). Approximately one-third of these cells are lymphoid-plasmacytoid–derived type and two-thirds are myeloid-derived type.
- Blood dendritic cell counts decrease with aging and increase with surgical stress (and presumably other stressful reactions) in relation to plasma cortisol levels.
- Fluctuations in blood dendritic cells are often independent of changes in blood monocyte counts.

For a more detailed discussion, see Marshall A. Lichtman: Monocytosis and Monocytopenia. Chapter 71, p. 1041 in *Williams Hematology*, 8th ed.

CHAPTER 37
Inflammatory and Malignant Histiocytosis

- The terms *histiocyte* and *macrophage* are synonyms for the mature cell of the monocyte-macrophage system. The latter is the preferred term in discussions of cell biology and immunology, but the former term continues to be used by pathologists and in textbooks for diseases of macrophages because of its entrenchment in the medical literature.
- A classification of the histiocytoses most relevant to hematologists is shown in Table 37–1. They have been classified based on whether they are monocyte-derived dendritic-cell-related, monocytes-macrophage-related, or neoplastic transformations of dendritic-cells or macrophages.
- Distinctions among the diseases of macrophages are made based on clinical findings, histopathology, immunophenotyping of surface antigen, cytochemistry, and cytogenetic or genetic features (Table 37–2).

TABLE 37–1	CLASSIFICATION OF HISTIOCYTIC DISORDERS

I. Disorders of varying biologic behavior, lacking cytologic atypia
  A. Dendritic-cell related*
    1. Langerhans cell histiocytosis
    2. Juvenile xanthogranuloma
    3. Erdheim-Chester disease
  B. Monocyte-macrophage related
    1. Hemophagocytic lymphohistiocytosis
      a. Familial and/or with identified dysfunctional gene mutation
    2. Secondary hemophagocytic syndromes
      a. Infection associated
      b. Malignancy associated
      c. Autoimmune associated
      d. Other
    3. Sinus histiocytosis with massive lymphadenopathy (Rosai-Dorfman disease)
    4. Solitary histiocytoma of macrophage phenotype

II. Malignant disorders
  A. Dendritic-cell related
  B. Histiocytic sarcoma
  C. Monocyte-macrophage related
  D. Leukemias
    1. Acute monocytic and, acute myelomonocytic (see Chap. 46)
    2. Chronic myelomonocytic leukemias (see Chap. 47)

*Here Langerhans cell histiocytosis is placed in relationship to monocyte-derived dendritic cell disorders. There is evidence that the dendritic cell proliferation in Langerhans cell histiocytosis is clonal and, thus, it is pathologically a neoplasm.
Source: *Williams Hematology*, 8th ed, Chap. 72, Table 72–2, p. 1048.

TABLE 37–2 DISTINCTIONS IN ANTIBODIES TO CELL-SURFACE EPITOPES AND MICROSCOPIC FINDINGS AMONG THE HISTIOCYTIC DISEASES

Clinical Findings	Langerhans Cell Histiocytosis	Malignant Histiocytosis	Erdheim-Chester Disease/ Juvenile Xanthogranuloma	Hemophagocytic Lymphohistiocytosis	Rosai-Dorfman Disease
	Langerhans cell	Interdigitating dendritic cell	Dermal dendritic cell	Monocyte-macrophage	Sinus histiocyte
HLH-DR	++	+	–	+	+
CD1a	++	–	–	–	–
CD14	–	–	++	++	++
CD68	+/–	+/–	++	++	++
CD163	–	–	–	++	++
CD 207 (Langerin)	+++	+	–	–	–
Factor XIIIa	–	–	++	–	–
Fascin	–	++	++	+/–	+
Birbeck granules	+	–	–	–	–
Hemophagocytosis	+/–	–	–	+/–	–
Emperipolesis	–	–	–	–	+

Source: *Williams Hematology*, 8th ed, Chap. 72, Table 72–1, p. 1048.

CLONAL HISTIOCYTOSES

Langerhans Cell Histiocytosis

Definition and History

- The term *Langerhans cell histiocytosis* includes disorders previously called histiocytosis X (eosinophilic granuloma, Letterer-Siwe disease, Hand-Schüller-Christian disease), self-healing histiocytosis, and Langerhans cell granulomatosis.
- Langerhans cells are macrophages with irregularly shaped nuclei present in epidermis, mucosa, lymph nodes, thymus, and spleen.
- As all macrophages types, they originate in marrow from a multipotential hematopoietic cell.
- Identified by unique racquet-shaped ultrastructural inclusions (Birbeck bodies) and by immunoreactivity to neuroprotein S-100, neuronal specific enolase, and surface antigen CD1a and CD207 (Langerin). Birbeck bodies, CD1a expression, and strong CD207 expression are pathognomonic for Langerhans cells.
- Principal function is to process antigen and present it to T cells.

Etiology and Pathogenesis

- Although long thought to be an inflammatory or immunologic disorder, it is now known to be a clonal disease, and, therefore, a neoplastic disorder with localized and disseminated forms.
- X-chromosome–linked, DNA probes found clonal CD1a+ histiocytes in all lesions tested whether solitary or widespread and whether the lesional cells studied are in one organ or another. In contrast, the T lymphocytes are polyclonal.
- The disease simulates inflammation because the neoplastic Langerhans cell, a dendritic histiocyte, makes up a very small fraction of most lesions ≤1 percent.
- The lesion is composed largely of accompanying inflammatory cells (e.g., eosinophils, T lymphocytes, macrophages), and is often xanthomatous, fibrotic, or granulomatous, simulating inflammation or infection.

Epidemiology

- Approximately 6 cases per million children less than age 15 years.
- Disease appears before age 10 years in 75 percent and before age 30 years in 90 percent of patients.
- Median age of presentation is 30 months, but disease can present in adults of any age.
- Males frequently have localized disease; 90 percent of cases with multisystem involvement occur before age 20 years.

Pathogenesis

- Langerhans cell histiocytosis could be a neoplasm based on the compelling evidence in several laboratories for a monoclonal pattern. Studies of adult solitary pulmonary involvement have not found clonal Langerhans cells. Array comparative genomic hybridization did not identify gene mutations in CD207+ cells (presumptive Langerhans cells).
- The Langerhans cells in this disorder behave as an immature dendritic cell and does not stimulate primary T-cell responses effectively. They present antigen poorly and proliferate at a low rate.

Clinical Findings

- Patients may present with single or multiorgan involvement.
- Lesions often involve bone (especially skull and facial bones), skin, lungs, lymph nodes, spleen, thymus, pituitary, and hypothalamus.
- Disease may be localized to a bone or soft tissue site, multifocal in bone only, or multifocal in bone and other sites.

- The disease can occur in any bone. The skull, femur, ribs, vertebrae (esp. cervical) and humerus are the most frequent sites involved.
- In children, the most frequent site is a lytic lesion of the skull, either painful or not.
- Bony involvement in the face bones has a several-fold risk of central nervous system involvement and diabetes insipidus.
- Diabetes insipidus may appear early or late in the course and is the most frequent sign of central nervous system involvement.
- Diabetes insipidus is the presenting symptom in approximately 4 percent of patients and 15 to 20 percent will develop diabetes insipidus during the course of the disease.
- Uncommonly, other central nervous system effects of the disease occur (e.g., mass lesions in gray or white matter, neurodegeneration with dysarthria, ataxia, dysmetria). Magnetic resonance imaging may show significant brain changes years before onset of clinical manifestations.
- Cervical lymph nodes most common lymphatic site involved. The thymus and mediastinal nodes may be enlarged.
- Infants may have fever, otitis media, or mastoiditis, with enlargement of liver, spleen, and lymph nodes, or self-limited skin lesions of head and neck.
- Skin lesions can have seborrheic or eczematoid features, and in infants, can be mistaken as prolonged "cradle cap" and in adults as dandruff.
- Skin lesions commonly affect skin flexures in groin, perianal area, the ears, the neck, the armpits, and below the breasts.
- Skin lesions in older children and adults may appear as red papules. Lesions may ulcerate.
- Skin lesions may precede more diffuse disease.
- Oral mucosal lesions include gingival hypertrophy, ulcers on the soft or hard palate, tongue, or lips can develop.
- Children and adolescents often have pain, tenderness, swelling caused by lytic bone lesion(s); bleeding from gastrointestinal tract; polydipsia; and polyuria as a result of hypothalamic involvement.
- Adult males may have primary pulmonary involvement causing chronic nonproductive cough, chest pain, dyspnea, wheezing. High frequency of associated lung cancer.
- Young women may have localized involvement of the genital tract or it may be part of multicentric involvement. Pregnancy is associated with exacerbation of diabetes insipidus.
- High-risk of severe disease sites include liver, spleen, lung, marrow.
- Massive splenomegaly can result in cytopenias.
- Liver enlargement can lead to dysfunction with low albumin, hyperbilirubinemia, and clotting factor deficiencies. Sclerosing cholangitis as a result of bile duct injury is a very serious complication.
- Lung involvement is far more common in adults than children and is associated with cigarette smoking. Chest radiographs show an interstitial infiltrate but computed tomography uncovers cystic and nodular pattern characteristic of Langerhans cell histiocytosis. Later fibrosis can lead to severe pulmonary insufficiency.
- Marrow involvement may be associated with hemophagocytic macrophages as a result of cytokine activation but bone or skin involvement and biopsy results should discriminate between hemophagocytic lymphohistiocytosis and Langerhans cell histiocytosis.
- Low-risk of severe disease sites includes skin, bone, lymph nodes, and pituitary gland singly or in any combination.

Laboratory Findings

- Neutrophilia, increased erythrocyte sedimentation rate, increased serum alkaline phosphatase level and other abnormalities indicative of liver disease may occur.

- Biopsy of involved tissue demonstrates pathologic Langerhans cells: abundant in proliferative lesions, scarce in fibrotic lesions. Langerhans cells express CD1a and CD207.
- Radiographs, computer tomograms, or positron emission tomograms can identify bone lesions. The later technique is useful to measure healing of bone after therapy.

Differential Diagnosis

- Depending on site of involvement, includes chronic granulomatous infections, various infections, lymphoma, collagen vascular disease, pneumoconiosis, amyloidosis.
- Reactive Langerhans cells may be present in biopsies of Hodgkin lymphoma, malignant lymphoma, and chronic lymphocytic leukemia.

Treatment

- Treatment of **skin disease** is dictated in part by extent of involvement. Topical glucocorticoids usually do not induce a satisfactory response. Oral methotrexate (20 mg/m^2), once weekly, for 6 months or oral thalidomide, 50 to 200 mg, nightly, can be beneficial. Topical nitrogen mustard may benefit those not responding to oral agents, if the disease is not widespread. Psoralen with ultraviolet A light (PUVA) has been used.
- Patients with **skull lesions of mastoid, temporal, or orbital bones** have a risk of developing diabetes insipidus and should receive 6 months of treatment with vinblastine, 6 mg/m^2, intravenously, weekly for 7 weeks, and then every 3 weeks, if a good response, coupled with prednisone, 40 mg/m^2, orally, daily, for 4 weeks, then tapered to zero over next 2 weeks. Thereafter, prednisone is given at 40 mg/m^2, orally, daily for 5 days, every 3 weeks with vinblastine injections.
- Patients with **femoral or vertebral lesions at risk of collapse** require orthopedic and neurosurgical evaluation. Radiation therapy and a stabilizing orthopedic or neurosurgical procedure, respectively, may be required.
- Patients with **bone lesions or combinations of skin, lymph node, or pituitary gland involvement with or without bone lesions** should receive (a) 6 months of treatment with vinblastine, 6 mg/m^2, intravenously, weekly for 7 weeks, and then every 3 weeks, if a good response, coupled with prednisone, 40 mg/m^2, orally, daily, for 4 weeks, then tapered to zero over next 2 weeks. Thereafter, prednisone is given at 40 mg/m^2, orally, daily for 5 days, every 3 weeks with vinblastine injections. Single drug treatment is insufficient in this setting and has a high relapse rate.
- Patients with spleen, liver, marrow, or lung (with or without skin, bone, lymph node, or pituitary gland involvement) should receive multidrug therapy as shown in Table 37–3.
- Patients with **central nervous system mass lesions** have received cladrabine in doses ranging from 5 to 13 mg/m^2 at various frequencies. Also, various other drug combinations have been reported for treatment of neurodegenerative disease associated with Langerhans cell histiocytosis.
- Optimal treatment of children with recurrent or refractory, or progressive disease has not been determined.
- Blood component therapy may be needed for severe cytopenias.
- Splenectomy for massive symptomatic splenomegaly and transfusion dependence (hypersplenism).
- Allogeneic hematopoietic stem cell transplantation has been beneficial in some patients with multisystem disease who were refractory to multidrug regimens. Non-myeloablative conditioning has been used successfully.
- Specific approaches have not yet been developed in clinical trials for refractory or recurrent disease and depends on the organ(s) involved and the duration of the prior remission.

- For isolated bone disease that recurs 6 months or more after the end of treatment, the same treatment program with vinblastine and prednisone can be reused (see above discussion on treatment of bone lesions).
- For high-risk organ disease, a multidrug program akin to that used for acute myelogenous leukemia or aggressive lymphoma, which includes cytarabine and cladrabine, can be used. Allogeneic stem cell transplantation should be incorporated into the latter treatment plan in eligible patients.
- Cladrabine and pentostatin have been used in relapsed patients and have frequent salutary effect in those with skin, bone, and lymph node involvement but less so in patients with liver, marrow, spleen or lung involvement.

Course and Prognosis

- Good prognosis is associated with isolated bone lesions.
- Poor prognosis is associated with onset of disease during first 2 years of life, fever not explained by infection, blood cytopenias, and abnormal liver function or pulmonary function tests.
- Refractory multisystem disease is defined as progression on therapy during first 6 weeks or no response to therapy by 12 weeks. Children in this category have approximately a 10 percent chance of long-term survival.
- Long-term survival (cure) in patients treated with vinblastine and prednisone for low-risk disease is very high, if treatment extends well beyond 6 months.
- Long-term survival in high-risk patients is dependent on a multidrug regimen (see Table 37–3), but many can enter long-term remissions. Long-term remissions are in the range of 80 percent following allogeneic hematopoietic stem cell transplantation.
- About 25 percent of children with low-risk disease treated successfully have long-term sequelae of therapy. Those with diabetes insipidus are at risk for hypopituitarism (up to 55 percent with growth hormone deficiency at 10 years follow-up) and should be monitored carefully for growth and development.

TABLE 37–3   COMPARISON OF RESULTS OF INTENSIVE MULTIDRUG THERAPY IN HIGH-RISK PATIENTS WITH LANGERHANS CELL HISTIOCYTOSIS

	Protocol Used			
	DAL-HX	LCH-I	LCH-II	JLCHSG-96
No. patients	63	143	193	59
Median age at diagnosis (years)	0.9	1.5	1	0.9
Therapy duration (months)	12	6	6	7.5
Response (% of patients)	79	53	63*, 74[†]	76
Reactivation (% of patients with a response)	30	50	47	45
Survival (% at 3 years)	94	93	88	97

DAL, Deutsche Arbeitsgemeinschaft für Leukaemieforschung und therapie in Kindersalter; LCH-I and LCH-II: Histiocyte Society, Langerhans cell histiocytosis treatment protocols I and II; JLCHSG, Japan Langerhans Cell Histiocytosis Study Group.
For example, the LC-II protocol included treatment with vinblastine, etoposide, prednisone, and 6-mercaptopurine. A protocol used by the JLCHSG included cytarabine, prednisolone, or methotrexate or daunorubicin, cyclophosphamide, vincristine, and prednisolone, if a prior poor response.
*Arm A (Vinblastine, prednisone, 6-mercaptopurine).
[†]Arm B (Vinblastine, prednisone, etoposide, 6-mercaptopurine).
Source: *Williams Hematology*, 8th ed, Chap.72, Table 72–3, p. 1052.

- About 75 percent of patients treated for high-risk disease have long-term problems. Orthopedic problems, hearing loss, neurologic abnormalities, and cognitive defects are among the sequelae seen. Secondary malignancies after intensive multidrug therapy, pulmonary insufficiency, sclerosing cholangitis, and marrow insufficiency may develop.

Special Characteristics in Adults with Langerhans Cell Histiocytosis
- Manifestations very similar to childhood cases.
- The disease has a median age of presentation of approximately 45 years.
- Isolated adult pulmonary disease has an association with smoking.
- In adults, chest pain may indicate a pneumothorax, which can be the presenting sign of pulmonary disease.
- Long periods before a diagnosis is made.
- Presenting symptoms in order of frequency are: dyspnea or tachypnea, polydipsia and polyuria, bone pain, weight loss, masses in lymph node areas, fever, gum problems, ataxia, and memory problems.
- Presenting signs in order of frequency are: skin rash, scalp nodules, soft-tissue swelling near bone lesions, lymphadenopathy, gingival hypertrophy, hepatosplenomegaly.
- Eighty percent of adult patients presenting with diabetes insipidus had other organ involvement develop over time (e.g., bone, skin, lung, lymph nodes).
- Adults have more frequent involvement of the mandible than children (30 versus 7%) and less frequent involvement of the skull than children (21 versus 40%).

Malignant Histiocytosis
Definition
- A rare, rapidly fatal disorder associated with jaundice, lymphadenopathy, refractory anemia, leukopenia, and hepatosplenomegaly.
- Malignant histiocytosis has been confused with large cell lymphomas. The term *malignant histiocytosis* should be restricted to neoplasms in which the cells have the immunophenotype of histiocytes.

Clinical Features
- Median age of onset is 35 years.
- Fever, weakness, weight loss, malaise, and sweating are frequent if disease is widespread (see Table 37–4).
- Generalized lymphadenopathy, hepatomegaly, and splenomegaly are frequent.
- Skin, central nervous system, and lung involvement may be associated.
- Localized disease may appear in skin, intestines, or isolated lymph node group.

Laboratory Features
- Anemia and thrombocytopenia present at time of diagnosis in virtually all patients; leukopenia is frequent.
- Marrow examination occasionally shows hemophagocytic macrophages, which are not an important diagnostic feature.
- Increased levels of serum bilirubin and lactic acid dehydrogenase often present. Liver-derived enzymes usually not significantly elevated.
- Elevated serum levels of tumor necrosis factor (TNF)-α, interleukin (IL)-6, IL-1α receptor, α_1-antitrypsin, and lysozyme, and angiotensin-converting enzyme are often present.

Diagnosis
- Diagnosis requires lymph node biopsy, marrow aspiration/biopsy, or biopsy of another involved site and unequivocal demonstration of macrophage phenotype and exclusion of lymphocyte phenotype.

TABLE 37–4 **CLINICAL FEATURES OF MALIGNANT HISTIOCYTIC DISEASES**

Histological type	Signs and symptoms	Comments
Dendritic or Langerhans cell sarcoma	Fever, weight loss, erythematous nodules or a skin rash. May involve bone, lymph nodes, lung, liver, brain.	May evolve from follicular (B-cell) lymphoma
Extranodal histiocytic sarcoma	Affect soft tissues of extremities (painless masses), gastrointestinal tract (painful masses), nasal cavity, lung and regional lymph nodes.	Most present as stage I or II tumors.
Interdigitating dendritic cell sarcoma	May be extranodal or lymph nodal. Extranodal cases can involve vertebrae, gastrointestinal tract, marrow, chest wall, pelvic space.	About 50% present with extranodal disease.
Follicular Dendritic cell sarcoma	Nodal and extranodal sites can be involved. Slow growing and painless tumors. Cervical, supraclavicular, and axillary nodes most commonly involved, but mediastinal or mesenteric nodes can be less often.	Metastasis uncommon but can involve lungs.

- Neoplastic histiocytes are positive for nonspecific esterase but not for peroxidase reactions, cytochemically.
- Usually can be distinguished by immunophenotype (Table 37–5). In addition, may variably express monocyte-macrophage surface antigens (e.g., CD11b, CD11c, CD14, CD15, CD33, CD36).
- Negative for T- and B-lymphocyte surface markers and do not have immunoglobulin or T-cell–receptor gene rearrangements.

TABLE 37–5 **MORPHOLOGIC AND IMMUNOPHENOTYPIC DISTINCTIONS AMONG MALIGNANT HISTIOCYTIC AND DENDRITIC TUMORS**

Phenotypic Feature	Histiocytic Sarcoma (18)	Langerhans Cell Tumor/ Sarcoma (26)	Follicular Dendritic Cell Tumor/ Sarcoma (13)	Interdigitating Cell Sarcoma (4)
Birbeck granules	Absent	Present	Absent	Absent
Desmosomes	Absent	Absent	Present	Present
Complex cellular junctions	Absent	Absent	Absent	Present
CD1a	0%	100%	0%	0%
S-100 protein	33%	100%	54%	100%
CD21	0%	0%	100%	0%
CD35	0%	0%	100%	0%
CD68	100%	96%	61%	50%

Parentheses indicate number of cases studied. Desmosomes (syn. macula adherens) are anchoring cell-to-cell junctions that form particularly strong intercellular bonds.
Source: *Williams Hematology*, 7th ed, Chap. 72, Table 72–5, p. 1001.

Differential Diagnosis

- Anaplastic large cell lymphomas, which are usually positive for CD30 and may express T-cell or, less often, B-cell antigens; Hodgkin lymphoma, and malignant fibrous histiocytoma, a myofibroblastic tumor that had masqueraded as a histiocytoma on morphologic grounds before marker studies were available.
- Related to other monocyte-macrophage neoplasms. Monoblastic leukemia without maturation, if extramedullary involvement is present and marrow is only partially involved. Generally, marrow involvement becomes extensive and leukemia becomes obvious in a short time.
- Langerhans cell sarcoma and follicular dendritic cell tumors are rare malignancies that have been characterized as macrophagic tumors.

Treatment

- No systematic drug trials because of infrequency of this tumor.
- Multidrug regimens, similar to those used for large-cell lymphomas (e.g., cyclophosphamide, doxorubicin, vincristine, and prednisone; also bleomycin, teniposide, mechlorethamine hydrochloride, and procarbazine are drugs that have been included in some multidrug programs) given at monthly intervals for variable periods.
- Remissions are infrequent but occasional long responses (~5 to 7 years) have been observed.
- Allogeneic hematopoietic stem cell transplantation should be considered in eligible patients.

INFLAMMATORY DISORDERS OF HISTIOCYTES

Hemophagocytic Lymphohistiocytosis

Definition

- A progressive and potentially fatal syndrome resulting from inappropriate activation of lymphocytes and macrophages.
- The pathologic hallmark is macrophages engulfing all types of blood cells in marrow, lymph nodes, spleen, or liver.
- Also known as autosomal recessive familial lymphohistiocytosis, familial erythrophagocytic lymphohistiocytosis, viral-associated hemophagocytic syndrome, or infection-related hemophagocytic syndrome.
- The designation primary hemophagocytic lymphohistiocytosis has been proposed for very young cases with known gene mutations or a family history and secondary or acquired hemophagocytic lymphohistiocytosis for older children, young adults, or those without known gene mutations or for infection-associated cases.
- The overarching term *hemophagocytic lymphohistiocytosis* has been proposed for all because (a) the same mutation may be seen in primary and secondary cases, (b) there is no rapid or definitive gene-testing diagnostic approach, (c) the clinical presentations are the same, and (d) in the acute setting, the distinction is not useful. Both forms should be diagnosed promptly and treated aggressively.

Epidemiology

- In Sweden, annual incidence 0.12/100,000 children or 1/50,000 live births.
- Males and females affected equally.
- Affects neonates and infants; 90 percent of cases are children younger than 2 years of age.
- Two-thirds of cases are in siblings; frequent parental consanguinity.

Pathogenesis

- Defect in natural killer (NK) and cytotoxic T-cell function lead to inappropriate activation of T cells and macrophages, which secrete proinflammatory cytokines: interferon-γ, TNF-α, IL-6, IL-10, IL-12, soluble IL-12R-α (sCD25).

- Hypercytokinemia ("cytokine storm") results in potentially fatal, severe multiorgan dysfunction.
- Mutation in perforin gene (*PRF1*) that leads to decreased perforin elaboration by NK cells and cytotoxic T-lymphocytes. This decreases apoptosis in target cells resulting in sustained inflammatory response.
- Mutations in other genes in NK and cytotoxic T cells (e.g., granzyme B) acting to decrease apoptosis of target cells, fostering failure to modulate inflammatory reactions.
- Syndromes with high frequency of hemophagocytic lymphohistiocytosis (e.g., Chédiak-Higashi syndrome, Hermansky-Pudlak syndrome) have immune deficiencies associated with lysosomal trafficking.
- Epstein-Barr virus infection in setting of immune deficiency state (e.g., X-linked lymphoproliferative disorder) can result in hemophagocytic syndrome.

Clinical Findings

- In infants: fever (>90%), anorexia, vomiting, irritability, rash (43%).
- Enlarged liver (90%) and spleen (85%) very common.
- Lymphadenopathy (42%), jaundice, ascites, edema may occur with progression of disease.
- Meningitis, encephalitic features, seizures, hemiplegia, or coma may ensue.

Laboratory Findings

- Anemia, reticulocytopenia, and thrombocytopenia in most patients at onset; neutropenia less common but with progression of disease, pancytopenia is the rule (Table 37–6).
- Marrow eventually contains an increased number of macrophages with prominent phagocytosis of blood cells (hemophagocytic histiocytes). This finding is neither sufficient to make the diagnosis nor is it always present. It is absent in one-third of cases and, thus, is not required for the diagnosis (Table 37–6).
- Repeat marrow biopsies as disease progresses may be helpful in uncovering hemophagocytosis, if suspicion of this disease is high.
- Marrow may progress to be hypoplastic with few macrophages and little evident hemophagocytosis.

TABLE 37–6   CLINICAL CRITERIA FOR DIAGNOSIS OF HLH*

I. HLH diagnosis is established with at least five of the following:
   A. Fever
   B. Splenomegaly
   C. Cytopenias in at least two cell lines:
      1. Hemoglobin <90 g/L
      2. Platelets <100 × 10^9/L
      3. Neutrophils <1 × 10^9/L
   D. Hypertriglyceridemia and/or hypofibrinogenemia:
      Fasting triglycerides >3 mmol/L (>265 mg/dL)
      Fibrinogen <1.5 g/L
   E. Hemophagocytosis in marrow or spleen or lymph nodes
   F. Low or absent activity of natural killer cells (specialized laboratory test)
   G. Ferritin >500 μ/L
   H. Soluble cD25 (soluble IL-2 receptor) >2400 units/mL

*Five of these eight clinical or laboratory findings are sufficient to make the diagnosis of HLH. It is important to obtain serial measurements of ferritin as well as complete blood counts and coagulation, and liver function tests when evaluating a patient.
HLH, hemophagocytic lymphohistiocytosis.
Source: *Williams Hematology*, 8th ed, Chap. 72, Table 72–5, p. 1057.

- The spleen contains swollen macrophages engorged principally with red cells and sometimes leukocytes and platelets.
- Serum alanine aminotransferase (ALT), aspartate aminotransferase (APT), bilirubin, lactic dehydrogenase, and triglyceride levels often elevated.
- Coagulation assays (esp. fibrinogen, partial thromboplastin time, and prothrombin time) should be performed and if abnormal further factor assays may be necessary.
- Increased serum concentrations of interferon-γ, TNF, soluble CD8, and IL-6 suggest relationship with cytotoxic T cells and inflammatory cytokines.
- Highly elevated soluble CD25 (soluble IL-2 receptor) >2400 units/mL along with four other criteria shown in Table 37–6 can be used to make the diagnosis.
- Biopsy of liver or lymph nodes reveals lymphohistiocytic infiltrate with cytologically normal macrophages engorged with phagocytosed erythrocytes (and often leukocytes and platelets). Paracortical lymphoid depletion in lymph nodes is also present.
- Highly elevated ferritin (>500 μg/L) virtually always present and levels >10,000 μg/L provide 90 percent sensitivity and 96 percent specificity for the diagnosis of hemophagocytic lymphohistiocytosis.
- Increasing serial serum ferritin levels are strongly suggestive of lymphohistiocytic hemophagocytic syndrome.
- Highly elevated ferritin (>500 μg/L) along with four other criteria as shown in Table 37–6 can be used to make a diagnosis.
- Cerebrospinal fluid examination in patients with nervous system signs may reveal pleocytosis and elevated fluid protein, indicating central nervous system involvement.
- Perforin expression of NK and T cells is decreased.

Differential Diagnosis
- Moderate infections, sepsis, multiorgan dysfunction, hepatitis, other causes for anemia and thrombocytopenia, and autoimmune diseases such as disseminated lupus erythematosus or rheumatoid arthritis may present with features overlapping the diagnostic findings in hemophagocytic lymphohistiocytosis.
- Consider hemophagocytic lymphohistiocytosis if no clear diagnosis is established and the patient's condition is deteriorating.
- Identification of an underlying immunodeficiency, such as X-linked lymphoproliferative disease, Chédiak-Higashi syndrome, or Griscelli syndrome should increase suspicion of hemophagocytic lymphohistiocytosis.
- Epstein-Barr virus, cytomegalovirus, and other herpes viruses are the most frequent causes of hemophagocytic lymphohistiocytosis. A wide variety of bacterial and fungal infections have been associated with hemophagocytic lymphohistiocytosis.
- The macrophage activation syndrome describes the signs and symptoms of hemophagocytic lymphohistiocytosis in patients with juvenile rheumatoid arthritis or systemic lupus erythematosus.
- The macrophage activation syndrome may include fever, hepatosplenomegaly, mental status changes, cytopenias, coagulopathy with hypofibrinogenemia. Proliferation of T lymphocytes and macrophages occur and may include poor NK cell function and low perforin expression.

Therapy
- One useful regimen is induction therapy with etoposide and dexamethasone followed by continuous treatment with cyclosporine and pulses of dexamethasone and etoposide.
- Despite neutropenia, etoposide is important, if it can be continued, because it provides singular apoptotic effects on macrophages.
- Cyclosporine levels greater than 200 ng/mL in patients with hypertension or liver or renal disease are dangerous. Such patients may experience seizures and encephalopathy.

- Patients with central nervous system signs or cerebrospinal fluid abnormalities receive intrathecal methotrexate.
- Treatment is often less intense for patients with HIV-associated hemophagocytic lymphohistiocytosis and patients with juvenile rheumatoid arthritis or systemic lupus erythematosus with the macrophage activation syndrome.
- Anti-TNF-α agents (e.g., infliximab or etanercept) can prove useful.
- In patients with the macrophage activation syndrome, therapy should start with cyclosporine and glucocorticoids but not etoposide. The latter should be added only if there is no evidence of improvement after 48 hours of therapy.
- Patients may require support with red cell and platelet transfusions and fresh frozen plasma.
- Prophylactic therapy for *Pneumocystis jiroveci* with sulfamethoxazole and fungi with fluconazole is usually administered.
- Newly diagnosed patients should have HLA typing and a search for a potential related or unrelated donor.
- Allogeneic hematopoietic stem cell transplantation from a histocompatible sibling or unrelated matched donor should be considered in any patient who has resistant disease, relapses, or who has familial hemophagocytic lymphohistiocytosis or a documented relevant gene mutation.

Course

- Can be rapidly fatal. With current therapy, 3-year survival is approximately 55 percent.
- Some patients have an initial good response but then relapse as indicated by increase in serum ferritin, coagulation abnormalities, respiratory insufficiency, hypotension, and deteriorating renal function.
- Death is from infection, hemorrhage, or central nervous system abnormalities.

Infection-Induced, Disease-Induced, or Drug-Induced Hemophagocytic Histiocytosis

Etiology

- Usually associated with systemic viral infection; occasionally with bacterial, fungal, or protozoal infections.
- Appears to be an unusual, exaggerated inflammatory reaction to infection.
- Also may occur in association with malignancies.

Clinical Findings

- Fever, severe malaise, myalgias, lethargy.
- Enlargement of liver and spleen frequent in children, less so in adults.

Laboratory Findings

- Severe anemia (<90 g/L), leukopenia ($<2.5 \times 10^9$/L), thrombocytopenia ($<50 \times 10^9$/L), or combination of two cytopenias in nearly all cases.
- Interferon-γ, TNF-α, IL-6, and soluble IL-2 receptor plasma levels are markedly increased.
- Macrophages may be present in the blood film.
- Marrow may be hypocellular, with decreased erythropoiesis and granulopoiesis. Increased macrophages, which frequently contain phagocytosed erythrocytes and erythroblasts and occasionally platelets and neutrophils.

Treatment

- Stop or decrease immunosuppressive therapy in transplant patients.
- If underlying infection, administer appropriate antimicrobial agents.
- Cyclosporine A, antithymocyte globulin, gamma globulin, and etoposide use has been accompanied by improvement in Epstein-Barr virus–associated syndrome.
- In patients with Epstein-Barr virus, rituximab can be useful.

Course
- Patients are severely ill but often recover in weeks with complete disappearance of evidence of histiocytosis in months.
- Fatal outcome frequent in immunosuppressed patients.

Sinus Histiocytosis with Massive Lymphadenopathy (Rosai-Dorfman Syndrome)
Definition
- A unique entity with polyclonal (nonmalignant) proliferation of histiocytes with massive lymphadenopathy. It is often self-limited.

Epidemiology
- Usually occurs in first three decades of life (median age 21 years) but may occur at any age.
- Often occurs in children with immunologic disorder.

Clinical Findings
- Massive, painless, bilateral cervical lymphadenopathy characteristic (90% of patients).
- Axillary and inguinal adenopathy develop in half the patients.
- Some patients may have fever, night sweats, malaise, and weight loss.
- Extranodal involvement in about 50 percent of patients. Virtually every tissue may be affected (e.g., skin, sinuses, orbit, salivary glands, liver, kidney, bone, and others).
- Bilateral parotid or submandibular gland enlargement may be present.
- Approximately 20 percent of patients have a maculopapular rash, which can be reddish, bluish, or yellow as a result of xanthomatous involvement.
- Approximately 20 percent have nasal and paranasal sinus involvement with nasal airway obstruction, epistaxis, nasal septal displacement, or mass lesions invading sinuses.
- Approximately 10 percent have eyelid or orbital involvement with proptosis.
- Approximately 5 percent have central nervous system involvement: intracranial, epidural, or dural masses, or nerve palsies.

Laboratory Findings
- Signs of chronic inflammation, i.e., anemia, neutrophilia, elevated erythrocyte sedimentation rate, polyclonal hypergammaglobulinemia.
- Pathologic features in lymph node include:
  — Marked capsular fibrosis, distention of sinuses by phagocytic macrophages. Plasma cells are plentiful.
  — Macrophages with ingested intact lymphocytes are virtually diagnostic. Erythrophagocytosis by macrophages is often present.
  — Macrophages positive for CD14, CD68, CD163 but are negative for CD1a (Table 37–2).
  — Macrophages also express lysozyme, transferrin receptor, IL-2 receptor.
  — The macrophage proliferation is polyclonal.

Therapy
- Acyclovir therapy may be effective. Herpesvirus 6 identified in 7 of 9 cases so studied.
- Glucocorticoids, cytotoxic agents, radiotherapy, and antibiotics are ineffective.

Course and Prognosis
- Lymph node enlargement usually progresses for weeks to months and then recedes, with no residual evidence of disease after 9 to 18 months.
- Some patients have persistent adenopathy; others may have a fatal outcome.

Erdheim-Chester Disease

Definition and Epidemiology

- A disease resulting from infiltration of lipid-laden histiocytes that infiltrate bones and viscera, cause a fibroblastic reaction, and lead to organ failure.
- The disease affects individuals from childhood to old age and has a mean age of onset of 50 years.
- The etiology s unknown.
- Cells have been determined to be clonal in several cases and polyclonal in several others. Thus, its status as a neoplasm is uncertain.

Clinical Findings

- Fever, weakness, and weight loss are common presenting complaints.
- Osteosclerosis of long bones is a principal feature.
- Extraosseous involvement occurs in 50 percent of patients.
- Encasing masses around various organs are characteristic.
- Retroperitoneal and renal involvement causes abdominal pain, dysuria, and hydronephrosis.
- Pulmonary involvement results in dyspnea and pulmonary insufficiency.
- Circumferential sheathing of aorta and coronary arteries may cause cardiac failure.
- Involvement of the pericardium can lead to effusions and effects on myocardial function.
- Diabetes insipidus is a very common presenting disorder.
- Some patients have focal neurologic signs, notably cerebellar dysfunction.
- Bilateral painless exophthalmous may appear.
- Xanthomatous skin lesions may emerge appearing as reddish-brown papules.

Laboratory Findings

- No specific chemical findings.
- Radiographs show bilateral patchy osteosclerosis of the metaphysic and diaphysis of the femur, proximal tibia, and fibula; lytic bone lesions occur in one-third of patients.
- Computed tomography may show perirenal infiltration extending through perirenal fat giving the appearance of "hair kidneys."
- Computed tomography may show aortic and aortic branch vessel with circumferential encasement by fibrous tissue.
- The histopathology is distinctive: lipid laden histiocytes with foamy or eosinophilic cytoplasm infiltrating bone and other organs. A fibroblastic reaction is characteristic. The histiocytes express CD68 and factor XIIIa, but do not express CD1a and lack Birbeck granules, the latter specific for Langerhans cell histiocytosis.

Treatment and Course

- No specific regimen has been shown to be effective. Most series have relatively few patients.
- Interferon-α has resulted in significant improvement in some patients in small series and single case reports.
- Glucocorticoids (1 mg/kg per day) have decreased exophthalmous or constitutional symptoms in a small fraction of patients so treated.
- Sixty percent of patients die of their disease and about two-thirds of that 60 percent do so within 6 months of diagnosis.
- The mean survival is less than 3 years.
- Cardiac, pulmonary, and renal failure are the principal causes of death.

Juvenile Xanthogranuloma

- A disease of children usually seen in the first 5 years of life.
- A disorder of dermal dendrocytes forming multiple nodules that affect principally the skin of the head, neck, and trunk.

- They are usually skin colored but may be erythematous or yellowish.
- Extracutaneous involvement is rare and systemic symptoms are present only if viscera are involved. Virtually any organ can be affected: nervous system, heart, lung, liver, spleen, intestines, others. Marrow involvement may cause cytopenias. Pituitary involvement may cause diabetes insipidus.
- Histiocytes are CD14+CD68+ and express factor XIIIa (**Table 37–2**).
- In early disease, intermediate sized histiocytes in sheet-like infiltrations. These cells have small quantities of lipid in the cytoplasm and no Touton-type giant cells (lipid-laden histiocytes with multiple nuclei with a small amount of centrally located cytoplasm.
- Established disease has abundant foamy histiocytes with Touton giant cells interspersed. Also some lymphocytes and eosinophils.
- If single or few lesions, no therapy is usually needed. Excisional biopsy can be done, if disfiguring.
- In rare cases of systemic disease, a variety of multidrug programs have been used. Inclusion of a vinca alkaloid and a glucocorticoid is recommended.

For a more detailed discussion, see Kenneth L. McClain and Carl E. Allen: Inflammatory and Malignant Histiocytosis. Chapter 72, p. 1047 in *Williams Hematology,* 8th ed.

CHAPTER 38
Lipid Storage Disease

MECHANISM OF MACROPHAGE EXPANSION

In Gaucher and Niemann-Pick diseases, major clinical manifestations result from accumulation of glucocerebroside and sphingomyelin, respectively, in macrophages, leading to their massive expansion in tissues (see Fig. 38–1).

GAUCHER DISEASE

Etiology and Pathogenesis

- Glucocerebroside accumulates because of a deficiency of glucocerebrosidase (β-glucosidase).
- Very rarely a neuropathic form may be caused by a deficiency of saposin, a β-glucosidase cofactor.
- Inherited as an autosomal recessive disorder, with high gene frequency among Ashkenazi Jews.
- More than 100 different mutations have been reported, but the 5 mutations most common in Ashkenazi Jews account for more than 95 percent of mutations in that population.
- The most common mutation in the Jewish population is 1226G (N370S). It usually gives rise to mild disease in the homozygous form.

Clinical Features

- Three types of Gaucher disease are recognized:
  - Type 1 occurs in both children and adults, and is primarily caused by an accumulation of glucocerebroside-laden macrophages in liver, spleen, and marrow. Neurologic manifestations are rare and primarily affect the peripheral nervous system.
  - Type 2 is exceedingly rare and is characterized by rapid neurologic deterioration and early death.
  - Type 3, or juvenile Gaucher disease, is a subacute neuropathic disorder with later onset of symptoms and better prognosis than type 2.
- Type 1 may be asymptomatic, or symptoms may range from minimal to severe:
  - Chronic fatigue is common.
  - Hepatic and/or splenic enlargement may cause significant (mechanical) problems.
  - Thrombocytopenia is a common presenting finding.
  - Skeletal lesions are often painful. "Erlenmeyer flask" deformity of the femur is common. Aseptic necrosis of femoral head and vertebral collapse may occur.

Laboratory Features

- Blood count may be normal, but normocytic, normochromic anemia with modest reticulocytosis is often found. Thrombocytopenia is common, particularly in patients with significant splenomegaly and may be severe.
- Leukocytes are deficient in acid β-glucosidase activity.
- Gaucher cells are large cells found in marrow, spleen, and liver in varying numbers. They are characterized by small, eccentrically placed nuclei and cytoplasm with characteristic crinkles or striations. The cytoplasm stains with the periodic acid–Schiff (PAS) technique.

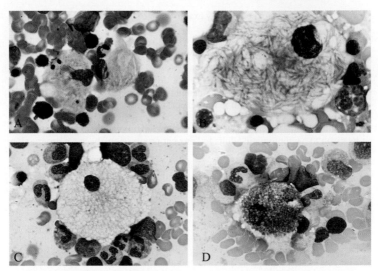

FIGURE 38-1 Marrow aspirates showing types of abnormal macrophages. **A.** Two Gaucher cells. These macrophages are engorged with glucocerebroside. Note the characteristically different cytoplasmic appearance from the Niemann-Pick cell in (C). The cytoplasm in the Gaucher cells have more cylindrical, not foamy, accumulations **B.** pseudo-Gaucher cell in a case of chronic myelogenous leukemia. A glucocerebroside-engorged macrophage resulting from the inability of the normal macrophage glucocerebrosidase content from handling the enormously increased substrate presented as a result of the very high granulocyte turnover rate. **C.** Niemann-Pick cell. Characteristic large macrophage with foam-like cytoplasm representing accumulation of sphingomyelin. **D.** Sea blue histiocyte. Note deep blue cytoplasmic granular appearance. These macrophages are laden with lipid, which stains blue with polychrome stains, such as Giemsa. *(Reproduced with permission from Lichtman's Atlas of Hematology, www.accessmedicine.com.)*

- Serum acid phosphatase, chitotriosidase, ferritin, and hexosaminidase activities are commonly increased.
- Biochemical abnormalities as a consequence of liver involvement may be found.
- Serum monoclonal Ig spikes have an increased incidence in Gaucher disease patients over the age of 50 years.
- Acquired coagulation factor deficiencies (isolated coagulation factors) have been reported.

Diagnosis
- Established by demonstrating β-glucosidase deficiency in leukocytes or cultured fibroblasts.
- The most widely used biomarker is chitotriosidase, which is elevated, often several thousand-fold, in patients with Gaucher disease. Deficiency of chitotriosidase occurs in 6 percent of the population.
- It is *not* necessary or desirable to perform a marrow examination or liver biopsy to demonstrate the presence of Gaucher cells. Cells indistinguishable from Gaucher cells are seen in other diseases, including chronic myeloproliferative disorders, Hodgkin lymphoma, myeloma, and AIDS.
- Demonstration of specific DNA abnormalities will establish the diagnosis, but negative studies do not rule it out unless the entire coding region is sequenced.

- Prenatal diagnosis can be made by examination of cells obtained by amniocentesis or chorionic villus biopsy.
- Heterozygosity may be assumed by assay of acid β-glucosidase activity in leukocytes or fibroblasts, but DNA analysis is the only reliable method.

Therapy

- Enzyme replacement therapy with recombinant human β-glucosidase (imiglucerase) has been successful. It is very expensive. New enzymes will come to the market soon.
- Notwithstanding the manufacturer's recommendations, the enzyme should not be given to asymptomatic adults to "prevent progression" because progression rarely occurs.
- The enzyme is usually infused at bi-weekly intervals, but weekly or monthly infusions can be effective as well.
- The total dose is usually 30 to 120 U/kg per month for type 1 patients. Higher doses relate to quicker responses, but are not needed for the majority of patients. Maintenance dose can be as low as 15 to 30 U/kg per month.
- Type 3 patients are treated with 60 to 120 U/kg per month. Enzyme replacement therapy does not affect neurologic disease. Type 2 should not be treated with enzyme replacement therapy.
- The response normally requires 6 months or more. The response can be monitored by an (impressive) reduction in liver and spleen size, and improvement or correction of cytopenias. The bone response is slower and less predictable.
- Chitotriosidase measurement is useful for monitoring both untreated patients, to assess stability *versus* deterioration, and treated patients, to assess response to therapy. A change in chitotriosidase levels rather than absolute values is used for monitoring.
- Escalation of doses to attempt to achieve a more rapid response is commonly recommended, but has not been demonstrated to be useful.
- In patients who are not suitable for enzyme replacement therapy, oral substrate reduction therapy using miglustat (an inhibitor of glucocerebroside synthase) may be considered.
- Future pharmacologic options consist of "chaperone therapy," stabilizing mutant (misfolded) glucocerebrosidase molecules that would otherwise be destroyed prior to their export from the endoplasmatic reticulum to the lysosome.
- Splenectomy (since introduction of enzyme replacement treatment less often performed) generally corrects anemia and thrombocytopenia caused by hypersplenism but may cause more rapid deposition of lipid in liver and marrow.
- Orthopedic procedures, particularly joint replacement, are useful in patients with severe joint damage.
- Hematopoietic stem cell transplantation is curative, but its use is limited by the risk.

Course and Prognosis

- There is often great variability in expression of the disease, even among siblings.
- Severity of the disease changes little after childhood, and progression does not occur or is gradual.
- Some adults with aggressive disease will have slow progression, measured over decades with a gradual fall in platelet count and new bone lesions.
- Pulmonary complications include infiltration of the lungs by Gaucher cells causing severe interstitial lung disease, usually in patients with severe liver disease and splenectomy. Pulmonary hypertension is rare and can be life-threatening and does not respond to enzyme replacement therapy.

- There is an increased incidence of malignancies in patients, particularly hemato-logic malignancies (multiple myeloma) and hepatocellular carcinoma. The latter is seen in cases with severe liver involvement with fibrosis following splenectomy.

NIEMANN-PICK DISEASE

Etiology and Pathogenesis

- Inherited as an autosomal recessive disorder.
- Types A and B disease are a consequence of acid sphingomyelinase (ASM) defi-ciency and are an infantile disease and a disease with later onset, respectively. They are now referred to as ASM deficiency.
- Type C disease is not a result of sphingomyelinase deficiency but rather of muta-tions in a gene designated *NPC1 or NPC2,* which is involved in cholesterol and glycolipid transport.
- The predominant lipid accumulating in tissues is sphingomyelin in types A and B, and of unesterified cholesterol and several glycolipids in type C.
- Characteristic *foam cells* are found in the lymphoid organs.

Clinical Features

- Type A disease has onset in infancy with poor growth and neurologic manifesta-tions.
- Type B disease usually presents with hepatosplenomegaly ordinarily in the first decade of life, but in mild cases not until adulthood. Neurologic findings are usually absent but pulmonary involvement is common.
- Type C disease is characterized by neonatal jaundice and dementia, ataxia, and psychiatric symptoms in later life.

Laboratory Features

Niemann-Pick Types A and B

- Mild anemia may be present.
- Blood lymphocytes typically contain small, lipid-filled vacuoles.
- Leukocytes are deficient in sphingomyelinase activity.
- Lipid profiles are always abnormal including high triglycerides and LDL-cholesterol in combination with low HDL cholesterol. The consequences for cardiovascular disease are unknown.

ASM Deficiency and Niemann-Pick Type C

- Large histiocytes containing small lipid droplets (foam cells) or sea-blue histio-cytes are demonstrable in many tissues, including marrow.

Diagnosis

- Types A and B disease diagnosed by demonstration that leukocytes or cultured fibroblasts are deficient in sphingomyelinase.
- Heterozygotes for types A and B cannot be reliably detected by measurement of sphingomyelinase activity. Genetic testing needs to be performed.
- Type C disease can be diagnosed by biochemical testing that demonstrates impaired cholesterol esterification and positive filipin staining in cultured fibro-blasts. Biochemical testing for carrier status is unreliable. Molecular genetic testing of the *NPC1* and *NPC2* genes detects disease-causing mutations in approximately 94 percent of individuals with NPC.

Treatment

- Enzyme replacement therapy is currently being developed for the treatment of Niemann-Pick type B disease.
- Some studies have suggested beneficial effects of miglustat in Niemann-Pick type C disease.

Course and Prognosis
- Patients with type A disease usually die before their third year of life.
- Most patients with type B disease reach adult life.
- Type C patients either die during infancy or have a protracted course with neurologic deterioration.

For a more detailed discussion, see Ari Zimran and Deborah Elstein: Lipid Storage Diseases. Chap. 73, p. 1065 in *Williams Hematology*, 8th ed.

PART V

PRINCIPLES OF THERAPY FOR NEOPLASTIC HEMATOLOGIC DISORDERS

CHAPTER 39
Pharmacology and Toxicity of Antineoplastic Drugs

BASIC PRINCIPLES OF CANCER CHEMOTHERAPY

- Knowledge of drug actions, pharmacokinetics, clinical toxicities, and drug interactions is essential for the proper and safe administration of cancer chemotherapy.
- Use established regimens, and recheck doses.
- Choice of a particular drug treatment program should depend on the disease, histology, and stage of the disease and on an assessment of individual patient tolerance.
- High-dose chemotherapy programs used in autologous and allogeneic hematopoietic stem cell transplantation result in additional organ toxicities that are not seen at conventional doses.
- Chemotherapy usually targets process of DNA replication.
- More recently, drugs have been introduced to target specific cellular processes, including receptor signaling, inhibition of oncoproteins, angiogenesis, and membrane cluster of differentiation antigens.

COMBINATION CHEMOTHERAPY

- Combination chemotherapy uses several drugs simultaneously based on certain empiric principles:
  - Each drug selected has demonstrable antitumor activity against the neoplasm for which it is used.
  - Each drug should have a different mechanism of action.
  - The drugs should not have a common mechanism of resistance.
  - Drug dose-limiting toxicities should not overlap.
  - Specific combinations chosen should be based on preclinical and clinical protocol-based evidence of synergistic activity.

CELL KINETICS AND CANCER CHEMOTHERAPY

- Cell cycle–specific agents, such as antimetabolites, kill cells as they traverse the DNA synthetic phase (S phase) of the cell cycle.
  - Diminished killing of resting cells.
  - Prolonged exposure to drug is useful for minimizing effects of asynchronous cell division.
  - High-dose regimens are the most useful.
- Non–cell cycle–dependent agents do not require cells to be exposed during a specific phase of the cell cycle.
  - Total dose of drug more important than duration of exposure.
  - Appropriate dose depends on: cell cycle dependence, toxicity to marrow and other tissues, pharmacokinetic behavior, interaction with other drugs, and patient tolerance.

DRUG RESISTANCE

- The basis for drug resistance is spontaneous occurrence of resistant cancer cell mutants and selection of drug-resistant cells under pressure of chemotherapy (clonal selection).
- Mechanisms such as additional mutations in mismatched repair genes and genes that block apoptosis also operate to impair treatment efficacy.
- Use of multiple drugs not sharing resistance mechanisms should be more effective than single agents.
- Multiple agents should be used simultaneously, as probability of double- or triple-resistant cells is the product of the probabilities of the independent drug-resistant mutations occurring simultaneously in the same cell.

DRUGS USED TO TREAT HEMATOLOGIC MALIGNANCIES

Cell Cycle–Active Agents

Methotrexate

- Methotrexate is used for maintenance therapy of acute lymphocytic leukemia, combination chemotherapy of lymphomas, and treatment and prophylaxis of meningeal leukemia.
- Inhibits dihydrofolate reductase, which leads to depletion of cellular folate coenzymes and to inhibition of DNA synthesis and cessation of cell replication.
- Acquired resistance is a result of increased levels of dihydrofolate reductase via gene amplification, defective polyglutamylation, and impaired cellular uptake.
- Is well absorbed orally in doses of 5 to 10 mg, but doses of more than 25 mg should be given intravenously.
- Excreted primarily unchanged by the kidney.
- Renal impairment is contradiction to methotrexate therapy.
- Dose-limiting toxicities are myelosuppression and gastrointestinal effects (mucositis, diarrhea, bleeding).
- Intrathecal methotrexate may produce acute arachnoiditis, dementia, motor deficits, seizures, and coma. Leucovorin cannot prevent or reverse CNS toxicities.
- Leucovorin intravenously will reverse acute toxicity of methotrexate, except for CNS toxicity.

Cytarabine (Cytosine Arabinoside, Ara-C)

- Used primarily to treat acute myelogenous leukemia, in combination with an anthracycline antibiotic drug.
- Ara-C triphosphate (Ara-CTP) is formed intracellularly, inhibits DNA polymerase, and causes termination of strand elongation.

- Acquired resistance is a result of a loss of deoxycytidine kinase, the initial activating enzyme of Ara-C, decreased drug uptake, or increased deamination.
- Cytarabine is not active orally and must be given parenterally.
- High CSF concentration achieved (50% of plasma level).
- Cytarabine may be given intrathecally for meningeal leukemia.
- At usual doses (100 to 150 mg/m^2, intravenously, q 12 h for 5 to 10 days), myelosuppression is dose-limiting toxicity.
- High-dose cytarabine therapy, 1 to 3 g/m^2, intravenously, at q 12 h for 6 to 12 doses, is especially effective in consolidation therapy of acute myelogenous leukemia.
- At the higher doses (g/m^2), neurologic, hepatic, and gastrointestinal toxicities may occur. Patients older than 50 years of age may develop cerebellar toxicity (ataxia, slurred speech), which can progress to confusion, dementia, and death. Severe conjunctivitis may also occur, but may be prevented or reduced by glucocorticoid eye drops.

Gemcitabine
- Although primarily used for solid tumors, gemcitabine, a 2′-2′-difluoro analogue of deoxycytidine, has significant activity against Hodgkin lymphoma.
- Its mechanism of action is similar to cytarabine, in that, as a nucleotide, it competes with deoxycytidine triphosphate for incorporation into the elongating DNA strand, where it terminates DNA synthesis.
- Gemcitabine achieves higher nucleotide levels in tumor cells than does Ara-CTP, and has a longer intracellular half-life. Standard schedules use 1000 mg/m^2 infused over 30 minutes.

5-Azacytidine and Decitabine (5-aza-2′-deoxycytidine)
- Cytidine analogues that display cytotoxic activity and that may induce differentiation at low doses.
- These drugs are used primarily in patients with myelodysplasia.
- Their differentiation actions result from their incorporation into DNA and subsequent covalent inactivation of DNA methyltransferase. The resulting inhibition of methylation of cytosine bases in DNA leads to enhanced transcription of otherwise silent genes. For example, the differentiating effects of 5-azacytidine are the basis for the induction of fetal hemoglobin synthesis in patients with sickle cell anemia and thalassemia.
- The usual doses of 5-azacytidine are 75 mg/m^2 per day for 7 days, repeated every 28 days, whereas decitabine is used in doses of 20 mg intravenously every day for 5 days every 4 weeks.
- Responses become apparent in patients with myelodysplasia after two to five courses.
- Their principal clinical toxicities are reversible myelosuppression, severe nausea and vomiting, hepatic dysfunction, myalgias, fever, and rash.

Purine Analogues: 6-Mercaptopurine (6-MP) and 6-Thioguanine (6-TG)
- Both 6-MP and 6-TG are converted to nucleotides by the enzyme hypoxanthine-guanine phosphoribosyl transferase (HPRT). Cell death correlates with incorporation of the 6-MP or 6-TG nucleotides into DNA.
- Both 6-MP and 6-TG are given orally.
- Equivalent myelosuppression occurs with 6-MP or 6-TG.
- Metabolism of 6-MP is inhibited by allopurinol; 6-TG metabolism is not affected.
- Thiopurine inactivating enzyme activity decreased in 10 percent of persons of European descent. May need dose adjustment.
- Myelotoxic with peak neutropenia and thrombocytopenia at about 7 days; moderate nausea and vomiting; mild, usually reversible hepatotoxicity.

Fludarabine Phosphate

- Fludarabine has outstanding activity in chronic lymphocytic leukemia (CLL). It is strongly immunosuppressive, like the other purine analogues, and is frequently used for this purpose in nonmyeloablative allogeneic hematopoietic stem cell transplantation and in the treatment of collagen vascular diseases.
- Administered intravenously, and eliminated mainly by renal excretion.
- The recommended oral dose is 40 mg/m^2 per day. In CLL, the recommended doses are 25 mg/m^2 per day for 5 days given as 2-hour infusions and repeated every 4 weeks. When administered at these doses, fludarabine causes only moderate myelosuppression.
- At recommended doses, moderate myelosuppression and opportunistic infection are major toxicities. Peripheral sensory and motor neuropathy may also occur.
- Tumor lysis syndrome may occur with treatment of patients with large tumor burdens. Thus, patients should be well hydrated and their urine alkalinized prior to beginning therapy.

Cladribine (2-Chlorodeoxyadenosine)

- A purine analogue active in hairy cell leukemia, low-grade lymphomas, and CLL. A single course of cladribine, typically 0.09 mg/kg per day for 7 days by continuous intravenous infusion, induces complete response in 80 percent of patients with hairy cell leukemia, and partial responses in the remainder.
- Administered intravenously and eliminated mainly by renal excretion.
- Cladribine is eliminated primarily (>50%) by renal excretion. In a patient with renal failure, continuous flow hemodialysis effectively cleared the drug and prevented serious myelosuppression.
- Cladribine retains effectiveness in at least a fraction of hairy cell leukemia patients resistant to deoxycoformycin or fludarabine.
- Myelosuppression, fever, and opportunistic infection are major toxicities.
- Repeated doses may produce thrombocytopenia.

Clofarabine (2-Chloro-2′Fluoro-Arabinosyladenine)

- This analogue has halogen substitutions on both the purine ring and arabinose sugar, resulting in a ready uptake and activation, to a highly stable intracellular triphosphate, which terminates DNA synthesis, inhibits ribonucleotide reductase, and induces apoptosis.
- As a single agent, the drug is well tolerated by elderly acute myelogenous leukemia (AML) patients in whom it produces remission rates of 30 percent.
- The usual adult dose of 52 mg/m^2 given as a 2-hour infusion daily for 5 days.
- The primary route of clofarabine clearance is through renal excretion, and dose adjustment according to creatinine clearance is recommended for patients with abnormal renal function.
- Toxicities include myelosuppression; uncommonly, fever, hypotension, and pulmonary edema, suggestive of capillary leak caused by cytokine release; hepatic transaminitis; hypokalemia; and hypophosphatemia.

Nelarabine (6-Methoxy-Arabinosylguanine)

- The only guanine nucleoside analogue, nelarabine has relatively specific activity as a secondary agent for T-cell lymphoblastic lymphoma and acute T-cell leukemias.
- Its mode of action is similar to the other purine analogues, in that it becomes incorporated into DNA and terminates DNA synthesis.
- Its selective action for T cells may relate to the ability of T cells to activate purine nucleosides and the lack of susceptibility of this drug to purine nucleoside phosphorylase, a degradative reaction.
- Usual doses are an intravenous 2-hour infusion of 1500 mg/m^2 for adults on days 1, 3, and 5, and a lower dose of 650 mg/m^2 per day for 5 days for children.

- The primary toxicities are myelosuppression and abnormal liver function tests, but the drug may cause a spectrum of neurologic abnormalities, including seizures, delirium, somnolence, and the Guillain-Barré syndrome of ascending paralysis.

Pentostatin (2-Deoxycoformycin)

- A purine analogue that inhibits adenosine deaminase, resulting in accumulation of intracellular adenosine and deoxyadenosine nucleotides, which are probably responsible for the cytotoxicity.
- Biweekly doses of 4 mg/m^2 are extremely effective in inducing pathologically confirmed complete responses in hairy cell leukemia.
- Severe depletion of T lymphocytes occurs and opportunistic infections are common.
- The drug is eliminated entirely by the kidney.

Hydroxyurea

- Hydroxyurea inhibits ribonucleotide reductase, which converts ribonucleotide diphosphates to deoxyribonucleotides.
- Hydroxyurea is used to treat polycythemia vera, essential thrombocythemia and primary myelofibrosis, the hyperleukocytic phase of chronic myelogenous leukemia (CML), and to reduce rapidly rising blast counts in the acute phase of CML or in hyperleukocytic AML.
- The drug has also become the standard agent for preventing painful crisis and reducing hospitalization in patients with sickle cell disease and in patients with hemoglobin (Hgb) SC.
- Its anti-sickling activity results from induction of Hgb F through its activation of a specific promoter for the γ-globin gene. It may also exert anti-sickling activity and decrease occlusion of small vessels through its generation of the vasodilator nitric oxide or through suppression of neutrophil production and expression of adhesion molecules, such as L-selectin.
- The dose of hydroxyurea is determined empirically; patients are usually started on 500 mg per day, and titrated upward to balance disease control and gastrointestinal toxicity in patients with myeloproliferative diseases, and to the limit of mild neutropenia in patients with sickle cell disease.
- Resistance occurs as a result of increases in ribonucleotide reductase activity or from development of a mutant enzyme that binds the drug less avidly.
- Well absorbed when administered orally.
- Renal excretion is major source of elimination.
- Major toxicities are leukopenia and induction of megaloblastic changes in marrow blood cells. Approximately 30 percent of individuals cannot tolerate hydroxyurea due to gastrointestinal symptoms or skin ulcers.
- May increase probability of evolution to acute myelogenous leukemia transformation when used to treat chronic clonal myeloid diseases, although this is controversial. There has been no report of enhanced leukemogenesis in patients treated with hydroxyurea for sickle cell diseases, despite over 20 years of use.

Vinca Alkaloids (Vincristine and Vinblastine)

- Vinca alkaloids bind to microtubules and inhibit mitotic spindle formation.
- Resistance occurs by acquisition of multidrug resistance phenotype or development of microtubules with decreased vinca alkaloid binding.
- Vincristine and vinblastine are both administered intravenously. The average single dose of vincristine is 1.4 mg/m^2 and that of vinblastine 8 to 9 mg/m^2. Sequential doses of the drugs are usually given weekly or every 2 weeks during a cycle of therapy.
- Approximately 70 percent of vincristine is metabolized in the liver. The site of vinblastine metabolism is unidentified. Liver disease, but not renal disease, requires a reduction in dose. In general, although specific guidelines for dose reduction have not been developed, a 50 percent decrease in dose is recommended

for patients presenting with a bilirubin level of 1.5 to 3 mg/dL and a 75 percent reduction for levels greater than 3 mg/dL.
- Very useful in Hodgkin or non-Hodgkin lymphomas and acute lymphocytic leukemia.
- The dose-limiting toxicity of vincristine is neurotoxicity, which may begin with paresthesias of fingers and lower legs and loss of deep-tendon reflexes. Constipation is common. Other severe neurologic effects can occur.
- Severe weakness of extensor muscles of hands and feet may occur with continued use.
- Marrow suppression is not a common side effect of vincristine, but a primary toxicity of vinblastine is leukopenia.
- Both vincristine and vinblastine are potent vesicants upon extravasation during administration.
- Neither vincristine nor vinblastine can be given intrathecally.

Taxanes (Paclitaxel and Docetaxel)
- Antimitotic drugs that bind to microtubules, although the taxanes differ in their mechanism and toxicity profile from the vinca alkaloids.
- Modest activity in lymphoma.
- Both drugs are cleared primarily by hepatic CYP metabolism, although by different isoenzymes (paclitaxel predominantly by CYP 2B6 and docetaxel by CYP 3A4) and are thus cleared more rapidly in patients treated with phenytoin (Dilantin) and other CYP-inducing drugs such as ketoconazole.
- Formulated in lipid-based solvents that can cause hypersensitivity reactions; therefore, both are administered after pretreatment with antihistamines and glucocorticoids to decrease risk of allergic reaction.
- Toxicities principally leukopenia, thrombocytopenia, and mucositis.
- Peripheral neuropathy, cardiac arrhythmias, and fluid retention can occur.

Campothecins (Irinotecan, Topotecan)
- Targets topoisomerase I, preventing resealing of single-strand DNA breaks.
- Irinotecan has activity against some lymphomas.
- Irinotecan, 125 mg/m^2, is administered intravenously once each week for 4 weeks with repetition at 6-week intervals.
- Irinotecan should be used with caution in patients with hepatic dysfunction.
- Topotecan, 1.5 mg/m^2 per day for 5 days, may be useful in oligoblastic leukemia, especially subacute myelomonocytic leukemia.
- Topotecan dose should be reduced if renal or hepatic impairment, including patients with Gilbert syndrome.
- Topotecan toxicity principally myelosuppression and mucositis.

Anthracycline Antibiotics
- Anthracycline antibiotics act by forming a complex with both DNA and the DNA repair enzyme topoisomerase II, resulting in double-stranded DNA breaks.
- Doxorubicin is a mainstay of treatment for Hodgkin disease, and non-Hodgkin lymphoma, in combination with a number of other agents (e.g., adriamycin/bleomycin/vinblastine/dacarbazine [ABVD] and cyclophosphamide/hydroxydaunorubicin (doxorubicin)/oncovin/prednisone [CHOP], respectively).
- Daunorubicin and idarubicin are used in combination with Ara-C for acute myelogenous leukemia.
- Mitoxantrone is used for acute myelogenous leukemia.
- The anthracyclines are usually given every 3 to 4 weeks. Schedules that avoid high-peak plasma levels may reduce cardiac toxicity.
- Idarubicin is the only anthracycline that has reasonable oral bioavailability.
- Doxorubicin and daunorubicin are metabolized in the liver. It is wise to begin therapy of patients with elevated serum bilirubin levels at 50 percent doses of doxorubicin or daunorubicin, and adjust according to tolerance.

- Myelosuppression is the major acute toxicity from anthracyclines. Nausea and vomiting may occur.
- Anthracyclines generate intracellular oxygen free radicals, which may cause cardiac toxicity.
- Doxorubicin may produce mucositis.
- All these drugs can produce reaction in previously irradiated tissues.
- All can produce tissue necrosis if extravasated.
- Dose-related chronic cardiac toxicity is a major side effect of doxorubicin and daunorubicin.
- Acute cardiac effects are arrhythmias, conduction disturbances, and pericarditis-myocarditis syndrome.
- Chronic cardiac effects are diminished ejection fraction and clinical congestive heart failure with high mortality.
- Children receiving anthracyclines may show abnormal cardiac development and late congestive heart failure as teenagers.
- Resistance to anthracyclines occurs with increased activity of the MRP protein and the P-glycoprotein transport system, and with altered topoisomerase II activity.

Epipodophyllotoxins

- Two semisynthetic derivatives of podophyllotoxin, VP-16 (etoposide) and VM-26 (teniposide), inhibit topoisomerase II and have significant clinical activity in hematologic malignancies.
- Etoposide is used in combination regimens for Hodgkin lymphoma, large cell lymphomas, leukemias, and various solid tumors, and is a frequent component of high-dose chemotherapy regimens.
- Binds to DNA and induces double-stranded breaks.
- Resistance is a result of expression of multidrug resistance phenotype or diminished drug binding.
- May be given orally or intravenously.
- Clinical activity is schedule dependent. Single conventional doses are ineffective; daily doses for 3 to 5 days are required.
- Hypotension may occur with rapid (>30 minutes) intravenous administration.
- Major toxicity is leukopenia; thrombocytopenia is less common.
- In high-dose protocols, mucositis is common and hepatic damage may occur.
- Etoposide may induce secondary acute myelogenous leukemias.

Bleomycin

- Bleomycin is used in combination chemotherapy programs for Hodgkin disease, aggressive lymphomas, or germ cell tumors.
- Antitumor activity is caused by formation of single- and double-stranded DNA breaks.
- Resistance is a result of accelerated drug inactivation, enhanced DNA repair capacity, or decreased drug accumulation.
- Administered intravenously or intramuscularly for systemic effects, and may be instilled intrapleurally or intraperitoneally to control malignant effusions.
- Eliminated largely by renal excretion. May need dose reduction with renal dysfunction.
- Has little effect on normal marrow.
- A major toxicity is pulmonary fibrosis, which is dose related and is usually irreversible.
- Skin changes, also a major toxicity, are dose related, and include erythema, hyperpigmentation, hyperkeratosis, and ulceration.
- Fever and malaise commonly occur.

L-Asparaginase

- L-Asparaginase is used in the treatment of lymphoid neoplasms.
- Neoplastic lymphoid cells require exogenous L-asparagine for growth. L-Asparaginase destroys this essential nutrient.

- L-Asparaginase is given either intravenously or intramuscularly.
- Hypersensitivity reactions vary from urticaria to anaphylaxis. Skin testing with drug may help confirm hypersensitivity. Intramuscular administration may result in fewer hypersensitivity reactions. Patients should be observed carefully after dosing, and epinephrine should be available to reverse acute hypersensitivity reaction.
- Hypoalbuminemia may result from inhibition of hepatic protein synthesis.
- Decreased antithrombin, protein C, and protein S levels may result in arterial or venous thrombosis. Preexisting clotting abnormalities, such as antiphospholipid antibodies or factor V Leiden, may predispose to thromboembolic complications.
- Decreased levels of fibrinogen and factors II, VII, IX, and X may result in bleeding.
- Inhibition of insulin production may result in hyperglycemia.
- High doses of L-asparaginase may cause cerebral dysfunction manifested by confusion, stupor, and coma, and may also cause nonhemorrhagic pancreatitis.
- L-Asparaginase can be used to prevent marrow suppression if given after high-dose methotrexate.

Non-Cell Cycle–Active Agents
Alkylating Drugs
- Used as single agents or in combination with other drugs to treat hematologic neoplasms.
- All form covalent bonds with electron-rich sites on DNA.
- Myelosuppression and mucositis are the major acute toxicities.
- Pulmonary fibrosis and secondary leukemias are the major delayed toxicities.
- Clinical basis of resistance to alkylating drugs is not fully understood.
- Rapidly eliminated by chemical conjugation to sulfhydryl groups or by oxidative metabolism.
- Cyclophosphamide and ifosfamide produce a toxic metabolite (acrolein) that is excreted in the urine and can cause hemorrhagic cystitis. Acrolein may be detoxified by sodium 2-mercaptoethane sulfonate (mesna) given simultaneously.
- Nitrogen mustard is a potent vesicant.
- Marrow toxicity is cumulative and is a function of the total dose.
- The incidence of secondary leukemias is related to the total dose administered and to the drugs used. Procarbazine is especially potent in inducing secondary leukemia.
- Dose-limiting toxicity of dacarbazine is nausea and vomiting.
- Nitrosoureas produce delayed myelosuppression, with nadir of blood counts 4 to 6 weeks after the dose, and can also cause nephrotoxicity.
- All alkylating agents can produce pulmonary fibrosis. Busulfan and nitrosoureas are the most likely to do so.

High-Dose Alkylating Agent Therapy
- High-dose chemotherapy programs use one or several alkylating agents because of the strong relationship between dose and cytotoxicity of these drugs.
- With autologous or allogeneic hematopoietic stem cell infusions, doses of alkylating agents can be increased 2- to 18-fold until extramedullary toxicities become limiting.

Thalidomide and Lenalidomide
- Thalidomide and lenalidomide have established value in treating myeloma refractory to first-line chemotherapy and are now being considered for use as first-line therapy in combination with other biological agents (e.g., proteasome inhibitors).
- When used in doses of 25 mg/day for 21 of 28 days, lenalidomide is dramatically effective in normalizing hematologic parameters in the subset of patients with myelodysplasia who have a 5q–deletion on cytogenetics.

- Lenalidomide produces dramatic tumor responses in patients with CLL, including a tumor flare and tumor lysis syndrome, a potentially fatal complication, even in patients with disease refractory to conventional agents.
- In CLL, the drug is equally effective in patients with poor prognostic cytogenetics (chromosomes 11 and 17 deletions).
- To avoid acute tumor responses, lenalidomide should be used in low doses (beginning at 2.5 to 5 mg/day and escalating thereafter).
- The mechanism of action of thalidomide and the newer analogue, lenalidomide, acts through a number of different mechanisms, including a prominent antiangiogenic effect against tumors, immune modulation, and inhibition of cytokine (e.g., tumor necrosis factor) secretion.
- The dose of thalidomide is 50 to 400 mg. There is no evidence for induction of metabolism on a daily dosing regimen. The major pathways for elimination including spontaneous hydrolysis of the imide esters, and further CYP-mediated metabolism by the liver. Less than 1 percent of the drug is excreted unchanged in the urine.
- Lenalidomide is well absorbed orally in doses up to 400 mg. Approximately 70 percent of administered drug is excreted unchanged by the renal route. Dose adjustments are recommended for patients in moderate (10 mg/day for creatinine clearance of 30–50 mL/min) or severe (10 mg every other day for creatinine clearance < 30 mL/min) renal failure.
- Lenalidomide causes much less sedation, constipation, and neurotoxicity than thalidomide, but it does cause prominent myelosuppression in 20 percent of patients.

Cell-Maturing (Terminal-Differentiating) Agents All-*Trans*-Retinoic Acid and Arsenic Trioxide

- Chemical agents, such as carotenes, retinoids, vitamin D, and some cytotoxic drugs, can cause maturation of human neoplastic granulocytic cells.
- All-*trans*-retinoic acid (ATRA) may induce a complete response in acute promyelocytic leukemia (APL) by causing maturation and apoptosis of leukemic promyelocytes.
- ATRA is given orally.
- ATRA used without an accompanying anthracycline antibiotic is associated with relapse.
- ATRA used with an anthracycline antibiotic has increased remission rates and duration of remission in APL.
- Toxicities of ATRA include dry skin, cheilitis, mild but reversible hepatic dysfunction, bone tenderness, hyperostosis on x-ray, and, occasionally, pseudotumor cerebri.
- The "retinoic acid syndrome" may occur, with respiratory failure, pleural and pericardial effusions, and peripheral edema usually associated with a rapid increase in the number of blood neutrophilic cells induced to mature from leukemic promyelocytes.
- High-dose glucocorticoid therapy may reverse the syndrome if the white blood cell count is rising rapidly. Otherwise, prompt administration of cytotoxic chemotherapy may prevent the syndrome.
- Arsenic trioxide induces apoptosis of leukemic cells in APL. Its mechanism of action probably stems from its ability to promote free radical production.
- Useful in refractory APL for reinduction of remission.

Histone Deacetylase Inhibitors

- This family of enzymes removes acetyl groups from amino groups of the lysines found in chromatin, thus promoting the compacting of chromatin and DNA and preventing gene expression.
- The most recent addition to the list of differentiating agents approved for clinical use against hematologic malignancies is vorinostat, or SAHA (suberoylanilide hydroxamic acid).

- Vorinostat causes partial or complete responses in 30 percent of patients with refractory cutaneous T cell lymphoma (CTCL).
- The drug causes minimal toxicity: mild to moderate fatigue, diarrhea, anemia, and minor decreases in the platelet count. Clinically significant thrombocytopenia occurs in 6 percent.

SMALL MOLECULES WITH SPECIFIC MOLECULAR TARGETS

c-ABL Kinase Inhibitors

- The first molecularly targeted drug to make a major impact on cancer treatment was imatinib mesylate (Gleevec), an inhibitor of ABL tyrosine kinase activity and notably the mutant ABL characteristic of the BCR-ABL fusion protein in CML.
- The drug has been impressively successful in inducing remission in chronic phase CML, and to lesser degrees in accelerated and blast crisis phases of the disease. However, many patients ultimately develop resistance to imatinib.
- Like imatinib, nilotinib and dasatinib are also inhibitors of the BCR-ABL kinase, as well as the c-KIT kinase and the platelet-derived growth factor receptor kinase. Dasatinib also inhibits the Src family kinases, an important secondary target in CML.
- Both dasatinib and nilotinib are more potent than imatinib. Nilotinib has been modified to overcome 32 of the 33 point mutations in the ABL portion of BCR-ABL that can cause resistance to imatinib. Dasatinib is unique in that it is able to bind BCR-ABL in both the open and closed configuration, which may be one of the mechanisms that allows it to overcome resistance.
- The BCR-ABL kinase inhibitors are all well absorbed by the oral route and subject to clearance by hepatic CYP 3A4 metabolism. Dasatinib's absorption is pH dependent and may be affected by the use of H_2-blockers or proton pump inhibitors.
- Imatinib, dasatinib, and nilotinib have modest toxicity, including gastrointestinal distress (diarrhea, nausea, and vomiting), fluid retention (edema and pleural effusions). Nilotinib causes a unique prolongation of the QT interval. All three drugs can induce neutropenia and anemia and hepatotoxicity.

Bortezomib

- Bortezomib inhibits the chymotryptic-like activity of the 20S subunit of the proteasome, thereby altering the balance of intracellular expression of regulators of proliferation and survival in a manner conducive to rapid and irreversible commitment of susceptible cells to their death.
- The drug is highly effective as a single agent in myeloma, due to multiple mechanisms including the induced accumulation of IκB, a proteasomal substrate, and the ensuing IκB inhibition of nuclear factor-κB which play an important role in myeloma cell survival.
- Bortezomib has now become a key component of many regimens in which it is combined with other agents, such as prednisone, melphalan, lenalidomide, or thalidomide.
- The standard schedule of bortezomib administration is an intravenous injection at a maximum tolerated dose of 1.3 mg/m^2 administered twice weekly with a 10-day rest period (days 1, 4, 8, 11, 22, 25, 29, and 32).
- The most common side effects are thrombocytopenia and painful sensory neuropathy.

THERAPEUTIC MONOCLONAL ANTIBODIES AND OTHER IMMUNOLOGICALLY BASED AGENTS

- Monoclonal antibodies used alone can block access to important growth promoting cell surface molecules; induce apoptosis upon binding; promote antibody dependent cellular cytotoxicity; and when coupled to toxic moieties, target cells for enhanced concentrations of the appended molecule.

Rituximab

- Rituximab was the first monoclonal to receive approval by the US Food and Drug Administration.
- It is a chimeric antibody containing the human immunoglobulin G1 and κ constant regions with murine variable regions that target the B-cell antigen CD20 expressed on the surface of normal B cells and on more than 90 percent of B-cell neoplasms.
- Rituximab induces programmed cell death upon binding to CD20.
- While initially approved for use as a single agent in indolent non-Hodgkin lymphoma, rituximab is now a component of multi-agent chemotherapy for a wide range of lymphomas and other B-cell neoplasms.
- Rituximab is infused intravenously both as a single agent and in combination with chemotherapy at a dose of 375 mg/m^2. As a single agent, it is given weekly for 4 weeks with maintenance doses every 3 to 6 months.
- Rarely, rituximab infusion leads to severe mucocutaneous skin reactions (Stevens-Johnson syndrome). Pretreatment with antihistamines, acetaminophen, and glucocorticoids have become a standard measure to modulate infusion reactions.
- Rituximab, as a result of immune suppression, may reactivate hepatitis B infection; patients should be screened for hepatitis B infection prior to initiation of therapy. It may also lead to progressive and fatal multifocal leukoencephalopathy caused by Jacob-Creutzfeldt virus. Hypogammaglobulinemia and delayed neutropenia may appear 1 to 5 months after administration.
- Resistance to rituximab may occur by down regulation of CD20, impaired ADCC, decreased complement activation, limited effects on signaling and induction of apoptosis, or inadequate blood levels.

Alemtuzumab

- Alemtuzumab (Campath) is a humanized monoclonal antibody targeted against the CD52 antigen present on the surface of normal neutrophils and lymphocytes as well as most B- and T-cell lymphomas.
- The drug can induce tumor cell death through ADCC and complement-dependent cytotoxicity. The antibody is most useful in treating low-grade lymphomas and CLL, particularly in patients with disease refractory to fludarabine.
- The most concerning side effects are acute infusion reactions and depletion of normal neutrophils and T cells.

Denileukin Diftitox

- Denileukin diftitox (Ontak, DAB389 IL-2) combines IL-2 and the catalytically active fragment of diphtheria toxin. The toxin fragment crosses into the target cell, carried in with its fusion partner which binds with high affinity to the human IL-2 receptor.
- Malignant T- and B-cell tumors express the high affinity form of the IL-2R, which is not expressed on normal resting T cells but is upregulated by antigen activation. The limited tissue expression of the high-affinity IL-2R makes this a selective target for cancer treatments.
- Denileukin diftitox causes hypersensitivity reactions, a vascular leak syndrome, and constitutional toxicities including fever, chills, and fatigue; glucocorticoid premedication significantly decreases toxicity.

Gemtuzumab Ozogamicin

- Gemtuzumab ozogamicin (Mylotarg), a humanized mouse antibody covalently linked to a potent chemical toxin, calicheamicin. The antibody recognizes CD33, an antigen expressed by more than 90 percent of AML cells but not expressed on normal marrow hematopoietic stem cells (although it is expressed on myeloid progenitor cells).

- The antibody conjugate produced a 30 percent complete response rate in relapsed AML, when administered at a dose of 9 mg/m^2 for up to three doses at 2-week intervals. Most patients require two to three doses to achieve remission.
- The drug is currently approved for use in older adults (>60 years) with acute myelogenous leukemia in first relapse.
- Its primary toxicities include myelosuppression in all patients treated, and hepatocellular damage in 30 to 40 percent of patients, manifested by hyperbilirubinemia and enzyme elevations. Patients may manifest a syndrome that resembles hepatic venoocclusive disease when they subsequently undergo myeloablative therapy, or when gemtuzumab ozogamicin follows high-dose chemotherapy.

Radioimmunoconjugates Tositumomab and Ibritumomab Tiuxetan

- The beta-emitter ^{90}yttrium (^{90}Y) has emerged as an attractive alternative to ^{131}I coupled monoclonal antibodies, based on its higher energy and longer path length, and effectiveness in larger tumors. It also has a short half-life and remains tightly conjugated to antibody, even after endocytosis, providing a safer profile for outpatient use.
- Murine anti-CD20 antibodies with either ^{131}I (tositumomab or Bexxar) or ^{90}Y (ibritumomab tiuxetan or Zevalin) have impressive responses rates of 65 to 80 percent in relapsed lymphomas.
- The administration of either ibritumomab tiuxetan or tositumomab requires two steps: first, a test dose to determine biodistribution and allow dose calculation, and a second step of actual therapeutic dosing. In each step, unlabeled antibody is first administered to saturate non-tumor binding sites. Use of these agents requires careful coordination between oncologist and a nuclear medicine specialist.

For a more detailed discussion, see Bruce A. Chabner, Jeffrey Barnes, James Cleary, Andrew Lane, Constantine Mitsiades, and Paul Richardson: Pharmacology and Toxicity of Antineoplastic Agents. Chap. 20, p. 283 in *Williams Hematology,* 8th ed.

CHAPTER 40
Principles of Hematopoietic Stem Cell Transplantation

SOURCES OF HEMATOPOIETIC STEM CELLS (HSCs)

Marrow

- Marrow for hematopoietic stem cell transplantation (HSCT) is typically aspirated by repeated placement of large bore needles into the posterior iliac crest, generally 50 to 100 aspirations simultaneously on both sides, while under regional or general anesthesia.
- The lowest cell dose to ensure stable long-term engraftment has not been defined with certainty, and a standard collection contains more than 2×10^8 nucleated marrow cells/kg recipient body weight.
- Current guidelines indicate that a volume of up to 20 mL/kg donor body weight should be effective.
- Seventy percent of donors fully recover by 2 weeks and the risk of serious complications is 1.2 percent.

Mobilized Peripheral Blood Stem Cells (PBSC)

- The most common method to harvest autologous and allogeneic PBSCs is by using granulocyte colony-stimulating factor (G-CSF) with or without chemotherapy. This procedure is safe and in a review of 5930 normal donors, serious side effects were uncommon (< 1%). Splenic rupture has been reported with an estimated incidence of 1 in 10,000.
- Randomized clinical trials have indicated that engraftment is more rapid with PBSC than with marrow-derived stem cells.
- The measurement of the absolute number of CD34+ cells/kg recipient body weight collected is a reliable and practical method for determining the adequacy of the PBSC product. A minimum of 2×10^6/kg CD34+ cells is usually recommended, although at this dose, 10 to 20 percent of autologous collections lead to suboptimal (slow or more rarely, no) engraftment. Platelet recovery is most sensitive to borderline collection numbers.
- Although the number of T cells in PBSC graft is 10-fold greater than in marrow, the incidence of acute graft-versus-host disease (GVHD) does not appear higher, probably because G-CSF influences the proportion of immune tolerizing T_{reg} cells in the apheresis product. However, the risk of chronic GVHD has been found to be about 10 percent higher in PBSC at most major transplant centers.
- The use of G-CSF to mobilize stem cells in patients with sickle cell anemia is contraindicated, since an acute increase in neutrophil counts can precipitate a catastrophic sickle cell occlusive crisis.

Umbilical Cord Blood

- Umbilical cord blood (UCB) collected from the umbilical vessels in the placenta at the time of delivery is a rich source of HSCs.
- Because these cells are immunologically relatively naïve, recipients may have satisfactory outcomes, even when crossing major histocompatibility barriers.
- An analysis of approximately 100 UCB transplants showed that recipients who received $< 1.7 \times 10^7$ cells/kg body weight had a high rate of graft failure. For adults, this usually requires the use of two closely and suitably matched cord bloods providing a higher CD34+ and CD3+ cell dose.

DEGREE OF MATCHING

HLA Matched Related Donor

- HLA matched sibling donors were the most common source of HSCT products prior to the establishment of sufficiently diverse unrelated stem cell donor banks. The experience with these transplants for any given disease always serves as the major comparison group for alternative SCT donor sources.

HLA Haploidentical Related Donor

- Because nearly every patient requiring HSCT has a haploidentical family donor (on average half of one's siblings and every parent or child), immune depletion of such stem cell products to reduce the inevitable fatal GVHD has been explored.
- Numerous studies document the feasibility of this approach, with acceptable rates of a GVHD, and control of the underlying leukemia, the widespread acceptance of haploidentical SCT remains hampered by the prolonged immune reconstitution and a high risk of serious infection experienced in these patients.

HLA Matched Unrelated Donor (MUD)

- The establishment of diverse banks of individuals willing to donate stem cells should their HLA type be required elsewhere in the world has greatly expanded the likelihood of obtaining a donor for the 60 percent or greater proportion of individuals for whom a suitable sibling donor cannot be identified (a percentage that approaches 100% in China). However, the likelihood of obtaining a MUD for persons of African or Hispanic descent is substantially lower.
- The only drawbacks to MUD transplants are moderately higher rates of GVHD, secondary to minor histocompatibility antigens less likely to match the transplant recipient if derived from an unrelated rather than a sibling donor, the longer time required to identify a suitable MUD, and the greater possibility (than for a family member) that once identified, a MUD might decline to donate.

HLA Partially Matched Cord Blood Donor

- Because of the immunologic naivete of UCB cells, two or greater HLA mismatches are often tolerated for transplantation, resulting in a similar frequency and severity of GVHD as seen using fully matched donors.
- Compared to adult sources of HSCs, UCB transplants engraft more slowly, especially the slow restitution of platelet counts.

Autologous HSCs

- Autologous HSCT is associated with the lowest rate of nonrelapse morbidity and mortality of any SCT strategy.
- The purpose of the infusion of autologous HSCs (referred to as autologous HSCT, although not crossing transplantation barriers and is not transplantation in the classic sense) is to permit the administration of very high dose, potentially lethal therapy, to induce remission and cure tumors such as leukemia, myeloma, or lymphoma. The autologous HSC infusion restores hematopoiesis and makes mortality from cytotoxic therapy–induced severe and prolonged marrow aplasia unlikely.
- One problem with autologous HSCT is the presence in the product of residual tumor cells contaminating the patient's marrow or blood. One approach to this issue is purging tumor cells from the HSC product before infusion. Controversy still exists as to whether purging is a requirement in most cases because the process often reduces the stem cell numbers.
- A number of *ex vivo* chemical-based purging strategies for autologous stem cell products failed, mostly because they damaged HSCs and reduced engraftment.

- A number of immunologic purging methods have been tested, both negative selection of tumor cells and positive selection of stem cells, and have provided mixed results. Perhaps the most common is selection and administration of CD34+ cells.
- While the administration of CD34+ graft products results in relatively rapid engraftment, with demonstrated reduction in tumor cell contamination by *in vitro* methods, ultimate relapse rates are not substantially improved and the risk of infection is greater because of immune cell depletion.
- Instead, *in vivo* purging has been widely applied to autologous transplantation. The use of chemotherapy and immunotherapy just prior to mobilization of HSCs reduces tumor cell contamination of the collected PBSC product, and simultaneously provides a reduction in total tumor burden in the patient prior to his/her high-dose conditioning regimen.

Purification of HSCs from Any Source

- In humans, the combination of positive selection for CD34, Thy-1, and negative selection for lineage markers, identified a homogenous HSC population.
- The goal is to purify HSC and thereby reduce the risk of occult malignant cells since marrow or blood mononuclear cells are often contaminated by malignant cells in patients with hematologic malignancies. These efforts present technical challenges primarily because of the rarity of HSC in marrow and G-CSF mobilized blood; however, adequate numbers of HSCs can be isolated free of contaminating tumor cells, in a majority of patients.
- The time to neutrophil and platelet recovery following purified HSC infusion is comparable to engraftment times using unmanipulated marrow as a graft source, but there is a significant delay in T-cell recovery, especially of CD4+ T cells, of up to 6 months in almost all patients.
- A number of patients develop unusual infections (i.e., severe cases of influenza, respiratory syncytial virus, cytomegalovirus, and *Pneumocystis* pneumonia), which raises concern using a "pure" HSC product as the sole source of hematopoietic reconstitution in clinical transplantation.
- Although too few patients were transplanted to evaluate whether the infusion of a product free of contaminating tumor cells impacted outcomes on event-free and overall survival, results appeared favorable.

Graft-versus-Tumor Effect

- Compared with autologous transplantation, allogeneic HSCT involves more pre-transplantation preparation, poses a greater risk of complications to the patient, is associated with a significantly higher nonrelapse morbidity and mortality, and the period of intensive posttransplantation follow-up is considerably longer. However, unlike autologous stem cell products, there is no risk of tumor contamination in allogeneic HSC products.
- Since tumor cells are host derived, and allogeneic immune cells recognize them as foreign, the potential exists for the graft to attack the residual tumor cells present in the patient following conditioning therapy. The evidence that allogeneic HSCT outcomes are greatly affected by this graft-versus-tumor effect is summarized in Table 40–1.

CONDITIONING REGIMENS

- A major obstacle to successful allogeneic HSCT is the immune competence of the recipient, providing the ability to reject the graft.
- This potential to reject infused donor cells is mediated predominantly through residual host T and NK cells.
- In addition to reducing residual tumor burden in transplant recipients, conditioning regimens must reduce or eliminate this immunologic barrier to successful HSCT.

TABLE 40-1	EVIDENCE FOR GRAFT-VERSUS-TUMOR EFFECT IN ALLOGENEIC HEMATOPOIETIC CELL TRANSPLANTATION

Temporal association between immune suppression drug withdrawal and disease remission.

Leukemia relapse rate is lower after allogeneic HCT than after syngeneic HCT.

Leukemia relapse is lower in patients who develop GVHD than in those who do not.

Leukemia relapse rate is lower after allogeneic HCT without GVHD than after syngeneic HCT.

Leukemia relapse rate is higher after T-cell–depleted allogeneic HCT than after unmodified HCT.

Donor lymphocyte infusions induce remission of leukemia that recurred after allogeneic HCT.

Allogeneic HCT after reduced-intensity conditioning induce long lasting remission of leukemia and lymphoma.

GVHD, graft-versus-host disease; HCT, hematopoietic cell transplantation.
Source: *Williams Hematology*, 8th ed, Chap. 21, Table 21–2, p. 319.

Total Body Irradiation (TBI)

- TBI has been a primary therapeutic modality included in autologous and allogeneic SCT regimens for patients with hematologic malignancies.
- TBI has excellent therapeutic effect against a variety of hematolymphoid malignancies, including leukemia that is resistant to chemotherapy, has sufficient immunosuppressive properties, and is able to treat tumor cell sanctuary sites like the testicles and the central nervous system.
- Most groups employ fractionated dose schedules to a total of 1200–1320 cGy.
- TBI is almost always used in conjunction with high-dose chemotherapy (e.g., cyclophosphamide) in full-dose conditioning regimens.
- An alternate form of irradiation is radioimmunotherapy, which involves the use of antibodies to CD33 or CD45 to deliver locally acting radionucleotides to sites of disease, notably in the marrow.
- Radiation toxicities include later development of cataracts, treatment-related malignancies, and growth impairment in children.

High-Dose Chemotherapy

- A number of chemotherapy regimens that are both effective for the tumor under treatment and are sufficiently immunologically ablative to allow successful HSC engraftment has been tested in patients undergoing autologous and allogeneic SCT for leukemia and lymphoma.
- For example, BCNU, VP-16 and cyclophosphamide alone, busulfan and cyclophosphamide (BuCy), and adjusted dose BuCy in which monitoring of Bu levels reduces its toxicity.

Reduced-Intensity Conditioning (RIC) Regimens

- The demonstration that immune-mediated mechanisms are critical in controlling minimal residual disease challenged the concept that relatively toxic full-dose chemoradiation is required for cure following allogeneic HSCT.
- Transplantation regimens that use significantly lower doses of chemoradiation yet that are sufficiently immunosuppressive to allow full donor hematopoietic cell engraftment, have shifted the burden of tumor eradication to graft-versus-tumor effects.
- RIC is better tolerated than traditional full-dose regimens and is particularly useful in older patients and in those individuals who have comorbid medical

conditions that preclude them from aggressive myeloablative regimens, and for patients without malignancy, in whom it is critical only to allow engraftment of a new immune system.

- One regimen came from detailed studies in a canine model and uses TBI at 2 Gy followed by immunosuppression with mycophenolate mofetil and cyclosporine in an attempt to prevent the recipient T cells from rejecting the graft.
- The addition of fludarabine to low-dose TBI or cyclophosphamide also reduces the risk of graft rejection to less than 5 percent.
- The risk of GVHD is not reduced by RIC.
- Because host hematopoiesis is not ablated when the patient receives his/her donor HSCs, marrow cells are chimeric soon after transplantation with RIC regimens. However, because host HSCs are at a competitive disadvantage, as they have been irradiated or subjected to toxic drugs during conditioning, over time the donor HSCs progressively populate the entire marrow.

EVALUATION AND SELECTION OF CANDIDATES FOR TRANSPLANTATION

- Patients considered for transplantation require in-depth counseling by experienced transplantation physicians, nurses, and social workers.
- Information regarding the prior course, including initial diagnostic studies, previous drug and radiation treatments, and responses to these interventions, as well as a psychosocial assessment of the patient and their caregivers, are important.
- Table 40–2 highlights the issues and topics that should be addressed during the counseling meetings with transplantation candidates and their families or friends.

TABLE 40–2   TOPICS ADDRESSED DURING COUNSELING MEETINGS WITH TRANSPLANT CANDIDATE AND CARE PROVIDER

I.	Rationale for why transplantation is a therapeutic option
II.	How the transplantation is performed Autologous Allogeneic—choice for full-dose versus RIC
III.	Source of cells Marrow versus blood versus other source
IV.	Risks of procedure
V.	Graft failure and graft rejection
VI.	Risk of GVHD Acute and chronic forms, compatibility of graft Likelihood for long-term immune suppression medication
VII.	Nonrelapse mortality at 100 days and 1 year
VIII.	Risks of relapse
IX.	Timing of transplant
X.	Projected result
XI.	Requirement for dedicated care provider
XII.	Other Financial implications Durable power of attorney Banking of sperm, *in vitro* fertilized eggs Duration of stay near the transplantation center Return to home and work Sexual activity Quality-of-life issues Habits such as smoking, alcohol, and drug addiction

GVHD, graft-versus-host disease; RIC, reduced-intensity conditioning.
Source: *Williams Hematology*, 8th ed, Chap. 21, Table 21–3, p. 321.

DISEASE STATUS AT THE TIME OF TRANSPLANTATION

- Disease status at the time of transplantation is the best predictor of long-term disease-free survival following allogeneic and autologous SCT.
- Attempts at salvaging patients with advanced disease who have failed multiple therapies are rarely successful and if transplantation is to be considered, it is best to consider early in the course of therapy.

AGE AND COMORBID CONDITIONS AT THE TIME OF TRANSPLANTATION

- Among adult and pediatric patients, older age at the time of transplantation is an important determinant that adversely affects nonrelapse mortality following autologous and full-dose allogeneic transplant conditioning.
- Comorbid medical conditions (e.g., diabetes mellitus, renal insufficiency) can have a significant impact on transplantation outcomes.
- Routine screening of heart and lung function to detect occult abnormalities is important, especially in older patients.
- Evaluation of liver and kidney function, as well as exposures to potential pathogens such as hepatitis B, hepatitis C, herpes viruses and HIV should be performed in all patients.

DISEASES TREATED WITH STEM CELL TRANSPLANTATION

- In general terms, autologous transplantation is recommended for patients whose malignancy exhibits chemosensitivity to conventional dose therapy and does not extensively involve the marrow.
- In contrast, allogeneic transplantation is generally pursued for hematologic malignancies and disorders that primarily originate in the marrow, such as acute and chronic leukemia, aplastic anemia, and the myelodysplastic and myeloproliferative syndromes.
- A variety of acquired nonmalignant and congenital disorders can be successfully treated with HSCT. Most notable is allogeneic HSCT for patients with severe aplastic anemia, for which outstanding results have been achieved for those individuals who have an HLA-matched sibling donor; upwards of 80 to 90 percent of these patients have a complete hematologic remission and a long-term disease-free course. HSCT for patients with clinically significant hemoglobin disorders, such as thalassemia major, has been successful, especially in patients without significant liver disease. Likewise, allogeneic HSCT is considered a treatment option for young patients with severe forms of sickle cell disease.
- Table 40–3 lists disorders commonly treated by transplantation.

SELECTED RESULTS OF STEM CELL TRANSPLANTATION

Acute Myelogenous Leukemia (AML)

- Hematopoietic SCT has a significant role in the treatment of AML patients. Many studies have consistently demonstrated that relapse rates are decreased by allogeneic transplantation. In particular, the likelihood of long-term survival is superior in patients with primary refractory disease, *de novo* AML with unfavorable cytogenetics at any stage of their disease, or with intermediate or favorable cytogenetics at first relapse or subsequent stages. Patients at first presentation with favorable cytogenetics should be treated with subtype specific chemotherapy. Whether patients with intermediate prognosis cytogenetics should be treated with allogeneic transplantation in first remission is controversial.

Acute Lymphocytic Leukemia (ALL)

- Virtually all adults with ALL and standard or high-risk features (including Ph + ALL) should be treated with allogeneic transplantation in first remission.

TABLE 40–3	**LIST OF DISEASES TREATED BY HEMATOPOIETIC CELL TRANSPLANTATION**	
Disease/Condition	Allogeneic HCT	Autologous HCT
Malignant disease		
Acute myelogenous leukemia	+	+
Acute lymphoblastic leukemia	+	–
Chronic myelogenous leukemia	+	+
Chronic lymphocytic leukemia	+	+
Myelodysplastic syndromes	+	–
Myeloproliferative syndromes	+	–
Non-Hodgkin lymphoma	+	+
Hodgkin lymphoma	+	+
Myeloma	+	+
Amyloidosis	–	+
Waldenström macroglobulinemia	+	+
Hairy cell leukemia	+	–
Selected solid tumors (testicular cancer, pediatric tumors)	–	+
Neuroblastoma	–	+
Nonmalignant diseases		
Acquired aplastic anemia	+	–
Congenital pure red cell aplasia	+	–
Fanconi anemia	+	–
Thalassemia	+	–
Sickle cell anemia	+	–
Paroxysmal nocturnal hemoglobinuria	+	–
Severe combined immunodeficiency	+	–
Wiskott-Aldrich	+	–
Congenital leukocyte dysfunction	+	–
Osteopetrosis	+	–
Familial erythrophagocytic lymphohistiocytosis	+	–
Glanzmann disease	+	–
Hereditary storage diseases	+	–
Selected autoimmune diseases	+	+

Source: *Williams Hematology*, 8th ed, Chap. 21, Table 21–4, p. 323.

Myeloma

- Autologous HSCT within the first year of initiating treatment has been the standard of care for patients younger than 70 years of age with newly diagnosed myeloma. Although neither chemotherapy nor autologous HSCT produces a cure, event-free and overall survival are prolonged following transplantation when compared to treatment with conventional chemotherapy alone. However, with the introduction of lenalidomide and bortezomib, and the ensuing markedly prolonged remissions they induce, the role of HSCT is being reexamined.

Non-Hodgkin Lymphoma

- Patients with chemosensitive moderate- and high-grade lymphoma beyond first complete remission have an improved overall survival with high-dose therapy followed by autologous HSCT compared to best-of-care salvage chemotherapy. Improvement in survival for patients with B-cell non-Hodgkin lymphoma may further be achieved with inclusion of rituximab as an *in vivo* purging strategy and perhaps in the posttransplantation setting. Relapse of lymphoma after autologous transplantation is the major reason for treatment failure. Several phase II studies reported that patients who suffer a relapse of lymphoma after autologous transplantation could still be salvaged and experience long-term survival of greater than 45 percent using RIC and allogeneic transplantation from matched related and unrelated donors.

COMPLICATIONS OF STEM CELL TRANSPLANTATION

- The first 100 days following the cell infusion is typically the time of greatest risk for recipients of autologous and allogeneic HSCT.
- The most common complications of HSCT are listed in Table 40–4.

TABLE 40–4   **COMPLICATIONS OF HEMATOPOIETIC CELL TRANSPLANTATION**

Vascular access complications
Graft failure
Blood group incompatibilities and hemolytic complications
Acute GVHD
Chronic GVHD
Infectious complications
   Bacterial infections
   Fungal infections
   Cytomegalovirus infection
   Herpes simplex virus infections
   Varicella-zoster virus infections
   Epstein-Barr virus infections
   Adenovirus, respiratory viruses, HHV-6, -7, -8, and other viruses
Gastrointestinal complications
   Mucosal ulceration/bleeding
   Nutritional support
Hepatic complications
   Sinusoidal obstructive syndrome
   Hepatitis: infectious versus noninfectious
Lung injury
   Interstitial pneumonitis: infectious versus noninfectious
   Diffuse alveolar hemorrhage
   Engraftment syndrome
   Bronchiolitis obliterans
Kidney and bladder complications
Endocrine complications
Drug–drug interactions
Growth and development
Late onset nonmalignant complications
   Osteoporosis/osteopenia, avascular necrosis, dental problems, cataracts, chronic fatigue, psychosocial effects, and rehabilitation
Secondary malignancies
Neurologic complications
   Infectious, transplant conditioning and immune suppression medication toxicities
Thrombotic thrombocytopenic purpura

GVHD, graft-versus-host disease; HHV, human herpes virus subtypes.
Source: *Williams Hematology*, 8th ed, Chap. 21, Table 21–5, p. 326.

Graft Failure

- Graft failure is defined as the lack of hematopoietic cell engraftment following autologous and allogeneic HSCT.
- Criteria are predominantly operational and graft failure is divided into primary (early) and secondary (late) phases.
- The consequences of graft failure are significant and include a high risk of mortality, often as a consequence of infection and hemorrhage related to cytopenias.

Graft Rejection

- Graft rejection is the immune-mediated rejection of allogeneic donor cells by residual host effector cells that occurs because of the genetic disparity between the recipient and the donor.
- The determination of graft rejection requires analysis of blood or marrow for chimerism as graft rejection is defined as the inability to detect a meaningful percentage of donor hematopoietic elements.
- Allogeneic HSCT following RIC is associated with incomplete eradication of host hematopoietic elements.

Sinusoidal Obstructive Disease (Veno-occlusive Disease)

- Sinusoidal obstructive syndrome (SOS) is a clinical syndrome of tender hepatomegaly, fluid retention, weight gain, and elevated serum bilirubin that follows autologous or allogeneic HSCT.
- The incidence of SOS varies significantly with the intensity of the regimen; from less than 10 percent with RIC to as high as 50 percent following regimens that use cyclophosphamide combined with TBI of greater than 14 Gy.

Infections

- Two important measures for reducing infections in immunocompromised transplant recipients are an effective hand-washing policy, and a strategy for preventing transmission of respiratory infections.
- Screening the blood supply has reduced the incidence of transfusion-related infections, especially hepatitis C virus and cytomegalovirus in seronegative recipients.
- The duration of neutropenia and severity of oral and gastrointestinal mucosal damage from the conditioning regimen are risk factors for infection before neutrophil recovery has occurred.
- Following neutrophil recovery, the persistent B- and T-cell–mediated immune deficiency increases susceptibility to opportunistic infections.
- Patients who require ongoing immunosuppressive therapy for the control of chronic GVHD are at risk for recurrent bacteremia with encapsulated bacteria and sinopulmonary infections.
- Fungal infections can be serious complications following HSCT and are more commonly observed in recipients of allografts as a result of the requirement for posttransplantation immunosuppression medication. Fluconazole prophylaxis decreases the incidence of invasive and superficial *Candida albicans* infections and may decrease the 100-day mortality in allogeneic HSCT recipients.
- Infection from the herpesvirus family members can cause significant morbidity and mortality and is a common phenomenon following HSCT. Most of the infections are a result of reactivation and the temporal pattern of reactivation follows a relatively predictable course.
- During the first 100 days after transplantation, patients with viremia are at high risk for developing cytomegalovirus pneumonitis or gastroenteritis. First-line therapy for patients with cytomegalovirus pneumonia or gastroenteritis is ganciclovir combined with intravenous immunoglobulin.

Acute GVHD

- Acute GVHD remains one of the most serious and challenging complications following allogeneic HSCT. The most important risk factor for the development of acute GVHD is the degree of HLA disparity between donor and recipient.
- Acute GVHD occurs prior to day 100 (although there are clearly exceptions) and primarily affects the skin, gastrointestinal tract, and liver. The severity score ranges between grades 0 and IV and is defined by involvement of each organ system.
- Acute GVHD, grades II to IV, is considered clinically significant because it is moderately severe, and usually consists of multiorgan disease. Grade II acute GVHD is not typically associated with a poor outcome; however, grades III and IV acute GVHD is associated with a high risk of mortality and decreased patient survival.
- The mainstay of acute GVHD prevention is prophylaxis with immunosuppressive drugs, and all patients undergoing allogeneic HSCT with a T-cell–replete graft require prophylaxis. Primary prophylaxis with cyclosporine-methotrexate or FK506 (tacrolimus)-methotrexate is the commonly used standard to prevent acute GVHD.
- The most common agent used to treat acute GVHD is a glucocorticoid, usually methylprednisolone or prednisone at a dose of 1 to 2 mg/kg per day with subsequent tapering once disease activity resolves. Glucocorticoids alone are effective in 50 percent of patients.
- A variety of other approaches have been explored in the treatment of acute GVHD, including the use of other immunosuppressive agents, antibody-based therapies either to T-cells or cytokines, and photopheresis, all administered in combination with prednisone.

Chronic GVHD

- The clinical manifestations of chronic GVHD are broad and share overlapping features with a variety of autoimmune disorders, such as scleroderma, lichen planus, and dermatomyositis. Chronic GVHD most commonly occurs beyond day 100.
- If generalized scleroderma occurs, it may lead to joint contractures and debility.
- Elevations in alkaline phosphatase and serum bilirubin are often the first indication of hepatic involvement with chronic GVHD. Damage to the bile ducts has a similar histopathology to that seen in primary biliary cirrhosis. Liver biopsies are often helpful in establishing a diagnosis.
- The mainstay of treatment for established chronic GVHD continues to be prednisone. Because of the chronic nature of this disease, long-term treatment is often required. Alternate-day dosing has been found to help reduce some of the toxicity associated with prolonged glucocorticoid use.

For a more detailed discussion, see Robert Lowsky and Robert S. Negrin: Principles of Hematopoietic Cell Transplantation. Chap. 21, p. 313 in *Williams Hematology,* 8th ed.

PART VI

THE CLONAL MYELOID DISORDERS

CHAPTER 41
Classification and Clinical Manifestations of the Clonal Myeloid Disorders

PATHOGENESIS

- Result from a mutation(s) of DNA within a single pluripotential marrow hematopoietic cell or very early progenitor cell. Mutations disturb the function of the gene product.
- Overt cytogenetic abnormalities can be found in 80 percent of cases of acute myelogenous leukemia (AML) in experienced laboratories (see *Williams Hematology*, 8th ed, Chap. 11, Fig. 11–3, p. 153).
  — Translocations (e.g., t(15;17)) and inversions of chromosomes (e.g., inv16) can result in the expression of fusion genes that encode fusion proteins that are oncogenic.
  — Overexpression or underexpression of genes that encode molecules critical to the control of cell growth or programmed cell death, often within signal transduction pathways or involving transcription factors occur.
  — Deletions of all or part of a chromosome (e.g., 5q- or -7) or duplication of all or part of a chromosome may be evident (e.g., trisomy 8).
- An early multipotential hematopoietic cell undergoes clonal expansion but retains the ability to differentiate and mature, albeit with varying degrees of pathologic features, into various blood cell lineages.
- The result is often abnormal blood cell concentrations (either above or below normal), abnormal blood cell structure and function; the abnormalities may range from minimal to severe.
- Resulting disease phenotypes are numerous and varied because of the nine differentiation lineages from a multipotential hematopoietic cell.
- Neoplasms that result can be grouped, somewhat arbitrarily, by the degree of loss of differentiation and maturation potential and by the rate of disease progression.
- Most patients can be grouped into the classic diagnostic designations listed in Table 41–1.

TABLE 41-1 **NEOPLASTIC (CLONAL) MYELOID DISORDERS**

I. Minimal-deviation neoplasms (no leukemic blast cells are evident in marrow)
   A. Underproduction of mature cells is prominent
      1. Clonal (refractory) sideroblastic anemia[a] (see Chap. 42)
      2. Clonal (refractory) nonsideroblastic anemia[a] (see Chap. 42)
      3. Clonal bi- or tricytopenia[a] (see Chap. 42)
      4. Paroxysmal nocturnal hemoglobinuria (see Chap. 45)
   B. Overproduction of mature cells is prominent
      1. Polycythemia vera (see Chap. 43)
      2. Essential thrombocythemia (see Chap. 44)

II. Moderate-deviation neoplasms (small proportions of leukemic blast cells usually present in marrow)
   A. Chronic myelogenous leukemia (see Chap. 47)
      1. Ph chromosome-positive, *BCR* rearrangement positive (~90%)
      2. Ph chromosome-negative, *BCR* rearrangement positive (~6%)
      3. Ph chromosome-negative, *BCR* rearrangement negative (~4%)
   B. Primary myelofibrosis[b] (chronic megakaryocytic leukemia) (see Chap. 48)
   C. Chronic eosinophilic leukemia (see Chaps. 34 and 47)
      1. *PDGFR* rearrangement positive
      2. *FGFR1* rearrangement-positive
   D. Chronic neutrophilic leukemia (see Chap. 47)
   E. Chronic basophilic leukemia (see Chap. 47)
   F. Systemic mastocytosis (chronic mast cell leukemia) (see Chap. 35)
      1. KIT^{D816V} mutation-positive (~90%)
      2. KIT^{V560G} mutation-positive (rare)

III. Moderately severe deviation neoplasms (moderate concentration of leukemic blast cells present in marrow)
   A. Oligoblastic myelogenous leukemia (refractory anemia with excess blasts)[a] (see Chap. 42)
   B. Chronic (syn. subacute) myelomonocytic leukemia (see Chap. 47)
      1. *PDGFR* rearrangement-positive (rare)
   C. Juvenile myelomonocytic leukemia (see Chap. 47)

IV. Severe deviation neoplasms (leukemic blast or early progenitor cells frequent in the marrow and blood)
   A. Phenotypic variants of acute myelogenous leukemia (see Chap. 46)
      1. Myeloblastic
      2. Myelomonocytic
      3. Promyelocytic
      4. Erythroid
      5. Monocytic
      6. Megakaryocytic
      7. Eosinophilic[c]
      8. Basophilic[d]
      9. Mastocytic[e]
      10. Histiocytic or Dendritic[f]

B. High-frequency genotypic variants of acute myelogenous leukemia [t(8;21), Inv16 or t(16;16), t(15;17), or (11q23)][g]
C. Myeloid sarcoma
D. Acute biphenotypic (myeloid and lymphoid markers) leukemia[h]
E. Acute leukemia with lymphoid markers evolving from a prior clonal myeloid disease.

---

[a]The World Health Organization includes these four disorders under the rubric of the "Myelodysplastic Syndromes," the classification of which is discussed in Chap. 42.
[b]The World Health Organization includes these three disorders under the rubric of the "Myeloproliferative Syndromes," the classification of which is discussed in Chaps. 43, 44, and 48.
[c]Acute eosinophilic leukemia is rare. Most cases are subacute or chronic and formerly were included in the category of the hypereosinophilic syndrome (see Chaps. 34, 46, and 47).
[d]Rare cases of acute basophilic leukemia are Ph-negative and are variants of acute myelogenous leukemia. Most cases have the Ph chromosome and evolve from chronic myelogenous leukemia (see Chaps. 35, 43, and 45).
[e]See Chap. 35.
[f]See Chap. 37.
[g]The World Health Organization has designated these cytogenetic subtypes as separate entities even though they also have phenotypes listed under phenotypic variants.
[h]Approximately 10% of cases of acute myeloblastic leukemia may be biphenotypic (myeloid and lymphoid markers on individual cells) when studied with antimyeloid and antilymphoid monoclonal antibodies (see Chap. 44).
Source: *Williams Hematology*, 8th ed, Chap. 85, Table 85–1, p. 1212.

MINIMAL TO MODERATE DEVIATION CLONAL MYELOID DISORDERS

- High degree of differentiation and maturation within the clone usually permit life spans measured in decades without treatment or with minimally toxic treatment approaches.

Ineffective Hematopoiesis (Precursor Apoptosis) is Prominent

- Clonal anemia, bicytopenia, or pancytopenia is the usual manifestation.
- Cytopenias resulting from ineffective hematopoiesis (exaggerated apoptosis) are the most characteristic feature.
- Striking dysmorphogenesis of blood cells.
- Altered size (macrocytosis and microcytosis).
- Altered shape (poikilocytosis).
- Altered nuclear or organelle structure of blood cells and their precursors (pathologic sideroblasts, acquired Pelger-Hüet neutrophil nuclear malformation, hypogranulation or hypergranulation, abnormal platelet granulation).
- Increase in leukemic blast cells in marrow or blood are not evident in these syndromes.
- Blast cells above an upper limit of 2 percent combined with multilineage abnormalities indicate the presence of oligoblastic myelogenous leukemia (synonym: refractory anemia with excess blasts). The often arbitrary use of a 5 percent blast threshold is not based on classical pathologic diagnostic decisions in which the presence of tumor (leukemic blast) cells is the principal basis for the diagnosis.
- These disorders have a propensity to evolve into polyblastic myelogenous leukemia (e.g., AML).

Overproduction of Precursor and Mature Cells Prominent

- Polycythemia vera and essential thrombocythemia.
- Leukemic blast cells not present in the marrow or blood.

- Differentiation and maturation in clone is maintained resulting in functional blood cells.
- Regulation of blood cell concentration is faulty with increased concentrations of some combination of red cells, granulocytes (especially neutrophils), and platelets.
- Survival of cohorts of patients with these diseases only slightly less than expected for age- and gender-matched persons.

MODERATE TO MODERATELY SEVERE DEVIATION CLONAL MYELOID DISORDERS

- Chronic myelogenous leukemia (CML) and primary myelofibrosis.
- Blast cells are slightly increased in marrow and blood in most patients with these disorders.
- Median life span is usually measured in years but is significantly decreased when compared with age- and gender-matched unaffected cohorts. The introduction into standard therapy of inhibitors of the BCR-ABL oncoprotein (tyrosine kinase inhibitors) has prolonged median survival significantly in most patients with CML.
- Although polycythemia vera and primary myelofibrosis have similar *JAK2* V617 mutational burdens, on average primary myelofibrosis is a more morbid disease with a significantly shorter life expectancy than polycythemia vera.

MODERATELY SEVERE DEVIATION CLONAL MYELOID DISORDERS

- Oligoblastic myelogenous leukemia (e.g. refractory anemia with excess myeloblasts).
- Chronic myelomonocytic leukemia.
  — Leukemic states that have low or moderate concentration of leukemic blast cells in marrow and often blood.
  — Anemia, often thrombocytopenia, and prominent monocytic maturation of cells.
  — Disorders fall into a group that progress less rapidly than AML and more rapidly than CML.
  — These subacute syndromes produce more morbidity than do the chronic syndromes and patients have a shorter life expectancy.
- Oligoblastic myelogenous leukemia comprises about 30 to 50 percent of the cases that have been grouped under the designation *myelodysplastic syndromes*.
- Atypical clonal myeloid syndromes are uncommon syndromes with trilineage abnormalities that do not fall easily into classifiable designations. Usually seen in patients older than 65 years of age.

SEVERE DEVIATION CLONAL MYELOID DISORDERS

AML and Its Subtypes

- There is an unlimited possibility for phenotypic variation based on the matrix of differentiation of the leukemic multipotential hematopoietic cell and the maturation of leukemic progenitor cells (**Fig. 41–1**).
- Subtype alerts the physician to special epiphenomena:
  — Hypofibrinogenic hemorrhage with promyelocytic or monocytic leukemia.
  — Tissue and central nervous system infiltration in monocytic leukemia.

Differentiation Variants

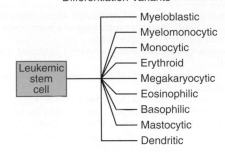

Leukemic stem cell
- Myeloblastic
- Myelomonocytic
- Monocytic
- Erythroid
- Megakaryocytic
- Eosinophilic
- Basophilic
- Mastocytic
- Dendritic

A

Maturation Variants

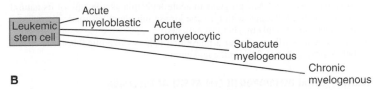

Leukemic stem cell
- Acute myeloblastic
- Acute promyelocytic
- Subacute myelogenous
- Chronic myelogenous

B

FIGURE 41-1 Phenotypic subtypes of acute myelogenous leukemia. Acute myelogenous leukemia has variable morphologic expression and a variable degree of maturation of leukemic cells into recognizable precursors of each blood cell type. This phenotypic variation results because the leukemic lesion resides in a multipotential cell capable of all the commitment decisions present normally. **A.** Morphologic variants of AML can be considered differentiation variants in which the cells derived from one of the options of commitment accumulate prominently, although not exclusively (e.g., leukemic erythroblasts, leukemic monocytes, leukemic megakaryocytes). In promyelocytic leukemia and in some cases of acute leukemia in younger individuals, the somatic mutation(s) may arise in a more differentiated progenitor. **B.** Acute myeloblastic leukemia, promyelocytic leukemia, subacute myelogenous leukemia, and chronic myelogenous leukemia can be considered maturation variants in which blocks at different levels of maturation are present in leukemic progenitor cells. Chronic myelogenous leukemia is an example of a leukemia in which differentiation to all lineages occurs and maturation to functional mature cells in each lineage occurs.
(Source: *Williams Hematology,* 8th ed, Chap. 85, Fig. 85–3, p. 1217.)

- Subtype identification requires some or all of the following:
  - Morphology of cells on stained films of blood and marrow.
  - Identification of cell antigenic phenotype (CD array) by flow analysis.
  - Histochemical characteristics of marrow and blood cells.
  - Cytogenetic or molecular diagnostic techniques for recurring genotypes.
  - Cytogenetic subclassification is more restricted because most cases have any of a variety of infrequently observed abnormalities making this approach complex.
  - Cytogenetic and molecular findings are very useful for determining treatment approach, estimating prognosis, and measuring minimal residual disease by polymerase chain analysis especially in cases in which the cells contain t(8;21), t(15;17), Inv 16, t(16;16), or 11q-.

TRANSITIONS AMONG CLONAL MYELOID DISEASES

- Patients with minimal, moderate, and moderately severe clonal myeloid disorders have an increased likelihood of progressing to a more severe syndrome or to florid AML, with a frequency ranging from:
  - About 1 percent of patients with paroxysmal nocturnal hemoglobinuria develop AML.
  - About 10 percent of patients with clonal anemia (e.g., refractory sideroblastic anemia) progress to AML.
  - About 35 percent of patients with clonal pancytopenia progress to florid AML.
  - About 1 percent of patients with polycythemia vera not treated with ^{32}P or an alkylating agent (larger proportion of those so treated) develop AML.
  - About 15 percent of patients with polycythemia vera evolve to a syndrome indistinguishable from primary myelofibrosis.
  - About 5 percent of patients with essential thrombocythemia progress to AML.
  - About 15 percent of patients with primary myelofibrosis evolve to AML.
- Most patients with CML progress to acute leukemia as a feature of its natural history. (Current therapy with tyrosine kinase inhibitors has markedly delayed the onset of acute leukemia in most patients.)
- Patients with CML may enter a phase that behaves like oligoblastic leukemia before progression to florid acute leukemia.

MULTIPOTENTIAL HEMATOPOIETIC CELL AS SITE OF THE LESION

- Proto-oncogene mutations develop in a multipotential hematopoietic or pluripotential lymphohematopoietic cell and result in most of the clonal myeloid diseases, especially in older patients.
- In CML, the mutation is in a pluripotential lymphohematopoietic cell.
- In other syndromes, the evidence for involvement of B- and T-lymphocyte lineages or multiple myeloid lineages is inconsistent.
- In AML, there is evidence for three levels of onset: pluripotential, multipotential, and bipotential progenitor cells.

PROGENITOR CELL LEUKEMIA

- Leukemic transformation in some (young) patients can occur in progenitor cells [e.g., colony-forming unit, granulocyte-macrophage (CFU-GM)] and can result in a true acute "granulocytic" leukemia without apparent intrinsic involvement of erythroid and megakaryocytic lineages.
- In t(15;17) promyelocytic AML, a subset of patients with acute monocytic leukemia, and a subset of patients with t(8;21) AML, the leukemia derives from the transformation of a granulocyte progenitor cell without intrinsic involvement of erythroid and megakaryocytic lineages.

CLINICAL MANIFESTATIONS

Deficiency, Excess, or Dysfunction of Blood Cells

- Abnormal blood cell concentrations are the primary manifestation of clonal myeloid diseases.
- Clonal myeloid diseases may have overt qualitative abnormalities of blood cells.
- Abnormal red cell shapes, red cell enzyme activities, or red cell membrane structures.
- Abnormal neutrophil granules, bizarre nuclear configurations, disorders of neutrophil chemotaxis, phagocytosis, or microbial killing.
- Giant platelets, abnormal platelet granules, and disturbed platelet function.

EFFECTS OF LEUKEMIC BLAST CELLS

Extramedullary Tumors

- Myeloid sarcomas (synonym: granulocytic sarcomas, chloromas, myeloblastomas, or monocytomas) are discrete tumors of leukemic myeloblasts or occasionally leukemic monocytes:
  — Develop in skin and soft tissues, periosteum and bone, lymph nodes, gastrointestinal tract, pleura, gonads, urinary tract, central nervous system, and other sites.
  — Uncommonly may be the first manifestation of AML, preceding the onset in marrow and blood by months or years.
  — Mistaken for large cell lymphomas by microscopy because of the similarity of the histopathology in biopsy specimens from soft tissues.
  — Immunohistochemistry should be used on such lesions to identify myeloperoxidase, lysozyme, CD117, CD61, CD68/KP1, and other relevant CD markers of myeloid cells. One of four histopathologic patterns usually is evident by immunocytochemistry: myeloblastic, monoblastic, myelomonoblastic, or megakaryoblastic.
  — May usher in the accelerated phase of CML.
- Ph-positive lymphoblastomas are the tissue variant of the capability of CML to transform into a terminal deoxynucleotidyl transferase-positive lymphoblastic leukemia in 20 to 30 percent of cases.
- Monocytomas are collections of leukemic promonocytes or monoblasts that may invade the skin, gingiva, anal canal, lymph nodes, or central nervous system.

RELEASE OF PROCOAGULANTS AND FIBRINOLYTIC ACTIVATORS

- Hemorrhage from disseminated intravascular clotting or exaggerated fibrinolysis feature of acute promyelocytic leukemia.
- Hemorrhage from procoagulant-fibrinolytic state sometimes occurs in other forms of acute leukemia, especially hyperleukocytic monocytic leukemia.
- The plasma levels of protein C activity, free protein S, and antithrombin are decreased in some patients with AML, notably but not exclusively with acute promyelocytic leukemia.
- Leukemic cells may express a procoagulant tissue factor or a plasminogen activator (e.g., annexin II on leukemic promyelocytes).
- Microvascular thrombosis is characteristic of the procoagulant effect. Large vessel thrombosis occurs and can result in stroke or loss of parts of extremities, but is uncommon.

HYPERLEUKOCYTIC SYNDROMES

- Five percent of patients with AML and 15 percent with CML have extraordinarily high blood leukocyte counts at diagnosis.
- In AML, leukemic cell counts over 100×10^9/L and in CML, leukemic cell counts over 300×10^9/L are usually present when the hyperleukocytic syndrome manifests itself.
- Metabolic effects (especially elevated serum uric acid and marked uricosuria) can result when massive numbers of leukemic cells in blood, marrow, and tissues are simultaneously killed by cytotoxic drugs. This can result in obstructive uropathy and renal failure.
- Leukostasis in AML and CML may be associated with effects in the pulmonary, central nervous system, special sensory, or penile circulation (see Table 41–2).
- Sudden death can occur in patients with hyperleukocytic acute leukemia as a result of intracranial hemorrhage.
- A respiratory distress syndrome attributed to pulmonary leukostasis occurs in some patients with acute promyelocytic leukemia after all-*trans*-retinoic acid therapy. The syndrome is usually, but not always, associated with prominent neutrophilia.

TABLE 41–2	CLINICAL FEATURES OF THE HYPERLEUKOCYTIC SYNDROME

I. Pulmonary circulation
   A. Tachypnea, dyspnea, cyanosis
   B. Alveolar–capillary block
   C. Pulmonary infiltrates
   D. Postchemotherapy respiratory dysfunction

II. Predisposition to tumor lysis syndrome

III. Central nervous system circulation
   A. Dizziness, slurred speech, delirium, stupor
   B. Intracranial (cerebral) hemorrhage

IV. Special sensory organ circulation
   A. Visual blurring
   B. Papilledema
   C. Diplopia
   D. Tinnitus, impaired hearing
   E. Retinal vein distention, retinal hemorrhages

V. Penile circulation
   A. Priapism

VI. Spurious laboratory results
   A. Decreased blood partial pressure of oxygen (Po_2); increased serum potassium
   B. Decreased plasma glucose; increased mean corpuscular volume, red cell count, hemoglobin, and hematocrit

Source: *Williams Hematology*, 8th ed, Chap. 85, Table 85–2, p. 1219.

THROMBOCYTHEMIC SYNDROMES: HEMORRHAGE AND THROMBOPHILIA

- In polycythemia vera, essential thrombocythemia, and primary myelofibrosis, the height of the white cell count is a predictor of thrombosis and the height of the platelet count correlates with likelihood of bleeding (platelet count $>1000 \times 10^9$/L increases bleeding risk).
- Hemorrhagic or thrombotic episodes can occur initially or can develop during the course of thrombocythemia.
- Procoagulant factors, such as the content of platelet tissue factor and blood platelet neutrophil aggregates, are higher in patients with essential thrombocythemia than normal persons and are higher among patients with the V617F *JAK2* mutation than patients with the wild-type gene.
- Arterial vascular insufficiency and venous thrombosis are the major vascular manifestations of thrombocythemia.
- Peripheral vascular insufficiency with gangrene and cerebral vascular thrombi can occur in thrombocythemia.
- Mesenteric, hepatic, portal, or splenic venous thrombosis can develop.
- Thrombotic complications occur in about one-third of patients with polycythemia vera.
- Gastrointestinal hemorrhage and cutaneous hemorrhage, the latter especially after trauma, are most frequent, but bleeding from other sites can also occur.
- Thrombosis of the veins of the abdomen, liver, and other organs are characteristic complications in approximately half the patients with paroxysmal nocturnal hemoglobinuria. Thrombosis is more common in the purely hemolytic type than in the type associated with marrow aplasia.

- A syndrome of splanchnic venous thrombosis associated with endogenous erythroid colony growth, the latter characteristic of polycythemia vera, but without blood cell count changes indicative of a myeloproliferative disease, has accounted for a high proportion of patients with apparent idiopathic hepatic or portal vein thrombosis. These cases may have blood cells with the Janus kinase 2 (*JAK2*) gene mutation without a clinically apparent myeloproliferative phenotype.

SYSTEMIC SYMPTOMS

- Fever, weight loss, and malaise may occur as an early manifestation of AML.
- Fever during cytotoxic therapy, when neutrophil counts are extremely low, is nearly always a sign of infection.
- Weight loss occurs in nearly one-fifth of patients with AML at the time of diagnosis.

METABOLIC SIGNS

- Hyperuricemia and hyperuricosuria are very common manifestations of AML and CML.
- Acute gouty arthritis and hyperuricosuric nephropathy are less common.
- Saturation of the urine with uric acid accentuated by cytotoxic therapy can lead to precipitation of urate, formation of gravel or stones, and obstructive uropathy.
- Hyponatremia can occur in AML, and in some cases, is a result of inappropriate antidiuretic hormone secretion.
- Hypokalemia is commonly seen in AML.
- Hypercalcemia occurs in about 2 percent of patients with AML.
- Lactic acidosis has also been observed in association with AML.
- In some cases, hypophosphatemia may occur because of rapid utilization of plasma inorganic phosphate in cases of myelogenous leukemia with a high blood blast cell count and a high fraction of proliferative cells.
- Hypoxia can result from the hyperleukocytic syndrome as a consequence of pulmonary vascular leukostasis.

FACTITIOUS LABORATORY RESULTS

- Elevations of serum potassium levels from the release of potassium in clotted blood if there is an extreme elevation of platelets or, less often, leukocytes.
- Glucose can be falsely decreased if autoanalyzer techniques omit glycolytic inhibitors in collection tubes in cases with high leukemic cell counts.
- Factitious hypoglycemia can also occur as a result of red cell utilization of glucose in polycythemic patients.
- Large numbers of leukocytes can lower blood oxygen content spuriously as a result of its utilization *in vitro* during measurement.

SPECIFIC ORGAN INVOLVEMENT

- Infiltration of the larynx, central nervous system, heart, lungs, bone, joints, gastrointestinal tract, kidney, skin, or virtually any other organ may occur in AML.
- Splenic enlargement in about one third of cases of AML and is usually slight in extent.
- Splenomegaly is present in a high proportion of cases of primary myelofibrosis (100%), CML (90%), and polycythemia vera (80%).
- In essential thrombocythemia, splenic enlargement is present in about 60 percent of patients.
  — Splenic vascular thrombi, microinfarctions, and splenic atrophy lower the frequency of splenic enlargement in thrombocythemia.

- Early satiety, left upper-quadrant discomfort, splenic infarctions with painful perisplenitis, diaphragmatic pleuritis, and shoulder pain may occur in patients with splenomegaly, especially in the acute phase of CML and in primary myelofibrosis.
- In primary myelofibrosis the spleen can become enormous, occupying the left hemiabdomen.
- Blood flow through the splenic vein can be so great as to lead to portal hypertension and gastroesophageal varices. Usually, reduced hepatic venous compliance also contributes to these changes.
- Bleeding and, occasionally, encephalopathy can result from the portosystemic venous shunts in primary myelofibrosis.

For a more detailed discussion, see Marshall A. Lichtman: Classification and Clinical Manifestation of the Clonal Myeloid Diseases. Chap. 85, p. 1211 in *Williams Hematology*, 8th ed.

CHAPTER 42
Myelodysplastic Syndromes (Clonal Cytopenias and Oligoblastic Myelogenous Leukemia)

DEFINITION

- Myelodysplasia is the term used, as a generalization, to encompass a diverse group of myeloid neoplasms that have in common (a) their origin in a somatically mutated multipotential hematopoietic cell, (b) ineffective hematopoiesis (late precursor apoptosis) leading to cytopenias despite a normocellular or hypercellular marrow, and (c) a propensity to undergo clonal progression to acute myelogenous leukemia (AML).
- Spectrum ranges from (a) indolent disorder with mild or moderate anemia to (b) more troublesome multicytopenias without morphologic evidence of leukemic cells to (c) oligoblastic (subacute) myelogenous leukemia with leukemic blast cells in the marrow and blood (Table 42–1).
- Clonal cytopenia refers to disorders without increased leukemic blast cells in the marrow. The manifestations vary from isolated anemia with a nearly normal marrow to severe multicytopenias with hypercellular marrow and with dysmorphia of marrow precursors and blood cells.
- Oligoblastic or subacute myelogenous leukemia (synonym: refractory anemia with excess blasts) refers to patients with cytopenias and with marrow containing 2 to 19 percent leukemic blast cells. (The World Health Organization [WHO] uses the range 5 to 19%.)
- If the marrow blast cell count is 20 percent or higher, the disease is considered acute myelogenous leukemia and so treated.
- The use of <5 percent marrow blasts as a demarcation is an anachronism dating from a decision made in 1955, at which time the first definition of remission in childhood acute lymphoblastic leukemia used <5 percent marrow blasts (and other salutary changes) to avoid additional cytotoxic treatment in an era without platelet transfusion, potent wide-spectrum antibiotics, or other support for children treated with multidrug regimens. Also, only light microscopy was available to distinguish nonleukemic lymphocytes in treated marrows from residual leukemic lymphoblasts. This, so-called, "5 percent rule" is irrelevant at the time of diagnosis, especially in the case of myeloblasts, but it has been ensconced.
- The use of 19 versus 20 percent blasts to distinguish oligoblastic myelogenous leukemia (refractory anemia with excess blasts) from AML is, of course, arbitrary and without pathobiologic foundation. The physician should determine management of the case by several factors (e.g., physiologic age, severity of cytopenias, transfusion requirements, frequency and severity of infections) not principally whether a patient with myelogenous leukemia has 15, 20, or 25 percent blast cells.

ETIOLOGY AND PATHOGENESIS

- The fundamental alteration is a somatically mutated multipotential hematopoietic cell, resulting in trilineage blood cell abnormalities in most cases. Even in clonal anemia in which the neutrophils count and platelet count are within the normal range, evidence of dysmorphia in neutrophil and megakaryocyte-platelet lineages may be evident on careful examination.

TABLE 42–1	**CLASSIFICATION OF THE MYELODYSPLASTIC SYNDROMES (CLONAL CYTOPENIAS AND OLIGOBLASTIC LEUKEMIA)**

1. Clonal (refractory) anemia (with or without pathologic sideroblasts).*
2. Clonal bicytopenia or tricytopenia (overt multilineage dysmorphic cytopenias).
3. Oligoblastic myelogenous leukemia (refractory anemia with excess myeloblasts).
4. Classic 5q–syndrome.
5. Apparent clonal myeloid disease that does not fit in any category shown above (e.g., chronic clonal monocytosis; Clonal isolated neutropenia or thrombocytopenia are rare occurrences as initial manifestations of a clonal myeloid disease and their inclusion by the WHO without a clonal chromosome or gene marker is arguable, unless at least subtle involvement of other lineages is evident. Non-clonal diseases should not be in this category.

*The WHO classification distinguishes refractory "nonsideroblastic" from sideroblastic anemia based on whether the case has ≥15% or <15% pathologic (ringed) sideroblasts in marrow erythroid cells. No basis exists for distinguishing the anemia based on proportion of pathologic sideroblasts because most patients with clonal anemia have pathologic sideroblasts, and the manifestations and course of the disease are virtually identical in patients with a high or low prevalence of pathologic sideroblasts. Given the relatively crude nature of quantification of pathologic sideroblasts and the biologic illegitimacy of such distinctions in any case, it is unnecessary to consider them two different diagnostic categories. Indeed, recent survival studies have collapsed the two groups into one category and the WHO should do so, also. The WHO also separates refractory anemia with excess blasts (oligoblastic myelogenous leukemia) into type 1 and type 2 if the blast percentage in the marrow at diagnosis is 5–9% or 10–19%, respectively. These distinctions are questionable in an individual case because of the inexactitude of marrow sampling but may have implications in large groups in which the error variance may be cancelled out. In any case, this factor is put in play in the prognostic scoring system, discussed later in this chapter, in which blast percentage is a variable. Other acute and chronic clonal myeloid diseases are categorized in Table 41–1.
Source: *Williams Hematology*, 8th ed, Chap. 88, Table 88–1, p.1250.

- Epigenetic gene modification contributes to the hematopoietic abnormalities and has become a target for therapy.
- Overt cytogenetic abnormalities are found in about 10 to 15 percent of patients with clonal anemia, but these abnormalities increase in prevalence to about 70 percent in patients with oligoblastic myelogenous leukemia.
- High-dose, prolonged benzene exposure is rare in countries with workplace regulations; DNA-damaging chemotherapeutic agents (esp. alkylating agents and topoisomerase II inhibitors) or high-dose radiation can result in myelodysplasia (as well as AML).
- Exaggerated apoptosis of late hematopoietic precursors results in blood cytopenias in the face of active marrow hematopoiesis.

PREVALENCE OF MAJOR CATEGORIES OF MYELODYSPLASIA

- This variable differs among different studies; however, Table 42–2 gives a reasonable representation of the frequency of each syndrome and the median survival of patients so categorized.
- These data were accumulated before the widespread use of agents such as lenalidomide and 5-azacytadine. This therapy may increase median survival in less severe categories.
- The proportion of patients among subtypes is dependent on the blast cell count threshold used. In essence, about 60 percent of patients have a clonal cytopenia or multicytopenia and 40 percent have oligoblastic myelogenous leukemia using the WHO blast count threshold of <5 percent marrow blasts.

TABLE 42–2 **DISTRIBUTION OF FIVE PRINCIPAL CATEGORIES OF MDS AMONG 374 PATIENTS**

MDS Subtype	% of Patients	% Marrow Blasts Median (Range)	Median Survival (Months)
Clonal anemia with low (<15%)[1] or high (≥15%)[2] proportion of pathologic sideroblasts	30	3 (0–4)	108
Clonal multicytopenias[3]	25	4 (0–4)	49
Oligoblastic myelogenous leukemia[4]	35	11 (5–19)	24
5q–syndrome[5]	7.5	4 (2–4)	Not statistically different from clonal anemia; DNS
Unclassifiable[6]	2.5	3 (2–4)	DNS

DNS, data not shown. WHO classification: [1]refractory anemia; [2]refractory sideroblastic anemia; [3]refractory anemia with multicytopenia; [4]refractory anemia with excess blasts types 1 and 2; [5]5q—syndrome; [6]unclassifiable category. Among the oligoblastic myelogenous leukemia patients, the survival was better the lower the diagnostic marrow blast count.
Source: *Williams Hematology*, 8th ed, Chap. 88, Table 88–2, p. 1260.

- Prognostic stratification, discussed later, may be a better assessment of distribution of patients by severity of disease and prognosis (see "Risk Categories" section below).

EPIDEMIOLOGY

- Incidence increases exponentially from age 40 (0.2/100,000 persons) to age 85 years (45 per 100,000 persons) in the United States.
- In younger adults, the onset is often preceded by chemotherapy or irradiation (secondary myelodysplasia) for another neoplasm.
- Male:female ratio about 1.5:1 (except in 5q- syndrome in which females predominate).
- Children 0.5 to 15 years have incidence rate of 0.1 per 100,000/year.
- Children usually have more advanced types (oligoblastic myelogenous leukemia).
- Childhood cases may evolve from predisposing inherited syndromes such as Fanconi anemia.

CLINICAL FEATURES

- May be asymptomatic if mild anemia is the principal feature, with little or no reductions in platelet and neutrophil counts.
- If moderate or severe anemia and/or granulocytopenia and thrombocytopenia develop, loss of sense of well being, pallor, dyspnea on exertion, easy bruising, and slow healing of minor cuts may be evident. The presence and intensity of these manifestations are a function of the gradient from mild anemia to severe pancytopenia to oligoblastic leukemia.
- Hepatomegaly or splenomegaly are uncommon findings (<10%).
- Hypothalamic malfunction with loss of libido and diabetes insipidus, neutrophilic dermatosis (Sweet syndrome), and inflammatory syndromes mimicking lupus erythematosus are each uncommon associated findings.

LABORATORY FEATURES

- Anemia occurs in more than 85 percent of patients and may be macrocytic, with rare circulating nucleated red cells. Misshapen cells (e.g., elliptocytes, other poikilocytes), anisochromia, and basophilic stippling are hallmarks of the dysmorphia in the blood film (see **Fig. 42–1**).
- Hemoglobin F levels may be increased; hemoglobin H may be present, rarely (with red cell shape and inclusions simulating α-thalassemia); red cell enzyme activities may be abnormal.
- Neutropenia occurs in at least 50 percent of cases. Coarse chromatin, nuclear hyposegmentation (acquired Pelger-Huët abnormality), and decreased cytoplasmic granulation of neutrophils commonly occur.
- Monocytosis often found and rarely may be the principal abnormality.
- Thrombocytopenia or occasionally thrombocytosis may be present. The later is especially notable in the 5q- syndrome. Platelets may be large, with decreased or fused granules. Platelet aggregation tests may be abnormal. Micromegakaryocytes may enter the blood.
- Marrow abnormalities include (a) hypercellularity, (b) delayed nuclear maturation of red cell precursors, (c) abnormal cytoplasmic maturation of red cell and neutrophil precursors, (d) pathologic sideroblasts (e.g., ringed sideroblasts), (e) megakaryocytes with unilobed or bilobed nuclei or odd number of nuclear lobes, (f) micromegakaryocytes, and (g) an increased proportion of myeloblasts. In approximately 10 percent of patients, the marrow may be hypocellular, simulating aplastic anemia. Careful search may show clusters of dysmorphic hematopoietic precursors and cytogenetic analysis may uncover a clonal abnormality, either or both indicative of myelodysplasia. Test to rule out paroxysmal nocturnal hemoglobinuria should be done in this setting (see Chap. 45).
- Chromosomal abnormalities occur in up to 70 percent in patients oligoblastic myelogenous leukemia of patients by G-banding or fluorescent *in situ* hybridization. The most common abnormalities (very similar to those in AML) are 5q-, -7/7q-, +8, -18/18q-, and 20q- but innumerable other less common clonal cytogenetic changes may be present. Occasional patients with thrombocytosis may have an abnormality of chromosome 3. Common translocations such as t(8;21), t(15;17), t(16;16) seen in AML are not features of the cells in myelodysplastic syndromes.
- Ferritin levels are often increased at diagnosis as a result of a shift in erythron iron to the storage compartments in proportion to the degree of anemia and increased iron absorption.

FIGURE 42–1 Blood and marrow films from patients with clonal cytopenias (MDS). **A.** Blood film. Anisocytosis. Poikilocytosis with occasional fragmented cells. Marked anisochromia with marked hypochromia, mild hypochromia and normochromic cells. **B.** Blood film. Marked anisocytosis. Mild anisochromia. Poikilocytes with occasional fragmented cells and oval and elliptical cells. Two polychromatophilic macrocytes. **C.** Blood film. Striking anisocytosis with giant macrocytes and microcytes. Poikilocytes with tiny red cell fragment and elliptocyte. **D.** Blood film. Mild anisocytosis. Ovalocytes and elliptocytes. Dacryocyte. Hyposegmented neutrophil with poor cytoplasmic granulation. **E.** Blood film. Marked anisocytosis (macrocytes and microcytes). Ovalocytes and elliptocytes. Acquired Pelger-Huët nuclear anomaly (classic pince-nez shape) in neutrophil. **F.** Blood film. Mild anisocytosis. Abnormal neutrophil with ring nucleus. **G.** Blood film. Anisochromia. Stomatocytes. Abnormal neutrophil nuclei with hyperlobulation and hyperchromatic staining. Note abnormal elongated nuclear bridge in neutrophil on left. **H.** Blood film. Atypical platelets. Two macrothrombocytes with excess cytoplasm and atypical central granules. Anisocytosis (conspicuous microcytes). Anisochromia (conspicuous hypochromic cells). Poikilocytosis with occasional fragmented red cells. **I.** Marrow film. Wright stain. Trilobed megakaryocyte. Wright stain. Macroerythroblasts. **J.** Marrow films. Prussian blue stain. Ringed sideroblasts. Wright stain. Erythroid hyperplasia with macroerythroblasts. **K.** Marrow film. Prussian blue stain. Ringed sideroblasts. **L.** Marrow film. Wright stain. Trilobed megakaryocytes. *(Reproduced with permission from Lichtman's Atlas of Hematology, www.accessmedicine.com.)*
(Source: *Williams Hematology,* 8th ed, Chap. 88, Fig. 88–2, p. 1254.)

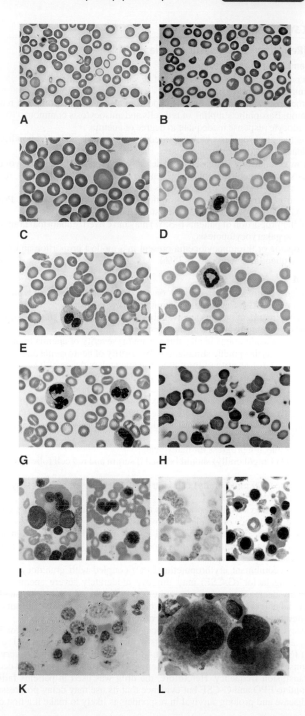

SPECIFIC SYNDROMES

Clonal (Refractory) Sideroblastic Anemia

Clinical and Laboratory Features

- Most patients are older than 50 years of age and have anemia.
- Anemia may be mild to severe.
- Macrocytosis with anisochromia (hypochromia and normochromia) of red cells common. Basophilic stippling of red cells and anisocytosis common.
- Reticulocyte response inadequate to degree of anemia.
- Ineffective erythropoiesis with impaired heme synthesis and mitochondrial iron overload are characteristic findings.
- Marrow cellularity is increased, with defective cytoplasmic maturation of erythroblasts, and ringed sideroblasts present. (The WHO, quite arbitrarily, requires ≥15% ringed [pathologic] sideroblasts for this designation.)
- Serum iron, ferritin levels, and saturation of transferrin are increased. Prussian blue stain of marrow shows increased storage iron.
- A smaller proportion of patients (~35%) may have overtly abnormal granulopoiesis or megakaryocytopoiesis.
- Neutropenia or thrombocytopenia present in a modest proportion and may not be consequential functionally (~35%).

Treatment

- Treatment options are predicated on specific abnormalities and prognostic category (see "Risk Categories" section below).
- The same treatment options are available for patients in any subtype of myelodysplasia depending on morbid manifestations.
- The main considerations in all subtypes are (a) severity of anemia (demethylating agents, erythropoietic stimulants), (b) severity of neutropenia and infections (antibiotics), (c) severity of thrombocytopenia and evidence of bleeding (platelet transfusion), (d) special case of hypoplastic marrow (immunosuppressive therapy), (e) evidence of progressive leukemic hematopoiesis (blast level) requiring acute leukemia type cytotoxic therapy or allogeneic hematopoietic stem cell transplantation. See following details.
- Asymptomatic patients without evidence of progression may not require treatment.
- Disorder may not progress for many years.
- Folic acid (1 mg/d orally) should be used if serum and red cell folic acid content are low.
- Pyridoxine (200 mg/d orally) can be tried if sideroblastic anemia is symptomatic, but success is rare.
- Danazol (200 to 400 mg/d orally) has occasionally increased platelet count or decreased frequency of platelet transfusion.
- In uncommon patients with clonal cytopenia and hypoplastic marrows, cyclosporine and antithymocyte globulin have resulted in improvement in hematopoiesis (see Chap. 3).
- Human recombinant erythropoietin (EPO) coupled with granulocyte-colony-stimulating factor (G-CSF) may improve moderately severe anemia or may markedly decrease transfusion requirements. This combination is usually not beneficial unless (a) the serum EPO level is <500 units/L and (b) the transfusion requirement is less than 2 units of red cells per month.
- 5-Azacytidine, 75 mg/m^2 per day, subcutaneously (or intravenously) for 7 days every 28 days can be useful in patients with symptomatic anemia and requirement for frequent transfusions. About 40 percent of patients have a very good response as judged by the increase in hemoglobin levels or a significant decrease in transfusion frequency. Heretofore, the drug was used in patients failing to respond to EPO and G-CSF but evidence that its use may delay progression of the disease and prolong survival in responders is likely to make it a first choice

in such patients, administered before the results of EPO+G-CSF are evident. Although 5-azacytidine is an antimetabolite, its benefit is thought to be related principally to its demethylating effects (reversing deleterious epigenetic effects).

- 5-Azacytidine may initially cause a fall in blood cell counts, even in responders, and transfusion requirements may increase during the first one to several weeks of therapy. It may take 4 to 5 cycles of therapy to achieve a response and maximum responses may not occur for 9 to 10 cycles.
- Decitabine, another cytotoxic agent with demethylating effects, has been approved for use in lieu of 5-azacytidine. One regimen proposed is 20 mg/m^2 intravenously over 1 hour daily for 5 days to be repeated every 4 weeks for a total of three cycles. Worsening of cytopenias may occur initially but some experts recommend that unless a complication of cytopenia develops or other serious side effects occur, the treatment program should not be modified.
- Red cell transfusion may be necessary if severe anemia or if coincidental ischemic diseases (e.g., angina or heart failure) are present with moderate anemia.
- Some patients with high red cell transfusion requirements develop iron-overload and should receive iron chelation therapy. Oral desferasirox, 20 mg/kg per day, has been approved by the FDA for this purpose. It can produce nausea, vomiting, abdominal pain, skin rash, and other adverse effects (see Chap. 9).
- One guideline for use of iron chelator therapy requires three criteria to be met: (a) probable survival for at least 1 year, (b) receipt of more than 20 units of red cells, (c) a serum ferritin of ≥1000 μg/L.
- Some patients do not progress or may live for many years before progression occurs. Others may have worsening hematopoiesis, more severe cytopenias and have morbidity and mortality from recurrent severe infections or hemorrhage.
- On average a normal or only slightly abnormal neutrophil and platelet count suggests a better prognosis. A mild anemia not requiring transfusions also portends a better outcome on average.
- About 10 percent of patients progress to AML over a 10-year period of observation.
- Median survival is about 7 to 9 years in different studies.

Clonal (Refractory) Nonsideroblastic Anemia

- Similar to refractory sideroblastic anemia in all respects but without pathologic sideroblasts in the marrow. (The WHO, quite remarkably, defines this category as having ≤15% ringed [pathologic] sideroblasts. In other words, clonal anemia with ≤15% pathologic sideroblasts is called nonsideroblastic in its classification.)
- This distinction in sideroblasts prevalence is irrelevant because there is no difference in the behavior of these two categories and prognosis and treatment criteria are the same in clonal nonsideroblastic or sideroblastic anemia. These categories should be collapsed into one subtype of "clonal anemia."

Clonal Multicytopenia with Hypercellular Marrow

- These patients present with clonal cytopenias with neutropenia and/or thrombocytopenia, as well as anemia.
- The blood and marrow findings are as described for clonal anemia, although neutropenia and/or thrombocytopenia are more prominent. Dysmorphic neutrophils (acquired Pelger-Huët nuclear and/or granule abnormalities) and platelets (giant size, abnormal granulation) may be evident in the blood. Dysmorphic neutrophil precursors and megakaryocytes with nuclear and cytoplasmic abnormalities are usually evident (e.g., abnormal neutrophil precursor granulation and nuclear hyposegmentation or hypersegmentation, hypolobulated or hyperlobulated megakaryocyte nuclei, micromegakaryocytes).

- Marrow and blood picture can be seen in patients with AIDS, but progression to acute leukemia is not a feature.
- Fever, especially in the setting of neutropenia, should be evaluated promptly and a suspected infection treated with broad-spectrum antibiotics, unless and until culture results permit more specific therapy.
- Therapy is as described in more detail in the section "Clonal (Refractory) Sideroblastic Anemia: Treatment" above. One or more of the following may be required: (a) EPO and G-CSF, (b) 5-azacytidine or decitabine, (c) red cell and platelet transfusions.
- In patients with severe morbidity and a suitable donor, allogeneic hematopoietic stem cell transplantation may be considered (using either myeloablative or non-myeloablative conditioning depending on patient age, comorbid conditions, and other individual factors).
- Median survival is about 2.5 to 4 years in different studies. AML develops in about 50 percent of patients, and about 25 percent die of infection or hemorrhage.
- Patients with complex cytogenetic patterns have a worse prognosis

The 5q-Syndrome
- Patients have a refractory anemia, with marrow abnormalities of dyserythropoiesis, erythroid multinuclearity, and hypolobulated, small megakaryocytes.
- Most patients do not have consequential neutropenia or thrombocytopenia.
- A proportion of patients have thrombocytosis ($>450 \times 10^9$/L). About 40 percent of patients with clonal anemia and thrombocytosis have hematopoietic cells carrying the Janus Kinase 2 (*JAK 2*) mutation. This variant seems to have a favorable prognosis.
- The syndrome is most common in older women but occurs in children.
- Marrow cells have deletion of long arm of chromosome 5 (5q-). In contrast to the 5q- lesion associated with other subtypes of myelodysplasia or acute myelogenous leukemia the break is between q13-q31, whereas in the other cases it is between q22-q33.
- Some patients do not require treatment at the time of diagnosis.
- Significant or symptomatic anemia is improved or ameliorated in about 85 percent of patients treated with lenalidomide, 10 mg/d orally, until improvement occurs or toxicity requires cessation. Improvement ranges from disappearance of signs of the disease, including the 5q-abnormality, to a decrease in transfusion requirements. The maximal response occurs on an average after approximately 5 weeks of treatment.
- Refractory patients with significant anemia may require red cell transfusions. Iron chelation therapy should be instituted based on the three criteria discussed under "Clonal (Refractory) Sideroblastic Anemia: Treatment" above.
- Median survival is approximately 10 years.
- The risk of progression to AML is about 5 to 10 percent over a protracted period of observation.

Monosomy 7-Associated Syndromes
- A frequent chromosomal abnormality in patients with myelodysplasia.
- Often seen in patients who develop disorder after chemotherapy or high-dose radiotherapy.
- Transformation to florid AML common.
- Usually not associated with special clinical features in adults.
- Children often have associated atypical myeloproliferative disease, subacute myelomonocytic leukemia, or juvenile myelomonocytic leukemia that rapidly progresses to AML (see Chap. 47).

OLIGOBLASTIC MYELOGENOUS LEUKEMIAS

Clinical Features

- Patients have 2 to 19 percent leukemic blasts in the marrow and 0 to 10 percent in the blood and may survive for months or years without specific or effective antileukemic therapy.
- Also known as smoldering leukemia, pauciblastic leukemia, subacute myelogenous leukemia, or refractory anemia with excess blasts.
- Patients are usually older than 50 years of age, with cytopenias or qualitative cellular abnormalities, as in the clonal cytopenias.
- Thrombocytopenia and/or neutropenia virtually always accompany anemia.
- Evolves into overt acute (polyblastic) myelogenous leukemia in approximately 50 percent of cases.
- Median survival is about 14 to 24 months in different studies and individual survival in large studies has ranged from 1 to 160 months, highlighting the heterogeneity of disease progression.
- High blast cell proportions in marrow or blood, high transfusion requirements, and complex cytogenetics are poor prognostic indicators.

Treatment

- Therapy should be individualized to the morbidity present and the evidence of progression. Some patients may not require treatment initially.
- Periodic patient evaluations are used to detect deteriorating blood counts in a timely manner.
- 5-Azacytidine or decitabine may be used to improve anemia or decrease red cell transfusion requirements. The very good response rate is below 30 percent of patients treated (see "Clonal (Refractory) Sideroblastic Anemia: Treatment" above for dosing details).
- Therapy with red cell transfusion often is required. If so, iron-chelation therapy should be used if the three criteria (endogenous EPO level, frequency of red cell transfusion needed, and ferritin level) specified in the treatment of "Clonal (Refractory) Sideroblastic Anemia: Treatment," above, are met (see Chap. 9).
- Platelet transfusion may be required for (a) platelet counts under 5.0×10^9/L, (b) evidence of exaggerated mucocutaneous bleeding, or (c) other significant bleeding episodes.
- ϵ-Aminocaproic or tranexamic acid, both antifibrinolytic agents, may be used to decrease the amount of thrombocytopenic bleeding.
- Thrombopoiesis-stimulating agents (e.g., thrombopoietin receptor agonists) are under study for their utility in ameliorating thrombocytopenia in patients with myelodysplasia. Results in a study in low-risk patients have shown effectiveness of romiplostin in half of those treated with platelet counts $<30 \times 10^9$/L. Long-term safety and effects in higher-risk patients in which thrombocytopenia is a more severe and more frequent problem are not yet reported.
- Neutropenic fever should be treated promptly with broad-spectrum antibiotics after appropriate cultures for bacteria and fungi are performed.
- If the disease progresses to frank AML, standard therapy for AML can be considered (see Chap. 46), although the remission rate is low and long-term responses are unusual in most patients and especially in patients over age 60 years.
- In patients older than 70 years or who have comorbid conditions or other frailties, attenuated AML therapy can be considered (see Chap. 46).
- In patients not suitable for standard or attenuated standard therapy, a variety of approaches, including low-dose cytarabine, 5-azacytidine or decitabine, etoposide, hydroxyurea, glucocorticoids, singly or in combination, have been tried with limited success.

- The response rate to most therapies is in the 5 to 20 percent range. One or another approach accomplishes improvement in different patients, making a standardized approach difficult at this time.
- Allogeneic hematopoietic stem cell transplantation can be curative. The younger the patient the better the results are with transplantation. The transplant physician involved should make an assessment of all related variables: patient's age, comorbid conditions, prior cytotoxic therapy, probability of a salutary outcome with the disease characteristics in question, patient's level of understanding and interest in the procedure, and others.

RISK CATEGORIES

- Patients with myelodysplastic syndrome have wide variations in manifestations within a subtype and among subtypes. For example, the number of cytopenias and severity of cytopenias are quite varied among patients.
- Some patients in the same diagnostic subtype do not require treatment whereas others have highly morbid manifestations, which are life-threatening.
- In order to accommodate this variation among and within subtypes, patients with myelodysplasia have been stratified into prognostic or risk categories using three variables: (a) marrow blast percentage, (b) prognostic category of their cytogenetic findings (good risk, intermediate risk, poor risk), and (c) number of cytopenias from 1 to 3 (see Tables 42–3 and 42–4).
- In the aggregate, these prognostic categories predict the requirement for therapy and median survival.
- The summation of prognostic category scores is a strong determinant of survival (Table 42–3). Adding age at diagnosis to the risk assessment further strengthens the prognostic utility of the categorization (Table 42–5).
- Details of therapeutic approaches based on prognostic score can be found in *Williams Hematology,* 8th ed, Chap. 86, p. 1263. These approaches use the same therapy described in this chapter under the subtypes of myelodysplasia: red cell transfusion, iron-chelation, immunosuppression, DNA-methylating agents, platelet transfusions, antibiotics, AML therapy, allogeneic hematopoietic stem cell transplantation, and experimental therapies.

THERAPY-RELATED MYELODYSPLASTIC SYNDROME

- Usually follows chemotherapy, radiation therapy, or combined modality therapy for solid tumors or lymphomas. Conditioning regimens for autotransplantation in lymphoma and myeloma result in secondary myelodysplasia.
- These cases have a poorer prognosis than *de novo* cases and are excluded from the calculations of prognostic indices.

TABLE 42–3	INTERNATIONAL PROGNOSTIC SCORING SYSTEM FOR MYELODYSPLASTIC SYNDROMES			
	Score Value			
Prognostic Variable	**0**	**0.5**	**1.0**	**1.5**
Marrow Blast (%)	<5	5–10	—	11–20
Karyotype	Good	Intermediate	Poor	—
Cytopenias	0,1	2,3	—	—

Risk groups: Low, 0; INT-1, 0.5–1.0; INT-2, 1.5–2.0; High, ≥2.5.
Karyotype: Good score, -Y, del(5q); poor score, complex abnormalities and chromosome 7 abnormalities; intermediate score, other abnormalities.
Source: *Williams Hematology,* 8th ed, Chap. 88, Table 88–3, p. 1262.

TABLE 42-4 **SURVIVAL OF PATIENTS WITH CLONAL CYTOPENIAS AND OLIGOBLASTIC MYELOGENOUS LEUKEMIA BASED ON THE IPSS**

IPSS Score at Diagnosis	No. of Patients	2-Year Survival	5-Year Survival	10-Year Survival	15-Year Survival
Low	267	85%	55%	28%	20%
Intermediate-1	314	70%	35%	17%	12%
Intermediate-2	179	30%	8%	0	—
High	56	5%	0	—	—

IPSS, International Prognostic Scoring System.
Data are expressed as percent of all patients in that risk category surviving at the time interval shown. These data were extrapolated from curves in Fig. 6 of Greenberg P, Cox C, LeBeau MM, et al: International scoring system for evaluating prognosis in myelodysplastic syndromes. *Blood* 89:2079, 1997.
Source: *Williams Hematology* 8th ed, Chap. 88, Table 88–4, p. 1262.

- Therapy is very difficult because the patient often has another cancer, has gone through periods of intensive cytotoxic therapy, may have other comorbidities, and a high proportion is of advanced age.
- Allogeneic hematopoietic stem cell transplantation may be useful in younger patients with a suitable donor and without comorbidities.

TRUE PRELEUKEMIC SYNDROMES

- In the 1950s through the early 1980s, myelodysplastic syndromes were erroneously described as preleukemia. This descriptive categorization, largely, has been discarded. Since these syndromes are clonal, they are neoplastic, and the vital and most critical transition in cell pathology has occurred from polyclonal to monoclonal hematopoiesis.

TABLE 42-5 **SURVIVAL OF PATIENTS WITH CLONAL CYTOPENIAS AND OLIGOBLASTIC MYELOGENOUS LEUKEMIA BASED ON THE IPSS STRATIFIED BY AGE**

IPSS Score and Age	2-Year Survival	5-Year Survival	10-Year Survival	15-Year Survival
Low ≤60 years	95%	80%	65%	30%
Low >60 years	80%	45%	18%	18%
Intermediate-1 ≤60 years	85%	50%	37%	18%
Intermediate-1 >60 years	62%	30%	12%	ND
Intermediate-2 ≤60 years	50%	15%	ND	—
Intermediate-2 >60 years	25%	5%	0	—
High ≤60 years	0	—	—	—
High >60 years	7%	0		

IPSS, International Prognostic Scoring System; ND, no data.
These data were extrapolated from curves in Fig. 7 of Greenberg P, Cox C, LeBeau MM, et al: International scoring system for evaluating prognosis in myelodysplastic syndromes. *Blood* 89:2079, 1997. Data are expressed as percent of all patients in that risk category surviving at the time interval shown.
Source: *Williams Hematology* 8th ed, Chap. 88, Table 88–5, p. 1262.

- Many cases have leukemic hematopoiesis in the classic sense (evident leukemic myeloblasts in marrow and blood) and all are leukemic in the pathobiologic sense, since they are all a clonal (neoplastic) disorder originating in a multipotential hematopoietic cell.
- Some polyclonal syndromes are truly preleukemic in the pathobiologic sense, polyclonal disorders that have a propensity to evolve into AML or oligoblastic myelogenous leukemia (higher-risk myelodysplasia). Examples are inherited conditions, such as Fanconi anemia, and acquired conditions, such as aplastic anemia. These numerous polyclonal preleukemia states are listed in Chap. 46, Table 46–1.

END NOTE

The term "refractory" is an 80-year-old anachronistic designation, used before these diseases were known to be clonal (neoplastic) and should be retired. Sideroblastic and nonsideroblastic clonal anemia should be treated as one subtype. They behave identically and their management and prognosis are not significantly different. The distinction in blast count of 5 to 9 and 10 to 19 among cases with overt leukemic hematopoiesis is questionable based on one marrow examination. There are some distinctions in group data, but they are of little usefulness in individual cases in which one must evaluate the degree of abnormality of hematopoiesis globally; determine the patient's progress over time; and whether, when, or if to use some form of acute leukemia therapy for progressive disease.

For a more detailed discussion, see Jane L. Leisveld and Marshall A. Lichtman: Myelodysplastic Syndromes (Clonal Cytopenias and Oligoblastic Myelogenous Leukemia). Chap. 88, p. 1249; Josef T. Prchal and Jaroslav F. Prchal: Polycythemia Vera. Chap. 86, p. 1263 in *Williams Hematology,* 8th ed.

CHAPTER 43
Polycythemia Vera

- Polycythemia vera (PV) is a clonal disorder due to somatic mutations of a multipotential hematopoietic cell, in which blood cell production, notably erythropoiesis, is increased independent of cytokine regulation. This results in exaggerated proliferation and accumulation of erythrocytic, granulocytic, and megakaryocytic cells. PV is one of the chronic myeloproliferative disorders (MPDs): essential thrombocythemia (ET), primary myelofibrosis (PMF), and chronic myelogenous leukemia (CML); these disorders are also called myeloproliferative neoplasms (MPN).
- Three myeloproliferative neoplasms (PV, ET, PMF) share a common molecular abnormality/marker, the *JAK2* kinase V617F mutation.

ETIOLOGY AND PATHOGENESIS

- PV arises from the neoplastic transformation of a single hematopoietic multipotential cell, which provides both a selective growth and survival advantage that results in the cells produced in the clone suppressing and replacing normal polyclonal hematopoiesis.
- The *JAK2* kinase V617F mutation directly activates erythropoietin (EPO) receptor.
- *In vitro* erythroid colonies developing in the absence of added EPO are characteristic for PV.
- Karyotypic abnormalities are not specific; develop later in the disease, may portend transformation into myelofibrosis or myelogenous leukemia.
- Familial incidence of PV and/or other MPDs, occurs in about 5 percent of patients.
- Incidence ranges from 1 to 2.5 per 100,000 reported in different countries.

CLINICAL FEATURES

- PV usually has an insidious onset, most commonly during the sixth decade of life, although may occur at any age, including childhood.
- Presenting symptoms and signs: headache, plethora, pruritus, thrombosis (esp. Budd-Chiari syndrome), erythromelalgia, and gastrointestinal bleeding. Many patients diagnosed because of elevated hemoglobin and/or platelets on routine medical examination. Other cases may be uncovered during investigation for blood loss, iron-deficiency anemia (sometimes as a result of prior bleeding), or thrombosis. Symptoms are reported by at least 30 percent of patients with polycythemia at the time of diagnosis.
- Neurologic complaints include vertigo, diplopia, scotomata, and transient ischemic events.
- Associated disorders include peptic ulcer disease and gout.
- Thrombotic and hemorrhagic events are the most significant clinical manifestations of PV; they may occur prior to diagnosis of the disease.
- Thrombotic episodes are the most common and the most important complications, occurring in about one-third of the patients; these may be fatal, and include stroke, myocardial infarction, deep venous thrombosis, hepatic vein thrombosis, and pulmonary embolism.
- Bleeding and bruising are common complications of PV, occurring in about one-quarter of the patients in some series (generally when platelet count over

1000×10^9/L). Whereas such episodes (such as gingival bleeding, nose bleeding, or easy bruising) are usually minor, serious gastrointestinal bleeding (which may mask polycythemia) and other hemorrhagic complications with a fatal outcome also can occur.

- Patients with uncontrolled PV undergoing surgery have a high risk of bleeding and/or thrombosis. Phlebotomy should be used to decrease hematocrit prior to surgery to lessen risk.

LABORATORY FEATURES

- The most consistent is a mutation in exon 14 of *JAK2* kinase, present in >95 percent of PV patients. It is a single nucleotide change *JAK2* G1849T, referred to as the *JAK2* V617F mutation.
- The detection of the *JAK2* V617F mutation provides a qualitative diagnostic marker for the identification of PV (as well as ET and PMF) and its differentiation from congenital and acquired reactive polycythemic disorders.
- *JAK2* V617F is present in other MPDs. In general, PMF and PV patients have the higher level, and ET patients the lower *JAK2* V617F allelic burden. In virtually all PV *JAK2* V617F-positive patients, at least some progenitors exist that are homozygous for the *JAK2* V617F mutation by uniparental disomy acquired by mitotic recombination.
- The uncommon cases of PV negative for *JAK2* V617F often carry one of a number of mutations in the terminus of exon 12.
- Hemoglobin is typically elevated. In patients who have or have had hepatic vein thrombosis, gastrointestinal blood loss, or have been treated with phlebotomy, hemoglobin may be normal. Hypochromia, microcytosis, and other evidence of iron deficiency are often present as a result of prior chronic blood loss usually through the stool.
- Red cell mass is usually elevated, sometimes not in proportion to the level of hemoglobin, implying a concomitant increase in plasma volume.
- Nucleated red cells and teardrops (dacrocytes) are not present in the blood film early in the disease.
- Absolute neutrophilia occurs in about two-thirds of patients, with occasional myelocytes and metamyelocytes. Slight basophilia also occurs in about two-thirds of patients.
- The platelet count is increased in over 50 percent of patients and exceeds 1000×10^9/L in about 10 percent. Acquired von Willebrand disease may be present (see Chap. 80).
- Platelets also may have a characteristic functional defect in the primary wave of aggregation induced by epinephrine while spontaneous platelet aggregation is accelerated.
- Marrow is usually hypercellular, with absent iron stores. A mild degree of marrow reticulin fibrosis may be present, particularly in long-standing disease.
- Prothrombin time and partial thromboplastin time may be spuriously prolonged if the amount of anticoagulant used in the test is not adjusted for the decreased proportion of plasma.

DIAGNOSIS

- The most important diagnostic features of polycythemia vera include:
    — The presence of the *JAK2* V617F mutation in blood cells.
    — Erythrocytosis (elevated hemoglobin and or red cell mass).
    — Low serum EPO levels.
    — Leukocytosis (specifically neutrophilia).
    — Thrombocytosis.
    — Splenomegaly.

- Other helpful clinical features are:
  - — Pruritus, often provoked by a warm bath or shower.
  - — Elevated serum vitamin B_{12} level.
  - — Elevated serum uric acid level.
  - — Normal or near-normal arterial oxygen saturation.
- Another test of value, if available, is demonstration of erythroid colony growth *in vitro* in absence of added EPO.
- Some consider the measurement of red cell mass to be the *sine qua non* for diagnosis of PV, but others believe this study should be reserved for special circumstances, such as in the case of unexplained thrombocytosis, splenomegaly, or a *JAK2* mutation and a normal hemoglobin concentration. If the hemoglobin concentration is greater than 16.5 g/dL in a woman or greater than 18.5 g/dL in a man, the probability of an elevated red cell mass is very high.

DIFFERENTIAL DIAGNOSIS

- The diagnostic task has been facilitated by the discovery of the *JAK2* kinase mutation that is present in >95 percent of all PV patients.
- Diagnostic criteria recently established by the World Health Organization are helpful in most cases (see Table 43–1). They are yet to be validated by prospective clinical studies.
- A *V617F*-negative patient may have PV and require a search for other *JAK2* mutations or they may have another type of polycythemia.
- A *V617*-positive patient may have another MPD.

THERAPY

- The mainstay of therapy for PV remains nonspecific myelosuppression, which many practitioners supplement with phlebotomies. Anagrelide may be added to control thrombocytosis (see Table 43–2).
- Additional measures are medications to prevent thrombotic events (i.e., aspirin) and to relieve symptoms; aspirin should not be used when platelet count is higher than 1000×10^9/L because it increases risk of bleeding.
- Promising therapies are pegylated interferon preparations, which are better-tolerated than non-pegylated preparations, and JAK2 inhibitors, which are being evaluated mainly in the post PV-myelofibrotic stage.
- It is useful to consider treatments in the plethoric and the spent phases separately.

TABLE 43–1	WORLD HEALTH ORGANIZATION CRITERIA FOR THE DIAGNOSIS OF POLYCYTHEMIA VERA	
	Major Criteria	**Minor Criteria**
A1	Hgb >18.5 g/dL (men) >16.5 g/dL (women) or Hgb >17 g/dL (men), or >15 g/dL (women) if associated with a sustained increase of ≥2 g/dL from baseline that cannot be attributed to correction of iron deficiency	Marrow trilineage myeloproliferation
A2	Presence of *JAK2 V617F* or similar mutation	Subnormal serum EPO level
		Endogenous (EPO-independent) erythroid colony growth

EPO, erythropoietin; Hgb, hemoglobin.
Diagnosis satisfied if both major and 1 minor or first major and 2 minor criteria are present.
Source: *Williams Hematology,* 8th edition 86-1, Chap. 86, Table 86-1, p. 1229)

TABLE 43–2	TREATMENT OF POLYCYTHEMIA VERA	
Treatment	Advantages	Disadvantages
Phlebotomy	Low risk. Simple to perform.	Does not control thrombocytosis or leukocytosis.
Hydroxyurea	Controls leukocytosis and thrombocytosis. Low leukemogenic risk.	Continuous therapy required.
Busulfan	Easy to administer. Prolonged remissions. Risk of leukemogenesis probably not high.	Overdose produces prolonged marrow suppression. Risks of leukemogenesis, long-term pulmonary and cutaneous toxicity.
^{32}P	Patient compliance not required. Prolonged control of thrombocytosis and leukocytosis.	Expensive and relatively inconvenient. Moderate leukemogenic risk.
Chlorambucil	Easy to administer. Good control of thrombocytosis and leukocytosis.	High risk of leukemogenesis.
Interferon	Low leukemogenic potential. Effect on pruritus.	Inconvenient, costly, frequent side effects.
Anagrelide	Selective effect on platelets.	Selective effect on platelets.

Source: *Williams Hematology,* 8th ed, Chap. 86, Table 86–3, p. 1230.

Plethoric Phase

- The treatment of patients in the plethoric phase of the disease is aimed at ameliorating symptoms and decreasing the risk of thrombosis or bleeding by reducing the blood counts. This is accomplished by myelosuppressive drugs and, additionally in some patients, phlebotomies, platelet-reducing agents, or interferon-α therapy.
- Treatment should be individualized according to risk factors:
  - *High risk* – patients with previous thrombosis and/or transient ischemic attacks.
  - *Intermediate risk* – patients over 60 years of age.
  - *Low risk* – the remaining patients.
- *High risk* and *intermediate risk* patients require interferon or other myelosuppressive therapy.
- The absolute leukocyte count strongly correlates with thrombotic complications, and this laboratory parameter is now being evaluated in the therapeutic decision-making process as are additional risk factors, including hypertension, smoking, and diabetes.
- Myelosuppression
  - Myelosuppressive therapy decreases blood counts, decreases the risk of vascular events, and ameliorates symptoms, and increases an overall sense of well-being. While there is also a clinical impression that it increases a patient's long-term survival, there are no clinical studies to document this.
  - At present, hydroxyurea at doses of 500 to 2500 mg daily is the preferred drug.

— Hydroxyurea's suppressive effect is of short duration. Thus, continuous rather than intermittent therapy is required. Because it is short acting, it is relatively safe to use, even when excessive marrow suppression occurs, since the blood counts rise within a few days of decreasing the dose or stopping the drug.

— Because it is not an alkylating agent, hydroxyurea has less potential for causing leukemic transformation.

— Busulfan (Myleran) or P^{32} may be used in selected cases.

- Phlebotomy
  — Is best used in conjunction with myelosuppression; it is also used as the initial treatment by some physicians.

  — Most patients of average size can tolerate initial phlebotomy of 450 to 500 mL about every 4 days until the target hemoglobin level is reached.

  — Contributes to iron deficiency. Iron supplementation is counterproductive and may result in rapid reappearance of polycythemia, but a short course of oral iron therapy is often helpful in amelioration of fatigue.

  — Phlebotomy alone is associated with a higher incidence of thrombotic events, especially in older patients, those with a high phlebotomy requirement, and those with a prior thrombotic event.

- Summary of therapeutic approach for patients not participating in clinical trials:
  — Myelosuppression with hydroxyurea daily, both as initial therapy (1500 mg qd) and long-term treatment (500 to 2000 mg qd), aiming to maintain neutrophil counts at low-normal levels. In addition, some patients require the use of phlebotomies and/or anagrelide to maintain the hemoglobin and platelet levels in normal ranges.

  — Aspirin at a dose 80 to 100 mg qd is given to all patients without histories of major bleeding or gastric intolerance and when platelet count is not over $1000 \times 10^9/L$).

  — Allopurinol for elevated uric acid levels and medication to control pruritus is used when required.

  — Judicious phlebotomies with isovolemic replacement in patients with hematocrits >55 percent (others recommend keeping hematocrtit <45 for men and <43 for women) and in patients who report immediate improvement of symptoms after phlebotomy. The symptoms that may be related to hyperviscosity are headaches, difficulty concentrating, and fatigue.

  — Pegylated interferon preparations are being used increasingly with excellent results reported in pilot studies.

  — JAK2 tyrosine kinase inhibitors are also being evaluated.

Spent Phase

- Sometimes after only a few years and usually after 10 or more years (but not in all patients), erythrocytosis in patients with PV gradually abates, phlebotomy requirements decrease and cease, and anemia develops. During this "spent" phase of the disease, marrow fibrosis becomes more marked and the spleen often becomes greatly enlarged. The condition (post-PV PMF) is indistinguishable from PMF (see Chap. 48). Patients typically have teardrops and leukoerythroblastic morphology, may have leukocytosis or leukopenia, thrombocytosis or thrombocytopenia, and immature leukocytes (including blasts) in the blood.

- Nonmyeloablative allogeneic stem cell transplantation should be considered for eligible patients as only a curative therapy.

- For patients not eligible for transplantation, the treatment is symptomatic/supportive only. It consists of any of:
  — JAK2 inhibitors.
  — Gentle myelosuppression with low doses of hydroxyurea.
  — Red cell transfusion and/or erythropoiesis stimulating agents.
  — thalidomide and its derivatives

— androgens
— experimental therapies
— General comfort measures and analgesics.
— Splenectomy may be considered for significant cytopenias, recurrent infarctions.

COURSE AND PROGNOSIS

- See Table 43–3 for criteria that define a patient's response to therapy.
- Thrombotic complications discussed in the preceding sections are the dominant cause of morbidity and mortality in patients with PV.
- In addition, and in contrast to other polycythemic disorders, PV has an increased risk of evolution to acute leukemia. While several clinical stages of PV are recognized (plethoric or proliferative phase, stable phase, spent phase or post-polycythemic myelofibrosis phase, and acute leukemia), it is not clear that these stages represent a sequential progression of the disease.
- PV is a disease that is compatible with normal or near-normal life for many years and many patients may not need any therapy while most would benefit from aspirin. However, most studies agree that there is excess mortality attributable to thrombotic complications and acute leukemia transformation as a direct consequence of PV.

TABLE 43–3	DEFINITION OF CLINICAL AND HEMATOLOGIC RESPONSE IN POLYCYTHEMIA VERA

Complete Response:
1. Hematocrit <45% without phlebotomy *and*
2. Platelet count ≤400 × 10⁹/L *and*
3. White blood cell count ≤10 × 10⁹/L, *and*
4. Normal spleen size on imaging, *and*
5. No disease-related symptoms

Partial Response:
Patients who do not fulfill the criteria for complete response, hematocrit <45% without phlebotomy, or response in three or more of the other criteria.

Barosi G, Birgegard G, Finazzi G, et al: Response criteria for essential thrombocythemia and polycythemia vera: result of a European LeukemiaNet consensus conference. Blood. 2009 113:4829, 2009).
Source: *Williams Hematology,* 8th ed, Chap. 86, Table 86–2, p. 1230.

For a more detailed discussion, see Josef T. Prchal and Jaroslav F. Prchal: Polycythemia Vera. Chap. 86, p. 1223 in *Williams Hematology,* 8th ed.

CHAPTER 44
Primary and Familial Thrombocythemia

- The upper limit of a normal platelet count is usually between $350 \times 10^9/L$ and $450 \times 10^9/L$ depending on the clinical laboratory and specific method used.
- Table 44–1 presents the major causes of elevation of the platelet count above the normal limit.

ESSENTIAL THROMBOCYTHEMIA (CLONAL THROMBOCYTOSIS)

Pathophysiology
- Essential thrombocythemia is a clonal disorder of multipotential hematopoietic progenitor cell and is a chronic myeloproliferative disorder related to polycythemia vera and primary myelofibrosis.
- Approximately 50 percent of patients express a mutant form of the *Janus (JAK)2* signaling kinase (*JAK2* V617F) found in several myeloproliferative disorders (polycythemia vera, primary myelofibrosis, rare cases of myelodysplastic syndromes). The mutant allele is almost invariantly found in one copy per cell in patients with essential thrombocythemia, and leads *in vitro* and *in vivo* to hematopoietic growth factor hypersensitivity, a hallmark of the disease.
- A smaller fraction of patients display other mutations of *JAK2*, or of the thrombopoietin receptor, c-Mpl. Nearly one-half of patients fail to express one of these mutations, and usually display lower hemoglobin concentrations than patients with *JAK2* V617F.

Clinical Features
- The criteria used for the diagnosis of essential thrombocythemia are shown in Table 44–2.
- Usually develops between ages 50 and 70. Sex distribution is slightly skewed toward women, especially in younger patients.
- Because platelet counts are now often done routinely, the disorder is being discovered in younger individuals and in patients who are asymptomatic.
- Rare familial cases have been reported.
- Constitutional or hypermetabolic symptoms are very uncommon.
- Mild splenomegaly is found in 40 to 50 percent of patients.
- Patients may have ecchymoses and bruising due to functional platelet deficiencies, or due to acquired von Willebrand disease if platelet counts are very high.
- Bleeding and thrombotic complications are major causes of morbidity and mortality. Table 44–3 summarizes the risks of thrombosis or bleeding.
- Bleeding is common and is characteristic of platelet or vascular disorders: mucosal, gastrointestinal, cutaneous, genitourinary, and postoperative.
- Use of aspirin may occasionally lead to serious bleeding complications, especially when platelet counts are above $1500 \times 10^9/L$ due to acquired von Willebrand disease.
- Thrombosis, more often arterial than venous, is most common in cerebral, peripheral, and coronary arteries.
- Twenty-five percent of all thrombotic events are lower-extremity deep venous thrombosis.

TABLE 44–1	MAJOR CAUSES OF THROMBOCYTOSIS

Clonal thrombocytosis
Essential thrombocythemia
Polycythemia vera
Primary myelofibrosis
Chronic myeloid leukemia
Refractory anemia with ringed sideroblasts and thrombocytosis
5q-minus syndrome

Reactive (secondary) thrombocytosis
Transient thrombocytosis
Acute blood loss
Recovery from thrombocytopenia (rebound thrombocytosis)
Acute infection or inflammation
Response to exercise
Response to drugs (vincristine, epinephrine, all-*trans*-retinoic acid)
Sustained thrombocytosis
Iron deficiency
Splenectomy or congenital absence of spleen
Malignancy
Chronic infection or inflammation
Hemolytic anemia

Familial thrombocytosis

Spurious thrombocytosis
Cryoglobulinemia
Cytoplasmic fragmentation in acute leukemia
Red cell fragmentation
Bacteremia

Source: *Williams Hematology,* 8th ed, Chap. 87, Table 87–2, p. 1240.

- Thrombosis in the myeloproliferative disorders often occur in unusual locations, such as hepatic artery (Budd-Chiari), sagittal venous sinus, upper extremity.

Erythromelalgia and Digital Microvascular Ischemia
- Caused by vascular occlusion with platelet thrombi.
- Patients have intense burning or throbbing pain, especially in feet.
- Symptoms are exacerbated by heat, exercise, and dependency, and relieved by cold and elevation of the lower extremity.

TABLE 44–2	DIAGNOSTIC CRITERIA FOR ESSENTIAL THROMBOCYTHEMIA

Diagnosis requires A1 to A3 or A1 + A3 to A5

A1	Sustained platelet count $>450 \times 10^9$/L
A2	Presence of an acquired pathogenic mutation (e.g., in *JAK2* or *MPL*)
A3	No other myeloid malignancy, especially PV, PMF, CML, or myelodysplastic syndrome
A4	No reactive cause for thrombocytosis and normal iron stores
A5	Marrow studies showing increased megakaryocytes displaying a spectrum of morphology with prominent large hyperlobulated forms; reticulin is generally not increased

Source: *Williams Hematology,* 8th ed, Chap. 87, Table 87–1, p. 1240.

TABLE 44-3	**RISKS OF THROMBOHEMORRHAGIC COMPLICATIONS IN ESSENTIAL THROMBOCYTHEMIA**	
	Thrombosis	Bleeding
Increased risk	Previous history of thrombosis	Use of aspirin and other nonsteroidal antiinflammatory drugs
	Associated cardiovascular risk factors (especially smoking)	Extreme thrombocytosis (platelet count $>2 \times 10^9$/L)
	Advanced age (>60 years)	
	Inadequate control of thrombocytosis (in high-risk patients)	
Not associated with risk	Degree of thrombocytosis *In vitro* platelet function	Prolonged bleeding time *In vitro* platelet function

- Painful vascular insufficiency may lead to gangrene and necrosis with normal peripheral pulses and patent major vessels on angiography.
- These problems often respond dramatically and promptly to small doses of aspirin and/or reduction of platelet count.

Cerebrovascular Ischemia
- Symptoms may be nonspecific (headache, dizziness, decreased mental acuity), and signs may be focal (transient ischemic attacks, seizures, or retinal artery occlusion).

Recurrent Abortions and Fetal Growth Retardation
- Multiple placental infarctions may lead to placental insufficiency with recurrent spontaneous abortions, fetal growth retardation, premature deliveries, and abruptio placentae.
- May require use of aspirin during pregnancy, but avoid at least 1 week prior to delivery to reduce risk of maternal or neonatal bleeding complications.

Hepatic and Portal Vein Thrombosis
- Usually occur with polycythemia vera but may occur with essential thrombocythemia.

Blood and Marrow Findings
- Platelet counts may range from only slightly above normal to several million platelets per microliter.
- Platelets may be large, pale blue–staining, and hypogranular. Nucleated megakaryocyte fragments having a lymphoblastoid appearance may be seen occasionally in the blood film.
- Some patients may have mild leukocytosis with hemoglobin concentration ranging from normal to mild anemia.
- The leukocyte differential count is usually normal, without nucleated red cells.
- Pseudohypokalemia may occur with extreme thrombocytosis or leukocytosis.
- Marrow shows increased cellularity with megakaryocytic hyperplasia and masses of platelet debris ("platelet drifts"). Megakaryocytes are frequently giant, with increased ploidy, and occur in clusters. Significant megakaryocytic dysplasia is uncommon.
- Some patients who have otherwise typical essential thrombocythemia will have the Philadelphia chromosome or the *BCR/ABL* gene rearrangement.

Clinical Tests of Hemostasis

- Abnormal tests serve as a marker for the disease but do not predict bleeding and/or thrombosis and, thus, are rarely of clinical utility.
- The bleeding (closure) time is prolonged in less than 20 percent of patients.
- Platelet aggregation abnormalities are variable:
    — Total loss of responsiveness to epinephrine is characteristic.
    — Reduced responses to collagen, ADP, and arachidonic acid occur in less than one-third of patients.
    — Patient platelets may display hyperaggregability or spontaneous aggregation *in vitro*.

Differential Diagnosis

- The diagnosis is made by genetic testing for *JAK2* V617F, another *JAK2* or *c-Mpl* mutation, or in their absence by exclusion because there is no specific marker for the disease. The following should be demonstrated:
    — The platelet count is usually greater than 600×10^9/L, on at least two occasions separated by 3 months, but some patients have platelet counts in the normal range or only slightly elevated.
    — The patient is not iron deficient or afflicted by an inflammatory condition.
    — There is no other recognizable cause for secondary thrombocytosis.
    — The Philadelphia chromosome is absent.
    — There is no evidence for myelofibrosis.

Therapy

Asymptomatic Patients

- The need to treat asymptomatic patients is controversial.

Symptomatic Patients

- Lowering the platelet count in patients with active bleeding and/or thrombosis is beneficial.
- Prompt reduction is especially warranted in patients with microvascular digital or cerebrovascular ischemia.

Treatment Options

- Urgent platelet count reduction can be achieved by plateletpheresis, but the benefit is short-lived, often with a rebound increase in platelet count.
- Hydroxyurea is highly effective as initial therapy. The usual starting dose is 10 to 30 mg/kg per day orally. Blood counts should be checked within 7 days of initiating therapy and frequently thereafter, seeking a maintenance dose that will maintain the platelet count at less than 400×10^9/L. The major side effects of hydroxyurea are gastrointestinal upset and reversible painful leg ulcers, occurring in approximately 30 percent of patients.
- Aspirin should be added in nearly all patients requiring treatment, unless contraindicated by bleeding, allergic complications, or extremely high platelet counts.
- A large randomized study of hydroxyurea plus aspirin vs. anagrelide plus aspirin demonstrated the superiority of the hydroxyurea plus aspirin arm in reducing complications.
- Anagrelide inhibits marrow megakaryocyte maturation and is effective alternative second-line therapy for patients who do not tolerate hydroxyurea. The starting dose is 0.5 mg orally four times daily or 1 mg orally twice daily. Dosage adjustments should be made weekly, depending on the blood count. The maintenance dose is usually 2.0 to 3.0 mg/d. Side effects include neurologic and gastrointestinal symptoms, palpitations, and fluid retention in approximately 25 percent of patients.
- Recombinant interferon-α is also effective therapy. It suppresses the abnormal megakaryocyte clone. The starting dose is 3 million units subcutaneously daily

with subsequent adjustments based on tolerance and response. Two major side effects are flu-like symptoms and psychiatric disturbance, especially in older patients. It has been recommended for patients less than 45 years because it is free from teratogenic or leukemogenic effects.

Course and Prognosis

- The major cause of morbidity and mortality are thrombosis and hemorrhage.
- Rarely, essential thrombocythemia may convert to another myeloproliferative disorder, or spontaneously convert to acute leukemia.

FAMILIAL THROMBOCYTOSIS

- A rare disorder usually inherited as an autosomal dominant trait.
- The disorder is occasionally due to mutations of the thrombopoietin gene, which lead to markedly increased serum thrombopoietin levels, or due to activating mutations of the thrombopoietin receptor.

For a more detailed discussion, see Philip A. Beer and Anthony R. Green: Essential Thrombocythemia. Chap. 87, p. 1237 in *Williams Hematology*, 8th ed.

CHAPTER 45
Paroxysmal Nocturnal Hemoglobinuria (PNH)

DEFINITION

- An acquired hematopoietic stem cell disorder characterized by deficiency of glycosyl phosphatidylinositol-anchored proteins (GPI-APs) on the surface of hematopoietic cells. Two complement regulatory proteins (CD55 and CD59) are GPI-anchored, and deficiency of these two proteins leads to the complement-mediated intravascular hemolysis that is the clinical hallmark of the disease. Marrow failure and thrombophilia also complicate the disease.
- It is the only hemolytic anemia caused by an acquired intrinsic defect of the red cell.

ETIOLOGY AND PATHOGENESIS

- The disorder is a consequence of somatic mutation of *PIGA*, a gene on the X chromosome that encodes a glycosyl transferase required for synthesis of the GPI anchor.
- Women and men are equally affected because *PIGA* is subject to X inactivation in somatic tissues of females.
- The somatic mutation arises in one or more hematopoietic stems cells, and as a consequence, all of the progeny of the mutant stem cell are deficient in all GPI-APs.
- More than 20 GPI-APs have been found to be deficient on the hematopoietic cells of PNH, but only deficiency of the complement regulatory proteins CD55 and CD59 has been shown conclusively to contribute to disease pathology.
- Appears to arise as a monoclonal or oligoclonal abnormality of stem cells. Several populations of cells of different sensitivity to complement have been identified in some patients, and molecular analysis shows that the complement-sensitivity phenotype is determined by *PIGA* mutant genotype, confirming that the disease is oligoclonal in some patients.
- The oligoclonal nature of PNH suggests that a specific selection pressure is applied to the marrow that favors outgrowth of *PIGA* mutant stem cells present in the marrow when the selective pressure is applied. The association of PNH with aplastic anemia suggests that the selection pressure may be immune-mediated. The basis of the clonal selection and clonal expansion of the *PIGA* mutant cells is not known.
- The extent to which the mutant clone or clones expands varies greatly among patients. In some patients, a mutant clone may account for >90 percent of hematopoiesis, while in other patients, <10 percent of the blood cells are derived from a mutant clone. In general, the severity of the disease is directly related to the size of the mutant clone.

CLINICAL FEATURES

- Overt hemoglobinuria occurs irregularly in most patients, precipitated by a variety of events including infection, surgery, trauma, and stress.
- Nocturnal hemoglobinuria is relatively uncommon as a presenting symptom.
- Patients have chronic intravascular hemolytic anemia, which may be severe depending on the size of the mutant clone.
- Modest splenomegaly is observed in some patients.

- Iron deficiency is common as a consequence of iron loss in the urine, resulting from intravascular hemolysis.
- Marrow failure of varying degrees is present in all patients with PNH.
- PNH is closely associated with aplastic anemia and may be seen less commonly in association with low-risk myelodysplastic syndromes.
- Bleeding may occur secondary to thrombocytopenia.
- Thrombophilia is a prominent feature and accounts for most of the mortality.
- Venous thromboses affecting unusual sites (e.g., dermal veins, splanchnic vessels including Budd-Chiari syndrome, cerebral veins) is characteristic of the thrombophilia of PNH.
- Arterial thromboses also occur.
- Pulmonary hypertension may develop secondary to thromboses in the pulmonary microvasculature.
- Pregnancy in PNH patients may be associated with abortion and venous thromboembolism.
- Renal manifestations include:
  — Hyposthenuria.
  — Abnormal tubular function.
  — Acute and chronic renal failure.
- Neurologic manifestations:
  — Headaches.
  — Cerebral venous thrombosis is uncommon.

LABORATORY FEATURES

- Anemia may be severe, with hemoglobin levels of less than 5 g/dL.
- Macrocytosis may be present because of mild to moderate reticulocytosis.
- The complement-mediated hemolysis of PNH is an intravascular process, and the concentration of serum lactic acid dehydrogenase (LDH) is markedly elevated in patients with clinically significant hemolysis.
- The anemia may be hypochromic and microcytic because of iron deficiency.
- Low leukocyte count, as a consequence of marrow failure, is characteristic.
- Decreased leukocyte alkaline phosphatase activity is observed because leukocyte alkaline phosphatase is a GPI-AP.
- Low platelet count, due to marrow failure, is common; normal in about 20 percent of patients.
- Marrow examination usually shows erythroid hyperplasia; marrow cellularity is not greatly increased. The marrow in some cases is very hypocellular, simulating aplastic anemia.
- Urine findings include:
  — Hemoglobin sometimes present.
  — Hemosiderinuria is a constant feature and the Prussian blue stain of urine sediment is thus positive. Use first-voided morning urine for hemosiderin assessment.
- The diagnosis is made by flow cytometric analysis of GPI-linked CD59 expression on peripheral blood cells. Both erythrocytes and neutrophils should be analyzed. Analysis of the erythrocytes provides information on the different phenotypes while analysis of neutrophils is the best way to quantify the size of the PNH clone.

DIFFERENTIAL DIAGNOSIS

- Consider PNH in patients with pancytopenia, particularly when accompanied by evidence of intravascular hemolysis (reticulocytosis and a high serum LDH concentration).
- PNH should be included in the differential diagnosis of patients with thrombosis at unusual sites (e.g., intra-abdominal veins), especially if there is concurrent evidence of intravascular hemolysis.

- Laboratory tests, which if abnormal in the presence of anemia or multicytopenia, may suggest a diagnosis:
  — Serum LDH concentration, reticulocyte count, analysis of iron stores, Prussian blue stain of urine sediment for hemosiderinuria.
- Definitive test:
  — Flow cytometric analysis for deficiency of CD55 and CD59 on erythrocytes and CD55, CD59 and other GPI-APs on granulocytes is sensitive and specific.

TREATMENT

- Transfusion for anemia.
- Oral iron therapy for iron deficiency.
- Eculizumab (Soliris) is a humanized monoclonal antibody that binds to and inhibits the function of complement C5, one of the components of the cytolytic membrane attack complex of complement. By blocking formation of the membrane attack complex, eculizumab inhibits the complement-mediated intravascular hemolysis of PNH. Eculizumab does not inhibit C3 activation on PNH erythrocytes. Consequently, the opsonized cells are destroyed extravascularly by the mononuclear phagocyte system.
- Steroid hormones:
  — Some patients respond dramatically to treatment with androgens. Synthetic androgens such as danazol may be preferable to naturally occurring androgens because of a more favorable toxicity profile.
  — Prednisone can be used to treat an exacerbation of the disease, but chronic use is not recommended because of adverse effects.
- Anticoagulants:
  — Prophylactic anticoagulation is controversial, but some studies suggest that the risk of thrombosis is related to the size of the PNH clone. For patients with clone sizes ≥50 percent (based on flow cytometric analysis of expression of GPI-APs on peripheral blood neutrophils) prophylactic anticoagulation with warfarin should be considered.
  — Useful in management of thrombotic complications. Thrombolytic therapy and/or a transjugular portosystemic shunt (TIPS) procedure should be considered for patients who develop Budd-Chiari syndrome.
- Splenectomy not indicated.
- Allogeneic hematopoietic stem cell transplantation is curative. Outcomes for transplant for patients with PNH are similar to those for patients transplanted for other marrow failure syndromes.

COURSE

- Variable, but prior to eculizumab therapy most patients who were not successfully treated by hematopoietic stem cell transplantation succumbed to complications. Eculizumab, thus, may change the natural history of the disease.
- Acute leukemia, aplastic anemia, or myelodysplastic syndrome may develop in some patients.

For a more detailed discussion, see Charles J. Parker: Paroxysmal Nocturnal Hemoglobinuria. Chap. 40, p. 521 in *Williams Hematology*, 8th ed.

CHAPTER 46
The Acute Myelogenous Leukemias

- Acute myelogenous leukemia (AML) is a malignancy originating in a multipotential hematopoietic cell characterized by clonal proliferation of abnormal blast cells in the marrow and impaired production of normal blood cells, resulting in anemia; thrombocytopenia; and low, normal, or high white cell counts depending on the number of leukemic cells in the blood. It occurs in nine morphologic variants, each with characteristic cytologic, genetic, and sometimes clinical features.

ETIOLOGY AND PATHOGENESIS

- The chronic clonal myeloid diseases may progress to florid AML (e.g., polycythemia vera, Chap. 43; essential thrombocythemia, Chap. 44), clonal cytopenias, Chap. 42; chronic myelogenous leukemia, Chap. 47).
- AML may develop with increased frequency in patients with certain congenital (Down syndrome) or inherited abnormalities (e.g., Fanconi anemia, familial platelet syndrome) as shown in Table 46–1.
- Non-syndromic, familial occurrence, suggesting an inherited predisposition gene, has been documented but is uncommon.
- Most cases arise *de novo* and are associated with acquired cytogenetic changes, including translocation, inversions, deletions, and others. These changes lead to the mutation of protooncogenes and the formation of oncogenes. Frequently, the latter encode mutant transcription factors that result in disruption of cell signaling pathways that cause malignant transformation.
- AML results from a series of somatic mutations in a multipotential hematopoietic cell or, in a small proportion of cases, a more differentiated, lineage restricted progenitor cell. In acute promyelocytic leukemia (APL), some cases of monocytic leukemia, and some young persons with other forms of AML, the disease originates in a mutated granulocytic-monocytic progenitor cell.
- AML requires at least two types of mutation: a primary oncogenic mutation, such as involving core-binding factor subunit genes (CBF-β or $RUNX1$), and an activating mutation, in a hematopoietic tyrosine kinase, such as FMS-like tyrosine kinase 3 ($FLT3$). The mutations in AML result in deregulated signaling pathways that disrupt differentiation and maturation, regulation of proliferation and of cell survival in varying combinations.

EPIDEMIOLOGY

- AML accounts for 80 percent of acute leukemias in adults and 15 to 20 percent in children.
- AML is the most frequent leukemia in neonates. This results in a bimodal incidence curve with a peak at less than 1 year of age of approximately 2 per 100,000 infants, dropping to approximately 0.4 cases per 100,000 at age 7 years, and then increasing to 1.0 per 100,000 by age 25 years. Thereafter, incidence increases exponentially to 20 cases per 100,000 persons in octogenarians.
- An exception to the striking change in incidence with age in adults is found in APL in which the incidence by age does not vary significantly.
- Four exposures: high-dose radiation, chronic benzene exposure usually in an industrial setting, treatment of other cancers with alkylating agents, topoisomerase II inhibitors or other cytotoxic drugs, and prolonged tobacco smoking—have been established as causative factors. Numerous other possible environmental factors have been studied but are unproven as causal factors.

TABLE 46–1	CONDITIONS PREDISPOSING TO DEVELOPMENT OF ACUTE MYELOGENOUS LEUKEMIA

Environmental factors
　　Radiation
　　Benzene
　　Alkylating agents, topoisomerase II inhibitors, and other cytotoxic drugs
　　Tobacco smoke

Acquired diseases
　　Clonal myeloid diseases
　　　　Chronic myelogenous leukemia
　　　　Primary myelofibrosis
　　　　Essential thrombocythemia
　　　　Polycythemia vera
　　　　Clonal cytopenias
　　　　Paroxysmal nocturnal hemoglobinuria
　　Other hematopoietic disorders
　　　　Aplastic anemia
　　　　Eosinophilic fasciitis
　　　　Myeloma
　　Other disorders
　　　　Human immunodeficiency virus infection
　　　　Thyroid disorders
　　　　Polyendocrine disorders
Inherited or Congenital Conditions
　　Sibling with AML
　　Amegakaryocytic thrombocytopenia, congenital
　　Ataxia-pancytopenia
　　Bloom syndrome
　　Congenital agranulocytosis (Kostmann syndrome)
　　Chronic thrombocytopenia with chromosome 21q 22.12 microdeletion
　　Diamond-Blackfan syndrome
　　Down syndrome
　　Dubowitz syndrome
　　Dyskeratosis congenita
　　Familial (pure, nonsyndromic) AML
　　Familial platelet disorder
　　Fanconi anemia
　　Naxos syndrome
　　Neurofibromatosis 1
　　Noonan syndrome
　　Poland syndrome
　　Rothmund-Thomson syndrome
　　Seckel syndrome
　　Shwachman syndrome
　　Werner syndrome (progeria)
　　Wolf-Hirschhorn syndrome
　　WT syndrome

Source: *Williams Hematology*, 8th ed, Chap. 89, Table 89–1, p. 1278.

- The risk of AML in a nonidentical sibling is approximately 2.5-fold that of unrelated individuals under age 15 years in persons of European descent.
- The risk of AML appears to be increased in Jews of Eastern European descent and the APL subtype among Latinos.

CLASSIFICATION

- AML develops clinically in nine morphologic variants that can be identified by a combination of blood cell and marrow morphology on stained slides, immuno-phenotype (CD profile) measured by flow cytometry (Table 46–2), and his-tochemical analysis, if necessary. Cytogenetic analysis provides a second level of classification. The diversity of specific cytogenetic abnormalities (hundreds) makes this useful only for the few most prevalent chromosome alterations (see Laboratory Features section below).

CLINICAL FEATURES

- Frequent presenting symptoms and signs are those reflecting anemia: pallor, fatigue, weakness, palpitations, and dyspnea on exertion; or thrombocytopenia: ecchymoses, petechiae, epistaxis, gingival bleeding, conjunctival hemorrhages, and prolonged bleeding after minor cuts.
- Minor pyogenic infections of the skin are common. Major infections are uncom-mon at diagnosis, prior to cytotoxic therapy.
- Anorexia and weight loss may occur.
- Fever may be present at onset.
- Mild splenomegaly or hepatomegaly is present in about one-third of patients. Lymph node enlargement is uncommon, except with the monocytic variant.
- Leukemic cells may infiltrate any organ in the body, but consequent organ dys-function is unusual. Occasionally, large accumulations of myeloblasts (myeloid sarcoma) may develop in virtually any tissue. Monoblasts frequently infiltrate tissues, and these sites can be symptomatic (e.g., leukemia cutis, gingival hyper-plasia, and others).

LABORATORY FEATURES

- Anemia and thrombocytopenia are nearly always present at diagnosis. Half the patients with AML have a platelet count $< 50 \times 10^9$/L.
- Red cell morphology is mildly abnormal (anisocytosis and occasional mis-shapen cells), although in occasional cases, more marked dysmorphia occurs.
- Total leukocyte count is below 5.0×10^9/L in about one-half of patients, and the absolute neutrophil count is less than 1.0×10^9/L in more than one-half of patients at diagnosis. Mature neutrophils may be hypersegmented, hyposeg-mented, or hypogranular.

TABLE 46–2	IMMUNOLOGIC PHENOTYPES OF AML
Phenotype	Usually Positive
Myeloblastic	CD11b, CD13, CD15, CD33, CD117, HLA-DR
Myelomonocytic	CD11b, CD13, CD14, CD15, CD32, CD33, HLA-DR
Erythroid	Glycophorin, spectrin, ABH antigens, carbonic anhydrase I, HLA-DR
Promyelocytic	CD13, CD33
Monocytic	CD11b, 11c, CD13, CD14, CD33, CD65, HLA-DR
Megakaryoblastic	CD34, CD41, CD42, CD61, anti-von Willebrand factor
Basophilic	CD11b, CD13, CD33, CD123, CD203c
Mast cell	CD13, CD33, CD117
Myeloid dendritic cell	CD11C, CD80, CD83, CD86

Source: *Williams Hematology*, 8th ed, Chap. 89, Table 89–2, p. 1280.

- Myeloblasts comprise from 3 to 95 percent of the leukocytes in the blood, and a small percent of the blast cells may contain Auer rods.
- Marrow contains leukemic blast cells, identified as myelogenous by reactivity with cytochemical stains (e.g., peroxidase), presence of Auer rods, or reactivity with antibodies to epitopes specific for myeloblasts or derivative cells (Table 46–2).
- The World Health Organization defines AML as having ≥ 20 percent blasts in the marrow. This breakpoint is not based on rational biologic considerations. APL, acute monocytic leukemia, acute myelomonocytic leukemia, and AML with evidence of maturation may not and often do not have ≥ 20 percent blast in the marrow (see also Chap. 42). Moreover, patients with 10 to 20 percent blasts in the marrow may behave as AML or progress rapidly to such behavior and require treatment for AML. The physician should eschew medicine by algorithm. Some of these approaches may be required for multi-institutional clinical trials but should not be transposed to the care of individual patients.
- Overt cytogenetic abnormalities (aneuploidy or pseudodiploidy) are present in about three-quarters of patients. t(8;21), t(15;17), inv 16, and translocations involving 11q are the most common, but several hundred unique cytogenetic abnormalities have been described in the cells of AML patients. The most prevalent abnormalities are shown in Table 46–3.
- Serum uric acid and lactic acid dehydrogenase levels are frequently elevated.
- Electrolyte abnormalities are infrequent, but severe hypokalemia may occur, and spurious hyperkalemia may be found in patients with very high leukocyte counts.
- Patients with very high leukocyte counts may also have spurious hypoglycemia and hypoxia as a result of consumption by the blast cells after the specimen is obtained.
- Hypercalcemia and hypophosphatemia may be present.

TABLE 46–3	CLINICAL CORRELATES OF FREQUENT CYTOGENETIC ABNORMALITIES OBSERVED IN AML	
Chromosome Abnormality	Genes Affected	Clinical Correlation
Loss or Gain of Chromosome		
Deletions of part or all of chromosome 5 or 7	Not defined with certainty	Frequent in patients with AML occurring *de novo* and in patients with history of chemical, drug, or radiation exposure and/or previous hematologic disease.
Trisomy 8	Not defined	Very common abnormality in acute myeloblastic leukemia. Poor prognosis, often a secondary change.
Translocation		
t(8;21) (q22;q22)	*RUNX1 (AML1)– RUNX1T1 (ETO)*	Present in ~8% of patients <50 years old and in 3% of patients >50 years old with AML. Approximately 75% of cases have additional cytogenetic abnormalities, including loss of Y in males or X in females. Secondary cooperative mutations of *KRAS, NRAS, KIT* common. Present in ~40% of myelomonocytic phenotype. Higher frequency of myeloid sarcomas.

Chromosome Abnormality	Genes Affected	Clinical Correlation
t(15;17) (q31; q22)	*PML-RAR-α*	Represents ~6% of cases of AML. Translocation involving chromosome 17, t(15;17), t(11;17), or t(5;17) is present in most cases of promyelocytic leukemia.
t(9;11); (p22; q23)	*MLL (especially MLLT3)*	Present in ~7% of cases of AML. Associated with monocytic leukemia. 11q23 translocations in 60% of infants with AML and carries poor prognosis. Rearranges *MLL* gene. Many translocation partners for 11q23 translocation. *MLL1,MLL4,MLL10* may also result in AML phenotype.
t(9;22) (q34; q22)	*BCR–ABL*	Present in ~2% of patients with AML.
t(1;22)(p13;q13)	*RBMIS-MKL1*	<1% of cases of AML. Admixture of myeloblasts, megakaryoblasts, micromegakaryocytes with cytoplasmic blebbing, dysmorphic megakaryocytes. Reticulin fibrosis common.
Inversion		
Inv (16) (p13.1;q22) or t(16;16) (p13.1;q22)	*CBF-βMYH11*	Present in ~8% of patients <50 years of age and in ~3% of patients >50 years of age with AML; often acute myelomonocytic phenotype; associated with increased marrow eosinophils; predisposition to cervical lymphadenopathy, better response to therapy. Predisposed to myeloid sarcoma.
Inv(3)(q21q26.2)	*RPN1-EVI1*	~1% of cases of AML. Approximately 85% of cases with normal or increased platelet count. Marrow has increased dysmorphic, hypolobulated megakaryocytes. Hepatosplenomegaly more frequent than usual in AML.

Source: *Williams Hematology*, 8th ed. Chap. 89, Table 89–3, p. 1284.

MARROW NECROSIS

- One-quarter of cases occur as a complication of AML.
- Bone pain (80% of cases) and fever (70% of cases) the two most frequent signs.
- Marrow aspirate is watery and serosanguineous. Marrow cells are indistinct and lose staining characteristics with pyknotic cells exhibiting karyorrhexis.
- Prognosis most closely related to underlying disease.

HYPERLEUKOCYTOSIS

- Signs and symptoms due to extreme elevations of the leukocyte count, usually to greater than 100×10^9/L, appear in about 5 percent of patients.
- Leukostasis is most likely to occur (a) in the circulation of the central nervous system, leading to intracerebral hemorrhage; (b) in the lungs, resulting in pulmonary insufficiency; or (c) in the penis, causing priapism (see Chap. 41).

ATYPICAL PRESENTATIONS OF AML

• *Hypoplastic leukemia.* AML may present with pancytopenia and a hypoplastic marrow. Careful microscopic and cell flow analysis examinations usually identify leukemic blast cells in marrow.
• *Oligoblastic myelogenous leukemia.* The disease may present with anemia and thrombocytopenia and a lower proportion of blast cells in the blood and marrow. This presentation is often referred to as myelodysplasia (specifically, refractory anemia with excess blasts) and is discussed in Chap. 42. Although median survival without remission-induction therapy is measured at about 20 months, it may be morbidly symptomatic, be progressive soon after diagnosis, and in the appropriate patient require AML-type therapy, especially in cases in which the marrow blast percentage is 10 to 20 percent at the time of diagnosis.
• *Mediastinal germ-cell tumors* and *AML* may coexist, and there is evidence for a clonal identity of the neoplastic cells of the two tumors.

AML IN NEONATES

• *Transient abnormal myeloproliferation,* i.e., markedly elevated leukocyte count with blast cells in the blood and marrow, present at birth or appearing shortly thereafter and resolving slowly over weeks or months without treatment.
• Similar cases with a cytogenetic abnormality may resolve and then later reappear as acute leukemia. Such disorders have been referred to as *transient leukemia.* These events occur in approximately 10 percent of newborns with Down syndrome.
• Apparently phenotypically normal newborns may have *congenital leukemia* or develop *neonatal leukemia.* However, these syndromes are 10 times more common in infants with Down syndrome. The leukemia in Down syndrome is usually acute megakaryocytic leukemia and is very responsive to chemotherapy.

AML IN OLDER PATIENTS

• Higher frequency of unfavorable prognostic cytogenetic changes.
• Higher frequency of drug-resistant phenotypes.
• Higher frequency of comorbid conditions.
• Lower tolerance to intensive chemotherapy.
• Lower rate of remission and shorter survival with current therapeutic approaches.

HYBRID (BIPHENOTYPIC) LEUKEMIAS

• Leukemias in which individual cells may have both myeloid and lymphoid markers (chimeric), or in which individual cells may have either myeloid or lymphoid markers but appear to arise from the same clone (mosaic). In some cases, individual cells may have markers for two or more myeloid lineages, such as granulocytic and megakaryocytic.
• Myeloid-Natural Killer Cell and t(8;13) myeloid–lymphoid hybrids are two explicit syndromes representing this phenomenon.
• *Mixed leukemias* are rare entities in which myeloid and lymphoid cells are present simultaneously, each derived from a separate clone (e.g., chronic myelogenous leukemia and chronic lymphocytic leukemia occurring simultaneously).

MORPHOLOGIC VARIANTS OF AML

• Table 46–4 presents the features of the morphologic variants of AML.
• The most common variants have phenotypic features of granulocytic, monocytic, erythroid, or megakaryocytic cells.

TABLE 46-4 MORPHOLOGIC VARIANTS OF AML

Variant	Cytologic Features	Special Clinical Features	Special Laboratory Features
Acute myeloblastic leukemia (M0,M1, M2)	1. Myeloblasts range from 20 to 90% of marrow cells. Cytoplasm occasionally contains Auer bodies. Nucleus shows fine reticular pattern and distinct nucleolus (1 or 2 usually). 2. Blast cells are sudanophilic. They are positive for myeloperoxidase and chloroacetate esterase, negative for nonspecific esterase, and negative or diffusely positive for PAS (no clumps or blocks). 3. Electron microscopy shows cytoplasmic primary granules.	1. Most common in adults, and most frequent variety in infants. 2. Three morphologic-cytochemical types (M0, M1, M2)	1. Chromosomes +8, −5, −7, del(11q) and complex abnormalities common. RUNX1(AML1) and FLT3 mutations occur in approximately 20 to 25% of cases. 2. M0 type blast cells positive with antibody to myeloperoxidase and anti-CD34 and CD13 or CD33 coexpression. AML1 mutations in ~25%. 3. M1 expresses CD13 and CD33. Positive for myeloperoxidase by cytochemistry. 4. M2 AML with maturation often associated with t(8;21) karyotype. 5. M2 AML with t(6;9)(p23q34), an uncommon variant, is associated with marrow basophilia, a high blast count, a high frequency of FLT3-ITD, and a poor outcome.
Acute promyelocytic leukemia (M3, M3v)	1. Leukemic cells resemble promyelocytes. They have large atypical primary granules and a kidney-shaped nucleus. Branched or adherent Auer rods are common. 2. Peroxidase stain intensely positive. 3. A variant has microgranules (M3v), otherwise has the same course and prognosis.	1. Usually in adults. 2. Hypofibrinogenemia and hemorrhage common. 3. Leukemic cells mature in response to all-trans-retinoic acid.	1. Cell contains t(15;17) or other translocation involving chromosome 17 (RAR-α gene). 2. Cells are HLA-DR negative.

(continued)

TABLE 46–4 (CONTINUED)

Variant	Cytologic Features	Special Clinical Features	Special Laboratory Features
Acute myelomonocytic leukemia (M4, M4Eo)	1. Both myeloblastic and monoblastic leukemic cells in blood and marrow. 2. Peroxidase–, Sudan–, chloroacetate esterase–, and nonspecific esterase–positive cells. 3. M4Eo variant has marrow eosinophilia.	1. Similar to myeloblastic leukemia but with more frequent extramedullary disease. 2. Mildly elevated serum and urine lysozyme.	1. Leukemic cells in eosinophilic variant (M4Eo) usually have inversion or translocation of chromosome 16.
Acute monocytic leukemia (M5)	1. Leukemia cells are large; nuclear cytoplasmic ratio lower than myeloblast. Cytoplasm contains fine granules. Auer rods are rare. Nucleus is convoluted and cell simulates promonocytes (M5a) or may contain large nucleoli: monoblasts (M5b) and may simulate monoblasts (M5b) and contain large nucleoli. 2. Nonspecific esterase–positive inhibited by NaF; Sudan–, peroxidase–, and chloroacetate esterase–negative. PAS occurs in granules, blocks.	1. Seen in children or young adults. 2. Gum, CNS, lymph node, and extramedullary infiltrations are common. 3. DIC occurs. 4. Plasma and urine lysozyme elevated. 5. Hyperleukocytosis common.	1. t(4;11) common in infants. 2. Rearrangement of q11;q23 very frequent.
Acute erythroid leukemia (M6)	1. Abnormal erythroblasts are in abundance initially in marrow and often in blood. Later the morphologic findings may be indistinguishable from those of AML.	1. Pancytopenia common at diagnosis.	1. Cells reactive with antihemoglobin antibody. Erythroblasts usually are strongly PAS and CD71-positive, express ABH blood group antigens. 2. Cells reactive with anti–Rc-84 (antihuman erythroleukemia cell-line antigen).
Acute megakaryocytic leukemia (M7)	1. Small blasts with pale agranular cytoplasm and cytoplasmic blebs. May mimic lymphoblasts of medium to larger size. 2. Leukemic cells with megakaryocytic morphology may coexist with megakaryoblasts.	1. Usually presents with pancytopenia. 2. Markedly elevated serum lactic acid dehydrogenase levels. 3. Marrow aspirates are usually "dry taps" because of the invariable presence of myelofibrosis. 4. Common phenotype in the AML of Down syndrome.	1. Antigens of von Willebrand factor, and glycoprotein Ib (CD42), IIb/IIIa (CD41), IIIa (CD61) on blast cells. 2. Platelet peroxidase positive.

Acute eosinophilic leukemia	1. Mixture of blasts and cells with dysmorphic eosinophilic granules (smaller and less refractile).	1. Hepatomegaly, splenomegaly, lymphadenopathy may be prominent. 2. Absence of neurologic, respiratory, or cardiac signs or symptoms characteristic of chronic eosinophilic leukemia (clonal hypereosinophilic syndrome).	1. Cyanide-resistant peroxidase stains eosinophilic granules. TEM shows eosinophilic granules to be smaller and missing central crystalloid. 2. Biopsy may show Charcot-Leyden crystals in skin, marrow, or other sites of eosinophil accumulation.
Acute basophilic leukemia	1. Mixture of blast cells and cells with basophilic granules in blood and marrow.	1. Often has hepatomegaly and or splenomegaly; symptoms often present. 2. Rash with urticaria, headaches, prominent gastrointestinal symptoms.	1. CD9 + CD25 + CD33 + CD123+ cells are usually present. 2. Toluidine blue-positive cells. 3. Hyperhistaminemia and hyperhistaminuria. 4. Cells negative for tryptase but positive for histidine decarboxylase.
Acute mast cell leukemia	1. Mast cells in blood and marrow. Most contain granules but some are agranular and may simulate monocytes.	1. Fever, headache, flushing of face and trunk, pruritus may be present. 2. Abdominal pain, peptic ulcer, bone pain, diarrhea more common than other AML subtypes. 3. Hepatomegaly, splenomegaly common. 4. Hemorrhagic diathesis may be evident.	1. CD13, CD33, CD68, CD117 often positive. 2. Cells positive for tryptase staining and serum tryptase elevated. 3. Hyperhistaminemia and hyperhistaminuria.

DIC, disseminated intravascular coagulation; NaF, sodium fluoride; PAS, periodic acid-Schiff; TEM, transmission electron microscopy.

NOTE: Parentheses indicate French-American-British (FAB) designation M0 through M7.

Source: *Williams Hematology*, 8th ed, Chap. 89, Table 89–4, p. 1288.

- Acute eosinophilic, basophilic, mastocytic, or histiocytic leukemias arising *de novo* are rare forms of AML.
- Images of morphologic variants and features of leukemic cells are shown in Fig. 46–1.

DIFFERENTIAL DIAGNOSIS

- Extensive proliferation of promyelocytes in the marrow may occur upon recovery from agranulocytosis induced by drugs or bacterial infection and transiently may mimic APL. This blood and marrow appearance resolves spontaneously in several days and has been called *pseudoleukemia*.
- In patients with hypoplastic marrows, it may be difficult to differentiate acute leukemia from aplastic anemia. Careful, and sometimes repeated, evaluation of blood and marrow cytology should permit the correct diagnosis.

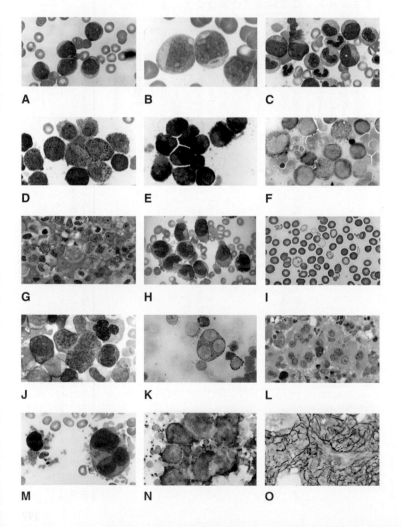

- Leukemoid reactions and nonleukemic pancytopenias do not have an increase in leukemic myeloblasts in the marrow or blood.

THERAPY, COURSE, AND PROGNOSIS

- Patient and the family should be informed about the nature of the disease, the treatment, and the potential side effects of the treatment.
- Treatment should be initiated as soon as possible after diagnosis, unless the patient is so frail or burdened by unrelated illness to make treatment inadvisable based on mutual understanding.
- Associated problems such as hemorrhage, infection, or anemia should be treated concurrently.
- Pretreatment laboratory studies should establish the specific diagnosis using immunologic, genetic, and molecular techniques, and assess the general condition of the patient, including blood chemistry tests, radiographic examinations, and cardiac studies, as indicated. Hemostasis should also be evaluated, in detail if screening tests show any abnormalities, if severe thrombocytopenia is present, or if the patient has APL or monocytic leukemia.
- An indwelling central venous catheter should be inserted prior to beginning treatment.
- Treatment with allopurinol, usually 300 mg daily orally, should be given if the serum uric acid level is greater than 7 mg/dL, if the marrow is hypercellular with increased blast cells, or if the blood blast cell count is moderately or markedly elevated. Intravenous uricase, a rapidly acting preparation, is also available for more urgent situations. Therapy may be discontinued after control of the uric acid level and cytoreduction.

FIGURE 46–1 Blood and marrow images of major subtypes of acute myelogenous leukemia (AML). **A.** Blood film of AML without maturation (acute myeloblastic leukemia). Five myeloblasts are evident. High nuclear-to-cytoplasmic ratio. Agranular cells. Nucleoli in each cell. **B.** Blood film. AML without maturation (acute myeloblastic leukemia). Three myeloblasts, one containing an Auer rod. **C.** Marrow film. AML with maturation. Three leukemic myeloblasts admixed with myelocytes, bands, and segmented neutrophils. **D.** Blood film. Acute promyelocytic leukemia. Majority of cells are heavily granulated leukemic promyelocytes. **E.** Blood film. Acute promyelocytic leukemia. Myeloperoxidase stain. Intensely positive. Numerous stained (black) granules in cytoplasm of leukemic progranulocytes. **F.** Blood film. Acute myelomonocytic leukemia. Double esterase stain. Leukemic monocytic cells stained dark blue and leukemic neutrophil precursors stained reddish-brown. **G.** Marrow film. AML with inv16. Note high proportion of eosinophils in field. Note myeloblasts with very large nucleoli at upper right. Also, intermediate leukemic granulocytic forms. **H.** Blood film. Acute monocytic leukemia. Leukemic cells have characteristics of monocytes with agranular gray cytoplasm and reniform or folded nuclei with characteristic chromatin staining. This case had hyperleukocytosis as evident by leukemic monocyte frequency in blood film. **I.** Blood film. Acute erythroid leukemia. Note population of extremely hypochromic cells with scattered bizarre-shaped poikilocytes admixed with normal-appearing red cells. **J.** Marrow film. Acute erythroid leukemia. Giant erythroblasts with multilobulated nuclei. **K.** Marrow film. Acute erythroid leukemia. Note giant trinucleate erythroblast and other leukemic erythroblasts with periodic acid-Schiff–positive cytoplasmic staining (reddish granules). **L.** Marrow section. Acute megakaryoblastic leukemia. Marrow replaced with atypical two- and three-lobed leukemic megakaryocytes with bold nucleoli. **M.** Marrow film. Acute megakaryoblastic leukemia. Marrow replaced with atypical megakaryocytes and megakaryoblasts with cytoplasmic disorganization, fragmentation, and budding. **N.** Marrow film. Acute megakaryoblastic leukemia. Marrow replaced with atypical megakaryocytes and megakaryoblasts staining for platelet glycoprotein IIIA (reddish-brown). Platelets in background also stained. **O.** Marrow section. Acute megakaryoblastic leukemia. Argentophilic (silver) stain shows marked increase in collagen, type III fibrils (marrow reticulin fibrosis), characteristic of this AML subtype. (*Reproduced with permission from Lichtman's Atlas of Hematology, www.accessmedicine.com.*)
(Source: *Williams Hematology*, 8th ed, Chap. 89, Fig. 89–1, p. 1283.)

• Exposure to pathogenic infectious agents should be minimized by hand washing by attendants, meticulous care of the intravenous catheter, assignment to an unshared room. Raw seafood and exposure to plants should be avoided.

Remission Induction Therapy
AML Variants Other than APL

• Cytotoxic chemotherapy is based on the concept that the marrow contains two competing populations of stem cells (leukemic monoclonal and normal polyclonal) and that profound suppression of the leukemic cells, such that they can no longer be detected morphologically in marrow aspirates or biopsies, is necessary in order to permit recovery of normal hematopoiesis (Fig. 46–2).

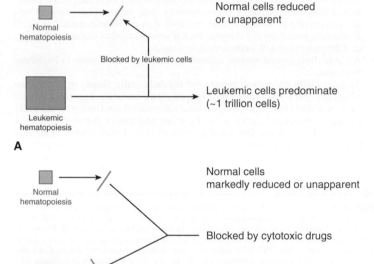

Normal hematopoiesis

Blocked by leukemic cells

Normal cells reduced or unapparent

Leukemic hematopoiesis

Leukemic cells predominate (~1 trillion cells)

A

Normal hematopoiesis

Blocked by cytotoxic drugs

Normal cells markedly reduced or unapparent

Leukemic hematopoiesis

Leukemic cells unapparent (<1 billion cells)

Iatrogenic aplastic pancytopenia provides opportunity for reemergence of normal hematopoiesis

B

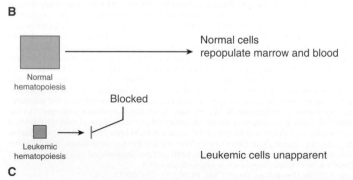

Normal hematopoiesis

Blocked

Normal cells repopulate marrow and blood

Leukemic hematopoiesis

Leukemic cells unapparent

C

- Therapy is usually initiated with two drugs, including an anthracycline antibiotic or anthraquinone and cytosine arabinoside (Table 46–5).
- Remission is inversely correlated with a patient's age and blood blast count. Those who have AML induced by prior chemotherapy or radiotherapy, and those who evolved to AML from an antecedent predisposing clonal myeloid disease, have lower remission rates than patients with *de novo* AML.
- Patients with leukocyte counts of $100 \times 10^9/L$ or more should be treated to achieve more rapid cytoreduction using hydroxyurea 1.5 to 2.0 g, orally, every 6 hours for about 36 hours with downward titration of dose as blast count diminishes. Leukapheresis (coupled with hydroxyurea) can further accelerate reduction of the white cell count (see Chap. 94). Hydration sufficient to maintain urine flow of at least 100 mL/h is necessary during the first several days of cytotoxic therapy.
- Severe neutropenia and other factors resulting from cytotoxic therapy frequently result in infection and require cultures and rapid institution of broad-spectrum antibiotic therapy until cultures results are known. If an organism is identified, antibiotic therapy can be tailored to its sensitivity spectrum.
- Red cell and platelet transfusions are often required. Patients should receive leukoreduced blood products to avoid allergic reactions and allosensitization and those who are candidates for allogeneic hematopoietic stem cell transplantation should receive irradiated blood products.
- Patients with evidence of intravascular coagulation or excessive fibrinolysis should be treated for those conditions (see Chaps. 86 and 87). If findings are equivocal, monitor patients with fibrinogen, D-dimer, and coagulation assays. These complications are of highest prevalence in patients with APL and acute monocytic leukemia but may occur uncommonly with other subtypes.

Treatment for APL

- About 80 percent of patients with APL develop complete remissions when treated with all-*trans*-retinoic acid (ATRA) (45 mg/m^2 per day orally, divided into two doses) and an anthracycline antibiotic (sometimes coupled with cytosine arabinoside) administered concurrently.
- The use of ATRA has markedly decreased the frequency of the hemorrhagic complications of APL. However, the lethal complication of intracerebral hemorrhage still occurs in about 5 to 10 percent of patients, despite effective therapy. ATRA should be started urgently on the suspicion that the acute leukemia is APL.
- Arsenic trioxide is being studied to determine its role in the initial therapy of APL. Arsenic trioxide coupled with ATRA is an effective regimen.

FIGURE 46–2 Remission–relapse pattern of acute myelogenous leukemia. **A.** Acute myelogenous leukemia at diagnosis or in relapse. Monoclonal leukemic hematopoiesis predominates. Normal polyclonal stem cell function is suppressed. **B.** Following effective cytotoxic treatment leukemic cells are unapparent in marrow and blood. Severe pancytopenia exists as a result of cytotoxic therapy. The reduction in leukemic cells can release inhibition of normal polyclonal stem cell function. **C.** If reconstitution of normal hematopoiesis ensues, a remission is established and blood cells return to near normal as a result of the recovery of polyclonal hematopoiesis. This relapse–remission pattern has not been seen in the subacute and chronic myeloid leukemias because it has not been possible to minimize the leukemic cell population with cytotoxic therapy to a point at which polyclonal hematopoiesis is restored. The only exception is the effect of BCR-ABL inhibitor therapy in which suppression of BCR-ABL–positive cells in chronic myelogenous leukemia can be achieved with return of polyclonal hematopoiesis. Uncommon examples of tyrosine kinase inhibitor responses in myeloid neoplasms with *PDGFR* or certain *KIT* mutations may also show this pattern. In a proportion of cases, BCR-ABL transcripts (minimal residual disease) can be detectable along with normal, polyclonal hematopoiesis. (Reproduced with permission from Lichtman MA. Stem Cells 18(5):304, 2000. Alpha Med Press.)

(Source: *Williams Hematology*, 8th ed, Chap. 85, Fig. 85–4, p. 1218.)

TABLE 46–5 REMISSION INDUCTION FOR AML: EXAMPLES OF CYTOSINE ARABINOSIDE AND ANTHRACYCLINE ANTIBIOTIC COMBINATIONS

Cytarabine	Anthracycline Antibiotic ± Another Agent	No. of Patients	Age Range in Years (Median)	Complete Remissions (%)	Year of Report
100 mg/m², days 1–7	DNR 45 mg/m², days 1–3	330	17–60 (47)	57	2009
100 mg/m², days 1–7	DNR 90 mg/m² days 1–3	327	18–60 (48)	71	2009
200 mg/m², days 1–7	DNR 60 mg/m², days 1–3	200	16–60 (45)	72	2004
200 mg/m², days 1–7	DNR 60 mg/m², days 1–3 Cladribine 5 mg/m², days 1–5	200	16–60 (45)	69	2004
200 mg/m² twice per day for 10 days (some in this report received FLAG-Ida vs. H-DAT)	DNR 50 mg/m², days 1, 3, 5 Thioguanine 100 mg/m² twice per day, days 10–20 Gemtuzumab ozogamicin 3 mg/m², day 1	64	18–59 (46.5)	91	2003
3 g/m² every 12 h for 8 doses	60 mg/m² DNR daily for 2 days	122	Adults	80	2000
100 mg/m² daily for 7 days (2 courses always given)	IDA 12 mg/m² daily for 3 days	153	NR	63	2000
500 mg/m² by continuous infusion, days 1–3, 8–10	Mitoxantrone 12 mg/m² for 3 days Etoposide 200 mg/m² IV, days 8–10	133	15–70 (43)	60	1996
100 mg/m² daily for 7 days	DNR 45 mg/m² for 3 days	113	NR (55)	59	1992
100 mg/m² daily for 7 days	IDA 13 mg/m² for 3 days	101	NR (56)	70	1992

DNR, daunorubicin; FLAG, fludarabine, cytarabine, and granulocyte colony-stimulating factor; H-DAT, hydroxydaunorubicin, cytarabine, and thioguanine; IDA, idarubicin; NR, not reported.

NOTE: The reader is advised to consult the original reports for details of induction and ancillary therapy and consolidation or continuation therapy, which may vary from protocol to protocol. The citations can be found in *Williams Hematology*, 8th ed, p. 1295.

Source: *Williams Hematology*, 8th ed, Chap. 89, Table 89–5, p. 1295.

Remission Maintenance Therapy

- Intensive postremission therapy results in longer duration of remission.
- There is no agreement on best current postremission therapy, in part because the age, cytogenic alteration, morphologic subtype, and other factors may dictate different options.
- Three principal modalities are available:
  — Intensive cytotoxic drug therapy (e.g., high-dose cytarabine).
  — Very intensive chemotherapy and autologous stem cell infusion.
  — Pretransplant conditioning regimen (e.g., chemoradiation) followed by allogeneic hematopoietic stem cell transplantation in patients deemed suitable for this approach based on availability of a suitable donor, age, comorbidities, probability of a salutary outcome, the patient's agreement, and other factors evaluated by the responsible transplant physician.

Relapsed or Refractory Patients

- Chemoradiation followed by allogeneic stem cell transplantation in patients with AML in second remission can induce long-term survival in about 25 percent so treated. Treatment with chemotherapy alone in this group is unlikely to result in long-term remission.
- Patients who relapse more than 12 months after initial chemotherapy can be given the same treatment again.
- Another therapy for relapsed patients is high-dose cytosine arabinoside with or without additional drug(s), such as mitoxantrone, amsacrine, or etoposide. Several options are shown in Table 46–6.
- Patients with APL who relapse may respond to arsenic trioxide treatment and chemotherapy.
- Chemoradiation followed by allogeneic hematopoietic stem cell transplantation may be used in refractory patients. Approximately 10 percent of such AML patients may be cured, and approximately 25 percent may achieve remissions of at least 3 years with marrow transplantation.

Special Therapeutic Consideration

- It may be necessary to reduce the dose of cytotoxic drugs administered to patients older than 60 years of age if concurrent illnesses (e.g., heart disease, diabetes) or other factors so dictate.
- Treatment of pregnant patients in the first trimester with antimetabolites increases the risk of congenital anomalies in the infant. However, babies born after intensive chemotherapy administered in the late second and third trimesters may develop normally.
- Intensive multidrug chemotherapy has been used successfully in patients younger than 17 years of age in whom long-term remission rates are in the 40 to 50 percent range. Infants younger than 1 year of age with neonatal AML do not respond well to chemotherapy and should be considered for allogeneic hematopoietic stem cell transplantation.

Special Nonhematopoietic Adverse Effects of Treatment

- Skin rashes develop in over 50 percent of the patients with AML during chemotherapy, often caused by one of the following drugs: allopurinol, β-lactam antibiotics, cytosine arabinoside, trimethoprim-sulfamethoxazole, miconazole, and ketoconazole.
- Cardiomyopathy may develop in patients receiving anthracycline antibiotics and other agents. The adverse effect on the heart may be quite delayed developing decades after therapy.
- Systemic candidiasis syndrome presents with fever, abdominal pain, and hepatomegaly and is associated with multiple hepatic candidiasis lesions detected radiographically or by ultrasound. May respond to prolonged therapy with antifungal agents, such as azoles or echinocandins.

| TABLE 46–6 | EXAMPLES OF CHEMOTHERAPY USED FOR RELAPSED OR REFRACTORY PATIENTS |

Regimen	No. of Patients	% of Patients Entering a Complete Remission (Median Duration)	Year
Gemtuzumab ozogamicin 6 mg/m^2 IV, days 1 and 13 Idarubicin 12 mg/m^2, days 2–4 Cytarabine 1.5 g/m^2, days 2–5	15	21 (27 weeks)	2003
Mitoxantrone 12 mg/m^2, days 1–3 Cytarabine 500 mg/m^2, days 1–3 Followed (at count recovery) by Etoposide 200 mg/m^2, days 1–3 Cytarabine 500 mg/m^2, days 1–3	66	36 (5 months)	2003
Cladribine 5 mg/m^2, days 1–5 Cytarabine 2 g/m^2, days 1–5 2 h after 2-CdA G-CSF 10 μg/kg/day, days 1–5	58	50 (29% disease-free at 1 year)	2003
Fludarabine 30 mg/m^2, days 1–5 Cytarabine 2 g/m^2, days 1–5 Idarubicin 10 mg/m^2 days 1–3 G-CSF 5 μg/kg per day, day +6 until neutrophil recovery	46	52 (13 months)	2003
Gemtuzumab ozogamicin 9 mg/m^2, days 1 and 15	43	9	2002
Mitoxantrone 4 mg/m^2, days 1–3 Etoposide 40 mg/m^2, days 1–3 Cytarabine 1 g/m^2, days 1–3, ± PSC-833	37	32	1999
Fludarabine 30 mg/m^2, days 1–5 Cytarabine 2 g/m^2, days 1–5± Idarubicin 12 mg/m^2, days 1–3 G-CSF 400 μg/m^2 daily until complete remission	85	66	1995

DNR, daunorubicin; FLAG, fludarabine, cytarabine, and granulocyte colony-stimulating factor; H-DAT, hydroxydauorubicin, cytarabine, and thioguanine; IDA, idarubicin; NR, not reported. NOTE: The reader is advised to consult the original reference for details of chemotherapy regimen administration. The citations may be found in *Williams Hematology*, 8th ed, p. 1301. Source: *Williams Hematology*, 8th ed, Chap. 89, Table 89–6, p. 1301.

- Patients receiving intensive cytotoxic therapy may develop necrotizing inflammation of the cecum (typhlitis), which can simulate appendicitis, and may require surgical intervention.
- Fertility may be sustained or be recovered in men and women undergoing intensive cytotoxic therapy, but infertility can occur especially after intensive regimens used for hematopoietic stem cell transplantation.

Results of Treatment

- By using current therapeutic approaches, remission rates approach 90 percent in children, 70 percent in young adults, 60 percent in the middle aged, and 25 percent in older patients.

TABLE 46–7	ACUTE MYELOGENOUS LEUKEMIA: FIVE-YEAR RELATIVE SURVIVAL RATES (1996–2006)
Age (Years)	Acute Myelogenous Leukemia*
<45	52.1
45–54	33.0
55–64	19.7
65.74	8.7
>75	1.9
<65	37.9
>65	5.1

*Rates expressed as number of cases per 100.
Source: SEER Cancer Statistics, TABLE XIII-13.16, National Cancer Institute, Washington, DC. Available at http://seer.cancer.gov/csr/1975_2007/browse_csr.php? section=13&page =sect_13_table.16.html

- Median survival of all patients in the full age-range is about 18 months because of the high proportion of patients over 65 years of age. The influence of age on survival of patients with AML is shown in Table 46–7.
- Relapse or development of a new leukemia has occurred rarely after 8 years in adults and 16 years in children.

Features Influencing the Outcome of Therapy

- Both the probability of remission and the duration of response decrease with increasing age at the time of diagnosis.
- Cytogenetic abnormalities such as inv(16), t(16;16), del(16q), t(8;21), or t(15;17) indicate a better prognosis, while –5, del(5q), –7, del(7q), t(9;22), and others indicate a poorer prognosis. A normal karyotype, +6, +8, and others are intermediate in outlook.
- Table 46–8 indicates frequency of better prognosis chromosome abnormalities with age at diagnosis. These are relative prognostic projections, and a better prognosis may not be an excellent prognosis. They may also influence the decision as whether to use allogeneic hematopoietic stem cell transplantation in first remission.
- AML that develops after prior cytotoxic therapy for another disease or after a clonal cytopenia or oligoblastic leukemia (myelodysplastic syndromes) has a significantly lower remission rate and shorter remission duration on average than *de novo* AML.

TABLE 46–8	FREQUENCY OF CYTOGENETIC FINDINGS WITH A MORE FAVORABLE PROGNOSIS BY AGE GROUP				
Age (Years)	No. of Cases Studied	t(8;21) (No. of Cases)	t(15;17) (No. of Cases)	Inv16/t (16;16) (No. of Cases)	Total (No. of Cases)	Favorable Karyotypes (% of All Cases)
10–39	307	27	38	33	98	32
40–59	584	36	28	28	92	16
60–69	579	18	25	21	63	11
70–79	381	5	7	5	17	4.5
≥80	45	1	2	0	3	6.6
Total	1896	87	100	87	273	22

Source: *Williams Hematology*, 8th ed, Chap. 89, Table 89–7, p. 1308.

- A leukocyte count greater than $30 \times 10^9/L$ or a blast cell count greater than $15 \times 10^9/L$ decreases the probability and the duration of remission.
- Many other laboratory findings are correlated with decreased remission rate or duration (see *Williams Hematology*, 8th ed, Table 89–9, p. 1310).

For a more detailed discussion, see Jane L. Liesveld and Marshall A. Lichtman: Acute Myelogenous Leukemia. Chap. 89, p. 1277 in *Williams Hematology*, 8th ed.

CHAPTER 47
The Chronic Myelogenous Leukemias

- *BCR-ABL*-positive chronic myelogenous leukemia (CML) results from a somatic mutation in a pluripotential lymphohematopoietic cell.
- CML is characterized by granulocytic leukocytosis, granulocytic immaturity, basophilia, anemia, and often thrombocytosis in the blood, intense leukemic granulocytic precursor expansion in the marrow, and splenomegaly.
- The natural history of the disease is to evolve into an accelerated phase in which cytopenias develop and response to chronic phase therapy is lost; it often terminates in acute leukemia.

ETIOLOGY

- Exposure to high-dose ionizing radiation increases the incidence of CML, with a mode of increased incidence that ranges from 4 to 11 years in different exposed populations.

PATHOGENESIS

Genetic Abnormality

- CML is the result of an acquired genetic abnormality that induces a malignant transformation of a single pluripotential lymphohematopoietic cell.
- The proximate cause is a translocation between chromosome 9 and 22 [t(9;22)]. This alteration juxtaposes a portion of the *ABL* protooncogene from chromosome 9 to a portion of the *BCR* gene on chromosome 22.
- The resulting gene fusion, *BCR-ABL,* creates an oncogene that encodes an elongated protein tyrosine phosphokinase (usually p210) that is constitutively expressed. This mutant protein disrupts cell signal pathways and results in the malignant transformation.
- The genetic alteration is present in erythroid, neutrophilic, eosinophilic, basophilic, monocytic, megakaryocytic, and marrow B- and T-lymphocytic cells, consistent with its origin in a pluripotential cell.
- The Philadelphia (Ph) chromosome specifically refers to chromosome 22 with a shortened long arm and is evident by light microscopy of cell metaphase preparations in approximately 90 percent of cases. Fluorescence *in situ* hybridization (FISH) can identify the fusion *BCR-ABL* gene in approximately 95 percent of cases.

Hematopoietic Abnormalities

- There is a marked expansion of granulocytic progenitors and a decreased sensitivity of the progenitors to regulation resulting in an inexorable increase in white cell count.
- Megakaryocytopoiesis is often expanded. Erythropoiesis is usually moderately deficient.
- Function of the neutrophils and platelets is nearly normal; infection and bleeding are not a feature of the chronic phase.

EPIDEMIOLOGY

- CML accounts for approximately 15 percent of all cases of leukemia and approximately 3 percent of childhood leukemias.
- Males are affected at approximately 1.5 times the rate of females.

- The age-specific incidence rate increases exponentially from late teen age (0.2 cases/100,000) to octogenarians (10 cases/100,000).
- Familial occurrence is vanishingly rare, and there is no concordance in identical twins.
- Neither chemical agents, including benzene, cytotoxic drugs, nor combusted tobacco smoke have a causal relationship with CML.

CLINICAL FEATURES

- Approximately 30 percent of patients are asymptomatic at the time of diagnosis. The disease is discovered coincidentally when an elevated white count is noted at a medical evaluation.
- Symptoms are gradual in onset and may include easy fatigability, malaise, anorexia, abdominal discomfort and early satiety, weight loss, and excessive sweating.
- Less frequent symptoms are those of hypermetabolism, such as night sweats, heat intolerance, and weight loss, mimicking hyperthyroidism; gouty arthritis; priapism, tinnitus, or stupor from leukostasis as a consequence of hyperleukocytosis; left upper-quadrant and left shoulder pain because of splenic infarction; diabetes insipidus; and urticaria as a result of histamine release.
- Physical signs may include pallor, splenomegaly, and sternal tenderness.

LABORATORY FEATURES

Blood Findings

- The hemoglobin concentration is decreased in most patients at the time of diagnosis. Occasional nucleated red cells can be seen on the stained blood film. Rare patients may have a normal or slightly increased hematocrit at the time of presentation.
- The leukocyte count is elevated, usually above 25×10^9/L, and often above 100×10^9/L (see **Fig. 47–1**). Granulocytes at all stages of development are present in the blood, but segmented and band neutrophils predominate (see **Table 47–1** and **Fig. 47–2**). Hypersegmented neutrophils are often present.

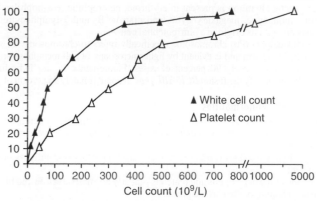

FIGURE 47-1 Total white cell count and platelet count of 90 patients with CML at the time of diagnosis. The cumulative percent of patients is on the *ordinate*, and the cell count is on the *abscissa*. Fifty percent of patients had a white cell count greater than 100×10^9/L and a platelet count greater than approximately 300×10^9/L at the time of diagnosis. Hematology Unit, University of Rochester Medical Center.

(Source: *Williams Hematology*, 8th ed, Chap. 90, Fig. 90–6, p. 1339.)

TABLE 47-1	WHITE BLOOD CELL DIFFERENTIAL COUNT AT THE TIME OF DIAGNOSIS IN 90 CASES OF Ph-CHROMOSOME–POSITIVE CHRONIC MYELOGENOUS LEUKEMIA

Cell Type	Percent of Total Leukocytes (Mean Values)
Myeloblasts	3
Promyelocytes	4
Myelocytes	12
Metamyelocytes	7
Band forms	14
Segmented forms	38
Basophils	3
Eosinophils	2
Nucleated red cells	0.5
Monocytes	8
Lymphocytes	8

NOTE: In these 90 patients, the mean hematocrit was 31 mL/dL, mean total white cell count was 160×10^9/L, and mean platelet count was 442×10^9/L at the time of diagnosis. Hematology Unit, University of Rochester Medical Center.
Source: *Williams Hematology*, 8th ed, Chap. 90, Table 90–1, p. 1340.)

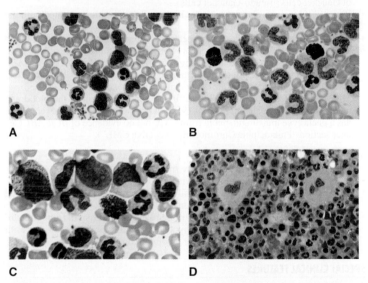

FIGURE 47-2 Blood and marrow cells characteristic of chronic myelogenous leukemia. **A.** Blood film. Elevated leukocyte count. Elevated platelet count (aggregates). Characteristic array of immature (myelocytes, metamyelocytes, band forms) and mature neutrophils. **B.** Blood film. Elevated leukocyte count. Characteristic array of immature (myelocytes, metamyelocytes, band forms) and mature neutrophils. Two basophils in the field. Absolute basophilia is a constant finding in CML. **C.** Blood film. Elevated leukocyte count. Characteristic array of immature (promyelocytes, myelocytes, metamyelocytes, band forms) and mature neutrophils. Basophil in the field. Two myeloblasts in upper center. Note multiple nucleoli (abnormal) and agranular cytoplasm. **D.** Marrow section. Hypercellular. Replacement of fatty tissue (normally approximately 60% of marrow volume in adults of this patient's age) with hematopoietic cells. Intense granulopoiesis and evident megakaryocytopoiesis. Decreased erythropoiesis.
(Reproduced from Lichtman's Atlas of Hematology, *www.accessmedicine.com, with permission.)*
(Source: *Williams Hematology*, 8th ed, Chap. 90, Fig. 90–7, p. 1339.)

- An increase in the absolute basophil count is found in virtually all patients. Basophils usually comprise less than 10 percent of leukocytes in the chronic phase, but occasionally make up a higher proportion. The absolute eosinophil count may also be increased.
- The platelet count is normal or increased at diagnosis but may increase during the course of the chronic phase, sometimes reaching $1000 \times 10^9/L$ and uncommonly as high as $5000 \times 10^9/L$ (see Fig. 47–1).
- Neutrophil alkaline phosphatase activity is low or absent in over 90 percent of patients. It may also be low in paroxysmal nocturnal hemoglobinuria, hypophosphatasia, with androgen therapy, and in about 25 percent of patients with primary myelofibrosis. It has been largely replaced as a diagnostic marker by cytogenetic and molecular analysis (see below).
- Whole blood histamine is markedly increased (mean = 5000 ng/mL) compared with normal levels (mean = 500 ng/mL) and is correlated with the absolute basophil count. Occasional cases of pruritus, urticaria, and gastric hyperacidity occur.

Marrow Findings and Cytogenetics

- The marrow is markedly hypercellular, primarily because of granulocytic hyperplasia. Megakaryocytes may be increased in number. Occasionally, sea-blue histiocytes and macrophages engorged with glucocerebroside from exaggerated cell turnover may be present. The latter cells mimic the appearance of Gaucher cells (pseudo-Gaucher cells).
- Reticulin fibrosis rarely is prominent in the marrow and is correlated with the expansion of megakaryocytes.
- The Ph chromosome is present in metaphase preparations of marrow cells in approximately 90 percent of patients. Some of the remaining patients have variant or cryptic translocations (see Fig. 47–3). FISH identification of *BCR-ABL* fusion and reverse transcriptase polymerase chain reaction (RT-PCR) to detect *BCR-ABL* mRNA transcripts are the two most sensitive diagnostic tests used.
- Molecular evidence of the *BCR-ABL* fusion gene is present in the blood and marrow cells of virtually all patients (95%) with apparent CML. The remainder has a phenotype indistinguishable from CML but no evidence of *BCR-ABL* (see later section "Philadelphia Chromosome-Negative CML").

Serum Findings

- Hyperuricemia and hyperuricosuria are frequent.
- Serum lactic acid dehydrogenase activity is elevated.
- Serum vitamin B_{12}-binding protein and serum vitamin B_{12} levels are increased in proportion to the total leukocyte count.
- Pseudohyperkalemia may be a result of the release of potassium from granulocytes in clotted blood, and spurious hypoxemia and hypoglycemia may result from cellular utilization in blood under laboratory analysis.

SPECIAL CLINICAL FEATURES

Hyperleukocytosis

- Approximately 15 percent of patients present with leukocyte counts of $300 \times 10^9/L$ (see Fig. 47–1) or higher and may have signs and symptoms of leukostasis from impaired microcirculation in the lungs, brain, eyes, ears, or penis.
- Patients may have tachypnea, dyspnea, cyanosis, dizziness, slurred speech, delirium, stupor, visual blurring, diplopia, retinal vein distention, retinal hemorrhages, papilledema, tinnitus, impaired hearing, or priapism.

Ph Chromosome-Positive or *BCR-ABL*-Positive Thrombocythemia

- Some patients (approximately 5%) present with the features of essential thrombocythemia (elevated platelet count and megakaryocytosis in marrow without

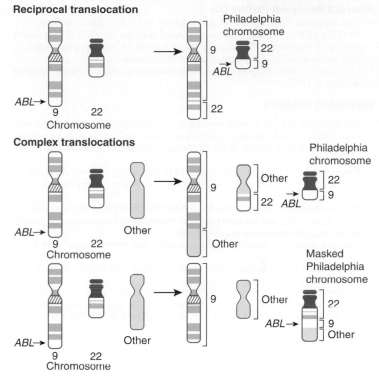

FIGURE 47-3 Translocations involved in chronic myelogenous leukemia. The positions of the *ABL* gene in each of the chromosomes before and after the translocation are noted. The origin of the chromosomal segments in each of the translocated chromosomes is indicated by a *bracket* on the side of the chromosome.
(Reproduced with permission from Rosson D, Reddy EP: *Mutat Res* May 195(3):231–243, 1988.)
(Source: *Williams Hematology,* 8th ed, Chap. 90, Fig. 90–8, p. 1341.)

significant change in hemoglobin or white cell count) but have the Ph chromosome and *BCR-ABL* fusion gene or no Ph chromosome but a *BCR* gene rearrangement.
* These patients later develop clinical CML or blast crisis. This presentation is considered a forme fruste of CML.

Neutrophilic CML
* This is a rare variant of *BCR-ABL*-positive CML in which the leukocytosis is composed of mature neutrophils.
* The white cell count is lower on average (30 to 50 × 10^9/L), blood basophilia and myeloid immaturity are absent, and splenic enlargement may not be evident.
* These patients have an unusual breakpoint in the *BCR* gene between exons 19 and 20, which leads to a larger BCR-ABL fusion oncoprotein (230kDa compared to the classic 210 kDa fusion protein).
* This variant tends to have an indolent course, perhaps because of the very low levels of p230 in the cells.

Minor-BCR Breakpoint-Positive CML

- This variant of CML has the BCR breakpoint at the first intron, resulting in a 190 kDa BCR-ABL fusion protein compared with the classic 210 kDa fusion protein. In this variant, the white cell count is lower on average, monocytosis is seen, and basophilia and splenomegaly are less prominent.
- This variant usually progresses to acute leukemia more rapidly on average than in classical CML.

DIFFERENTIAL DIAGNOSIS

- The diagnosis of CML is made on the basis of neutrophilic granulocytosis with some immature cells (promyelocytes, myelocytes), basophilia, and splenomegaly, coupled with detection of the Ph chromosome and/or the *BCR-ABL* fusion gene.
- Polycythemia vera is usually distinguished by the elevated hemoglobin concentration, white cell count less than 25×10^9/L, and absence of myeloid immaturity in the blood film.
- Primary myelofibrosis has distinctive red cell morphologic changes (poikilocytosis, anisocytosis, and teardrop red cells), invariable splenomegaly, and usually intense reticulin fibrosis on marrow biopsy.
- Essential thrombocythemia rarely has a white cell count greater than 25×10^9/L.
- In each of the other chronic clonal myeloid diseases, the absence of *BCR* rearrangement is a key distinction from CML.
- Extreme reactive leukocytosis (leukemoid reaction) may occur in patients with an inflammatory disease, cancer, or infection but is not associated with basophilia, significant granulocytic immaturity, or splenomegaly. The clinical setting usually distinguishes a leukemoid reaction. *BCR* gene rearrangement is absent.

TREATMENT

Hyperuricemia

- Most patients have massive expansion and turnover of blood cells with accompanying hyperuricemia or the risk of hyperuricemia with therapeutic cytoreduction.
- Patients can receive allopurinol, 300 mg/day orally, and adequate hydration before and during therapy to control exaggerated hyperuricemia and hyperuricosuria. It takes several days to lower the uric acid level. Discontinue the drug when uric acid is under control to minimize toxicity, especially skin rashes.
- Rasburicase, a recombinant urate oxidase, is effective in hours but is given intravenously and is more expensive. The manufacturer recommends 5 days of use but that is usually unnecessary to lower the uric acid sufficiently. If the uric acid is very high (e.g., > 9 mg/dL), a single dose of 0.2 mg/kg of ideal body weight can be used with allopurinol on successive days for about 36 hours.

Hyperleukocytosis

- If the white cell count is very high > 300×10^9/L and especially if signs of hyperleukocytosis are present, hydroxyurea, 1 to 6 mg/day depending on the height of the white cell count may be used initially. The dose is decreased as the count decreases and is usually at about 1 g/day when the leukocyte count reaches 20×10^9/L.
- If needed, maintenance doses should be adjusted to keep the total white count at about 5 to 10×10^9/L.
- Blood counts should be followed and the drug should be stopped if the white count falls to 5×10^9/L or less.
- The major side effect of hydroxyurea is suppression of hematopoiesis, often with megaloblastic erythropoiesis.

- Hyperleukocytosis usually responds rapidly to hydroxyurea but, if necessary, because of compelling signs of hyperleukocytosis (e.g., stupor, priapism), leukapheresis can be instituted simultaneously. Leukapheresis removes large numbers of cells minimizing the metabolic effects of tumor lysis (e.g., exaggerating hyperuricemia, hyperphosphatemia) while hydroxyurea is killing and retarding production of leukemic cells.

Thrombocytosis

- In the uncommon circumstance in which thrombocytosis is so prominent that early platelet reduction therapy is warranted, hydroxyurea or anagrelide can be used.

Tyrosine Kinase Inhibitor Therapy

- Recent studies indicate either nilotinib or dasatinib has a significant, approximately 15 percent, increase in cytogenetic and molecular response and a more rapid response on average when compared to imatinib mesylate. Either of these two drugs has become favored as initial therapy. If a patient has had an excellent molecular response on imatinib mesylate it is reasonable to continue that therapy. It is too early to be absolutely certain that the long-term results will mimic that of imatinib but the probability is sufficiently high to use these second generation agents as initial therapy because of their improved initial effects.
- Patients with newly diagnosed CML should be started on a tyrosine kinase inhibitor (TKI). Three choices are approved by the FDA at this time. Dasatinib, 100 mg/day orally, nilotinib, 300 mg every 12 hours, orally, or imatinib mesylate (imatinib) 400 mg/day, orally. In cases with hyperleukocytosis, white cell reduction should precede start of a TKI to lower the risk of tumor lysis syndrome (see above "Hyperleukocytosis")
- The efficacy of a TKI is measured by three indicators of response: hematologic, cytogenetic, and molecular (see Table 47–2).
- The criteria for assessing the response to a TKI are shown in Table 47–3.
- As long as a patient is having continued reduction in the size of the leukemic clone as judged by cytogenetic or molecular measurements, the TKI is continued at the same dose.

TABLE 47–2	CRITERIA FOR EXTENT OF A TKI TREATMENT RESPONSE
Hematologic response	White cell count $<10 \times 10^9$/L, platelet count $<450 \times 10^9$/L, no immature myeloid cells in the blood, and disappearance of all signs and symptoms related to leukemia (including palpable splenomegaly) lasting for at least 4 weeks.
Major cytogenetic response	Less than 35% of cells containing the Ph chromosome by cytogenetic analysis of marrow cells.
Complete cytogenetic response	No cells containing the Ph chromosome by cytogenetic analysis of marrow cells.
Major molecular response	Blood cell BCR-ABL/ABL ratio $<0.05\%$ (3-log reduction in PCR signal from mean pretreatment baseline value).
Complete molecular response	Blood cell BCR-ABL levels undetectable (usually by nested RT-PCR method).

TKI, tyrosine kinase inhibitor Source: *Williams Hematology*, 8th ed, Chap. 90, Table 90–2, p. 1344.

TABLE 47–3	GUIDELINES FOR RESPONSE TO A TKI		

| | Disease Response | | |
Time of Observation (months)	Unsatisfactory	Suboptimal Response	Optimal Response
3	No HR	PHR	CHR
6	No mCyR	mCyR	MCyR
12	No MCyR	MCyR	CCyR
18	No CCyR	CCyR	MMR

CHR, complete hematologic response; CCyR, complete cytogenetic response; HR, hematologic response; mCyR, minor cytogenetic response; MCyR, major cytogenetic response; MMR, major molecular response; PHR, partial hematologic response.
NOTE: Response is defined in Table 47–2. These data are applicable to therapy with imatinib, 400 mg/day, as initial therapy in chronic phase. Data for dasatinib or nilotinib are not yet available but are likely to be similar. Unsatisfactory or suboptimal implies need to consider change in treatment approach, as appropriate for that patient. Usually this change is an increase in the dose, a shift to an alternative TKI, or as a later option an allogeneic hematopoietic stem cell transplantation, if eligible. These guidelines are approximate in that a patient showing continued response to a TKI can be continued on that therapy until a response plateau has been reached, at which time the response can be evaluated using the benchmarks noted. TKI, tyrosine kinase inhibitor.
Source: *Williams Hematology*, 8th ed, Chap. 90, Table 90–3, p. 1346.

- If the patient stops responding before a complete cytogenetic or complete molecular remission occurs, the dose may be increased and/or an alternative second generation TKI should be considered (nilotinib or dasatinib).
- Imatinib is generally well tolerated. The main side effects are fatigue, edema, nausea, diarrhea, muscle cramps, and rashes. Severe periorbital edema is occasionally observed. Hepatotoxicity occurs in about 3 percent of patients. There are numerous other uncommon side effects. The principal side effects of dasatinib include cytopenias and fluid retention, notably pleural effusion. The side effects of nilotinib include rash, hyperglycemia, increased serum lipase and amylase (pancreatitis), transaminitis, and hypophospatemia.
- Neutropenia and thrombocytopenia may occur early in TKI use. Dose reduction for side effects is not recommended. If absolutely necessary, cessation may be required. Often, the mild cytopenias improve with continued therapy.
- Guidelines to judge the response to a TKI based on duration of treatment is shown in Table 47–3. Continued response can be quite prolonged, stretching over several years.
- TKIs may be teratogenic. Women in the child-bearing age group can (a) use contraception during therapy, (b) use interferon-α until delivery if pregnant when diagnosed and then be placed on a TKI, or (c) if in a complete **molecular** remission, could have TKI therapy stopped until she conceives and be restarted after delivery.
- Leukapheresis may be useful as sole treatment in patients in early pregnancy when it may be necessary to control the white cell count and splenic enlargement without chemotherapy.
- In the case of TKI intolerance or resistance, the alternative second generation TKI can be tried: dasatinib, 100 mg/day, or nilotinib, 400 mg twice per day.
- Failure of TKI therapy during the course of the disease is often the result of a mutation in the *ABL* portion of *BCR-ABL*, which interferes with drug action.
- There are several mutations than can induce TKI resistance. Thus, PCR is impractical as a tool to find mutations. It is possible to sequence *ABL* and, by comparing the results to known mutations, determine the likelihood that a dasatinib-sensitive or nilotinib-sensitive mutation may be present.

TABLE 47–4   GUIDELINES FOR MONITORING OF PATIENTS IN CHRONIC PHASE WHO ARE UNDERGOING TKI THERAPY

1. At diagnosis, before starting therapy, obtain Giemsa-banding cytogenetics and measure BCR-ABL transcript numbers by quantitative PCR using marrow cells. If marrow cannot be obtained, use FISH on a blood specimen to confirm the diagnosis.
2. At 3, 6, 9, and 12 months after initiating therapy, perform FISH for t(9;22) on blood cells and quantitative PCR for BCR-ABL transcripts.
3. At 6 months, obtain marrow cytogenetics for cells with Ph chromosome. Repeat every 6 months until complete cytogenic response. If there is a CCyR at 6 months, this does not need to be done at 12 months.
4. Once CCyR is obtained, monitor quantitative PCR on blood cells every 3 months. Continue yearly marrow examination of marrow cytogenetics to identify clonal evolution, if indicated.
5. These guidelines presume continued response to the TKI until complete cytogenetic response achieved. If this does not occur, see text for approach.

CCyR, complete cytogenetic response; FISH, fluorescence *in situ* hybridization, TKI, tyrosine kinase inhibitor.
Reproduced with permission from www.nccn.org/professional/physicians_gls/PDF/cml.pdf
Source: *Williams Hematology*, 8th ed, Chap. 90, Table 90–5, p. 1353.

- If the T315I *ABL* mutation is found, allogeneic hematopoietic stem cell transplantation should be considered for eligible patients because that mutation is resistant to imatinib, nilotinib, and dasatinib. Third generation TKI inhibitors entering trial may be available for this situation in the future.

Other Drugs
- Under special circumstances several other second-line drugs can be considered: interferon-α, homoharringtonine, cytarabine, busulfan, and others. These are discussed in *Williams Hematology*, 8th ed, Chap. 90, p. 1348.

Allogeneic Hematopoietic Stem Cell Transplantation
- Transplantation has decreased markedly in frequency in chronic phase CML because of the very favorable prognosis of those treated with tyrosine kinase inhibitors who achieve a complete cytogenetic remission.
  — Should be considered in patients (a) who are eligible after all signs of continued improvement on tyrosine kinase inhibitors have stopped and a complete cytogenetic remission has not been achieved, (b) who are intolerant to tyrosine kinase inhibitors, or (c) who show progression of disease after using several tyrosine kinase inhibitors.
  — The early mortality rate in younger patients (younger than 40 years of age) without comorbid conditions is approximately 15 percent.
  — Engraftment and 5-year survival can be achieved in approximately 60 percent of patients in chronic phase, and some patients are cured. In patients over 50 years of age, the 5-year survival is somewhat decreased.
  — Some patients die of severe graft-versus-host disease and opportunistic infection in the first 5 years after transplant.
  — There is a 20 percent chance of relapse of CML in the 6 years after apparently successful transplant.
  — Donor T lymphocytes play an important role in successful suppression of the leukemia by initiating a graft-versus-leukemia reaction.
  — Disease status can be monitored by FISH (*BCR-ABL* fusion) or RT-PCR (*BCR-ABL* mRNA transcripts).

— Donor lymphocyte infusion can produce remission in transplanted patients who have relapse of their disease. Ten million mononuclear cells/kg body weight may be sufficient to induce a graft-versus-leukemia effect and a remission. Response rates to this treatment may be as high as 80 percent.

Radiation or Splenectomy

• Patients with marked splenomegaly and splenic pain or encroachment on the gastrointestinal tract who do not respond to drug therapy may benefit transiently from splenic radiation. Marked splenomegaly usually associated with acute transformation of the disease.
• Patients with focal extramedullary myeloid sarcomas with pain may benefit from local radiation.
• Splenectomy is of limited value but may be helpful in some patients, such as those with thrombocytopenia and massive splenomegaly, refractory to therapy. Postoperative complications are frequent.

COURSE AND PROGNOSIS

• The median survival has been greatly prolonged with tyrosine kinase inhibitors.
• As many as 90 percent of patients tolerant to TKIs may achieve a complete cytogenetic remission after 5 years of treatment.
• In a major study, the 7-year overall survival was 86 percent in those able to be maintained on imatinib. This finding may be improved with the use of second generation TKIs, nilotimib and dasatinib. Third generation TKIs are entering trials.
• Table 47–4 provides guidelines for monitoring patients in chronic phase of CML being treated with tyrosine kinase inhibitors.
• Table 47–5 provides the relative 5-year survival by age at diagnosis.
• A report of patients in CMR treated with imatinib with undetectable BCR-ABL transcripts (>5 log reduction) in whom imatinib therapy was stopped indicated that approximately 40 percent may have enduring remissions off TKI treatment. Importantly, those that relapsed were successfully retreated with imatinib.

ACCELERATED PHASE OF CML

• The natural history of CML is for patients to eventually become resistant to therapy at which point the disease enters a more aggressive phase characterized by severe dyshematopoiesis, refractory splenomegaly, extramedullary tumors, and, often, development of a clinical picture of acute leukemia—the "blast crisis."
• Although this evolution occurs in patients who are resistant or intolerant to tyrosine kinase inhibitors, the frequency per unit time has decreased markedly

TABLE 47–5	CHRONIC MYELOGENOUS LEUKEMIA: 5-YEAR RELATIVE SURVIVAL RATES (1996–2006)
Age (years)	**Percent of Patients**
<45	78.2
45–54	77.4
55–64	63.0
65–74	39.5
>75	24.7

NOTE: These data may underestimate the salutary effect of tyrosine kinase inhibitor treatment between 2006 and the current date.
Source: Data from Surveillance, Epidemiology, End Results Cancer Statistics, 5-Year Survival Rates, Table 13.6, All Races and Sexes by Age at Diagnosis. National Cancer Institute, Washington, DC. Available at www.seer.cancer.gov.

as a result of the prolonged remissions induced by these agents. It may take another decade to determine the rate of this event in persons who enter a complete cytogenetic remission after imatinib or its congeners and whether the nature of the accelerated phase mimics the one we have observed over the last 150 years.

- The Ph chromosome and *BCR* gene rearrangement persist in myeloid or lymphoid blasts in the accelerated phase, but additional chromosomal abnormalities often develop, such as trisomy 8, trisomy 19, isochromosome 17, or gain of a second Ph chromosome, and characteristic molecular genetic changes have been identified.

Clinical Features
- Unexplained fever, night sweats, weight loss, malaise, arthralgias.
- Development of new extramedullary sites of disease containing Ph chromosome-positive blast cells.
- Diminished responsiveness to previously effective drug therapy.

Laboratory Findings
Blood Findings
- Progressive anemia with increasing anisocytosis and poikilocytosis, increased numbers of nucleated red cells.
- An increasing proportion of blasts in the blood or marrow, which may reach 50 to 90 percent at the time of blastic crisis.
- Increase in the percentage of basophils (occasionally to levels of 30 to 80 percent).
- Appearance of hyposegmented neutrophils (acquired Pelger-Huët abnormality).
- Thrombocytopenia.

Marrow Findings
- Marked dysmorphic changes may be seen in any or all cell lineages, or florid blastic transformation may occur.

Blast Crisis
- Extramedullary blast crisis is the first sign of the accelerated phase in about 10 percent of patients. Lymph nodes, serosal surfaces, skin, breast, gastrointestinal or genitourinary tracts, bone, and the central nervous system are most often involved.
- Central nervous system involvement is usually meningeal. Symptoms and signs are headache, vomiting, stupor, cranial nerve palsies, and papilledema. The spinal fluid contains cells, including blasts, and the protein level is elevated.
- Acute leukemia develops in most patients in the accelerated phase. It is usually myeloblastic or myelomonocytic, but may be of any cell type.
- About one-third of patients develop acute lymphoblastic leukemia (ALL), with blast cells that contain terminal deoxynucleotidyl transferase, an enzyme characteristic of ALL, and surface markers typical of B cells.

Treatment of Patients with AML Phenotype
- Acute myelogenous leukemic transformation (any subtype can occur) is essentially incurable with chemotherapy presently available.
- The strategy that is most likely to result in a prolonged remission is allogeneic hematopoietic stem cell transplantation, albeit with a low long-term remission rate. Thus, drug therapy, in patients eligible for transplantation, is focused on a remission sufficiently long to accomplish transplantation in that state.
- One can start with dasatinib, 140 mg/day or 70 mg q 12 h or nilotinib, 400 mg q 12 hours, and then the alternative drug if the response is inadequate. Reports of good remissions with one but not another tyrosine kinase inhibitor have been

observed. Remission or reversion to chronic phase usually are short-lived and allogeneic hematopoietic stem cell transplantation from a histocompatible donor should be urgently considered for eligible patients.

* Tyrosine kinase therapy can be combined with mitoxantrone plus etoposide or cytarabine (an AML drug protocol) depending on patient's ability to tolerate such an approach (see Chap. 46).

Treatment of Patients with Acute Lymphocytic Leukemia Phenotype

* Start with dasatinib, 140 mg/day or 70 mg q 12 h or nilotinib, 400 mg q 12 h. If remission ensues, consider allogeneic stem cell transplantation if patient is eligible and a donor is available. These TKIs can induce remissions in the lymphoblastic acute leukemia crisis.
* If relapse after a TKI, consider ALL drug protocol such as vincristine sulfate, 1.4 mg/m^2 (to a maximum of 2 mg/dose) intravenously once per week, and prednisone, 60 mg/m^2 per day orally. A minimum of 2 weeks of therapy should be given to judge responsiveness.
* About one-third of patients will reenter the chronic phase with this treatment, but the median duration of remission is about 4 months, and relapse should be expected. Since acute lymphocytic blast crisis occurs in about 30 percent of cases, a 30 percent response represents about 9 percent of all patients entering ALL blast crisis.
* The response rate may be improved by more intensive therapy, similar to that used in *de novo* ALL, but not dramatically so. Most patients do not respond to repeat therapy.
* Allogeneic hematopoietic stem cell transplantation from a histocompatible donor may lead to prolonged remission in blast crisis. Thus, eligible patients who enter remission with therapy should be strongly considered for transplantation.

ACUTE LEUKEMIAS WITH THE PHILADELPHIA CHROMOSOME

* Philadelphia chromosome-positive AML appears, in some cases, to be instances of CML, presenting in myeloid blast crisis, while other cases appear to be unrelated to CML.
* Philadelphia chromosome-positive ALL represents about 3 percent of cases of childhood ALL and 20 percent of cases of adult ALL.
* In both adults and children, the prognosis is worse for those patients with leukemic cells containing the Ph chromosome.
* Some Ph chromosome-positive ALL patients have the same size BCR-ABL fusion oncoprotein (p210) that characterize CML and are believed to be patients with CML presenting in lymphoid blast crisis. The remaining patients have a p190 fusion protein and are thought to have *de novo* ALL.
* Treatment generally combines a tyrosine kinase inhibitor, as used for CML blast crisis, with intensive therapy for AML or ALL as described in Chaps. 46 and 55, respectively.

CHRONIC MYELOID LEUKEMIAS WITHOUT THE PH CHROMOSOME (TABLE 47-6)

Chronic Myelomonocytic Leukemia

* Approximately 75 percent of cases are over 60 years of age at onset.
* Male:female ratio 1.4:1.
* Onset insidious with weakness, exaggerated bleeding, fever, and infection most common.
* Hepatomegaly and splenomegaly occur in about 50 percent.
* Usually anemia and monocytosis ($>1.0 \times 10^9$/L) are present; less than 10 percent of cells in blood are myeloblasts.
* White cell count may be decreased, normal, or elevated and can reach levels of over 200×10^9/L.

TABLE 47–6 TYPES OF CHRONIC MYELOGENOUS LEUKEMIA

Type of Chronic Myelogenous Leukemia	Molecular Genetics	Major Clinical Features	Further Details in *Williams Hematology*, 8th ed
BCR rearrangement-positive chronic myelogenous leukemia	>95% p210$^{BCR-ABL}$; <5% p190 or p230	Splenomegaly in 80% of cases; WBC >25 × 10^9/L; blood blasts <5%; Ph chromosome in 90% of cases; *BCR* gene rearrangement in 100% of cases	Page 1338
Chronic myelomonocytic leukemia	Various cytogenetic abnormalities	Anemia, monocytosis >1 × 10^9/L; blood blasts <10%; increased plasma and urine lysozyme; *BCR* rearrangement absent; rare cases with *PDGFR*-β mutation respond to imatinib	Page 1356
Chronic eosinophilic leukemia	Various cytogenetic abnormalities	Blood eosinophil count >1.5 × 10^9/L; cardiac and neurologic manifestations common; a proportion of cases have *PDGFR*-α mutations and are responsive to imatinib mesylate	Page 1358
Chronic basophilic leukemia	Various cytogenetic abnormalities	Only 5 cases reported; hemoglobin 6–13 g/dL; basophilia of 3.4–41 × 10^9/L; 2 of 5 cases with splenomegaly; very cellular marrow (>90%) in each case with mild increase in type III collagen, and megakaryocytic dysmorphia; increase in marrow mast cells in 3 of 5 cases	Page 1359
Chronic monocytic leukemia	Various cytogenetic changes	Proportion of monocytes elevated; very rare form of leukemia	Page 1359
Juvenile myelomonocytic leukemia	Various cytogenetic changes	Infants and children < 4 years; eczematoid or maculopapular rash; anemia and thrombocytopenia; increased Hgb F in 70% of cases; neurofibromatosis in 10% of cases; abnormality of chromosome 7 (e.g., del 7, del 7q, etc.) in approximately 20% of patients; *BCR* rearrangement absent	Page 1360
Chronic neutrophilic leukemia	Various cytogenetic changes	Segmented neutrophilia >20,000/μL; splenomegaly >90% of cases; no blood blasts; platelets >100 × 10^9/L; 75% of cases have normal cytogenetics; *BCR* rearrangement absent	Page 1361
BCR rearrangement-negative chronic myelogenous leukemia	Various cytogenetic changes	Clinical findings indistinguishable from *BCR* rearrangement-positive CML; Ph chromosome and *BCR-ABL* fusion gene absent	Page 1362

Source: *Williams Hematology*, 8th ed, Chap. 90, Table 90–6, p. 1357.

- Marrow is hypercellular, with granulomonocytic hyperplasia.
- Myeloblasts and promyelocytes are increased but are less than 30 percent of cells in marrow.
- Approximately one-third of patients have an overt cytogenetic abnormality (e.g., monosomy 7, trisomy 8).
- Plasma and urine lysozyme concentrations are nearly always elevated.
- *RAS* gene mutations are frequent.
- Includes most cases of so-called Philadelphia chromosome-negative, BCR rearrangement-negative CML.
- A small percentage of patients have a translocation fusing the *PDGFR*-β gene with one of several gene partners (e.g., *TEL*). These cases may be associated with prominent eosinophilia.
- Several prognostic variables have been identified. Among the most compelling are height of blast cell count, severity of anemia, serum LDH, and spleen size at time of diagnosis.
- Median survival is approximately 12 months with a range of 1 to 60.
- Approximately 20 percent of patients progress to overt AML.

Treatment

- No standard or highly successful therapy has been developed. See *Williams Hematology,* 8th ed, Chap. 90, p.1356.
- Low-dose cytosine arabinoside, hydroxyurea, etoposide may induce occasional partial remissions for short periods of time (~0.5–1 year, usually).
- 5-Azacytidine or decitabine has resulted in improvement in some patients.
- Occasional patients with *PDGFR-partner* fusion oncogenes may respond to imatinib, 400 mg/day, orally.
- Other cytotoxic drugs, maturation-enhancing agents, interferons, and growth factors have been used.
- Marrow transplantation has yielded more favorable results than other therapies but the afflicted population has a median age of 70 years, making transplantation for most problematic.

Chronic Eosinophilic Leukemia

- A BCR-ABL negative chronic clonal myeloid disease manifest by prolonged exaggerated blood eosinophilia unexplained by parasitic or allergic disease.
- Fever, cough, weakness, easy fatigability, abdominal pain, maculopapular rash, cardiac symptoms, signs of heart failure, and a variety of neurologic symptoms may coexist in some combination.
- Eosinophilia is a constant finding. Anemia is often present. Platelet counts are normal or mildly decreased. Total white cell counts are normal or elevated in relationship to the degree of eosinophilia, which may be as high as 100×10^9/L.
- Marrow examination reveals markedly increased eosinophilic myelocytes and segmented eosinophils. Reticulin fibrosis may be present.
- Many different cytogenetic abnormalities can be found. Notably a high frequency of translocations involving chromosome 5 occur.
- Immunophenotyping and PCR do not show evidence of clonal T-cell population or T-cell receptor rearrangement.
- Pulmonary function studies may be consistent with fibrotic lung disease.
- Echocardiography may detect mural thrombi, thickened ventricular walls, and valvular dysfunction
- Skin, neural, brain biopsy, if indicated, shows intense eosinophilic infiltrates.
- A subset of patients with elevated serum tryptase (> 11.5 ng/mL), intensely hypercellular marrow eosinophilia with a high proportion of immature eosinophils, high serum B_{12} and IgE levels, more prone to pulmonary and endocardial fibrosis, the *FIL1L1-PDGFR*-α oncogene, are responsive to tyrosine kinase inhibitors (e.g., imatinib).

- In patients who are unresponsive to imatinib mesylate or its second generation congeners, should be considered for allogeneic hematopoietic stem cell transplantation if eligible and with an available donor.
- Other patients may be treated with glucocorticoids, hydroxyurea, anti-IL-5 antibodies in an effort to decrease the eosinophil count and ameliorate the eosinophil-induced deleterious tissue effects.
- If the patient is not imatinib-sensitive or eligible for transplantation, chronic eosinophilic leukemia is difficult to control. Occasional patients may progress to acute eosinophilic or myelogenous leukemia. Cardiac, pulmonary, and neurologic manifestations, if not stabilized, contribute to morbidity and mortality.

Juvenile Chronic Myelomonocytic Leukemia

- Occurs most often in children younger than 4 years of age.
- Twenty percent of patients have *RAS* mutations.
- Ten percent have neurofibromatosis and *NF1* mutations.
- Infants have failure to thrive; children present with fever, malaise, persistent infection, and skin and nasal bleeding.
- Fifty percent of patients have eczematoid or maculopapular skin lesions.
- Nearly all patients have splenomegaly.
- Anemia, thrombocytopenia, and leukocytosis are common.
- The blood contains monocytes up to 100×10^9/L; immature granulocytes, including blast cells; and nucleated red cells.
- Fetal hemoglobin concentration is increased in about two-thirds of the patients.
- The marrow shows granulocytic hyperplasia, with an increase in monocytes and leukemic blast cells.
- The disease has been refractory to chemotherapy. Four to six drug combinations have induced partial remissions in some patients and may extend survival although median survival is usually less than 36 months.
- Allogeneic hematopoietic stem cell transplantation can prolong survival, but cures, even with this approach, are few and far between.
- The median survival is less than 2 years, but occasional patients (usually infants) or massively treated patients survive for longer periods with the disease.

Chronic Neutrophilic Leukemia

- Characterized by a leukocyte count of 25,000 to 50,000/μL, with about 90 to 95 percent mature neutrophils.
- Neutrophil alkaline phosphatase activity is increased.
- Marrow shows granulocytic hyperplasia usually with a normal proportion of blasts.
- Ph chromosome and *BCR* gene rearrangement are absent.
- *JAK2*(V617F) mutation is present in a small proportion (~15 to 20%) of these patients.
- Liver and spleen are enlarged and are infiltrated with immature myeloid cells and megakaryocytes.
- There have been no systematic studies of treatment.
- Busulfan and hydroxyurea have been used with transient benefit.
- May terminate in typical AML.
- Median survival is 2 to 3 years.

Philadelphia Chromosome-Negative CML

- About 4 percent of patients with a phenotype indistinguishable from BCR-ABL-positive CML, do not have the Ph chromosome or *BCR* gene rearrangement on assiduous search.
- Median age is 66 years and ranges from 25 to 90 years.
- Median white cell count is lower (approximately 40×10^9/L) but the range is wide (11 to 296×10^9/L).

- The morphologic features in blood and marrow are characteristic of classic CML.
- Splenomegaly in only 50 percent at diagnosis.
- Disease progression marked by cytopenias. Median survival is 2 years and only 7 percent survive for more than 5 years.
- One-third of patients monitored until death developed AML.
- Occasional patients have extended complete responses to interferon-α. Hydroxyurea is often used to control the white cell count or decrease splenomegaly (palliative therapy).

For a more detailed discussion, see Jane L. Liesveld and Marshall A. Lichtman: Chronic Myelogenous Leukemias and Related Disorders. Chap. 90, p. 1331 in *Williams Hematology*, 8th ed.

CHAPTER 48
Primary Myelofibrosis

DEFINITION

- Primary myelofibrosis is a chronic clonal myeloid disorder that originates in mutations in a multipotential hematopoietic cell. The disease is characterized by (a) anemia, (b) splenomegaly, (c) increased CD34+ cells, immature granulocytes, erythroid precursors, and teardrop-shaped red cells in the blood, (d) marrow fibrosis and increased dysmorphic megakaryocytes, and (e) osteosclerosis.

EPIDEMIOLOGY

- Onset characteristically after age 50 years.
- Median age at diagnosis approximately 68 years.
- Adult males and females affected equally.
- Incidence about 1.0 case per 100,000 in persons of European descent.

PATHOGENESIS

- Origin in the neoplastic transformation of a multipotential hematopoietic cell.
- In approximately 50 percent of cases, the hematopoietic cells (blood cell lineages) contain the mutation *JAK2* V617F.
- In approximately 10 percent of cases, the hematopoietic cells contain a mutation in the *MPL* gene, which encodes the thrombopoietin receptor.
- Constitutive mobilization and circulation of CD34+ cells as a result of epigenetic methylation of the CXCR4 promoter, leading to decreased expression of CXCR4 on CD34+ cells and their enhanced migration from marrow to blood.
- CD34+ cells in this disorder generate about 24-fold the megakaryocytes in culture than do CD34+ cells from normal persons.

Fibroplasia

- Reticulin fibers (type III collagen), as detected by silver staining, are increased in the marrow in most patients. Fibrosis may progress to thick collagen bands (type I collagen) identified with the trichrome stain.
- Increased plasma concentrations of procollagen III amino-terminal peptide, prolylhydroxylase, and fibronectin are present.
- The extent of fibrosis is correlated with the prevalence of dysmorphic megakaryocytes and release of fibroblast growth factors from the megakaryocyte α granules (e.g., platelet-derived growth factor, basic fibroblast growth factor, epidermal growth factor, transforming growth factor-β, and others).
- The fibroblastic proliferation in the marrow is a reaction to the cytokines released by an increased density of dysmorphic megakaryocytes, not an intrinsic part of the clonal expansion of hematopoietic cells.
- Thicker bands of collagen fibrosis (type I collagen) may develop as the marrow fibrosis advances.

CLINICAL FEATURES

- The median age at diagnosis is approximately 68 years, but the disorder may occur at any age.
- The sex incidence is equal in adults, but twice as many females as males in young children.

- Rarely, myelofibrosis is preceded by extended exposure to benzene or very high-dose ionizing radiation.
- Approximately 25 percent of patients are asymptomatic at time of diagnosis.
- Fatigue, weakness, shortness of breath, palpitations, weight loss, night sweats, and bone pain are common presenting symptoms.
- Wasting, peripheral edema, or bone tenderness may occur.
- Left upper-quadrant fullness, pain or dragging sensation, left shoulder pain, and early satiety may result from splenic enlargement and/or infarction.
- Splenomegaly is present in virtually all patients at the time of diagnosis and is massive in one-third of cases.
- Hepatomegaly is present in two-thirds of patients.
- Neutrophilic dermatosis (Sweet syndrome) may be present.

SPECIAL CLINICAL FEATURES

Prefibrotic Stage

- Many experts believe that one can identify a prefibrotic stage of myelofibrosis in which early changes, such as slight anemia, slight neutrophilia, and thrombocytosis occur. The latter is a constant finding. The marrow biopsy may not show increased reticulin fibers at this stage. A constant feature, however, is an increase in marrow megakaryocytes, often with dysmorphic features. Large and small megakaryocytes are admixed. Use of a megakaryocyte marker, such as CD61, to stain the marrow, makes the increased megakaryocyte population very evident. The diagnosis may be considered essential thrombocythemia (see Chap. 44) until this stage progresses to develop the other classic findings of primary myelofibrosis (see Table 48–1).

Extramedullary Hematopoiesis and Fibrohematopoietic Tumors

- Present in liver and, especially, spleen, in this disorder and contributes to the organomegaly.

TABLE 48–1	DIAGNOSTIC FINDINGS IN PRIMARY MYELOFIBROSIS

Prefibrotic stage
  Anemia may be absent or mild
  Neutrophilia may be absent or slight
  Thrombocythemia very frequent
  BCR-ABL fusion gene absent
  If present, *JAK2* mutation indicative of diagnosis of myeloproliferative disease
  Cellular marrow with mild increase in granulopoiesis; increased megakaryocytes, clusters of very dysmorphic megakaryocytes and megakaryocytic nuclei; no to very slight increase in reticular fibers on silver stain
  Palpable splenomegaly infrequent
  Absent or slight anisopoikilocytosis including teardrop red cells
Fully developed stage
  Anisopoikilocytosis with teardrop red cells in every oil immersion field
  Immature myeloid cells in blood
  Increased CD34-positive cells in blood
  Erythroblasts in blood
  Marrow usually hypercellular but invariably has increased megakaryocytes, clusters of highly dysmorphic megakaryocytes, and megakaryocyte bare nuclei regardless of overall marrow cellularity
  Marrow reticulin fibrosis plus or minus collagen fibrosis
  BCR-ABL fusion gene absent
  JAK2 mutation in approximately 50% of patients
  Splenomegaly in virtually all patients

- Extramedullary hematopoiesis is not effective as a source of blood cell production.
- Hematopoietic foci are often present in adrenals, kidneys, lymph nodes, bowel, breast, lungs, and other sites.
- Hepatic extramedullary hematopoiesis worsens after splenectomy and leads to an enlarging liver, sometimes massive, and can result in hepatic failure.
- Identification of a mass on imaging, unexpected neurologic signs, or other unexpected findings should raise the consideration of a fibrohematopoietic tumor that can arise in any tissue or organ.
- Central nervous system sites of extramedullary hematopoiesis can be associated with subdural hemorrhage, delirium, increased cerebrospinal fluid pressure, papilledema, coma, motor and sensory impairment, and paralysis.
- Hematopoietic foci on serosal surfaces can cause effusions in the thorax, abdomen, or pericardial spaces.

Portal Hypertension and Esophageal Varices
- Strikingly increased splenoportal blood flow and decreased hepatic vascular compliance can lead to portal hypertension, ascites, esophageal and gastric varices, intraluminal gastrointestinal bleeding, and hepatic encephalopathy.
- The hepatic venous pressure gradient, normally <6 torr, is markedly elevated.
- Portal vein thrombosis may occur.

Pulmonary Artery Hypertension
- About one-third of patients with primary myelofibrosis have an elevated pulmonary artery pressure, the fraction that is symptomatic is relatively small.

Bone Changes
- Osteosclerosis may develop with increased bone density evident on radiographs and marrow biopsy.
- Periostitis may lead to severe bone pain.
- Increased bone blood flow (up to 25% of cardiac output) may contribute to the development or accentuation of congestive heart failure.

Immune Findings
- Various immune products may develop, such as anti-red cell, anti-neutrophil, antiplatelet antibodies, antinuclear antibodies, or antiphospholipid antibodies.
- Inflammatory cytokines including interleukin(IL)-1β, IL-6, IL-8, tumor necrosis factor-α are frequently elevated and may contribute to constitutional symptoms.

Thrombotic Arterial or Venous Events
- Incidence is elevated but not to the extent seen in polycythemia vera (see Chap. 43). Age, elevated platelet count, and coincident vascular disease are the three principal risk factors for thrombosis.
- Portal vein thrombosis may be presenting event in some patients.

LABORATORY FEATURES

Blood Findings
- Normocytic-normochromic anemia is found in most patients (mean = 105 g/L with a very wide range).
- Anisopoikilocytosis, and teardrop red cells (dacryocytes) are constant findings (see Fig. 48–1).
- Occasional nucleated red cells are seen in the blood film in most patients.
- Anemia may be worsened by an expanded plasma volume and/or splenic trapping of red cells.

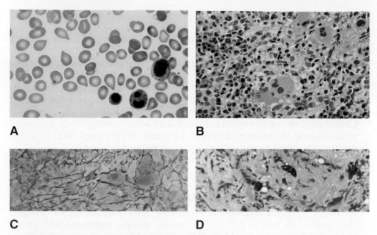

FIGURE 48-1 Blood film and marrow sections from patients with primary myelofibrosis. **A.** Blood film. Characteristic teardrop poikilocytes, a nucleated red cell, and a segmented neutrophil with a dysmorphic nucleus are evident. **B.** Marrow section. Low power. Hypercellular marrow with increased number of hypolobular megakaryocytes. **C.** Marrow section. Silver impregnation stain. Marked increase in argentophilic fibers representing collagen type III (reticulin). **D.** Marrow section. Collagen fibrosis with extensive replacement of marrow with swirls of collagen fibers. *(Reproduced with permission from* Lichtman's Atlas of Hematology, *www.accessmedicine.com.)*

- Reticulocyte count is variable but usually the absolute reticulocyte count is low for the degree of anemia.
- Hemolysis may be present and rarely may be autoimmune, with a positive antiglobulin (Coombs) test.
- Acquired hemoglobin H disease with hypochromic-microcytic red cells and red cell inclusions (hemoglobin H precipitates) staining with brilliant cresyl blue can occur rarely, admixed with typical white cell and platelet changes of myelofibrosis.
- Erythroid aplasia may coexist, rarely.
- The total leukocyte count averages approximately $12 \times 10^9/L$ in many studies and is usually less than $40 \times 10^9/L$, but may be as high as $200 \times 10^9/L$ with neutrophilic granulocytosis predominating.
- Neutropenia occurs in 15 percent at the time of diagnosis.
- Myelocytes and metamyelocytes are present in the blood of all patients, along with a low proportion of blast cells (0.5 to 5%).
- Neutrophils may have impaired phagocytosis, decreased myeloperoxidase activity, and other functional abnormalities.
- Basophils may be slightly increased in number.
- About 40 percent of patients have elevated platelet counts, and one-third has mild to moderate thrombocytopenia.
- Giant platelets, abnormal platelet granulation, and occasional circulating micro-megakaryocytes are characteristic.
- The bleeding (closure) time may be prolonged and platelet aggregation with epinephrine may be impaired along with depletion of dense granule ADP and decreased lipoxygenase activity in platelets.
- Pancytopenia occurs in 10 percent of patients at presentation, usually secondary to ineffective hematopoiesis coupled with splenic sequestration.
- The variable blood counts are a reflection of an unpredictable combination of effective or ineffective hematopoiesis, expanded hematopoiesis in one or another blood cell lineage, exaggerated late precursor apoptosis in one or another lineage, effect of splenomegaly on blood cell pooling or shortened survival, presence of

anti-blood cell antibodies, and other factors. Thus, (a) anemia, neutrophilia, and thrombocytosis, (b) anemia, neutropenia, and thrombocytosis, (c) anemia, neutrophilia, and thrombocytopenia, and (d) anemia, neutropenia, and thrombocytopenia may be present at diagnosis. The first pattern mentioned is the most common. Occasionally, anemia may not be present initially.

- Increased numbers of circulating multipotential, granulocytic, monocytic, and erythroid progenitor cells are found.
- Increased CD34+ cells in the blood is characteristic and >15 × 10^6/L is virtually diagnostic of primary myelofibrosis. Their frequency is roughly correlated with extent of disease and disease progression.
- Serum levels of uric acid, lactic acid dehydrogenase, alkaline phosphatase, and bilirubin are often elevated.
- Serum levels of albumin, cholesterol, and high-density lipoproteins are usually decreased.
- Immune manifestations include anti–red cell antibodies, antinuclear antibodies, anti–gamma globulins, antiphospholipid antibodies, and others may be found.

Marrow Findings
- See Fig. 48–1.
- Marrow aspiration is often unsuccessful because of fibrosis ("dry tap").
- Biopsy is often cellular, with variable degrees of erythroid, granulocytic, and megakaryocytic expansion.
- Silver stain shows increased reticulin, often extreme. Gomori trichrome stain may show collagen fibrosis, which can be extreme, along with osteosclerotic changes
- Megakaryocytes are prominent even in hypocellular, densely fibrotic specimens, and they are usually strikingly dysmorphic: giant or dwarf forms, abnormal nuclear lobulation, and naked nuclei.
- Increased marrow neoplastic megakaryocytopoeisis is the most constant and characteristic feature of the disease and accounts for several of the secondary manifestations (e.g., marrow fibrosis).
- Granulocytes may have hyperlobulation or hypolobulation, acquired Pelger-Huët anomaly, nuclear blebs, and nuclear-cytoplasmic asynchrony.
- Small clusters of blast cells may be present.
- Dilated marrow sinusoids are common, with intrasinusoidal immature hematopoietic cells and megakaryocytes.
- Increased marrow microvessel density is present (enhanced angiogenesis) in 70 percent of patients.

CYTOGENETICS
- Cytogenetic abnormalities are present in approximately 50 percent of cases. Aneuploidy (monosomy or trisomy) or pseudodiploidy (partial deletions and translocations) are common. These cytogenetic abnormalities are not seen in fibroblasts. Since marrow aspirates may be difficult to obtain because of the fibrosis, a panel of fluorescence *in situ* hybridization probes that reflect the most prevalent abnormalities seen may be used to search for cytogenetic abnormalities (see discussion in *Williams Hematology*, 8th ed, Chap. 91, p. 1388).

Magnetic Resonance Imaging
- Marrow fibrosis alters the T1-weighted images that normally result from marrow fat. As cellularity and fibrosis increase, hypointensity of T1- and T2-weighted images develop. Primary myelofibrosis cannot be distinguished from secondary, although the clinical and laboratory findings usually make the distinction evident. Osteosclerosis and vertebral changes (sandwich vertebrae) can be detected. Periosteal reactions also can be identified with this imaging technique.

DIFFERENTIAL DIAGNOSIS

- Chronic myelogenous leukemia: In CML, the white count is often greater than 100×10^9/L at presentation, red cell shape is usually approximately normal, and marrow fibrosis is minimal. The Philadelphia chromosome and/or *BCR-ABL* fusion gene are present in hematopoietic and blood cells.
- Myelodysplasia: Pancytopenia and maturation abnormalities may occur in both myelodysplasia and myelofibrosis. Teardrop-shaped red-cell frequency (every oil immersion field), prominent splenomegaly, and marrow fibrosis should help distinguish primary myelofibrosis from a myelodysplastic syndrome in most cases.
- Hairy cell leukemia may show findings consistent with primary myelofibrosis (anemia, splenomegaly, marrow fibrosis), but the presence of abnormal mononuclear (hairy) cells in marrow and blood with characteristic CD phenotype separates the two disorders (see Chap. 57).
- Disorders with reactive marrow fibrosis include metastatic carcinoma (e.g., breast, prostate), disseminated mycobacterial infection, mastocytosis, myeloma, renal osteodystrophy, angioimmunoblastic lymphadenopathy, gray platelet syndrome, systemic lupus erythematosus, polyarteritis nodosa, neuroblastoma, rickets, Langerhans cell histiocytosis, and malignant histiocytosis.
- Primary autoimmune myelofibrosis has no associated evidence of a connective tissue disease, especially systemic lupus erythematosus. Anemia and sometimes pancytopenia may be present, but neither the blood cell changes indicative of primary myelofibrosis (teardrop cells, anisopoikilocytosis) nor splenomegaly is present. Often responds to glucocorticoids.
- Coincidental disorders with myelofibrosis include lymphoma, chronic lymphocytic leukemia, hairy cell leukemia, macroglobulinemia, amyloidosis, myeloma, and monoclonal gammopathy, and virtually all cases of pulmonary hypertension.
- All clonal myeloid diseases may have increased reticulin in the marrow, but only primary myelofibrosis has collagen fibrosis.
- Acute megakaryocytic leukemia may show intense marrow fibrosis (acute myelofibrosis), but the characteristic red cell changes and splenomegaly are absent and blast cells and very dysmorphic micromegakaryocytes are more prominent in blood and marrow.

TRANSITIONS BETWEEN IDIOPATHIC MYELOFIBROSIS AND OTHER MYELOPROLIFERATIVE DISORDERS

- Polycythemia vera: approximately 15 percent of patients treated with phlebotomy or myelosuppression develop classic myelofibrosis (akin to primary myelofibrosis), usually in a progressive pattern over a period of many years.
- Apparent primary thrombocytosis may evolve into classic primary myelofibrosis.
- Acute leukemia develops in about 5 to 10 percent of patients with *de novo* primary myelofibrosis, and in about 20 percent of those with polycythemia vera who have transformed into primary myelofibrosis, especially those who have been treated with myelosuppressive agents. An oligoblastic myelogenous leukemia may precede the development of florid acute leukemia.

TREATMENT

- Some patients are asymptomatic for long periods of time and do not require therapy. There is currently no cure other than allogeneic hematopoietic stem cell transplantation, which may be difficult if fibrosis is extensive.
- Severe anemia may improve with androgen therapy in some patients (e.g., danazol, 600 mg/day, orally, may be less virilizing). Careful monitoring of hepatic function and periodic liver imaging with ultrasound to detect liver tumors are essential.

- Glucocorticoids (prednisone 25 mg/m^2 per day, orally, for a limited period) may occasionally be helpful in patients with significant hemolytic anemia. High-dose glucocorticoids have been reported to ameliorate primary myelofibrosis in children, but their secondary effects are severe and they should not be used for prolonged periods, if avoidable.
- Few patients have such inappropriately low serum erythropoietin as to indicate a recombinant human erythropoietin product would be useful.
- Decreases in splenic and hepatic size, improvement in constitutional symptoms (fever, bone pain, weight loss, night sweats), and improvement in blood counts (increase in hemoglobin, decrease in elevated platelet counts), and decreased marrow fibrosis can occasionally be obtained with low doses of oral hydroxyurea (e.g., 0.5 to 1.0 g/day or 1.0 to 2.0 g three times per week). Blood counts at appropriate intervals to allow dosage adjustment is important (every week, then every 2 weeks, then every month, for example).
- Patients with myelofibrosis tend to have a lower tolerance to chemotherapy than other patients with other clonal myeloid diseases and dosage should be lowered accordingly until tolerance determined.
- Interferon-α has been useful in treating splenic enlargement, bone pain, and thrombocytosis.
- Inhibitors of JAK2 can provide some benefits: most often they lead to a decrease in spleen size and a lessening of constitutional symptoms. Thrombocytopenia may be dose-limiting. They may benefit patients without a JAK2 mutation, perhaps because they inhibit JAK isoforms that contribute to cytokine release.
- Lenalidomide can induce marked improvement in hemoglobin concentration, increase in platelet count, and decrease in spleen size in about 25 to 30 percent of patients treated.
- Bisphosphonates (e.g., etidronate, 6 mg/day on alternate months) may relieve bone pain from osteosclerosis and periostitis and may improve hematopoiesis.
- Selective low-dose radiation therapy may be useful for:
  — Severe splenic pain or massive splenic enlargement (with contraindication to splenectomy such as thrombocytosis).
  — Ascites from peritoneal extramedullary hematopoiesis.
  — Focal areas of severe bone pain from periostitis or osteolysis of a fibrohematopoietic tumor).
  — Extramedullary tumors, especially of the epidural space.
- Allogeneic stem cell transplantation can be efficacious in patients with a suitable donor and features felt to be compatible with a good outcome from transplantation (e.g., acceptable age-range, absence of comorbidities, and other features).
- Nonmyeloablative allogeneic hematopoietic stem cell transplantation may increase age at which transplantation may be useful.
- Major indications for splenectomy:
  — Very painful, enlarged spleen unresponsive to drug or local radiation treatment.
  — Excessive red cell and/or platelet transfusion requirement.
  — Refractory hemolysis.
  — Severe, symptomatic thrombocytopenia.
  — Portal hypertension.
- Patients with prolonged bleeding times, prothrombin times, or partial thromboplastin times are at serious risk for bleeding during and after surgery. They require meticulous preoperative evaluation and replacement therapy, surgical hemostasis, and postoperative care.
- Postsplenectomy morbidity is about 30 percent and mortality about 10 percent.
- Splenectomy for primary myelofibrosis has special difficulties because of large size, the adherence to neighboring structures (e.g., inferior surface of diaphragm), prominent collateral circulation, and dilated splenoportal arteries.

- The morbidity and mortality from splenectomy and the minimal evidence for prolongation of life has led to conservatism in using this approach. It can, however, be helpful in carefully selected patients.
- Portal hypertension as a result of increased splenic blood flow may be improved by splenectomy, especially if the hepatic wedge pressure is elevated as a result of a large splenic blood flow to the liver. In patients with portal hypertension resulting from an intrahepatic block or hepatic vein thrombosis and a hepatic venous pressure gradient well above the normal of <6 torr, a splenorenal shunt can be performed. To avoid abdominal surgery, a transjugular intrahepatic portosystemic shunt can be used.
- Anagrelide may be useful for postsplenectomy thrombocytosis.

COURSE AND PROGNOSIS

- Median survival is approximately 5 years after diagnosis (range: 1 to 15 years).
- At least 16 variables have been associated with a less favorable prognosis.
- Six relatively consistent poor prognostic signs are (a) older age, (b) severity of anemia, (c) exaggerated leukocytosis ($>25 \times 10^9$/L) or leukopenia ($<4.0 \times 10^9$/L), (d) fever sweating or weight loss at the time of diagnosis, and (e) a higher proportion of blast cells in blood ($>1.0\%$), (f) cytogenetic abnormalities involving chromosomes 5, 7, or 17.
- Major causes of death are infection, hemorrhage, postsplenectomy mortality, and transformation into acute leukemia.
- Spontaneous remissions are rare.

For a more detailed discussion, see Marshall A. Lichtman and Ayalew Tefferi: Primary Myelofibrosis. Chap. 91, p. 1381 in *Williams Hematology*, 8th ed.

PART VII

THE POLYCLONAL LYMPHOID DISEASES

CHAPTER 49
Classification of the Polyclonal Lymphoid Disorders

CLASSIFICATION

- Polyclonal lymphocyte and plasma cell disorders can be classified into two major groups (Table 49–1):
  - Primary disorders that result from defects intrinsic to B lymphocytes (e.g., X-linked agammaglobulinemia), T lymphocytes (e.g., congenital thymic aplasia), and/or natural killer cells, the latter usually coupled with a B or T cell deficiency (e.g., interleukin (IL)-7 receptor α-chain deficiency) (see Chap. 51).
  - Acquired disorders that result from physiologic or pathophysiologic responses to extrinsic factors, usually infectious agents (e.g., Epstein-Barr virus or human immunodeficiency virus infection). (See Chaps. 50, 52, 53.)
- The monoclonal lymphoid disorders are classified in Chap. 54 and individual neoplastic lymphoid diseases are described in Chaps. 55–72.
  - Disparate disorders can have similar clinical manifestations, such as recurrent infections as a result of either B or T cell deficiency.
- Lymphocyte disorders can have clinical manifestations that are not restricted to cells of the immune system (e.g., leprosy or systemic lupus erythematosus).
- In some cases, classification is influenced by disease manifestations:
  - Diseases caused by production of pathologic autoantibodies; e.g., autoimmune hemolytic disease (see Chaps. 24–26), autoimmune thrombocytopenia (see Chap. 120), and systemic autoimmune diseases (e.g., myasthenia gravis).
  - Diseases caused by excess production of lymphocyte cytokines; e.g., chronic inflammatory disorders.

TABLE 49–1	**CLASSIFICATION OF NON-CLONAL DISORDERS OF LYMPHOCYTES AND PLASMA CELLS**

I. Primary disorders*
  A. B-lymphocyte deficiency or dysfunction
    1. Agammaglobulinemia
       a. Acquired agammaglobulinemia
       b. Associated with celiac disease
       c. X-linked agammaglobulinemia of Bruton
    2. Selective agammaglobulinemia
       a. IgM deficiency
          (1) Bloom syndrome
          (2) Isolated
          (3) Wiskott-Aldrich syndrome
       b. Selective IgG deficiency
       c. IgA deficiency
          (1) Isolated asymptomatic
          (2) Steatorrheic
       d. IgA and IgM deficiency
    3. Hyper-IgA
    4. Hyper-IgD
    5. Hyper-IgE
    6. Hyper-IgE associated with HIV infection
    7. Hyper-IgM immunodeficiency
    8. X-linked lymphoproliferative disease
  B. T-lymphocyte deficiency or dysfunction
    1. Cartilage-hair hypoplasia
    2. Lymphocyte function antigen-1 deficiency
    3. Thymic aplasia (DiGeorge syndrome)
    4. Thymic dysplasia (Nezelof syndrome)
    5. Thymic hypoplasia
    6. Wiskott-Aldrich syndrome
    7. ZAP-70 deficiency
    8. Purine nucleoside phosphorylase deficiency
    9. Interleukin-7 receptor deficiency
    10. Major histocompatibility complex class I deficiency
    11. Coronin-1A deficiency
    12. IPEX syndrome caused by mutations in FoxP3 that cause a deficiency of CD4+ regulatory T cells (T_{regs})
    13. APECED syndrome caused by mutations in the autoimmune regulator gene (AIRE) gene
    14. Autoimmune lymphoproliferative syndrome
    15. Calcium entry channel deficiency caused by mutations in *ORAI1* or *STIM1*
  C. Combined T- and B-cell deficiency or dysfunction
    1. Ataxia-telangiectasia
    2. Combined immunodeficiency syndrome
       a. Adenosine deaminase deficiency
       b. Thymic alymphoplasia
    3. Major histocompatibility complex class II deficiency—bare lymphocyte syndrome
    4. IgG and IgA deficiency and impaired cellular immunity (type I dysgammaglobulinemia)
    5. Immunodeficiency with thymoma
    6. Pyridoxine deficiency
    7. Reticular agenesis (congenital aleukocytosis)
    8. Omenn syndrome
    9. WHIM syndrome resulting from mutation in the CXCR4 gene
    10. Nijmegen breakage syndrome

II. Acquired disorders
  A. Acquired immunodeficiency syndrome
  B. Reactive lymphocytosis or plasmacytosis
    1. *Bordetella pertussis* lymphocytosis
    2. Cytomegalovirus mononucleosis
    3. Drug-induced lymphocytosis
    4. Epstein-Barr virus mononucleosis
    5. Inflammatory (secondary) plasmacytosis of marrow
    6. Other viral mononucleosis
    7. Polyclonal lymphocytosis
    9. Serum sickness
    10. *Toxoplasma gondii* mononucleosis
    11. Viral infectious lymphocytosis
  C. T-lymphocyte dysfunction or depletion associated with systemic disease
    1. Leprosy
    2. Lupus erythematosus
    3. Sjögren syndrome
    4. Sarcoidosis

*Further details of primary (inherited or congenital) immunodeficiency diseases can be found in Chap. 51, Primary Immunodeficiency Syndromes.
Source: *Williams Hematology*, 8th ed, Table 80–1, p. 1138.

CLINICAL MANIFESTATIONS

B-Lymphocyte Disorders

- Infection with any class of microorganism (e.g., bacteria, viruses, fungi) as a result of immunoglobulin deficiency and impaired opsonization and clearance of pathogen.
- Tissue or organ abnormality as a result of pathogenic autoantibodies (e.g., immune hemolytic anemia, immune thrombocytopenia, myasthenia gravis, thyroiditis)

T-Lymphocyte Disorders

- T-cell depletion results in immune deficiency.
- Clinical manifestations depend on the subset(s) of T cells involved:
  — *Depletion of T_H1-type $CD4^+$ T cells:* Impaired delayed type hypersensitivity can result in an increased risk of opportunistic infections (e.g., mycobacteria, listeria, brucella, fungi, or other intracellular organisms) as a result of the deficient cellular immune response to these organisms.
  — *Depletion of T_H2-type $CD4^+$ T cells:* Impaired secondary antibody response to bacteria, viruses and fungi.
  — *Depletion of $CD4^+$ regulatory T-cells:* Can result in systemic autoimmune diseases.
  — *Depletion of $CD4^+Th17$ in skin and gastrointestinal tract:* Can result in increased risk of infection in those sites.
- Graft-versus-host disease, mediated by T lymphocytes, usually secondary to allogeneic hematopoietic stem cell transplantation (see Chap. 40).
- Acquired immunodeficiency syndrome is a result of the lytic effect of the human immunodeficiency virus entry into $CD4^+$ T lymphocytes.

For a more detailed discussion, see Thomas J. Kipps: Classification and Clinical Manifestations of Lymphocyte and Plasma Cell Disorders, Chap. 80, p. 1137 in *Williams Hematology,* 8th ed.

CHAPTER 50
Lymphocytosis and Lymphocytopenia

LYMPHOCYTOSIS

Definition
- Adults: absolute lymphocyte count exceeds 4.0×10^9/L (see Chap. 1).
- Normal lymphocyte count in childhood is higher than adults (mean ~6.0×10^9/L) until about 3 years of age (see Chap. 1).
- Table 50–1 lists conditions associated with lymphocytosis.
- Examine blood film to determine if there is abnormal prevalence of:
  — Reactive lymphocytes, associated with infectious mononucleosis (see Chap. 53).
  — Large granular lymphocytes, associated with large granular lymphocyte leukemia (see Chap. 58).
  — Small lymphocytes and smudge cells, associated with chronic lymphocytic leukemia (CLL) (see Chap. 56).
  — Small cleaved lymphocytes, associated with low- or intermediate-grade lymphomas (see Chap. 62).
  — Blasts, associated with acute lymphocytic leukemia (see Chap. 55).
- Several key tests permit discrimination between polyclonal and monoclonal disorders. Flow cytometric immunophenotyping of cell surface markers (CD), serum protein electropheresis and immunofixation for monoclonal immunoglobulins, studies of T-cell–receptor gene rearrangement, or clonal cytogenetic findings can distinguish monoclonal lymphocytosis (B or T lymphocytic leukemia or lymphoma) from polyclonal (reactive) lymphocytosis.

Primary Clonal Lymphocytosis
- Neoplastic (monoclonal) proliferation of B cells, T cells, or natural killer (NK) cells.
- Monoclonal B-cell lymphocytosis (see Chap. 56).
  — No associated clinical manifestations.
  — Some patients may develop CLL or another type of progressive lymphoproliferative disease (see Chap. 56).
- Chronic natural killer (NK) cell lymphocytosis (see Chap. 58).
  — CD3−CD16+CD56+ lymphocytes
  — Approximately 60 percent of cases without other signs or symptoms.
  — Others may have blood cytopenias, especially neutropenia, neuropathy, splenomegaly.
- Acute and chronic lymphocytic leukemias and lymphomas with blood involvement (see Chap. 54).

Primary Polyclonal Lymphocytosis
- Persistent polyclonal lymphocytosis of B lymphocytes.
  — A high proportion of lymphocytes have bilobed nuclei or have other nuclear abnormalities (Fig 50–1).
  — Lymphocytes are "polyclonal" in their expression of immunoglobulin (Fig. 50–1).
  — Commonly associated only with mild splenomegaly and/or raised serum IgM but can have features that resemble those of patients with monoclonal B-cell malignancies.

TABLE 50–1   CAUSES OF LYMPHOCYTOSIS

I. Primary lymphocytosis
- A. Lymphocytic malignancies
  1. Acute lymphocytic leukemia (Chap. 55)
  2. Chronic lymphocytic leukemia and related disorders (Chap. 56)
  3. Prolymphocytic leukemia (Chap. 55)
  4. Hairy cell leukemia (Chap. 57)
  5. Adult T-cell leukemia (Chaps. 55 and 67)
  6. Leukemic phase of B-cell lymphomas (Chaps. 61, 62)
  7. Large granular lymphocytic leukemia (Chaps. 58, 67)
     a. Natural killer (NK) cell leukemia (Chap. 67)
     b. CD8+ T-cell large granular lymphocytic leukemia (Chap. 67)
     c. CD4+ T-cell large granular lymphocytic leukemia (Chap. 67)
     d. γ/δ T-cell large granular lymphocytic leukemia (Chap. 67)
- B. Monoclonal B-cell lymphocytosis (Chap. 56)
- C. Persistent polyclonal B cell lymphocytosis

II. Reactive lymphocytosis
- A. Mononucleosis syndromes (Chap. 53)
  1. Epstein-Barr virus
  2. Cytomegalovirus
  3. Human immunodeficiency virus
  4. Herpes simplex virus type II
  5. Rubella virus
  6. *Toxoplasma gondii*
  7. Adenovirus
  8. Infectious hepatitis virus
  9. Dengue fever virus
  10. Human herpes virus type 6 (HHV-6)
  11. Human herpes virus type 8 (HHV-8)
  12. Varicella zoster virus
- B. *Bordetella pertussis*
- C. NK cell lymphocytosis (see Chap. 58)
- D. Stress lymphocytosis (acute)
  1. Cardiovascular collapse
     a. Acute cardiac failure
     b. Myocardial infarction
  2. Staphylococcal toxic shock syndrome
  3. Drug-induced
  4. Major surgery
  5. Sickle cell crisis
  6. Status epilepticus
  7. Trauma
- E. Hypersensitivity reactions
  1. Insect bite
  2. Drugs
- F. Persistent lymphocytosis (subacute or chronic)
  1. Cancer
  2. Cigarette smoking
  3. Hyposplenism
  4. Chronic infection
     a. Leishmaniasis
     b. Leprosy
     c. Strongyloidiasis
  5. Thymoma

Source: *Williams Hematology*, 8th ed, Table 81–1, p. 1142.

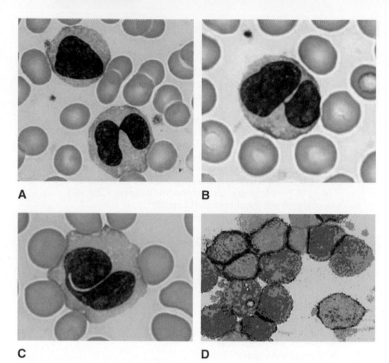

A   **B**

C   **D**

FIGURE 50-1 Persistent polyclonal lymphocytosis of B lymphocytes. Blood film. **A–C.** Examples of the nuclear abnormality of lymphocytes in this disorder. The lymphocyte nucleus may be bilobed or segmented although not fully bilobed. Some are monolobed. **D.** Light chain analysis. Immunoenzymatic method. Cytocentrifuge cell preparation. Antikappa immunoglobulin light chain tagged with peroxidase and anti-lambda light chain tagged with alkaline phosphatase. Note polyclonal reactivity of lymphocytes; some cells with surface kappa light chains (*brownish*) and some with surface lambda light chains (*reddish*). Molecular studies did not show immunoglobulin gene rearrangement. *(Reproduced with permission from Lichtman's Atlas of Hematology, www.accessmedicine.com. These Atlas images were generously provided by Dr. Xavier Troussard, Laboratoire d'Hématologie CHU Côte de Nacre, Caen, France.)*
(Source: *Williams Hematology,* 8th ed, Chap. 81, Fig. 81-1, p. 1143.)

— Most patients have small numbers of B cells with chromosomal abnormalities, most commonly involving chromosomes 3, 14 (at the immunoglobulin heavy chain locus), and 18 (at the *BCL-2* locus).
— Generally, not progressive, although some cases may evolve into a monoclonal lymphoproliferative disease.

Secondary (Reactive) Lymphocytosis

• Lymphocytosis secondary to a physiologic or pathophysiologic response to infection of B lymphocytes, toxins, cytokines, or unknown factors.

Infectious Mononucleosis

• Caused by Epstein-Barr virus infection.
• Lymphocytosis principally from a polyclonal increase in CD8$^+$ T lymphocytes.
• Characteristic reactive lymphocytes evident on blood film (see **Fig. 50–2**).
• See Chap. 53.

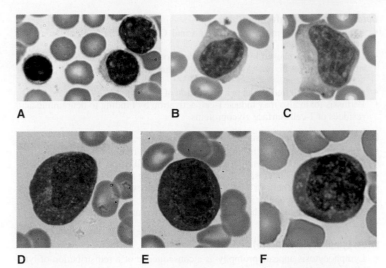

FIGURE 50-2 Blood films. **A.** Acute infectious lymphocytosis. The lymphocytosis in this disorder of childhood is composed of normal appearing lymphocytes, which may vary somewhat in size as shown in the blood of this case. Note typical small lymphocyte with dense chromatin pattern and scant rim of cytoplasm and somewhat two larger lymphocytes with less dense chromatin pattern. **B, C.** Reactive lymphocytes. Large lymphocytes with an increased proportion of cytoplasm with basophilic cytoplasmic edges, often engaging neighboring red cells. Nucleoli may occasionally be evident. This variation in lymphocyte appearance can occur in a variety of disorders that provoke an immunologic response, including viral illnesses. They are indistinguishable in appearance by light microscopy from the reactive lymphocytes seen in infectious mononucleosis, viral hepatitis, or other conditions such as Dengue fever. **D–F.** Plasmacytoid lymphocytes. In this type of reactive lymphocytosis, the lymphocytes are large and have deep blue-colored cytoplasm, approaching the coloration of plasma cell cytoplasm, but they retain the nuclear appearance, cell shape, and cell size of a medium-size lymphocyte, and they do not develop a prominent paranuclear clear zone or markedly eccentric nuclear position as do most plasma cells. They may be seen in a variety of situations including infections, drug hypersensitivity, and serum sickness-type reactions. *(Reproduced with permission from Lichtman's Atlas of Hematology, www.accessmedicine.com.)* (Source: *Williams Hematology,* 8th ed, Chap. 81, Fig. 81–2, p. 1144.)

Lymphocytosis Induced by other Infectious Diseases

- Usually viral (e.g., hepatitis A virus).
- Characterized morphologically by reactive lymphocytes (see Fig. 50–2).

Acute Infectious Lymphocytosis

- Disease of childhood, usually ages 2 to 10 years.
- Characterized by marked lymphocytosis of polyclonal morphologically normal T lymphocytes and NK cells (see Fig. 50–2).
- Infection of unknown etiology, but some cases have been associated with acute infection by coxsackievirus B2, toxoplasmosis, or falciparum malaria.
- Usually asymptomatic, but fever, abdominal pain, or diarrhea may be present for a few days.
- No enlargement of liver or spleen.
- Lymphocytosis usually 20 to 30 × 10^9/L but as high as 100 × 10^9/L.
- Lymphocytosis may persist for several weeks after clinical symptoms have subsided.
- Marrow shows variable increase in number of lymphocytes.
- Serum negative for heterophil antibodies.

Bordetella pertussis Infection

- Lymphocytosis of morphologically normal $CD4^+$ T cells, ranging from 8 to 70×10^9/L.
- Lymphocytosis caused by failure of lymphocytes to leave the blood because of pertussis toxin, an ADP-ribosylase that inhibits chemokine receptor signaling.
- Characteristic clefted nuclei in a proportion of lymphocytes usually evident.
- Pertussis toxin also may induce T-cell activation by binding to neuraminic acid residues of T-cell–surface glycoproteins.

Large Granular Lymphocytosis

- Can result from increase in NK cells, $CD8^+$ cells or, rarely, $CD4^+$ cells.
- Most common form is result of expansion of CD3-CD16+CD56+ NK cells.
- Termed NK lymphocytosis, NK cell counts, ranging from 4 to 15×10^9/L.
- Expansion of NK cells or T cells may represent an exaggerated response to systematic infections and/or immune deregulation.
- May be associated with rheumatoid arthritis (less than 1.0% of cases).
- See Chap. 58.

Stress Lymphocytosis (Acute)

- Lymphocytosis appears promptly as a consequence of a redistribution of lymphocytes induced by adrenaline.
- Lymphocytosis, often greater than 5×10^9/L, reverts to normal or low levels within hours.
- May be associated with trauma, surgery, acute cardiac failure, septic shock, myocardial infarction, sickle cell crisis, or status epilepticus.

Hypersensitivity Reactions

- Reactions to insect bites may be associated with a large granular lymphocytic lymphocytosis and lymphadenopathy.

Persistent Chronic Polyclonal Lymphocytosis

- Cancer:
  - Solid tumors.
  - Thymoma, probably a result of release of thymic hormones by neoplastic thymic epithelium.
- Postsplenectomy lymphocytosis.
  - Can persist for prolonged periods after splenectomy (e.g., > 50 months).
- Chronic inflammatory diseases:
  - In systemic diseases associated with inflammation; e.g., sarcoidosis, Wegener granulomatosis.
- Autoimmune diseases, e.g., rheumatoid arthritis.
  - In rheumatoid arthritis patients with Felty syndrome (associated neutropenia), it is important to rule out T-cell large granular lymphocytic leukemia (see Chap. 58).
- Cigarette smoking:
  - In smokers, a polyclonal increase in CD4 T cells and in B cells (some binuclear) may occur, especially in HLA-DR7-positive women.
  - Lymphocytosis may resolve upon cessation of smoking.

LYMPHOCYTOPENIA

Definition

- Absolute lymphocyte count is less than 1.0×10^9/L.
- Usually caused by a decrease in CD4+ (helper) T cells because this cell type accounts for about half of all blood lymphocytes.
- Table 50–2 lists the conditions associated with lymphocytopenia.

Inherited Causes

- Stem cell abnormality, either quantitative or qualitative, resulting in ineffective lymphopoiesis (see Chap. 51).
- Other abnormalities, such as the Wiskott-Aldrich syndrome, result in premature destruction of T cells because of cytoskeletal abnormalities (see Chap. 51).

Acquired Lymphocytopenia

Infectious Diseases

- AIDS; destruction of CD4$^+$ T cells infected with HIV-1 or HIV-2 (see Chap. 52).
- Other viral diseases such as influenza.

TABLE 50–2   CAUSES OF LYMPHOCYTOPENIA

I. Inherited causes
  A. Congenital immunodeficiency diseases (Chap. 51)
    1. Severe combined immunodeficiency disease
      a. Aplasia of lymphopoietic progenitor cells
      b. Adenosine deaminase deficiency
      c. Absence of histocompatibility antigens
      d. Absence of CD4+ helper cells
      e. Thymic alymphoplasia with aleukocytosis (reticular dysgenesis)
      f. Mutations in genes required for T-cell development
    2. Common variable immune deficiency
    3. Ataxia-telangiectasia
    4. Wiskott-Aldrich syndrome
    5. Immunodeficiency with short-limbed dwarfism (cartilage-hair hypoplasia)
    6. Immunodeficiency with thymoma
    7. Purine nucleoside phosphorylase deficiency
    8. Immunodeficiency with veno-occlusive disease of the liver
  B. Lymphopenia resulting from genetic polymorphism
II. Acquired causes
  A. Aplastic anemia (Chap. 3)
  B. Infectious diseases
    1. Viral diseases
      a. Acquired immunodeficiency syndrome (Chap. 52)
      b. Severe acute respiratory syndrome
      c. West Nile encephalitis
      d. Hepatitis
      e. Influenza
      f. Herpes simplex virus
      g. Herpes virus type 6 (HHV-6)
      h. Herpes virus type 8 (HHV-8)
      i. Measles virus
      j. Other
    2. Bacterial diseases
      a. Tuberculosis
      b. Typhoid fever
      c. Pneumonia
      d. Rickettsiosis
      e. Ehrlichiosis
      f. Sepsis
    3. Parasitic diseases
      a. Acute phase of malaria infection

(Continue)

TABLE 50–2   CONTINUED

  C. Iatrogenic
    1. Immunosuppressive agents
      a. Antilymphocyte globulin therapy
      b. Alemtuzumab (CAMPATH 1-H)
      c. Glucocorticoids
    2. High-dose psoralen plus ultraviolet A treatment
    3. Stevens-Johnson syndrome
    4. Chemotherapy
    5. Platelet or stem cell apheresis procedures
    6. Radiation
    7. Major surgery
    8. Extracorporeal bypass circulation
    9. Renal or marrow transplant
    10. Thoracic duct drainage
    11. Hemodialysis
    12. Apheresis for donor lymphocyte infusion
  D. Systemic disease associated
    1. Autoimmune diseases
      a. Arthritis
      b. Systemic lupus erythematosus
      c. Sjögren syndrome
      d. Myasthenia gravis
      e. Systemic vasculitis
      f. Behçet-like syndrome
      g. Dermatomyositis
      h. Wegener granulomatosis
    2. Hodgkin lymphoma (Chap. 59)
    3. Carcinoma
    4. Primary myelofibrosis
    5. Protein-losing enteropathy
    6. Renal failure
    7. Sarcoidosis
    8. Thermal injury
    9. Severe acute pancreatitis
    10. Strenuous exercise
    11. Silicosis
    12. Celiac disease
  E. Nutritional and dietary
    1. Ethanol abuse
    2. Zinc deficiency
 III. Idiopathic
  A. Idiopathic CD4+ T lymphocytopenia

Source: *Williams Hematology,* 8th ed, Table 81–2, p. 1146.

- Active tuberculosis; lymphocytopenia usually resolves 2 weeks after initiating appropriate therapy.

Iatrogenic
- Radiotherapy, chemotherapy, administration of antilymphocyte globulin or alemtuzumab (CAMPATH-1H).
- Treatment of psoriasis with psoralen and ultraviolet A irradiation may result in T-lymphocyte lymphopenia.
- Glucocorticoid therapy. Mechanism unclear, possibly redistribution as well as cell destruction.

- Major surgery. Mechanism may be redistribution of lymphocytes.
- Thoracic duct drainage. Lymphocytes are removed from the body.
- Platelet apheresis. Lymphocytes, as well as platelets, are removed from the body, resulting in transient lymphopenia.

Systemic Disease Associated with Lymphocytopenia

- Systemic lupus erythematosus. Probably mediated by autoantibodies.
- Sarcoidosis. Probably a consequence of impaired T-cell proliferation.
- Protein-losing enteropathy. Lymphocytes may be lost from the body.

Burns

- Profound T-cell lymphocytopenia caused by redistribution from blood to tissues.

Nutritional/Dietary Factors

- Zinc deficiency. Zinc is necessary for normal T-cell development and function.
- Excess alcohol intake may impair lymphocytic proliferation.

Idiopathic CD4$^+$ T Lymphocytopenia

- Defined as a CD4$^+$ T-lymphocyte count less than 3×10^8/L on two separate occasions without serologic or virologic evidence of HIV-1 or HIV-2 infection.
- Congenital immunodeficiency diseases, such as common variable immunodeficiency, should be excluded (see Chap. 51).
- Decrease of CD4$^+$ cell counts is generally gradual.
- More than half of reported cases had opportunistic infections indicative of cellular immune deficiency (e.g., *Pneumocystis jiroveci* pneumonia). Such patients are classified as having idiopathic CD4$^+$ T-lymphocytopenia and severe unexplained HIV-seronegative immune suppression. In contrast to patients infected with HIV, these patients generally have stable CD4$^+$ counts over time and reductions in other lymphocyte subgroups, and may experience complete or partial spontaneous reversal of the CD4$^+$ T lymphocytopenia.

For a more detailed discussion, see Thomas J. Kipps: Lymphocytosis and Lymphocytopenia. Chap. 81, p.1141 in *Williams Hematology*, 8th ed.

CHAPTER 51
Primary Immunodeficiency Syndrome

- Primary immune deficiency diseases (PIDDs) are characterized by increased susceptibility to infections and are determined by the failure of either the humoral or cellular arms of the immune system or both.
- The clinical features of PIDDs are listed in Table 51–1.
  — Characterized, principally by recurrent pyogenic bacterial infections, including sinusitis, furunculosis, and recurrent or chronic pneumonias that often terminate in bronchiectasis. These infections are initially responsive to antibiotics but soon relapse.
- Evaluation of serum immunoglobulin (Ig) levels and specific antibody responses in patients with recurring infections without an apparent predisposing cause should be made.
  — Baseline Ig levels are often low or virtually absent.
  — Antibody response to immunization is often inadequate.
- Abnormality of cellular immunity causes:
  — Susceptibility to viral, protozoal, and fungal infections.
  — Patients are often anergic. Rejection or clearance of allogeneic cells may be impaired.
  — There may be a secondary defect in humoral immunity because of T-cell dysfunction and loss of B-cell helper activity.
- Autoimmune diseases such as immune-mediated hemolytic anemia, thrombocytopenia, or rheumatoid arthritis-like conditions occur at a higher frequency in certain primary immunodeficiency states.
- The more severe primary immune deficiencies are usually present in infancy, although common variable immunodeficiency (CVID) often presents later in life.
- In Ig-deficient patients, treatment with intravenous immunoglobulin (IVIG) may decrease infectious events.
- The autosomal recessive syndromes are frequently the result of consanguineous marriages.

PREDOMINANT ANTIBODY DEFICENCIES

X-Linked and Autosomal Recessive Agammaglobulinemia
Definition and Genetic Features
- Caused by maturation defect in B-cell development.
- X-linked agammaglobulinemia is the result of a mutation in the Bruton tyrosine kinase (*BTK*) gene.
- Autosomal recessive agammaglobulinemia is the result of mutations in genes relevant to immunoglobulin heavy or light chains, i.e., *IGHM, IGLL1, CD79a, CD79b* or the B-cell adaptor molecule, *BLINK*.

Clinical Features
- X-linked and autosomal recessive agammaglobulinemia have similar clinical features: low Ig levels, decreased B cells, and recurrent infections.
- Normal levels of IgG at birth as a result of transfer from maternal circulation. Thus, usually asymptomatic for the first few months of life.
- Symptoms and signs vary and may be mild or severe (see Table 51–1). First develop between 4 and 12 months of age. First signs of the disease may not be apparent for several years in some patients.

TABLE 51–1	**CLINICAL FEATURES OF PRIMARY IMMUNODEFICIENCY DISORDERS**		
Neutrophils numerical or functional defects	Complement deficiencies	Antibody deficiencies	Combined immune deficiencies
Severe bacterial and fungal infections Skin or deep bacterial and fungal abscesses Infections sustained by unusual bacteria and fungi	Recurrent or severe infections sustained by encapsulated pathogens Recurrent *Neisseria meningitidis* infections Autoimmune manifestations (SLE-like) Atypical hemolytic uremic syndrome Recurrent angioedema (C1-INH deficiency)	Recurrent infections after 4–6 months of age Intestinal *Giardia lamblia* infection Enterovirus meningoencephalitis	Early-onset respiratory and gut infections Opportunistic infections Growth failure Persistent candidiasis Erythroderma

SLE, systemic lupus erythematosus.
Source: *Williams Hematology*, 8th ed, Chap. 82, Table 82–1, p. 1154.

- Otitis media, sinusitis, pyoderma, diarrhea are most frequent presenting findings.
- Pneumonia, meningitis, septicemia, osteomyelitis, and septic arthritis may occur later.
- Neutropenia may accompany X-linked agammaglobulinemia and increase the risk of recurrent or chronic infections.
- Most common pathogens: *Haemophilus influenzae*, *Streptococcus pneumoniae*, and *Staphylococcus aureus*.
- The response to many viral infections is often normal but usually susceptible to echovirus and coxsackie virus presenting as meningoencephalitis, dermatomyositis, or hepatitis. They are also unusually susceptible to poliovirus. Attenuated live polio vaccine can cause severe morbidity and mortality once maternal antibodies have disappeared.
- Gastroenteritis caused by *Giardia lamblia*, *Campylobacter* species, or rotavirus is common and may be associated with malabsorption.
- Patients have an increased incidence of aggressive rectosigmoid carcinoma.

Laboratory Features
- Reduced level of serum Ig is the hallmark; B cells are less than 1 percent of normal (tonsils are absent).
- B cell maturation arrest prevents plasma cell development and these cells are absent from marrow, gastrointestinal tract, and lymph nodes.
- Specific antibodies are also reduced or absent (Table 51–2).
- Flow cytometry can be used to measure the BTK protein in normal monocytes or platelets and female carriers can be identified.

TABLE 51–2 COMMON PRIMARY IMMUNODEFICIENCIES: LABORATORY AND CLINICAL FEATURES

	Lymphocytes			Cellular Immunity	Humoral Immunity						Common Infections
					Serum Immunoglobulins				Antibody Responses		
	B	T	NK		M	G	A	E			
Predominantly antibody deficiency											
X-linked agammaglobulinemia (BTK)	−	+	+	+	↓	↓	↓	↓	−		Bacteria, *Giardia lamblia*
Autosomal recessive (AR) agammaglobulinemia											
λ5, Igα, Igβ, or BLNK deficiency	−	+	+	+	↓	↓	↓	↓	−		Bacteria
Hypogammaglobulinemia (AR) ICOS, CD19, CD21, BAFF-R	−	+	+	+	↓	↓	↓	↓	−		Bacteria
Transient hypogammaglobulinemia of infancy	+	+	+	+	N/↓	N/↓	N/↓	N/↓	+/−		Bacteria
Selective IgA deficiency	+	+	+	+	N	N	↓	N	+/−		Bacteria, *G. lamblia*
Common variable immune deficiency	+	+	+	+	N/↓	↓	↓	↓	−		Bacteria, *G. lamblia*
IgG subclass deficiencies	+	+	+	+	N	N/↓	N/↓	N	+/−		Bacteria
Hyper-IgM syndrome											
Activation-induced cytidine deaminase deficiency	+	+	+	+	N/↑	↓	↓	↓	+/−		Bacteria
Uracil-DNA glycosylase deficiency	+	+	+	+	N/↑	↓	↓	↓	+/−		Bacteria
X-linked CD40 ligand deficiency	+	+	+	+	N/↑	↓	N/↓	↓	+/−		Bacteria, viruses, fungi
CD40 deficiency	+	+	+	+	N/↑	↓	N/↓	↓	+/−		Bacteria, viruses, fungi
X-linked IKK-γ (NEMO) deficiency	+	+	+	+	N/↑	↓	↓	↓	+/−		Bacteria, viruses, fungi
Severe combined immunodeficiency (SCID)											
Interleukin receptor γ-chain deficiency (X-linked SCID)	+	−	−	−	N	↓	↓	↓	−		Bacteria, viruses, fungi
Janus-associated kinase 3 (JAK3) deficiency	+	−	−	−	N	↓	↓	↓	−		Bacteria, viruses, fungi
Interleukin-7 receptor α-chain deficiency	+	−	−	−	N	↓	↓	↓	−		Bacteria, viruses, fungi

Immunodeficiency	NK	T	B		IgG	IgA	IgM	IgE		Characteristic Infections
Zap-70 tyrosine kinase deficiency	+	+/−	+	−	N	N/↓	N/↓	N/↓	+/−	Bacteria, viruses, fungi
Adenosine deaminase (ADA) deficiency	−	−	−	−	↓	↓	↓	↓	−	Bacteria, viruses, fungi
Purine nucleotide phosphorylase (PNP) deficiency	+	−	+	−	N	↓	↓	↓	+/−	Bacteria, viruses, fungi
Recombinase activating gene (RAG 1/2) deficiency	−	−	+	−	↓	↓	↓	↓	−	Bacteria, viruses, fungi
Artemis deficiency	−	−	+	−	↓	↓	↓	↓	−	Bacteria, viruses, fungi
Reticular dysgenesis (AK2 deficiency)	−	−	−	−	↓	↓	↓	↓	−	Bacteria, viruses, fungi
Primary T-cell deficiency										
Congenital thymic aplasia (DiGeorge syndrome)	+	−	+	−	N	N	N	N	+/−	Bacteria, viruses, fungi
Major histocompatibility complex (MHC) class II deficiency	+	+/−	+	+	N	N	N	↓	+/−	Bacteria, viruses, fungi
Transport-associated protein (TAP)-1 or TAP-2 deficiency (MHC class I deficiency)	+	+/−	+	−	N	N	N	N	+	Bacteria, viruses, fungi
Th1 deficiency										
Interferon-γ and interferon-γ receptor deficiency	−	+	+	+	N	N	N	N	+	Mycobacteria, *Salmonella*
Interleukin-12 and interleukin-12 receptor deficiency	−	+	+	+	N	N	N	N	+	Mycobacteria, *Salmonella*
Other well-defined immunodeficiency syndromes										
Ataxia-telangiectasia	+	+	+	+	N/↑	N/↓	N/↓	N/↓	+/−	Bacteria
Wiskott-Aldrich syndrome	+	+/−	+	+/−	↓	N	↑	N/↓	+/−	Bacteria

*Natural killer lymphocytes (NK), T cells (T), B cells (B).

Normal levels (+), reduced or absent levels (−); normal (N), elevated (↑), or reduced (↓) serum immunoglobulins.

Source: *Williams Hematology*; 8th ed, Chap. 82, Table 82–2, p. 1155.

- Analysis of mutations in the *BTK* gene can be used to make the diagnosis and to identify affected males *in utero*.

Treatment

- Treatment with intravenous IVIG: pooled plasma-derived preparation that contains IgG and IgA.
- Individualized doses that usually start at 400 to 600 mg/kg intravenously every 4 weeks.
- Prophylactic antibiotic therapy may be useful in certain circumstances, such as patients with chronic lung disease.

Course

- Treatment with IVIG markedly decreases enteroviral infections but some patients develop neurodegenerative disease or chronic ileitis (Crohn-like disease) despite treatment and without evidence of an infectious etiology.

Hyperimmunoglobulin M Syndromes
Definition and Genetics Abnormalities

- Characterized by recurrent infections associated with low serum levels of IgG, IgA, and IgE but normal or increased levels of IgM.
- Mutations affect genes involved in B-cell activation, class switch recombination (*CSR*), and somatic hypermutation (*SHM*).
- Mutations occur in genes encoding enzymes intrinsic to B cells, i.e., *AID*, *UNG*, and the *NEMO* gene, the latter crucial for nuclear factor-κB activation.

X-Linked Hyper-IgM as a Result of CD40L Deficiency

- Caused by mutations in *CD40L* distributed throughout the gene resulting in nonfunctional CD40L protein.
- Normally, CD40L on surface of CD4+ T lymphocytes interacts with CD40 expressed constituently on B lymphocytes.

Clinical Features

- Characterized by recurrent bacterial infections in infants. Often presents with interstitial pneumonia caused by *Pneumocystis jiroveci*.
- Fifty percent of affected males also develop neutropenia.
- High risk of developing chronic *Cryptosporidium* infections complicated by ascending cholangiolitis and chronic liver disease.
- Progressive neurodegeneration, as in X-linked agammaglobulinemia, can occur.

Laboratory Features

- Normal blood B cell subsets but B cells are naïve.
- Defective lymph node germinal center development and severe deficiency in follicular dendritic cells.
- Response to specific antigens reduced (see Table 51–2).
- Mild cases left untreated can lead to red cell aplasia as a result of chronic parvovirus B19 infection.

Treatment

- During infancy, treat with trimethoprim-sulfamethoxazole to prevent *P. jiroveci* pneumonia.
- IVIG doses are similar to X-linked agammaglobulinemia to prevent chronic infections including parvovirus.
- Allogeneic hematopoietic stem cell transplantation should be considered if an appropriate donor can be identified.
- Treat severe and persistent neutropenia with G-CSF.

Autosomal Recessive Hyper-IgM with CD40 Mutations

- Similar clinical features to those with CD40L mutations.

Autosomal Recessive Hyper-IgM Syndrome Caused by an Intrinsic Defect
- Mutations of the activation-induced cytidine deaminase gene (*AID*).
- Because of mild phenotype, often discovered later in life.

Clinical Features
- Recurrent bacterial infections that affect upper and lower respiratory tract.
- Enlarged tonsils and lymph nodes from marked follicular hyperplasia.
- T- and B-cell subset are normal but all $CD27^+$ memory B cells fail to switch isotypes and express IgM and IgD.
- Treatment with IVIG prophylaxis often associated with excellent long-term prognosis.

X-linked Anhydrotic Ectodermal Dysplasia with Immunodeficiency Caused by Mutations of NEMO
- Characterized by partial or complete absence of sweat glands, sparse hair growth, and abnormal dentition.
- Most patients present with bacterial infections, especially *S. pneumoniae S. aureus*, and atypical mycobacteria; 20 percent of infections are caused by viral infections.
- Approximately 20 percent of patients develop inflammatory bowel disease.
- Treatment with IVIG is useful but does not prevent the occurrence of serious complications.

Common Variable Immunodeficiency and Selective IgA Deficiency
- CVID is heterogeneous and may present at any age but usually occurs during adulthood.
- Characterized by hypogammaglobulinemia, impaired antibody responses, and recurrent bacterial infections.
- In conjunction with selective IgA deficiency, most common primary immunodeficiency syndrome.
- Selective IgA deficiency may be the initial presenting finding in later CVID.
- Familial concordance in approximately 20 percent of cases and CVID and IgA deficiency can occur in the same family.

Clinical Features and Treatment of CVID
- Characterized by recurring sinopulmonary infections and bacterial pneumonia.
- If untreated, may lead to bronchiectasis and chronic lung disease.
- Lymphadenopathy and splenomegaly are common.
- Caseating granuloma of lung, spleen, liver, skin, and other tissues are damaging to organ function.
- Frequent gastrointestinal complaints. Lymphoid hyperplasia of the small bowel results in a syndrome mimicking chronic inflammatory bowel disease.
- Bowel disease associated with *G. lambia* or *Campylobacter* infections.
- Autoimmune disorders are common and may resemble rheumatoid arthritis, dermatomyositis, or scleroderma.
- May develop autoimmune hemolytic anemia, autoimmune thrombocytopenia purpura, autoimmune neutropenia, pernicious anemia, and chronic active hepatitis.
- Despite normal B-lymphocyte levels and lymph node cortical follicles, patients have agammaglobulinemia that may be profound.
- Uncommonly, patients may have an associated thymoma.

Treatment and Course
- IVIG infusions and prophylactic antibiotics are beneficial but often insufficient to prevent serious complications.
- There is a marked increase in the risk of lymphoma, gastrointestinal cancers, and a variety of other cancers.

- Allogeneic hematopoietic stem cell transplantation is not recommended unless used to treat a secondary lymphoma.

Clinical Features and Treatment of Selective IgA Deficiency

- Characterized by less than 10 mg/dL of IgA.
- Differs greatly between ethnic groups: Highest frequency in Scandinavia and lowest in Asian populations.
- Fundamental defect is the failure of IgA-bearing B lymphocytes to mature into IgA-secreting plasma cells.
- Most persons remain healthy.
- If disease signs occur, they include recurrent sinopulmonary infections and atopic symptoms including allergic conjunctivitis, rhinitis, and eczema. Food allergies are common, and asthma is more refractory to symptomatic treatment.
- Symptomatic individuals have concomitant deficiency in IgG_2 and IgG_3 and poor responses to polysaccharide antigens.
- Chronic giardiasis, malabsorption, celiac disease, primary biliary cirrhosis, and pernicious anemia can occur.
- Higher incidence of rheumatoid arthritis, myasthenia gravis, thyroiditis, and systemic lupus erythematosus.
- No specific treatment is available.
- In patients with chronic pulmonary disease, selective prophylactic antibiotic therapy may be useful and where a defect in response to polysaccharide antigens is suspected or measured, prophylactic IVIG can be beneficial.

SEVERE COMBINED IMMUNODEFICIENCIES

Definition and History

- Heterogeneous group of genetic disorders that is characterized invariably by a severe impairment of T-lymphocyte development and function and a variable defect in either B or NK cells or both (see Fig. 51–1).

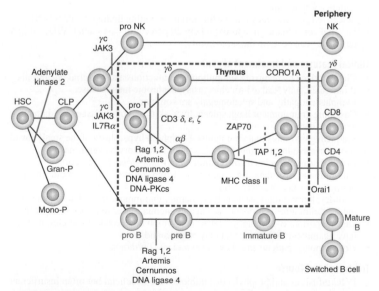

FIGURES 51-1 Disruption of the normal T-cell development by mutations of genes known to cause a severe combined immunodeficiency syndrome.
(*Source: Williams Hematology*, 8th ed, Chap. 82, Fig. 82–1, p. 1157.)

- Severe combined immunodeficiency (SCID) can be classified into four groups based on the associated immune cell deficiencies:
  — T−B+NK− SCID (Most common type)
  — T−B+NK+ SCID
  — T−B−NK+ SCID
  — T−B−NK− SCID
- Incidence rate is 1 in 50,000 births.
- Most common form is inherited as an X-linked trait.
- Reconstitution of a functioning immune system by transplantation of histocompatible allogeneic lymphohematopoietic stem cells may be lifesaving.

Molecular Defects and Pathogenesis of SCID

Resulting from Increased Apoptosis of Lymphocyte Progenitors

- Adenosine deaminase (ADA) deficiency:
  — Inherited as an autosomal recessive trait.
  — Characterized by the virtual absence of T lymphocytes as a result of absence of ADA resultant high intracellular levels of adenosine and deoxyadenosine and phosphorylated metabolites result in T-cell progenitor apoptosis.
  — Reduction in number of B cells, also.
- Purine nucleoside phosphorylase (PNP) deficiency
  — High levels of deoxyguanosine triphosphate cause destruction of immature thymocytes and neuronal toxicity.
  — Characterized by decreased T-cell counts. B and NK cells unaffected.
- Adenylate kinase 2 deficiency
  — Originally termed *reticular dysgenesis*. So named because absence of cells in lymphohematopoietic organs left a background of reticular cells and fibers and the inference was drawn, erroneously, that this stroma could not support immune and blood cell development.
  — Autosomal recessive SCID characterized by extreme lymphopenia, absence of neutrophils (loss of G-CSF responsiveness), and sensorineural deafness.
  — Severe sepsis early in infancy.
  — Successful treatment with allogeneic stem cell transplantation indicates it is a cellular and not stromal (reticular cell) disorder.

Result of defective signaling through the T-cell receptor (TCR)

- Defects of IL-7 receptor(R)-mediated signaling abrogate development of T cells and defects in IL-15R signaling affect development of NK cells resulting in SCID type T-B+NK-.
- X-linked *IL2Rγ* gene mutations account for 40 percent of all SCID cases and result in lack of T and NK cells (T-B+NK-). However, B-cell function is impaired by failure of T helper function and a non-functional common gamma chain shared by several other key interleukin receptors (e.g., 2R, 4R, 9R,15R, and 21R).
- JAK3 deficiency is an autosomal recessive disorder with a phenotype identical to X-linked SCID type T-B+NK-.
- Defects in V(D) J recombination affect both T and B cell development and causes T-B-NK+ SCID.
- RAG1 and RAG2 deficiencies causes T-B-NK+ SCID and account for 10 percent of all SCID cases.
- Defects of the CD3, δ, ε, or ζ chains affect signaling through the TCR and cause T-B+NK+ SCID.

Clinical Features of SCID

- Characterized by *P. jiroveci* pneumonia, cytomegalovirus (CMV), adenovirus, parainfluenza 2 virus, respiratory syncytial virus, chronic diarrhea, failure to thrive, and persistent candidiasis.

- Infections develop in first months of life.
- Hypoplastic lymphoid tissue (atrophic tonsils and lymph nodes).
- Absence of thymic shadow on chest radiograph.

Laboratory Features of SCID
- Lymphocyte count usually less than 2.0×10^9/L.
- In infants, marked blood T-cell deficiency. Blood CD3+ cells should be determined.
- Maternal T-cell engraftment and "leaky" SCID characterized by expression of CD45RA+ whereas infants T cells are CD45RA naïve and fail to respond to mitogens *in vitro*.
- Ig levels low in infants.
- Eosinophilia and elevated levels of IgE.
- Marrow abnormalities observed in ADA, PNP, XLF, and LIG4 deficiencies.
- ADA and PNP deficiency-related SCID, elevated levels of deoxyadenosine triphosphate, and deoxyguanosine triphosphate, respectively in red cells.

Therapy, Course, and Prognosis of SCID
- Fatal if untreated.
- High-dose intravenous sulfamethoxazole/trimethoprim (20 mg/kg) is effective in treating *P. jiroveci* pneumonia.
- CMV should be treated with ganciclovir.
- Adenoviral infections should be treated with cidofovir.
- IVIG and antimicrobial prophylaxis should be administered to reduce risk of infections.
- Survival is dependent on immune reconstitution by allogeneic hematopoietic stem cell transplantation.
- Enzyme replacement has benefited SCID patients with ADA deficiency and gene therapy has been successful in that variant of SCID without adverse events (e.g., acute leukemia from insertional mutagenesis).

OTHER COMBINED IMMUNODEFICIENCIES

Omenn Syndrome
- Mutations in *RAG1* and *RAG2* most common, which restrict T-cell maturation and function. For example, negative selection of autoreactive T cells is reduced and regulator T cell development is impaired.

Clinical Findings
- Severe infections.
- Early onset, diffuse rash, or generalized erythroderma.
- Alopecia.
- Lymphadenopathy and hepatosplenomegaly.
- A pattern of congenital anomalies occurs together more frequently than one would expect on the basis of chance.

Laboratory Findings
- Leukocytosis with eosinophilia.
- Hypoproteinemia with edema.
- Oligoclonal expansion of anergic, activated T lymphocytes that infiltrate and damage target tissues.
- Decreased serum IgG, M, and A levels, but elevated IgE.
- Distribution of blood CD4 and CD8 lymphocyte subsets are skewed.
- Lymphocyte production of IL-4 and IL-5 increased.
- Lymphocyte response to antigens nonexistent and response to mitogens is varied.
- Blood B and NK cell counts are abnormal in some patients.

Treatment
- Optimal approach is allogeneic hematopoietic stem cell transplantation.
- Patients require aggressive nutritional support, correction of hypoproteinemia, and treatment or prevention of infections with antibiotics, antifungals, and serum immunoglobulin replacement.
- Careful use of immunosuppression with glucocorticoids or cyclosporine A may mitigate T-cell induced tissue damage.

ZAP-70 Deficiency
- Form of SCID resulting from the inability to support positive selection of CD8+ lymphocytes in the thymus.

Clinical Features
- Severe infections.
- Palpable lymph nodes and thymic shadow is visible on the chest radiograph.
- CD8+ T cells reduced, but absolute lymphocyte count is normal.
- Response to mitogens *in vitro* reduced indicating CD4+ lymphocytes defective.
- Some, but not all patients, have severe hypogammaglobulinemia.

Treatment
- Optimal approach is allogeneic hematopoietic stem cell transplantation.

MHC Class I Deficiency
- Characterized by reduced expression of MHC class I molecules at the cell surface.
- Autosomal recessive trait, may be caused by mutations in *TAP1*, *TAP2,* or Tapasin genes, which defects interfere with intracellular transport of antigens and their loading onto MHC class I molecules and cell surface expression of the MHC complex.

Clinical Findings
- Low levels of CB8+ T cells and Ig levels are variable.
- Recurrent respiratory infections in children.
- Chronic inflammatory lung disease and skin lesions in patients with *TAP1* and *TAP2* deficiencies.
- Chronic lung disease is usually the cause of death.

Treatment
- Prophylactic and therapeutic measures used for cystic fibrosis are beneficial. Maintaining liquid pulmonary secretions, appropriate antibiotic use.

MHC Class II Deficiency
- Autosomal recessive inheritance.
- Characterized by lack of MHC class II expression.
- Found in North African populations.
- Four gene mutations are known: *CIITA, RFXANK, RFX5*, and *RFXAP.*
- These mutations encode defective transcription factors that normally control MHC class II antigen expression by binding to the proximal promoters of the MHC class II gene.

Clinical Features
- Blood CD4+ T cell count is reduced.
- Severe lung infections.
- Chronic diarrhea.
- Sclerosing cholangitis, often secondary to *Cryptosporidium* or CMV infection.

Treatment and Course
- Poor prognosis.
- Respiratory infections are predominant cause of death.
- Nutritional support is often needed and antibiotic prophylaxis and immunoglobulin replacement therapy are required, but with marginal impact on long-term prognosis.
- May be treated with allogeneic hematopoietic stem cell transplantation but overall results are unsatisfactory. Severe graft-versus-host disease is common.

Coronin-1A Deficiency
- Characterized by mutations affecting both alleles of the *CORO1A* gene, an actin regulator expressed principally in hematopoietic cells.
- Regulates release of T lymphocytes from thymus and trafficking of naïve T cells.
- Characteristic finding is T-cell lymphopenia with normal numbers of B and NK cells.
- Treatment by allogeneic hematopoietic stem cell transplantation is best approach if a donor available.

Signal Transducers and Activator 5b (STAT5b) Deficiency
- Autosomal recessive disease characterized by the association of growth hormone insensitivity and a highly variable degree of immune deficiency.
- Results in impaired transcriptions of genes involved in immune system function and other non-immune related genes.

Clinical Features
- Short stature in the face of normal or elevated levels of growth hormone but insulin growth factor is very low.
- Pulmonary infections including *P. jiroveci* pneumonia.
- Increased susceptibility to severe viral diseases.
- Lung fibrosis.
- Failure to respond to growth hormone replacement therapy.
- Glucocorticoids may be beneficial if there is evidence of lung fibrosis.

Ca^{2+} Entry Channel Deficiency
- Autosomal recessive disorder.
- Mutations of both *ORAI1* and *STIM1* genes, the products of which regulate the function of calcium channels in the cell membrane and endoplasmic reticulum, respectively.
- Clinical features resemble SCID.
- Additional features include nonprogressive myopathy, ectodermal dysplasia, hepatosplenomegaly, hemolytic anemia, and thrombocytopenia.
- In spite of hypergammaglobulinemia, specific antibody responses are defective and T cells do not respond to mitogens in part as a result of failure of calcium influx after stimulation.
- Allogeneic hematopoietic stem cell transplantation can correct the defect.

DEFECTIVE THYMIC DEVELOPMENT

DiGeorge Syndrome
- Developmental disorder caused by abnormal cephalic neural crest migration and differentiation in the third and fourth pharyngeal arches during embryonic development.
- Approximately 75 percent of persons with this phenotype have a deletion at band q11.2 on chromosome 22 (referred to as 22q11.2 deletion syndrome).

Clinical and Laboratory Features

- Phenotype varies but classically has the triad of (1) congenital cardiac defects, (2) hypocalcemia as a result of parathyroid insufficiency, and (3) immune deficiency as a consequence of aplasia or hypoplasia of the thymus.
- Fifty to 80 percent develop cardiac defects; 50 to 60 percent develop hypocalcemia.
- Mild to moderate immune deficiency involving T-cell maturation and function with T-cell numbers often less than 1.5×10^9/L.
- High incidence of autoimmune diseases, such as rheumatoid arthritis and thyroiditis.
- As young adults, develop social, behavioral, and psychiatric problems.
- Those with profound T-cell deficiency may develop B-cell lymphomas.
- If suspected, fluorescence *in situ* hybridization can be used to detect 22q11.2 deletion.

Treatment

- Cardiac defects and hypocalcemia require immediate attention.
- Patients may require antibiotic prophylaxis, IVIG therapy, and if T-cell function is absent, immune reconstitution by allogeneic hematopoietic stem cell transplantation if a donor is available.

PRIMARY IMMUNODEFICIENCY DISORDERS PRESENTING AS AUTOIMMUNE DISEASES

- The concept of a link between immune dysregulation and autoimmunity has been strengthened by the discovery of distinct single gene defects resulting in unusual susceptibility to autoimmune diseases.

IPEX Syndrome

- The acronym IPEX derives from the presence of **i**mmune dysregulation, **p**olyendocrinopathy, **e**nteropathy, and an **X**-linked inheritance.
- Characterized by early onset diarrhea secondary to autoimmune enteropathy.
- Multiple endocrinopathies including type 1 diabetes mellitus, thyroiditis, and, rarely, adrenal insufficiency.
- Autoimmune hemolytic anemia, thrombocytopenia, and neutropenia are common complications.
- Eczema or other chronic dermatitis may occur.
- Elevated serum IgA and IgE. Absence of CD4+CD25+FOXP3+regulatory T cells
- Cyclosporine A, tacrolimus, sirolimus, or glucocorticoids can provide temporary amelioration.

APECED Syndrome

- The acronym APECED derives from the presence of **a**utoimmune **p**olyendocrinopathy, **c**andidiasis, and **e**ctodermal **d**ystrophy.
- Autosomal recessive disorder also known as autoimmune polyglandular syndrome (APS) type I.
- Results from mutations in the *AIRE* gene, which causes a decrease in the expression of tissue restricted antigens, failure of negative selection of autoreactive T cells in the thymus, and a resultant release of autoreactive T cell clones to peripheral lymphatic tissues.
- Found in isolated populations such as Finns, Iranian Jews, and Sardinians.
- Patients present with chronic mucocutaneous candidiasis and endocrinopathies, predominantly involving the parathyroid and adrenal glands, less frequently the thyroid and the pancreas.
- Associated with ectodermal manifestations, such as dystrophic finger nails and dental enamel.

Autoimmune Lymphoproliferative Syndrome

- The acronym ALPS derives from the **a**utoimmune **l**ympho**p**roliferative **s**yndrome.
- Mutations are found in the genes required for "programmed cell death." Fas-mediated apoptosis pathway mutations account for about 85 percent of cases:
  - — Mutations in CD95 (ALPS type Ia)
  - — Mutations in CD95L (ALPS type Ib)
  - — Mutations in caspase 10 or caspase 8 (ALPS type II) (approximately 5% of cases)
  - — No mutations of Fas, FasL, or caspases (ALPS type III) (approximately 10% of cases)
- Phenotype caused by defective apoptosis of lymphocytes, resulting in polyclonal lymphadenopathy, hepatosplenomegaly, and autoimmune disorders, which most commonly include autoimmune hemolytic anemia, thrombocytopenia, and neutropenia.
- Spleen and lymph nodes show pronounced hyperplasia and the T-cell population includes a large proportion of TCRα/β+ CD4-CD8- cells.
- Treatment options include immunosuppressive therapy.
- Splenectomy is recommended in patients with large spleens.
- Long-term prognosis is poor.
- Lymphoma develops in about one of ten patients.

OTHER WELL-DEFINED IMMUNODEFICIENCY DISEASES

Wiskott-Aldrich Syndrome (WAS)

Definition

- X-linked disorder characterized by thrombocytopenia, small platelets, eczema, recurrent infections, immunodeficiency, and a high incidence of autoimmune diseases and malignancies (see Chap. 76).
- Phenotype is associated with null-mutations of the gene that encodes the WAS protein (WASP).
- Milder phenotype is called X-linked thrombocytopenia (XLT).
- Characterized by mild eczema and few problems.

Clinical and Laboratory Features

- Thrombocytopenia in the range of 20 to 60×10^9/L and microplatelets, but normal numbers of marrow megakaryocytes.
- Hemorrhagic manifestations may be mild.
- Classic WAS is characterized by bacterial, fungal, and viral infections.

Treatment

- May require antibiotic prophylaxis and IVIG.
- If autoimmune symptoms arise, immunosuppressive therapy may be required.
- Early allogeneic hematopoietic stem cell transplantation is treatment of choice; outcome is excellent if a matched-related or unrelated donor can be identified.
- Splenectomy ameliorates the bleeding tendency by increasing the number of blood platelets.
- XLT patients often have an excellent prognosis, but may develop complications, including serious bleeding, autoimmune diseases, and malignancies.
- Standard-conditioning for myeloablative transplantation (busulfan, cyclophosphamide, with or without antithymocyte globulin) is required.

The Hyperimmunoglobulin E Syndromes

Autosomal Dominant Hyper-IgE Syndrome (HIES)

- Autosomal dominant or sporadic multisystem immunodeficiency.
- Characterized by eczema, *S. aureus*-induced skin abscesses, recurrent pneumonia with abscess and pneumatocele formation, *Candida* infections, and skeletal and connective tissue abnormalities.

- Serum IgE levels greater than 2000 IU/mL and often much greater.
- Eosinophilia, neutrophil chemotactic defects and decreased lymphocyte proliferation to specific antigens.
- Treatment includes prophylactic antibiotic therapy to decrease the frequency of *S. aureus* pulmonary infections.
- Antifungal therapy is indicated to prevent recurrent *Candida* infections.
- Allogeneic hematopoietic stem cell transplantation has not been of clear benefit in the cases so treated.

Autosomal Recessive Hyper IgE Syndromes

- Characterized by elevated serum levels of IgE, recurrent bacterial, fungal, and viral infections including herpes simplex, therapy-resistant molluscum contagiosum, and recurrent varicella zoster.

Immunoosseous Dysplasias
Cartilage-Hair Hypoplasia

- Autosomal recessive characterized by short-limbed dwarfism, light colored hypoplasic hair, marrow cell dysplasia, Hirschsprung disease, and a variable degree of immunodeficiency from normal to severe, and increased susceptibility to malignancies.
- In the severe cases, allogeneic hematopoietic stem cell can correct the immune abnormalities.

Schimke Syndrome

- The disease is caused by a gene that encodes for a chromatin remodeling protein.
- Autosomal recessive condition characterized by dwarfism, microcephaly, cognitive and motor abnormalities, renal impairment leading to renal failure, facial dimorphisms, marrow failure, premature atherosclerosis, and immunodeficiency ranging from T-cell lymphopenia to SCID.
- Recurrent bacterial, fungal, and viral infections, including with opportunistic organisms occur in over half the patients.
- Combined allogeneic hematopoietic stem cell and renal transplantation has been used with success.

Warts, Hypogammaglobulinemia, Infections, and Myelokathexis Syndrome (WHIMS)

- Autosomal dominant disorder caused by a mutation in CXCL4 that disrupts the chemokine CXCL12 receptor involved in leukocyte trafficking.
- Retention and apoptosis of neutrophils in marrow (myelokathexis) causes severe neutropenia.
- Early onset of recurrent bacterial infections is common.
- Warts resulting from papillomavirus infection develop in second decade of life.
- Hypogammaglobulinemia, lymphopenia, and low B-cell counts are common.
- IVIG replacement therapy and antibiotics as required. Recombinant G-CSF can increase neutrophil count.
- Warts are resistant to local therapy and should be monitored for neoplastic transformation.

CHROMOSOMAL INSTABILITY SYNDROMES ASSOCIATED WITH IMMUNODEFICIENCY

- Characterized by increased spontaneous or induced DNA breaks, susceptibility to infections secondary to immune deficiency, and an increased risk of malignancies.
- Genes responsible for these diseases protect human genome integrity by contributing to the complex task of double-strand break repair

Ataxia-Telangiectasia (AT)

- A multisystem disorder, characterized by immunodeficiency, progressive neurologic impairment, and ocular and cutaneous telangiectasia.
- Immune deficiency is variable and may include cellular and humoral immunity.
- Thymus is small.
- Mutation in *ATM* gene results in inability to repair double-stranded DNA breaks.
- Common to have recurrent respiratory infections that result in chronic lung disease.
- Phenotype is low or absent IgA and IgE and is often combined with IgG_2 and IgG_4 deficiency.
- Clinical manifestations include cerebellar ataxia, which becomes evident when a child begins to walk. Involuntary movements become a handicap and most are wheelchair bound by age 10 years.
- Children do not develop normal speech patterns.
- Cortical cerebellar degeneration involves primarily Purkinje and granular cells; progressive changes to the central nervous system also occur.
- Cytogenetic abnormalities include chromosomal breaks, translocations, rearrangements, and inversions; these defects increase following *in vitro* exposure of cells to radiation.
- Elevation of serum α-fetoprotein is a very common and characteristic laboratory finding.
- Infections and cancer (lymphomas, usually T-cell type (50%), leukemias (25%), and solid tumors (25%) are the most common causes of death.

Ataxia-Telangiectasia-Like Disorder (ATLD)

- Similar clinical features to AT with progressive ataxia but a slower progression of disease.
- Characterized by mutations in the gene encoding the hMre11 protein, part of the DNA repair complex.

Nijmegen Breakage Syndrome (NBS)

- Characterized by short stature, microcephaly, a bird-like face, immunodeficiency, chromosomal instability, increased sensitivity to radiation and radiomimetic drugs (e.g., alkylating agents), and a high likelihood of developing malignancies.
- Absence of telangiectasia formation and of neurodegeneration.
- Development of respiratory infections is common.
- Humoral and cellular immunity is defective.
- Characterized by increased chromatid and chromosome breaks, rearrangements/translocations involving chromosomes 7 and 14, telomere fusions, radioresistant DNA synthesis, and hypersensitivity to radiation.
- High incidence of lymphoid malignancies and certain solid tumors (e.g., rhabdomyosarcoma).
- Prophylactic antibiotics and IVIG for patients with recurrent infections.
- Allogeneic hematopoietic stem cell transplantation has been successful.

Bloom Syndrome (BS)

- Caused by mutation in *BMS* gene that encodes a protein involved in sensing DNA damage and contributes to maintenance of genomic integrity during DNA replication or repair.
- Characterized by short stature, hypersensitivity to sunlight, increased susceptibility to infections, and a predisposition to early development of cancer, e.g., lymphoma and leukemia in first two decades of life and cancer of colon, skin, and breast at a later age.
- Fifty percent of patients develop cancer before the age of 25.

- Confirmed by demonstrating excessive numbers of sister-chromatid exchanges, increased chromatid gaps and breaks, and the presence of quadriradial configuration composed of two homologous chromosomes.
- Patients may benefit from antibiotic prophylaxis and IVIG therapy, if immune deficiency is documented. Because of increased radiation sensitivity, exposure to any form of irradiation should be restricted.

CYTOTOXICITY DISORDERS

Familial Hemophagocytic Lymphohistiocytosis (FHL)

- Characterized by uncontrolled proliferation of activated lymphocytes and histiocytes that secrete large amounts of proinflammatory cytokines (see Chap. 33).

Clinical and Laboratory Features

- Signs and symptoms appear within first year of life.
- Symptoms include high fever, severe hepatosplenomegaly, lymphadenopathy, hemorrhagic manifestations from thrombocytopenia, and edema. Also may have neurologic symptoms.
- Immunologic findings include persistently impaired cytolytic activity of NK cells and elevated levels of inflammatory cytokines (IFN-γ, IL-1, IL-6, tumor necrosis factor-γ) in the blood.
- The diagnosis of FHL forms that are characterized by reduced NK cell degranulation (such as *UNC13D* and *STX11* defects) may be facilitated by the analysis of membrane expression of the lysosomal marker CD107a.
- Without treatment FHL is fatal.
- If disease is active, treatments include antimicrobials, etoposide, immune suppression (antithymocyte globulin), cyclosporine A, and dexamethasone.
- Cure can be achieved by allogeneic hematopoietic stem cell transplantation.

X-Linked Lymphoproliferative Disease (XLP1 and XLP2)

- XLP1 is characterized by mutations in the *SH2D1A* gene that encodes the SLAM-associated protein (SAP) involved in T and NK cell signaling and impair T and NK cell cytotoxicity capability.
- XLP2 is characterized by mutations in the *XIAP* gene and also lack NK and T cells.

Clinical and Laboratory Features

- Fulminant Epstein-Barr virus (EBV) infectious mononucleosis in 60 percent of cases.
- Hypogammaglobulinemia can follow primary EBV infection.
- EBV-related lymphoma in 30 percent of cases (esp. Burkitt lymphoma).
- Flow cytometry can be used to detect lack of SAP protein expression in circulating T and NK lymphocytes.

Treatment and Prognosis

- If untreated, approximately 70 percent of patients die within 10 years of onset.
- Mortality rate is higher (approaches 100%) in patients who have fulminant infectious mononucleosis.
- Treatment of choice is allogeneic hematopoietic stem cell transplantation when performed early in life before EBV infection.
- Nonmyeloablative allogeneic hematopoietic stem cell transplantation may be useful after EBV infection supervenes in patients with severe organ toxicity.
- Use of anti-CD20 monoclonal antibody can reduce EBV load and improve clinical status.
- Igs can be used to reduce the risk of infections in patients with hypogammaglobulinemia.

- Anti-tumor necrosis factor-α therapy or etoposide may be useful in patients with active EBV infection and a severe systemic inflammatory response.

Chediak-Higashi Syndrome

- Autosomal recessive disorder characterized by immune dysregulation with impaired cellular cytotoxicity, partial oculocutaneous albinism, platelet functional abnormalities, and neurologic involvement (see Chap. 33).
- Caused by mutations in the *LYST* gene the encoded protein of which contributes to sorting lysosomal proteins and fusing lysosomal vesicles.
- Common features include bruises and bacterial and viral infections.
- "Accelerated phase" of syndrome is characterized by high fever, hepatosplenomegaly, coagulation abnormalities, increase of liver enzymes and bilirubin (with possible jaundice), edema, and neurologic symptoms.
- Morphologic hallmark of disease: abnormally large granules in lymphocytes, neutrophils, platelets, melanocytes, and neurons.
- Examination of the blood film permits detection of the enlarged and abnormal granules in blood cells.
- Allogeneic hematopoietic stem cell transplantation can ameliorate immune and cellular abnormalities but does not prevent progressive neurologic involvement.

Griscelli Syndrome Type 2 (GS2)

- Autosomal recessive syndrome characterized by immunodeficiency and hypopigmentation. Variable degree of neurologic involvement is also present.
- Caused by mutations in the *RAB27A* gene, which encodes a guanosine triphosphate involved in intracellular transport of granules.
- Susceptible to pyogenic infections.
- "Accelerated phase" of syndrome is characterized by high fever, hepatosplenomegaly, neutropenia, and thrombocytopenia.
- Hypopigmentation is a result of large clumps of melanin in the hair shafts.
- Allogeneic hematopoietic stem cell transplantation can ameliorate the manifestations of the disorder.

Hermansky-Pudlak Type 2

- Caused by mutations of the *AP3B1* gene, which encodes a protein that regulates sorting of lysosomal membrane proteins to the granules.
- Characterized by oculocutaneous albinism, bleeding tendency, recurrent infections, and moderate to severe neutropenia (see Chaps. 32 and 33).
- The bleeding tendency results from decreased platelet dense granules and faulty degranulation.
- Missorting of tyrosinase in melanocytes accounts for albinism.
- Bony anomalies (with dysplastic acetabulae), facial dysmorphism and development of pulmonary fibrosis are features.
- Control of infections is important to manage disease.
- G-CSF may improve chronic neutropenia.

IMMUNODEFICIENCIES WITH SELECTIVE SUSCEPTIBILITY TO PATHOGENS

Toll-Like Receptor (TLR)-Signaling Defects

- Deficiencies of IRAK-4. MyD88, TLR3, and UNC-93B proteins occur.
- Two phenotypes have been identified.
- TLR-signaling defects result in increased susceptibility to herpes simplex virus encephalitis (HSE) associated with mutations have been identified in the *UNC-93B1* gene.
- TLR-signaling defects with increased susceptibility to recurrent, invasive pyogenic infections associated with mutations in IRAK-4 and MyD88.

- Diagnosis can be suspected based on the history of infection associated with poor inflammatory responses.
- Defects involving other microbial pattern-recognition signaling pathways with increased susceptibility to fungal infections.

Mendelian Susceptibility to Mycobacterial Disease

- Defects occur along the JAK-STAT4 pathway.
- IL-12p40 deficiency is characterized increased risk of severe infections due to Calmette-Guerin and environmental mycobacteria.
  — Only genetically-determined cytokine deficiency known in humans.
  — Treatment with antibiotics and interferon-γ.
- IL-12Rβ_1 deficiency is characterized by infections with mycobacteria of low virulence and *Salmonella* species.
  — Treatment with antibiotics and IFN-γ is effective and prognosis is good.
- IFN-γR1 and IFN-γR2 deficiencies produce variable susceptibilities.
  — Persons with complete deficiencies develop severe infections with mycobacteria early in life with lack of granuloma formation.
  — Complete STAT1 deficiency causes increased susceptibility to mycobacterial disease with a severe clinical course.
  — Dominant partial STAT1 deficiency is caused by a heterozygous mutation that allows formation of the IFN-α/β-dependent ISGF3 transcription factor, but abrogates expression of the γ-activating factor, composed of STAT1 homodimers. Affected individuals have either a mild clinical course, characterized by selective susceptibility to mycobacterial infections or are asymptomatic.

GENETICALLY DETERMINED DEFICIENCIES OF THE COMPLEMENT (C) SYSTEM

- Mutations in the classic pathways (C1q, C1r/C1s, C4, C2, and C3) result in pyogenic infections and autoimmune diseases.
- Mutations in the alternative pathway (factors B, D, h, properidin) result in meningococcal and pneumococcal sepsis.
- Mutations in the terminal complement components (C5-C9) result in increased susceptibility to *Neisseria* species infections.
- Mutations in C1 esterase inhibitor (*C1-INH*) gene is the cause of hereditary angioedema.
- Diagnosis of a deficiency assesses the hemolytic function of CH50 and AH50.
  — If CH50 absent and AH50 normal, may be a C1, C4, or C2 defect.
  — If CH50 normal and AH50 absent, may be a properdin or factor D defect.
  — If CH50 and AH50 abnormal, may be a C3 to C8 defect.
  — CH50 usually at half normal in the case of C9 defects.
- Treatment is determined by the type of deficiency.

For a more detailed discussion, see Hans D. Ochs and Luigi D. Notarangelo: Immunodeficiency Diseases. Chap. 82, p. 1153 in *Williams Hematology*, 8th ed.

CHAPTER 52
The Acquired Immunodeficiency Syndrome

DEFINITION AND HISTORY

- Patients with serologic evidence of infection with the human immunodeficiency virus (HIV) can be diagnosed as having acquired-immunodeficiency syndrome (AIDS) based upon "clinical" or "immunologic" criteria (see Table 52–1).
  - Patients with AIDS diagnosed based on clinical criteria are classified as having "clinical AIDS."
  - Patients with AIDS diagnosed based on a blood CD4 T cell count of less than $200/\mu L$ are classified as having "immunological AIDS."
- Patients with HIV are living longer in the era of highly active antiretroviral therapy (HAART).
- United Nations estimated that 30 to 35 million people worldwide were living with HIV infection in 2007, with the majority being infected by heterosexual contact.

ETIOLOGY AND PATHOGENESIS

Human Immunodeficiency Virus 1

- The primary cause of AIDS is infection with HIV-1.
- HIV-1 is a member of the *Lentivirinae* subfamily of retroviruses.
  - Retroviruses are RNA viruses that induce a chronic cellular infection by converting their RNA genome into a DNA provirus that is integrated into the genome of the infected cell.
- Infection by these lenetviruses is characterized by long periods of clinical latency followed by gradual onset of disease-related symptoms.

Transmission of HIV

- The four main routes of HIV infection are:
  - *Sexual contact* with an infected partner.
    - The risk for HIV transmission through sexual contact may be increased in persons with other concurrent sexually transmitted diseases.
  - *Parenteral drug use*.
    - Sharing needles and syringes is the main mode of transmission.
  - *Exposure to infected blood or blood products*.
    - Ninety percent of those who receive a contaminated unit of blood become infected.
    - Risk of HIV transmission through transfusion of a unit of red blood cells tested negative for antibodies to HIV is approximately 1 in 493,000 transfusions.
  - *Perinatal exposure*.
    - HIV-1 may be transmitted *in utero*, intrapartum (at the time of delivery) or postpartum, through ingestion of HIV-1-infected mother's milk.
    - The risk of infection from mother to infant differs in various parts of the world, ranging from approximately 15 percent in Europe and approximately 40 to 50 percent in Africa.
    - The risk of perinatal transmission is increased from mothers with more advanced HIV disease, higher HIV-1 viral load in the plasma, or a history of cigarette smoking and/or active drug abuse.

TABLE 52–1	DEFINITION OF AIDS IN THE UNITED STATES

Clinical AIDS-defining conditions in persons infected with HIV
    Opportunistic infections
    Lymphomas (non-Hodgkin)
    Kaposi sarcoma
    Cervical cancer
    Wasting syndrome
    AIDS dementia syndrome
    Recurrent bacteria pneumonia ($\geq$2 episodes/yr)
    Mycobacterium infections
Immunologic AIDS
    CD4 cell counts <200/μL
    CD4 percent of lymphocytes <14%

Source: *Williams Hematology,* 8th ed, Chap. 83, Table 83–1, p. 1176.

- Antiretroviral agents in pregnancy and delivery, with subsequent administration to the infant for the first 6 weeks of life, has resulted in a dramatically reduced rate of transmission, from approximately 25 to 8 percent with zidovudine alone and even lower with use of HAART.

Pathogenesis of HIV Infection

- HIV infection results in aberrant immune regulation and immunodeficiency.
  - Defects include decreased lymphocyte proliferative response to soluble antigens *in vitro,* decreased helper response in immunoglobulin (Ig) synthesis, impaired delayed hypersensitivity, decreased interferon (IFN)-γ production, and decreased helper T-cell response of virally infected cells.
- Infection with HIV-1 results in a progressive loss of CD4+ T lymphocytes.
- Monocytes, macrophages, and follicular dendritic cells of the lymph nodes express CD4 antigen and can be infected by HIV.
- Macrophage-tropic (*M-tropic*) strains of HIV use the CCR5 chemokine receptor to infect both macrophages and CD4+ lymphocytes.
- Loss of follicular dendritic cells results in defective antigen processing in patients with advanced HIV disease.
- Pronounced polyclonal activation of B lymphocytes is common, especially during early stages of disease and results in hypergammaglobulinemia.
- Antigen-specific B-cell proliferation and antibody production are decreased in patients with AIDS.
- HIV infection is associated with an increase in autoimmune phenomena and an increase risk of B-cell lymphomas.
- Natural killer (NK) cell activity is decreased in the blood of HIV-infected individuals.

DIAGNOSIS OF HIV

- The primary diagnostic screening test is the enzyme-linked immunosorbent assay (ELISA) for detection of antibodies to HIV glycoproteins.
  - The median time from initial infection to first detection of HIV antibody is about 2 to 4 weeks.
- Testing by polymerase chain reaction (PCR) may detect the presence of HIV within 1 week of initial infection.

COURSE AND PROGNOSIS

- Infection by HIV-1 causes a gradual but progressive loss of immune function, leading to development of nonspecific symptoms and then specific infections and/or neoplastic disease.

— Without effective antiretroviral therapy, patients who develop AIDS generally experience relentless deterioration in physical health and ultimately die of one or more complications secondary to acquired immunodeficiency, organ dysfunction, and/or malignancy associated with HIV infection.

- Acute Retroviral Syndrome
  — An acute clinical illness often is associated with initial HIV infection.
  — Occurs in approximately 75 percent of patients.
  — Typically begins 1 to 3 weeks after primary infection and lasts for 1 to 2 weeks.
  — Symptoms include fatigue, malaise, headache, fever, rash, and photophobia lasting several weeks; myalgia and a morbilliform rash.
  — Generalized lymphadenopathy termed *persistent generalized lymphadenopathy* may occur toward the end of the acute retroviral syndrome and persist indefinitely.
- Early Asymptomatic HIV Disease
  — After resolution of the acute retroviral syndrome, the patient usually returns to a state of well being.
- Advanced symptomatic HIV disease can define the diagnosis of AIDS.
- The list of AIDS-defining clinical conditions is presented in Table 52–1.
- Laboratory Features of Disease Progression
  — Quantitation of plasma HIV RNA (viral load) and CD4+ lymphocyte count are the most useful parameters.

HEMATOLOGIC ABNORMALITIES

Anemia

- Anemia is common in HIV-infected individuals, occurring in approximately 10 to 20 percent at initial presentation and diagnosed in approximately 70 to 80 percent of patients over the course of disease.
- Numerous causes for anemia exist in HIV-infected patients (see Table 52–2).
- Anemia with a hemoglobulin of <10 g/dL may be associated with shorter survival.
- Recovery from anemia is independently associated with improved survival.
- HAART can correct or improve anemia associated with HIV infection.
- Erythropoietin can correct or improve anemia associated with HIV infection.
  — Low erythropoietin levels and blunted response to erythropoietin are extremely common in the setting of HIV infection.
  — Erythropoietin 100 to 200 U/kg weight can be administered subcutaneously three times per week until improvement of the hemoglobin concentration and then approximately once every week or every other week to maintain a hemoglobin concentration of approximately 11 to 12 g/dL.
  — Clinical trials have demonstrated the equivalent efficacy of 40,000 U of erythropoietin given weekly compared with the original thrice-weekly schedule in anemic HIV-infected patients.
  — Patients with a baseline endogenous erythropoietin level of 500 IU/L or less more likely to respond to erythropoietin therapy.

Neutropenia

- Neutropenia is reported in approximately 10 percent of patients with early, asymptomatic HIV infection and in more than 50 percent of individuals with more advanced HIV-related immunodeficiency.
  — Thus, the risk of bacterial infection increased 2.3-fold for HIV-infected individuals with absolute neutrophil counts (ANC) less than 1.0×10^9 cells/L and increased by 7.9-fold in those with ANC levels less than 500 cells/μL.
- The use of HAART can be associated with improvement of neutropenia.

Thrombocytopenia

- Thrombocytopenia ($<100 \times 10^9$/L) is relatively common during the course of HIV infection.

TABLE 52-2 MECHANISMS AND CAUSES OF ANEMIA IN HUMAN IMMUNODEFICIENCY VIRUS INFECTION

Mechanism of Anemia	Cause of Anemia
Decreased red cell production	Neoplasm infiltrating the marrow
	Lymphoma
	Kaposi sarcoma
	Other
	Infection
	Atypical *Mycobacterium* (*Mycobacterium avium intracellulare* or *Mycobacterium avium complex*)
	Mycobacterium tuberculosis
	Cytomegalovirus
	Parvovirus B19
	Fungal infection
	Medications
	HIV infection
	Abnormal growth of burst-forming unit–erythroid
	Anemia of chronic disease
	Blunted erythropoietin production and response
	Iron-deficiency anemia secondary to chronic blood loss
Ineffective production	Folic acid deficiency
	Vitamin B_{12} deficiency
Increased red cell destruction	Coombs-positive hemolytic anemia
	Hemophagocytic syndrome
	Thrombotic thrombocytopenic purpura
	Disseminated intravascular coagulation
	Medications and recreational drugs
	Sulfonamides, Dapsone
	Oxidant drugs in glucose-6-phosphate dehydrogenase deficiency
	Nitrite "poppers"

Source: *Williams Hematology*, 8th ed, Chap. 83, Table 83–2, p. 1179.

— The incidence of thrombocytopenia over 1 year was 9 percent in patients with clinical AIDS, 3 percent in patients with immunologic AIDS (<200 CD4+ cells/μL), and approximately 2 percent in patients with neither clinical nor immunologic AIDS.
— Thrombocytopenia is associated with history of:
— AIDS.
— Injection drug use.
— History of anemia or lymphoma.
— Being an American of African descent.
• Thrombocytopenia is associated with shorter survival.
• Persons with HIV infection have a high risk of secondary thrombocytopenia because of increased risk of other infections or treatment with myelosuppressive medicine.
• What has previously been described as HIV-associated immune thrombocytopenic purpura (ITP) is increasingly characterized as "primary HIV-associated thrombocytopenia (PHAT).
• In contrast to *de novo* ITP, PHAT is associated with a higher rate of splenomegaly, typically less severe thrombocytopenia, and a 20 percent spontaneous remission rate.

- Presence of platelet-specific antibodies, against both glycoprotein (GP) IIb and GPIIIa, have been detected in patients with PHAT.
- Antibodies against platelet GPIIb-IIIa have been demonstrated to be cross-reactive with HIV GP160/120.
- A further mechanism of antibody-induced destruction of platelets arises from the absorption of immune complexes against HIV.
- Mean platelet survival is decreased in patients with PHAT.
- Mean platelet production is decreased in patients with untreated PHAT.
- Reduced production of platelets in the setting of HIV infection may be direct due to infection of the megakaryocyte by HIV.
- The diagnosis of PHAT is clinical and requires the exclusion of secondary causes of thrombocytopenia and discontinuation of potentially myelosuppressive medications.
- Zidovudine may be effective in the treatment of patients with PHAT.
- HAART is effective for treatment of PHAT.
  — HAART was associated with a significantly increased platelet count after 3 months.
- Treatment with interferon-α (IFN-α) at 3,000,000 U given subcutaneously three times per week increases platelet counts after 3 weeks.
  — Platelet response was documented in 66 percent, with a mean increase of 60×10^9/L.
  — IFN-α was found to prolong platelet survival, whereas no significant increase in platelet production was noted.
- Treatment with high-dose intravenous immunoglobulin (IVIG) at 1,000 to 2,000 mg/kg may result in a significant rise in platelet counts within 24 to 72 hours.
  — IVIG often is reserved for use in patients who are acutely bleeding or require an immediate increase in platelet count.
- Use of anti-Rh immunoglobulin in nonsplenectomized Rh-positive patients with PHAT is another potential mode of therapy.
  — Requirements for effective therapy with anti-Rh (D) include presence of Rh+ red cells in the patient, a baseline hemoglobin level adequate to permit a 1- to 2-g decrease as a result of hemolysis, and presence of a spleen.
  — Patients were treated with 25 mg/kg intravenously over 30 minutes on 2 consecutive days.
  — Patients responded with a platelet count greater than 50×10^9/L with response first noted at approximately 4 days and median response duration of 13 days.
  — Maintenance therapy with anti-Rh immunoglobulin of 13 to 25 mg/kg intravenously administered every 2 to 4 weeks, resulted in a long-term response (>6 months) in 70 percent of patients.
  — Subclinical hemolysis due to the anti-Rh immunoglobulin occurred in all patients, with a decrease in hemoglobin of 0.4 to 2.2 g.
- Splenectomy has been used effectively to treat patients with intractable thrombocytopenia.
  — A complete response was seen in 92 percent of patients (platelet count >100×10^9/L).
  — No difference was found when the survival or rate of progression to AIDS in the 68 splenectomized patients was compared with the rate in the 117 patients who did not undergo the procedure, indicating that splenectomy was not associated with more rapid progression of HIV disease.
  — Approximately 6 percent of patients who underwent splenectomy in one series experienced fulminant infection.
- Prednisone at an oral dosage of 1 mg/kg per day has been associated with an 80 to 90 percent response rate in HIV-infected patients with thrombocytopenia secondary to intractable thrombocytopenia.
  — The potential development of fulminant Kaposi sarcoma in dually HIV-infected and human herpes virus (HHV)-8–infected patients after use of

glucocorticoids has dampened enthusiasm for the use of prednisone to treat thrombocytopenia in HIV-infected patients.

Venous Thrombosis

- There may be an increased incidence of venous thromboembolic disease in persons with HIV infection.
- The increased risk of thrombosis appears independent of concurrent malignancy.
- HIV infection may be associated with the development of a hypercoaguable state.
- Abnormalities of coagulation proteins observed in HIV-infected patients include acquired deficiencies in protein S, protein C, and heparin cofactor II.

Thrombotic Thrombocytopenia Purpura (TTP)

- Associated with advanced HIV positive.
- Factors associated with occurrence of TTP include higher HIV viral loads, lower CD4+ counts, and increased incidence of AIDS diagnoses, as well as infections with *Mycobacterium avium* complex and hepatitis C.
- The incidence of TTP is decreasing in the HAART era.

HIV-ASSOCIATED MALIGNANCIES

- More than 40 percent of all HIV-infected patients eventually are diagnosed with cancer.
- In the HAART era, malignancies account for 20 percent of deaths in persons with HIV-infection.
- Spectrum of neoplastic disease appears to be wider than initially thought.
- Three cancers currently considered AIDS-defining in HIV-infected persons are:
  — Kaposi sarcoma: associated with the epidemic from the onset in 1981.
  — Intermediate- or high-grade B-cell lymphoma: added to the case definition for AIDS in 1985.
  — Uterine cervical carcinoma: which became an AIDS-defining illness in 1993.
- There is increased risk of Hodgkin lymphoma among patients infected with HIV.

AIDS-Related Lymphoma

Epidemiology

- Patients with AIDS have a risk of developing lymphoma that is nearly 100 times greater than that of the general population.
- The incidence of lymphoma increases with time after infection and may approach 20 percent for patients with prolonged, far-advanced immunodeficiency.
- In the United States, the relative risk of developing lymphoma within 3 years of an AIDS diagnosis was increased by 165-fold compared to people without AIDS.
- Lymphomas have increased since the widespread use of HAART.
  — In contrast, HAART has led to a major and dramatic decline in the incidence of Kaposi sarcoma.
  — In both the pre-HAART and HAART periods, patients with lower CD4+ cell counts were more likely to develop lymphoma.
  — However, patients infected with HIV who maintain high CD4+ counts and good immune function with effective HAART therapy may have a reduced risk for developing lymphoma compared with HIV-infected patients with low CD4+ counts.

Pathology

- Over 80 percent of lymphomas associated with AIDS are intermediate- or high-grade B-cell tumors including immunoblastic or large B-cell types and small noncleaved or Burkitt lymphomas (see Table 52–3).

TABLE 52–3   CATEGORIES OF HIV-ASSOCIATED LYMPHOMAS: WORLD HEALTH ORGANIZATION CLASSIFICATION

Lymphomas also occurring in immunocompetent patients
  Burkitt lymphoma
    Classic
    With plasmacytoid differentiation
    Atypical
  Diffuse large B-cell lymphoma
    Centroblastic
    Immunoblastic
  Extranodal marginal zone B cell lymphoma of mucosa-associated lymphoid tissue (MALT) lymphoma (rare)
  Peripheral T-cell lymphoma (rare)
  Classic Hodgkin lymphoma
Lymphomas occurring more specifically in patients who are HIV positive
  Primary effusion lymphoma
  Plasmablastic lymphoma of the oral cavity
  Lymphomas occurring in other immunodeficiency states
  Polymorphic B-cell lymphoma

Source: *Williams Hematology,* 8th ed, Chap. 83, Table 83–3, p. 1187.

- The two most common histologic subtypes of lymphoma in HIV-infected patients are Burkitt lymphoma (see Chap. 65) and diffuse large B-cell lymphoma (see Chap. 61).

Burkitt Lymphoma
- In some cases, the cells have a plasmacytoid appearance, characterized by medium-size cells with abundant cytoplasm and eccentric nuclei.
- This type of Burkitt lymphoma is termed *Burkitt lymphoma with plasmacytoid differentiation* in the WHO classification, an entity unique to patients with HIV.

Diffuse Large B-cell Lymphoma
- In the World Health Organization classification, AIDS-related diffuse large B-cell lymphomas are divided into centroblastic and immunoblastic subtypes.
- Compared to the centroblastic subtype, the immunoblastic subtype more frequently involves extranodal sites, particularly the central nervous system (CNS), and is more commonly associated with Epstein-Barr virus infection.

Primary Effusion Lymphoma
- Primary effusion lymphoma and plasmablastic lymphoma of the oral cavity occur principally in patients with HIV infection.
- Primary effusion lymphoma is uncommon, representing only a small fraction of all AIDS-related lymphomas, and is caused by HHV-8.

T-Cell Lymphoma
- Patients with AIDS are at an increased risk for developing T-cell lymphomas.
- The prevalence of T-cell lymphomas among patients with AIDS-related lymphoma is approximately 3 percent.

Clinical Features
- B symptoms, such as fever, night sweats, and weight loss, are present at diagnosis in 80 to 90 percent of patients with AIDS-related lymphoma, and 61 to 90 percent have far-advanced disease presenting in extranodal sites.
- Virtually any anatomic site may be involved.

- The more common sites of initial extranodal disease include the CNS (17 to 42%), gastrointestinal tract (4 to 28%), marrow (21 to 33%), and liver (9 to 26%).
- Staging evaluation should include computed tomographic (CT) scanning of the chest, abdomen, and pelvis; a gallium-67 scan or positron emission tomography (PET) scan; marrow aspirate and biopsy; and other studies as clinically indicated.
- Lumbar puncture should routinely be performed because approximately 20 percent of patients have leptomeningeal lymphoma, even in the absence of specific symptoms or signs.
- Intrathecal methotrexate or cytosine arabinoside is often given to prevent isolated CNS relapse.

Primary CNS Lymphoma

- Approximately 75 percent of patients with primary CNS lymphoma have far-advanced HIV disease, with median CD4+ cell counts less than 50/μL, and a prior history of AIDS.
- Initial symptoms and signs may be variable, with seizures, headache, and/or focal neurologic dysfunction noted in most patients.
- Radiographic scanning reveals relatively large mass lesions (2 to 4 cm), which tend to be few in number (one to three lesions). Ring enhancement may be seen.
- There is no specific radiographic picture.
- PET scanning may be useful in differentiating cerebral lymphoma, which has a glucose uptake above that of the surrounding cortex. This is in contrast to toxoplasmosis which has a glucose uptake below that of the cerebral cortex.
- In addition, thallium-201 single-photon emission computerized tomography scanning may be useful, with a median T1 uptake index greater than 1.5 and a lesion size greater than 2.5 cm serving as independent predictors of primary CNS lymphoma.
- Pathologically, almost all such lymphomas are of diffuse large B-cell or immunoblastic subtypes and are uniformly associated with Epstein-Barr virus infection within malignant cells.
- Detection of Epstein-Barr virus DNA (Epstein-Barr nuclear antigen) in cerebrospinal fluid by PCR may be used as a diagnostic criterion.
- Use of cranial radiation is associated with a complete remission rate of only 50 percent and median survival of only 2 or 3 months.
- Use of HAART is associated with significantly prolonged survival.

T-Cell Lymphomas

- Systemic B symptoms, consisting of fever, drenching night sweats, and/or unexplained weight loss, are extremely common in patients with T-cell lymphomas.
- T-cell lymphomas also present with advanced lymphomatous disease, with stage IV disease confirmed in up to 90 percent.

Primary Effusion Lymphoma

- Outcome with polychemotherapy has generally been poor, with median survival of approximately 2 months.
- Studies reported complete remissions in patients treated with HAART alone.
- Palliative measures include draining effusions and therapeutic radiation to affected areas.

Prognostic Markers In AIDS-Related Lymphoma

- The age-adjusted international prognostic index (IPI) established for immunocompetent patients with intermediate grade lymphoma is also predictive of outcome in AIDS patients with lymphoma (see Chap. 61).
- High risk group and low CD4+ cell count are the two predictors of poor survival.
- Histology of Burkitt lymphoma was an independent poor prognostic factor for survival.

- Low IPI and postgerminal center differentiation were identified as independent prognostic factors for relatively long disease-free survival.
- Patients with systemic lymphoma with leptomeningeal involvement have decreased survival.

Treatment

- AIDS Clinical Trials Group in the United States compared standard-dose m-BACOD and GM-CSF support with reduced-dose m-BACOD without GM-CSF in 198 HIV infected patients with aggressive lymphomas.
  - No significant differences were found in either response rate (standard dose 52% vs. reduced dose 41%) or median survival (standard dose 6.8 months vs. reduced dose 7.7 months).
  - However, reduced dose m-BACOD was associated with a statistically significant lower toxicity.
- The EPOCH regimen consists of a 96-hour continuous infusion of etoposide, prednisone, vincristine, and doxorubicin, and a bolus of cyclophosphamide, which was dose adjusted based on the patient's CD4+ cell count and neutrophil count at the nadir.
  - The overall complete remission rate was 74 percent. Among patients with CD4+ cell counts greater than 100/μL, the complete remission rate was 87 percent, and the overall survival was 87 percent at 56 months.
  - A particular survival advantage in patients with CD4+ cell counts of less than 100/μL was reported by adding rituximab to EPOCH.
  - R-EPOCH (rituximab on days 1 and 5) was given to 21 subjects with AIDS-related lymphoma. Persons with CD4+ cell counts greater than 100/μL fared similarly after EPOCH with or without rituximab whereas, persons with CD4 cell counts less than 100/μL had survival of 57 percent with R-EPOCH versus 16 percent with EPOCH alone.
  - Rituximab increased the risk of severe and life-threatening infection when used in combination with chemotherapy in patients with AIDS.
- Concurrent use of HAART during administration of chemotherapy is generally tolerated.
  - Use of HAART is associated with improved survival in patients with AIDS-related lymphoma.
  - Delaying HAART until completion of chemotherapy is reasonable for patients with CD4+ counts greater than 100/μL, but does not appear to be necessary.
  - Including HAART therapy with chemotherapy in patients with CD4+ counts less than 100/μL cells clearly seems important given the poor survival rates in this group when HAART is not employed.
- With the advent of HAART and improvement in supportive care, HIV-infected patients with relapsed or refractory lymphoma now can be effectively retreated with high-dose chemotherapy and peripheral stem cell transplantation.

Hodgkin Lymphoma in the Setting of HIV Infection

- HIV-related Hodgkin lymphoma seems to be associated with more profound immunodeficiency.
- Paradoxically, the highest risk of HIV-related Hodgkin lymphoma is found in persons with CD4+ counts between 225 and 250 cells/μL, which are above the level required to establish an immunologic AIDS diagnosis.
- The risks decline with CD4+ cell counts both above and below that range with the lowest risks seen with counts less than 75 CD4+ cells/μL.
- HIV-related Hodgkin lymphoma is characterized by the preponderance of more aggressive histologic subtypes, with mixed cellularity Hodgkin lymphoma and lymphocyte depletion Hodgkin lymphoma diagnosed in 41 to 100 percent of patients.

- Another distinguishing feature of HIV-related Hodgkin lymphoma is its close association with Epstein-Barr virus.
- Systemic B symptoms such as fever, drenching night sweats, and/or weight loss occur in 70 to 100 percent of patients with HIV-related Hodgkin lymphoma compared with 30 to 60 percent of patients with *de novo* Hodgkin lymphoma.
- Marrow involvement is present in 50 percent of patients with underlying HIV infection, often presenting with pancytopenia and systemic B symptoms.
- Staging evaluation should include a thorough history; physical examination; standard laboratory tests; CT scans of the chest, abdomen, and pelvis; gallium or PET scans; and bilateral marrow biopsies.
- With the availability of HAART, better treatment outcomes with combination chemotherapy have been reported.
- Although improved outcomes have been reported in the HAART era, results still are inferior compared with those in HIV-negative patients with Hodgkin lymphoma, even among those with stage IV disease.

Multicentric Castleman Disease in the Setting of HIV Infection

- Multicentric Castleman disease (MCD) is a diffuse lymphoproliferative disorder.
- MCD is characterized histologically by angiofollicular hyperplasia and plasma cell infiltration.
- MCD manifests itself as a systemic syndrome with elevated IL-6 and C-reactive protein. The syndrome may flare for several days to weeks, resolving spontaneously at times.
- Clinical features include lymphadenopathy, splenomegaly, fevers, weight loss, hypotension, pancytopenia, hypoalbuminemia, and oligoclonal or monoclonal gammopathy.
- In the setting of HIV, persons with MCD are at increased risk for both Kaposi sarcoma and lymphoma.
- Neither HIV viral load nor CD4+ cell count has been predictive of the risk of developing MCD, MCD flares, or MCD-related lymphoma.
- MCD is universally associated with HHV-8.
- Improvements and exacerbations after initiating HAART have been described.
- MCD in patients infected with HIV is often progressive and potentially fatal.

 For a more detailed discussion, see Erin Gourley Reid: Hematologic Manifestations of Acquired Immunodeficiency Syndrome. Chap. 83, p. 1175 in *Williams Hematology,* 8th ed.

CHAPTER 53
The Mononucleosis Syndromes

DEFINITION

- Infectious mononucleosis is defined as any blood lymphocytosis induced in response to an infectious agent.
- Usually greater than 50 percent of the circulating white cells are lymphocytes, more than 10 percent of which have the morphology of reactive lymphocytes (see Fig. 53–1).
- Table 53–1 lists the etiologic agents that produce mononucleosis.
- Pharyngeal form:
  — Sore throat preceded by 1 to 2 weeks of lethargy.
  — Epstein-Barr virus (EBV) generally is the cause.
- Glandular form without pharyngitis:
  — Lymph node enlargement.
  — Usually caused by agents other than EBV, e.g., *Toxoplasma gondii*.
- Typhoidal form:
  — Lethargy with fever or diarrhea without pharyngitis, usually as a consequence of cytomegalovirus (CMV).

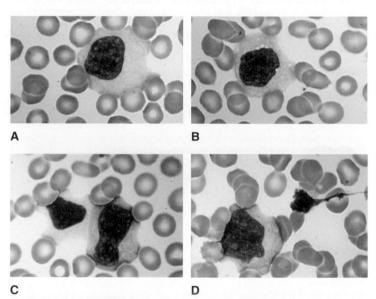

A **B**

C **D**

FIGURE 53-1 A–D. Blood films from patients with EBV-induced mononucleosis. These reactive lymphocytes exhibit the characteristic changes seen in patients with infectious mononucleosis: large lymphocytes with abundant cytoplasm. The cytoplasmic margin often spreads around (is indented by) neighboring red cells and the margin may take on a densely basophilic coloration. This type of reactive T lymphocyte may be seen in a variety of diseases and is not specific changes but are characteristic. (Reproduced with permission from *Lichtman's Atlas of Hematology,* www.access-medicine.com.)

(Source: *Williams Hematology,* 8th ed, Chap. 84, Fig. 84–1, p. 1202.)

TABLE 53–1	ETIOLOGIC AGENTS ASSOCIATED WITH MONONUCLEOSIS SYNDROME
Epstein-Barr virus	Hepatitis A
Cytomegalovirus	Adenovirus
Human immunodeficiency virus	*Toxoplasma gondii*
Human herpes virus-6	*Bartonella henselae*
Metapneumovirus	*Brucella abortus*
Rubella	

Source: *Williams Hematology*, 8th ed, Chap. 84, Table 84–1, p. 1200.

ETIOLOGY AND PATHOGENESIS

- Caused by two members of the herpes virus family: EBV or CMV.
- After the early phase of fever, which lasts for 3 to 7 days, laboratory abnormalities include a blood lymphocyte proportion greater than 50 percent, often with greater than 10 percent reactive lymphocytes.
- Table 53–2 lists other complications of EBV and CMV mononucleosis.

FEATURES OF MONONUCLEOSIS CAUSED BY EACH ETIOLOGIC AGENT

- Table 53–3 list the signs and symptoms associated with EBV and CMV mononucleosis.
- Target cell for EBV mononucleosis is the B lymphocyte.
- Target cell for CMV mononucleosis is the macrophage.
- The "mononucleosis" for both is the increase in reactive blood T lymphocytes.
- Hepatosplenomegaly common for both EBV and CMV mononucleosis.
- Incubation period for EBV or CMV is 30 to 50 days.

EBV MONONUCLEOSIS

Virology and Pathogenesis

- DNA virus of the *gammaherpsevirinae* subfamily.
- Infects 90 percent of the world population.
- Peak incidence occurs in the age group from 12 to 25 years and during the summer months.

TABLE 53–2	COMPLICATIONS IN PATIENTS WITH EBV OR CMV MONONUCLEOSIS	
	EBV	**CMV**
Hemolytic anemia	+ +	+
Thrombocytopenia	+	+
Aplastic anemia	+	−
Splenic rupture	+	−
Jaundice (> age 25 years)	+ +	+ +
Guillain-Barré*	+	+ +
Encephalitis*	+ +	+/−
Pneumonitis*	+/−	+
Myocarditis*	+	−
B-cell lymphoma	+	−
Agammaglobulinemia	+	−

*Can occur without mononucleosis syndrome. + +, common; +, infrequent; +/−, uncommon; −, not observed.
Source: *Williams Hematology*, 8th ed, Chap. 84, Table 84–2, p. 1200.

| TABLE 53–3 | SIGNS AND SYMPTOMS OF EBV AND CMV: EFFECT OF AGE (PERCENT OF PATIENTS) |

Signs and Symptoms	Percent of Subjects		
	EBV (Age 14–35 Years)	EBV (Age 40–72 Years)	CMV (Age 30–70 Years)
Fever	95	94	85
Pharyngitis	95	46	15
Lymphadenopathy	98	49	24
Hepatomegaly	23	42	N/A
Splenomegaly	65	33	3
Jaundice	8	27	24

Source: *Williams Hematology,* 8th ed, Chap. 84, Table 84–3, p. 1200.

- B lymphocytes are the initial target of EBV during primary infection.
- Surface receptor for EBV is CD21 on B cells.
- Initial infection causes polyclonal or oligoclonal B-cell proliferation.
- Neoantigen(s) on EBV-infected B cells induces a cytotoxic T-cell response.
- Most circulating lymphocytes are reactive T cells.
- Cytotoxic T cells destroy most EBV-infected B cells leading to disease resolution.
- Following infection, the virus persists throughout life in a latent form.

Epidemiology
- Transmission requires close mucocutaneous contact.
- In the developing world and in the lowest socioeconomic strata of the developed world, nearly everyone is subclinically infected by age 5 years and mononucleosis is rarely clinically apparent.
- In the upper socioeconomic strata of the developed world, persons avoid infection in infancy; instead, they become exposed to the virus between the ages of 12 and 25 years by contact with a latently infected asymptomatic individual.
- Individuals who are raised in more protected environments or in single-child families may reach an age of 30 years or older before they are infected.

Clinical Manifestations
- Vary by age:
  — When young children acquire infection with EBV, they develop a typical childhood illness of respiratory tract infection (43%), otitis media (29%), pharyngitis (21%), gastroenteritis (7%), or typical mononucleosis (<10%).
  — Age group 12 to 25 years, the earliest manifestations of disease—fever and lassitude—develop 30 to 45 days after patients become infected. Initial symptoms of pharyngitis, tonsillar enlargement, sometimes massive, and fever result from infection and proliferation of the B lymphocytes that are found in the pharyngeal of the Waldeyer ring of the lymph nodes.
- Liver function abnormalities, usually cholestatic, are frequently present.
- Maculopapular rash with EBV mononucleosis can be worsened by administration of ampicillin or amoxicillin.
- Group A streptococcus infection may occur coincidentally, but does not affect the disease and its usual course.
  — Penicillin or erythromycin indicated if group A streptococcus isolated from throat cultures of symptomatic patients.

- Complications caused by immune dysregulation or lymphocyte proliferation:
  — Immune thrombocytopenic purpura (ITP) or autoimmune hemolytic anemia.
  — Splenic rupture.
  — Acute airway obstruction resulting from exaggerated pharyngeal lymphadenopathy.
  — B-cell lymphoproliferative disorder/lymphoma in immunosuppressed patients.
- Disease abates with the occurrence of a T-cell-mediated counter-response to the virus-induced polyclonal B-cell proliferation and clinical improvement occurs within 24 to 48 hours in most cases.

Laboratory Findings

Table 53–5 lists the laboratory abnormalities for EBV and CMV mononucleosis.

Antibody Responses

- Heterophile antibody is positive only with EBV.
- Autoantibodies:
  — Cold agglutinins occur frequently with EBV infection.
- Antibody tests for EBV:
  — Antibodies to EBV do not react with CMV or with the heterophile antigen.
  — IgM and IgG antivirus capsid antigen (VCA) appear during acute illness (IgM persists for months, IgG for life).
  — Early antigen (EA) specific antibodies appear slightly later than IgG anti-VCA, and persist for years.
  — Antibodies to Epstein-Barr nuclear antigen (EBNA) do not develop until after the acute illness resolves and persist for life.
  — A presumptive diagnosis of EBV infectious mononucleosis may be made if the patient has antibodies specific for VCA, but not for EBNA.

Reactive Lymphocytes

- Expansion of cytotoxic T lymphocytes produces lymphocytosis. Reactive lymphocytes are larger than lymphocytes normally found in the blood (see Fig. 53–1).
- Reactive lymphocytes are a hematologic hallmark of infectious mononucleosis, but they are not always found and are not pathognomonic.

Other Blood Test Abnormalities

- Liver function abnormalities are common, predominantly elevated serum alkaline phosphatase and γ-aminotransferase activity with no or only slight elevation of bilirubin in most patients.

Course and Prognosis

Complications of EBV Mononucleosis

- Hematologic:
  — Occur infrequently, but include severe immune thrombocytopenia with petechiae, immune hemolytic anemia, immune-mediated agranulocytosis, and aplastic anemia.
- Neurologic:
  — Can occasionally develop encephalitis, acute disseminated encephalomyelitis (*Alice in Wonderland* syndrome), acute cerebellar ataxia, viral meningitis, Guillain-Barré syndrome, transverse myelitis, and cranial nerve palsies.
  — Other complications that may be associated are chronic fatigue, multiple sclerosis, systemic lupus erythematosus, rheumatoid arthritis, and chronic progressive EBV infection, T or NK lymphoproliferation, lymphoma, and hemophagocytic syndrome.

Other EBV-Associated Disease Processes
Neoplastic Potential of the Virus
- Has been associated Burkitt lymphoma and other tumors (see Table 53–4).
- Detectable in neoplastic B cells (Reed-Sternberg cells) of approximately 35 percent of patients with Hodgkin lymphoma; etiologic role uncertain.
- Because of the severe consequences of EBV infection, several approaches to preventing or treating these disorders are under way including:
  — Development of an EBV vaccine.
  — Adoptive transfer of activated cytotoxic T cells.
  — Development of peptides that inhibit viral replication.

CMV MONONUCLEOSIS

- Second most common cause of infectious mononucleosis.

Epidemiology
- Teenage mothers carrying CMV in their cervix transmit it to their newborn child, and transmission also occurs through breast milk.
- Transmission from contact with infected young children also plays a role.
- Sexual transmission.

Clinical Manifestations
- See Table 53–2 and 53–4 for a list of complications and clinical findings.
- The basic clinical disease is fever, often as high as 40 °C (104 °F), with a palpable spleen and laboratory abnormalities.
- Commonly occurs in older individuals, often those older than 50 years.
- Reactive lymphocytosis is a result of T cells reacting against CMV-infected monocytes/macrophages (see Table 53–4).

TABLE 53–4　SPECIAL PROBLEMS WITH EBV OR CMV	
Epstein-Barr Virus	**Cytomegalovirus**
Rare congenital infection	Congenital infection
Chronic progressive mononucleosis	Posttransplant primary infection
Hemophagocytic syndrome	Graft-versus-host disease association
X-linked B-cell lymphoma	Transfusion-related infection
Posttransplant lymphoproliferative disease	*Aspergillus* and/or *Pneumocystis* infection
T or NK lymphoproliferative disease	
African Burkitt lymphoma	
Approximately 20% of Burkitt lymphoma in the United States	
Approximately 35% of Hodgkin lymphoma	
Nasopharyngeal carcinoma	
Approximately 5% of gastric carcinoma	
Leiomyoma and leiomyosarcoma in HIV or immunosuppressed patients	
Oral hairy leukoplakia	

Source: *Williams Hematology,* 8th ed, Chap. 84, Table 84–4, p. 1203.

TABLE 53–5   **LABORATORY ABNORMALITIES IN MONONUCLEOSIS SYNDROME**

	Frequency	
	EBV	CMV
Heterophile antibody	+ + +	–
Lymphocytosis	+ + +	+ +
Reactive lymphocytes	+ + +	+ +
Abnormal liver function	+ +	+ +
Antinuclear factor	+	+
Cold agglutinins	+	+
Cryoglobulins	+	+
Decreased platelets	+ +	+

+ + +, Characteristic; + +, common; +, occurs.
Source: *Williams Hematology,* 8th ed, Chap. 84, Table 84–5, p. 1204.

Laboratory Findings

- See Table 53–5.
- Polyclonal antibody and heterophile antibody responses do not occur, but specific anti-CMV antibodies do develop.
- Because the incubation period ranges between 30 and 40 days, IgM and IgG antibodies to CMV usually are positive at presentation.
- Tests for CMV:
  — Primary infection diagnosed by fourfold rise in anti-CMV antibody titer.
  — Assay for CMV antigenemia more sensitive than anti-CMV antibody titer.
  — Polymerase chain reaction (PCR) for detection of CMV DNA is most sensitive.

Complications

- Hemolytic anemia and thrombocytopenia occur in primary CMV infection and are other factors that may lead the clinician initially to consider a diagnosis of lymphoma.
- Various neurologic complications can occur, but Guillain-Barré syndrome is the most frequent and is usually associated with CMV infection.

PRIMARY HIV INFECTION

- Mononucleosis can occur soon after primary infection (see Chap. 52).
- See Table 53–6 for the clinical findings.
- Mononucleosis symptoms are self-limited but may last for several weeks.

TABLE 53–6   **CLINICAL FINDINGS IN PRIMARY HIV INFECTION**

Finding	Frequency (%)
Fever	79
Pharyngitis	48
Oral ulcers	29
Lymphadenopathy	44
Splenomegaly	5
Hepatomegaly	<1
Reactive lymphocytes	Uncommon

Source: *Williams Hematology,* 8th ed, Chap. 84, Table 84–6, p. 1205.

- Leukopenia, thrombocytopenia, a relative increase in band neutrophils, and a small proportion of reactive lymphocytes usually can be identified on the blood.
- Lymphocytosis is uncommon.

OTHER AGENTS LINKED TO MONONUCLEOSIS SYNDROME

- Herpes virus-6
- Varicella zoster.
- Hepatitis A or B.
- Rubella.
- Adenovirus.
- *T. gondii:*
  — Only nonviral agent commonly identified as causing a mononucleosis syndrome.
  — Infection secondary to ingestion of cysts in raw meat or of oocysts in cat feces.
  — There is no documented person-to-person transmission.
  — Is usually asymptomatic or isolated lymphadenopathy without fever.
  — Patients do not commonly have pharyngitis.

DIFFERENTIAL DIAGNOSIS

- Acute pharyngitis can be caused by infection with β-hemolytic streptococcus, adenovirus, *Arcanobacterium haemolyticum*.
- Fever, lymphocytosis, and splenomegaly may raise consideration of lymphoma.
- CMV infection can be associated with presence of antinuclear antibodies similar to those of patients with new-onset systemic lupus erythematosus.
- Mononucleosis syndrome of toxoplasmosis can be distinguished from that caused by other infections by presence of high-titer antitoxoplasma antibodies.
- Patients with mononucleosis syndrome secondary to hepatitis virus infection generally have abnormal liver function tests.

THERAPY AND COURSE

- Disease is usually self-limited.
- Acetaminophen and/or gargling with saline for fever and pharyngitis.
- Prednisone 40 to 60 mg/day for 7 to 10 days, then taper dose over 1 week for severe or life-threatening complications, such as:
  — Imminent upper airway obstruction.
  — Immune thrombocytopenia purpura.
  — Immune hemolytic anemia.
  — Central nervous system involvement.
- Acyclovir generally is ineffective in the treatment of infectious mononucleosis.
- Ganciclovir may be beneficial for immunocompromised patients or in patients with severe, complicated primary EBV mononucleosis.
- Ganciclovir (5 mg/kg day for 14 days) is effective against CMV, but recommended only for patients with severe disease and/or who are immunocompromised.
- Antiretroviral therapy for primary HIV-1 infection can clear viremia and restore CD4 lymphocytes (see Chap. 52).

Mononucleosis in Pregnancy

- Abortion may be considered for any pregnant woman who develops infectious mononucleosis as a result of primary infection with EBV, CMV, or toxoplasmosis, especially during the first trimester.
- EBV mononucleosis during gestation can produce severe congenital anomalies, including microcephaly, hepatosplenomegaly, cataracts, mental retardation, or death.

- About half of the infants born to mothers who develop primary CMV infection during pregnancy will have congenital infection. Of these, about one-quarter will be symptomatic and/or have congenital anomalies.
- Primary toxoplasmosis infection in first trimester also can result in congenital abnormalities.
- Mothers with antitoxoplasmosis antibodies before pregnancy do not transmit the organism to the developing infant.
- HIV-1 can be transmitted to the infant during primary infection and should be treated with zidovudine alone or in combination with elective caesarean section to reduce the rate of maternal-infant HIV-1 transmission (see Chap. 52).

 For a more detailed discussion, see Robert F. Betts: Mononucleosis Syndromes. Chap. 84, p. 1199 in *Williams Hematology*, 8th ed.

PART VIII

THE CLONAL LYMPHOID AND PLASMA CELL DISEASES

CHAPTER 54
Classification and Clinical Manifestations of the Malignant Lymphoid Disorders

CLASSIFICATION

- Lymphocyte malignancies comprise a wide spectrum of different morphologic and clinical syndromes.
- The International Lymphoma Study Group proposed a new classification termed *R*evised *E*uropean–*A*merican *L*ymphoma classification, or *REAL* classification which was modified in 2001 and updated in 2008 by the World Health Organization (WHO) (see Table 54–1).
- The REAL/WHO classification makes use of the pathologic, immunophenotypic, genetic, and clinical features to define separate disease entities (Table 54–1).
- Distinctive cytogenetic abnormalities are also described in Table 54–1.
- Tumors are divided into two categories: indolent versus aggressive (Tables 54–2 and 54–3).

ASSOCIATED CLINICAL SYNDROMES

Abnormal Production of Immunoglobulin

- Neoplastic B cells can secrete monoclonal immunoglobulin proteins inappropriately (see Chap 68).
- If the monoclonal protein is IgM, IgA, or some subclasses of IgG (namely IgG3), this may increase the viscosity of the blood, impairing flow through the microcirculation (see Chaps. 69 and 70).
- The microcirculation can be impeded further by associated erythrocyte–erythrocyte aggregation (pathologic rouleaux) that often occurs when the blood concentration of immunoglobulin is high.
- Impaired circulation because of high blood viscosity and rouleaux can result in the "hyperviscosity syndrome" (see Chap. 70).

— Manifestations of the hyperviscosity syndrome include headache, dizziness, diplopia, stupor, retinal venous engorgement, and frank coma.
- Monoclonal immunoglobulins also can impair granulocyte or platelet function, or interact with coagulation proteins to impair hemostasis.
- Excessive excretion of immunoglobulin light chains can lead to several types of renal tubular dysfunction and renal insufficiency (see Chap. 69).
- Cryoglobulins (or immunoglobulins that precipitate at temperatures below 37°C) can result in Raynaud syndrome, skin ulcerations, purpura, or digital infarction and gangrene (see Chap. 25).
- Excessive production of monoclonal immunoglobulin can lead to formation of amyloid (see Chap. 72).

TABLE 54–1 INDOLENT LYMPHOMAS

Disseminated Lymphomas/Leukemias
    Chronic lymphocytic leukemia
    Hairy cell leukemia
    Lymphoplasmacytic lymphoma
    Splenic marginal zone B-cell lymphoma (with or without villous lymphocytes)
    Plasma cell myeloma/plasmacytoma
Nodal Lymphomas
    Follicular lymphoma
    Nodal marginal zone B-cell lymphoma (with or without monocytoid B cells)
    Small lymphocytic lymphoma
    Extranodal lymphomas
    Extranodal marginal zone B-cell lymphoma of mucosa-associated lymphoid
        tissue (MALT) type

Source: *Williams Hematology*, 8th ed, Chap. 92, Table 92–2, p. 1407.

TABLE 54–2 AGGRESSIVE LYMPHOMAS

Immature B-Cell Neoplasms
    B-lymphoblastic leukemia/lymphoma
Mature B-Cell Neoplasms
    Burkitt lymphoma/Burkitt cell leukemia
    Diffuse large B-cell lymphoma
    Follicular lymphoma grade III
    Mantle cell lymphoma
Immature T-Cell Neoplasms
    T-lymphoblastic lymphoma/leukemia
Peripheral T- and Natural Killer (NK) Cell Neoplasms
    T-cell prolymphocytic leukemia/lymphoma
    Aggressive NK cell leukemia/lymphoma
    Adult T-cell lymphoma/leukemia (associated with HTLV-1 [human T-cell
        leukemia virus type 1])
    Extranodal NK/T cell lymphoma
    Enteropathy-associated T-cell lymphoma
    Hepatosplenic T-cell lymphoma
    Subcutaneous panniculitis-like T-cell lymphoma
    Peripheral T-cell lymphomas, not otherwise specified
    Angioimmunoblastic T-cell lymphoma
    Anaplastic large cell lymphoma, primary, systemic

Source: *Williams Hematology*, 8th ed, Chap. 92, Table 92–3, p. 1407.

- Production of autoreactive antibodies in relationship to B-lymphocytic neoplasia may lead to:
  — Autoimmune hemolytic anemia (see Chaps. 24 and 25).
  — Autoimmune thrombocytopenia (see Chap. 74).
  — Autoimmune neutropenia (see Chap. 32).
- Autoantibodies directed against tissues are implicated in the etiopathogenesis of diseases such as autoimmune thyroiditis, adrenalitis, encephalitis, or other inflammation of other organs.
- Demyelinization can occur in patients with monoclonal immunoglobulin, resulting in peripheral neuropathies, or polyneuropathy (see Chaps. 68, 69, and 70).
- Occasionally, *p*olyneuropathy is associated with *o*rganomegaly, *e*ndocrinopathy, a *m*onoclonal protein, and *s*kin changes, resulting in *POEMS* syndrome (see Chap. 69).

Marrow and Other Tissue Infiltration
- Neoplastic lymphocytes may infiltrate the marrow extensively, impairing hematopoiesis.
- Malignant lymphocyte proliferation or infiltration may result in any combination of splenomegaly and lymphadenopathy of either superficial or deep lymph nodes.
- Malignant lymphocytes also can infiltrate extranodal sites:
  — T-cell lymphomas and leukemias frequently involve the skin, mediastinum, or central nervous system.
  — B-cell lymphomas may involve the salivary glands, endocrine glands, joints, heart, lung, kidney, bowel, bone, or other extranodal sites.
  — Marginal zone B-cell lymphoma of *m*ucosa-*a*ssociated *l*ymphoid *t*issue, or *MALT,* frequently involves the stomach, lung, and salivary glands.

Lymphokine-Induced Disorders
- Neoplastic lymphocytes may elaborate cytokines that contribute to the disease morbidity.
- Cutaneous T-cell lymphomas may elaborate T_H2-type cytokines (e.g., interleukins 4, 5, 10, and 13), causing eosinophilia or eosinophilic pneumonia (see Chaps. 66 and 67).
- Neoplastic plasma cells may secrete interleukin-1 (IL-1), a cytokine that can stimulate osteoclasts (leading to extensive osteolysis, severe bone pain, and pathologic fractures) and enhance production of antidiuretic hormone (leading to a syndrome of inappropriate secretion of antidiuretic hormone) (see Chap. 69).
- Dysregulated extrarenal production of calcitriol, the active metabolite of vitamin D, may underlie the hypercalcemia associated with Hodgkin lymphoma and other lymphomas (see Chap. 59).

Systemic Symptoms
- Lymphomas may produce "B symptoms," e.g., fever, night sweats, and weight loss (see Chaps. 59 and 61).
- Pruritus is common in Hodgkin lymphoma, and its severity parallels disease activity.
- Systemic symptoms may be present in Hodgkin lymphoma in the absence of obvious, bulky lymph node or splenic tumors.

Metabolic Signs
- Aggressive lymphomas and acute lymphocytic leukemias may have high-proportions of rapidly dividing and dying cells, causing hyperuricemia and hyperuricosuria.

TABLE 54-3   CLASSIFICATION OF LYMPHOMA AND LYMPHOID LEUKEMIA BY WORLD HEALTH ORGANIZATION

Neoplasm	Morphology	Phenotype	Genotype
B-Cell Neoplasms			
Immature B-Cell Neoplasms			
Lymphoblastic leukemia (see Chap. 55)	Medium to large cells with finely stippled chromatin and scant cytoplasm	TdT+, sIg–, CD10+, CD13+/–, CD19+, CD20–, CD22–, CD34+/–, CD33+/–, CD45+/–, CD79a+	t(1;19), t(9;22), and defects at 11q23-defects associated with poor prognosis
Lymphoblastic lymphoma (see Chap. 65)	Medium-sized cells with high nuclear to cytoplasmic ratio	See above	See above
Mature B-cell Neoplasms			
Leukemias			
Chronic lymphocytic leukemia (see Chap. 56)	Small cells with round, dense nuclei	sIg+ (dim), CD5+, CD10–, CD19+, CD20+ (dim), CD22+ (dim), CD23+, CD38+/–, CD45+, FMC-7–	IgR, trisomy 12 (~30%), del at 13q14 (~50%), 11q– (15%)
Prolymphocytic leukemia (see Chap. 56)	≥55% prolymphocytes	sIg+ (bright), CD5+/–, CD10–, CD19+, CD22+, CD23+/–, CD45+	IgR, trisomy 12 (~30%)
Hairy cell leukemia (see Chap. 57)	Small cells with cytoplasmic projections	sIg+ (bright), CD5–, CD10–, CD11c+(bright), CD19+, CD20+, CD25+, CD45+, CD103+, Annexin A+	IgR,
Lymphomas			
Small lymphocytic lymphoma (see Chap. 56)	Small round cells	sIg+ (dim), CD5+, CD19+, dim CD20+, CD23+, CD45+	IgR, trisomy 12 (~30%), del at 13q14 (~40%), 11q– (~15%)
Lymphoplasmacytic lymphoma (see Chap. 70)	Small cells with plasmacytoid differentiation	cIg+, CD5–, CD10–, CD19+, CD20+/– Plasma cell population: CD38+, CD138+, cIgM+	IgR, 6q– in 50% of marrow-based cases [the t(9;14) was proved to be wrong]
Mantle cell lymphoma (see Chap. 63)	Small- to medium-sized cells	sIgM+, sIgD+, CD5+, CD10–, CD19+, CD20+, CD23–, Cyclin D1+, FMC-7+	IgR, t(11;14)(q13;q32) (~100% by FISH), involving BCL1 and IgH

Type	Morphology	Immunophenotype	Genetics
Follicular lymphoma (follicle center lymphoma; see Chap. 62)	Small, medium, or large cells with cleaved nuclei	sIg, CD5−, CD10+, CD19+, bright CD20+, CD23−/+, CD38+, CD45+	IgR, t(14;18)(q32;q21) (~85%) involving BCL2 and IgH
Marginal zone B-cell lymphoma (see Chap. 64)	Small or large monocytoid cells	sIgM+, sIgD−, cIg + (~50%), CD5−, CD10−, CD11c+/−, CD19+, CD20+, CD23−, CD43+/−	IgR, commonly with trisomy 3 and/or t(11;18)(q21;q21) involving API2, MLT, or t(1;14)(p22;q32) involving BCL10
Mucosa-associated lymphoid tissue (MALT) type (see Chap. 64)	See above	See above	See above
Nodal type	See above	See above	IgR,
Splenic type	Small to large monocytoid and/or villous lymphocytes	sIgM+, sIgD−, CD5+/−, CD19+, CD20+, CD23−	
Diffuse large B-cell lymphoma (see Chap. 61)	Large, irregular cells that can resemble centroblasts, immunoblasts, multilobate cells, or even RS-like cells	sIgM+, sIgD+/−, CD5−/+, CD10−/+, CD19+, CD20+, CD45+, PAX5+	IgR, 3q27 abnormalities and/or t(3;14)(q27;q32) involving BCL6 (~40%) or t(14;18)(q32;q21) (~25%) involving BCL2
Primary mediastinal (thymic) large B-cell lymphoma (see Chap. 61)	Same as above	sIg−, CD5−, CD10−/+, CD15−, CD19+, CD20+, CD22+, CD30+/−, CD45+, CD79a+	Gain of 9q24 (75%), gain 2p15 (50%) Lack of rearrangements of BCL2, BCL6, or MYC
Burkitt lymphoma (see Chap. 65)	Medium-sized, round cells with abundant cytoplasm	sIgM+, CD5−, CD10+, CD19+, CD20+, CD23−, CD45+	t(8;14)(q24;q32), t(2;8)(q11;q24), or t(8;22)(q24;q11), involving Ig loci and C-MYC at 8q24
Burkitt-like lymphoma (see Chap. 65)	Medium-sized, round cells with abundant cytoplasm	Same as above except sIg −, cIg +/−, and CD10−	Same as above except more typically expresses high levels of BCL2 and ~30% have BCL2 rearrangements

(continued)

TABLE 54–1 (CONTINUED)

Neoplasm	Morphology	Phenotype	Genotype
B-Cell Neoplasms			
Plasma cell neoplasms Myeloma (see Chap. 69)	Plasma cells with occasional plasmablasts	cIg+, sIg–, CD5–, CD10–, CD19–, CD20–, CD38+(bright), CD45–/+, CD56–/+, CD117+/–(bright), CD138+(bright)	IgR, commonly with complex karyotypes and/or t(6;14) (p25;q32) involving *MUM1*. t(11;14)(q23;q32) can be found in 15–25% of cases
Plasma cell leukemia (see Chap. 69)	Plasmablastic cells with prominent nucleoli	Same as above except usually CD56–	Same as above
Plasmacytoma (see Chap. 69)	Plasma cells	Same as plasma cell myeloma	Same as above
Waldenström macroglobulinemia (see Chap. 70)	Lymphocytes, plasmacytoid cells, and plasma cells	CD5+/–, CD10–, CD19, CD20+, CD22+, CD38+/–	IgR, complex karyotypes common
Hodgkin Lymphoma (HL)			
Nodular lymphocyte predominant HL (see Chap. 59)	"Popcorn cells" with nuclei resembling those of centroblasts	BCL6+, CD19+, CD20+, CD22+, CD45+, CD79a+, CD15–, and rarely CD30+/–, Bob1+, Oct2+, PAX5+	IgR, with high-level expression of *BCL6*
Classic HL			
Nodular sclerosis HL	R-S cells and lacunar cells dispersed in reactive lymphoid nodules	R-S cells typically are CD15+, CD20+/–, CD30+, CD45–, CD79a–, PAX5+ (dim)	R-S cells generally express *PAX5* and *MUM1*, variable expression of *BCL6*, and have IgR, without functional Ig

Lymphocyte-rich HL	Few R-S cells with occasional "popcorn" appearance dispersed in lymphoid nodules	Same as above	Same as above
Mixed cellularity HL	R-S cells dispersed among plasma cells, epithelioid histiocytes, eosinophils, and T cells	R-S cells typically are CD15+, CD30+, CD45−, CD79a−	R-S cells generally express *PAX5* and *MUM1*, variable expression of *BCL6*, and have IgR, without functional Ig
Lymphocyte-depleted HL	Prominent numbers of R-S cells with effacement of the nodal structure	Same as above	Same as above

T-Cell Neoplasms

Immature T-Cell Neoplasms			
Lymphoblastic leukemia (see Chap. 55)	Medium to large cells with finely stippled chromatin and scant cytoplasm	TdT+, CD2+/−, cytoplasmic CD3+, CD1a+/−, CD5+/−, CD7+, CD10+/−, CD4/+CD8+ or CD4−/CD8−, CD34+/−	Abnormalities in *TCR* loci at 14q11 (TCR-α), 7q34 (TCR-β), or 7p15 (TCR-γ), and/or t(1;14)(p32–34; q11) involving *TAL1*
Lymphoblastic lymphoma (see Chap. 55)	Same as above	Same as above	Same as above
Mature T-Cell Neoplasms			
Leukemias			
T-cell prolymphocytic leukemia (see Chap. 67)	Small to medium size cells with cytoplasmic protrusions or blebs	TdT−, CD2+, CD3+, CD5+, CD7+, CD4+ and CD8− is more common than CD4− and CD8+, but can be CD4+ and CD8+	α/β TCR rearrangement, inv14(q11;q32)(∼ 75–80%)
T-cell large granular lymphocytic leukemia (see Chap. 58)	Abundant cytoplasm and sparse azurophilic granules	CD2+, CD3+, CD4 −/+, CD5+, CD7+, CD8+/−, CD16+/−, CD56−, CD57+/−	α/β TCR rearrangement, γ/δ rearrangement can be seen.

(continued)

TABLE 54–1 (CONTINUED)

Neoplasm	Morphology	Phenotype	Genotype
Lymphomas		T-Cell Neoplasms	
Extranodal T/NK-cell lymphoma, nasal type ("angiocentric lymphoma"; see Chaps. 58 and 67)	Angiocentric and angiodestructive growth	CD2+, cytoplasmic CD3+, CD4−, CD5−/+, CD7+, CD8−, CD56−, EBV+	TCR rearrangements variable, EBV present by *in situ* hybridization
Cutaneous T-cell lymphoma (mycosis fungoides; see Chap. 66)	Small to large cells with cerebriform nuclei	CD2+, CD3+, CD4+, CD5+, CD7+/−, CD8−, CD25−, CD26+	α/β TCR rearrangements
Sézary syndrome (see Chap. 66)	Same as above	Same as above	Same as above
Angioimmunoblastic T-cell lymphoma	Small to medium size immunoblasts with clear to pale cytoplasm around follicles and high endothelial venules	CD3+/−, CD4+, CD10+, CXCL13+, PD-1+, EBV+	α/β TCR rearrangement (75–90%), IgR, (25–30%), trisomy 3 or 5 noted
Peripheral T-cell lymphoma (not otherwise unspecified; see Chap. 67)	Highly variable	CD2+, CD3+, CD5+, CD7−, CD4+CD8− more often than CD4−CD8+, which is more often than CD4+CD8+	α/β TCR rearrangement
Subcutaneous panniculitis-like T-cell lymphoma	Variably-sized atypical cells with hyperchromasia infiltrating fat lobule	CD2+, CD3+, CD4−, CD5+, CD7−, CD8+, and cytoxic molecules (perforin, granzyme B, and TIA1)	α/β TCR rearrangement
Enteropathy-associated T-cell lymphoma	Small to large atypical lymphocytes	CD2+, CD3+, CD5−, CD7+, CD8−/+, CD4−, CD103+	β TCR rearrangement

Hepatosplenic T-cell lymphoma	Small to medium size cells with condensed chromatin and round nuclei	CD2+, CD3+, CD4−, CD5+, CD7+/−, CD8+/−	γ/β TCR rearrangement, rarely α/β TCR rearrangement, isochromosome 7q
Adult T-cell leukemia/lymphoma (see Chap. 55)	Highly pleomorphic with multilobed nuclei	CD2+, CD3+, CD5+, CD7−, CD25+, CD4+CD8− more often than CD4−CD8+	α/β TCR rearrangement, integrated HTLV-1
Anaplastic large-cell lymphoma	Large pleomorphic cells with "horseshoe"-shaped nuclei, prominent nucleoli, and abundant cytoplasm	TdT−, ALK1+, CD2+/−, CD3+/−, CD4−/+, CD5−/+, CD7+/−, CD8−/+, CD13−/+, CD25−/+, CD30+, CD33−/+, CD45+, HLA-DR+, TIA+/−	TCR rearrangement, t(2;5)(p23;q35) resulting in nucleophosmin–anaplastic lymphoma kinase fusion protein (NPM/ALK); other translocations involving 2p23 are also seen
Primary cutaneous CD30+ anaplastic large cell lymphoma	Anaplastic large cells as above in cutaneous nodules	TdT−, CD2−/+, CD3−/+, CD4+, CD5−/+, CD7+/−, CD25+/−, CD30+, CD45+	TCR rearrangement but without t(2;5)(p23;q35), therefore, ALK1

Natural Killer Cell Neoplasms

Large granular lymphocytic leukemia (see Chap. 58)	Abundant cytoplasm and sparse azurophilic granules	TdT−, CD2+, CD3−, CD4−, CD5−/+, CD7+, CD8−/+, CD11b/−, CD56+, CD57+/−	No TCR rearrangement
Aggressive NK-cell leukemia	Same as above	Same as above	No TCR rearrangement, EBV present
Extranodal NK-cell lymphoma, nasal-type ("angiocentric lymphoma")	Angiocentric and angiodestructive growth	CD2+, cytoplasmic CD3ε−, CD4−, CD5−/+, CD7+, CD8−, CD56+	No TCR rearrangement, EBV present

Source: *Williams Hematology*, 8th ed, Chap. 92, Table 92–1, p. 1405

- Cytotoxic therapy of bulky disease may cause extreme hyperuricemia, hyperuri-cosuria, hyperkalemia, and hyperphosphatemia, referred to as the *tumor lysis syndrome*.
- Precipitation of uric acid in the renal tubules and collecting system can lead to acute obstructive nephropathy and renal failure.
- Hypercalcemia and calciuria are common complications of plasma cell myeloma.

Extranodal Involvement
- May also involve skin, mediastinum, or the central nervous system.
- B cell lymphomas may involve the salivary glands, endocrine glands, joints, heart, lung, kidney, bowel, bone, or other extranodal sites (see Chap. 60).

For a more detailed discussion, see Thomas J. Kipps and Huan-You Wang: Classification of Malignant Lymphomas. Chap. 92, p. 1403 in *Williams Hematology,* 8th ed..

CHAPTER 55
The Acute Lymphocytic Leukemias

DEFINITION

- Acute lymphocytic (syn. lymphoblastic) leukemia (ALL) is a neoplastic disease of immature lymphocytes or lymphocyte progenitor cells of either the B- or T-cell lineage.
- The immune phenotype of the leukemia cells reflects the cell-lineage and differentiation stage of the transformed clone.
- At diagnosis the leukemia cells typically have replaced normal cells in the marrow and have disseminated to various extramedullary sites, accounting for many of the clinical manifestations.
- Treatment of ALL has progressed incrementally, beginning with the development of effective therapy for central nervous system (CNS) disease, followed by intensification of early treatment.
- Based on National Cancer Institute statistics, patients with ALL <45 years of age have a 5-year survival of 75 percent, which is heavily influenced by the approximately 80 percent cure rate in children with the disease. The 5-year survival is approximately 25 percent in the age group 45 to 54 and decreases in each succeeding decade to approximately 6 percent in patients over 65 years.

ETIOLOGY AND PATHOGENESIS

- Initiation and progression of ALL are driven by successive mutations that alter cellular functions, including an enhanced ability of self renewal, a subversion of control of normal proliferation, a block in differentiation, and an increased resistance to death signals (apoptosis).
- Chemical carcinogens have been studied for a potential role in causation but no unambiguous associations have been found.
- High-dose ionizing radiation, as experienced by atomic bomb survivors, may increase the risk for ALL.
- Nonionizing electromagnetic radiation is not a causal factor.

Incidence

- The age-adjusted incidence rate of ALL is 1.6 per 100,000 men and women per year in the United States.
  - It is estimated that 5430 cases (3220 males and 2210 females) were diagnosed with ALL in 2008 in the United States.
  - The median age at diagnosis for ALL is 13 years and approximately 61 percent are diagnosed before the age of 20 years.
  - ALL is the most common malignancy diagnosed in patients younger than age 15 years, accounting for 23 percent of all cancers and 76 percent of all leukemias in this age group.
- Only 20 percent of adult acute leukemias are ALL.
- Age-specific incidence patterns are characterized by a peak between the ages of 2 and 4 years, followed by falling rates during later childhood, adolescence, and young adulthood.
- Incidence rises again in the sixth decade and reaches a second, smaller peak in the elderly.
- The incidence of ALL differs substantially in different geographic areas.
  - Rates are higher among populations in northern and western Europe, North America, and Oceania, with lower rates in Asian and African populations.

- Hyperleukocytosis ($>100 \times 10^9$ white cells/L) occurs in 12 percent of white children, and 23 percent of black children and in 16 percent of adults.

Risk Factors

- Children with Down syndrome have a 10- to 30-fold increased risk of acute leukemias, including ALL.
  — *P2RY8-CRLF2* fusion and activating *JAK* mutations together contribute to leukemogenesis in approximately half of the cases of Down syndrome patients with ALL.
- Patients with genetic syndromes that affect genomic stability and/or DNA repair are at increased risk. These disorders include:
  — Ataxia-telangiectasia.
  — Nijmegen breakage syndrome.
  — Bloom syndrome.
- *In utero* (but not postnatal) exposure to diagnostic x-rays confers a slightly increased risk of ALL.

Prenatal Origins of Some Cases of ALL

- Germline single-nucleotide polymorphisms (SNPs) of *ARID5B* gene have been associated with childhood hyperdiploid B-cell precursor ALL.
- Retrospective identification of leukemia-specific fusion genes (e.g., *MLL-AF4*, *ETV6-RUNX1* [also known as *TEL-AML1*]) and development of concordant leukemia in identical twins indicate that some leukemias have a prenatal origin.
  — The coincidence of ALL among identical twins is about 20 percent overall, but approaches 100 percent if the index twin had developed ALL before the age of 1 year; the latter has been shown to be caused by metastasis within a shared placental circulation of ALL cells from one twin to the other *in utero*.
  — In identical twins with the t(4;11)/*MLL-AF4*, the concordance rate is nearly 100 percent, and the latency period is short (a few weeks to a few months).
  — The lower concordance rate in twins with the *ETV6-RUNX1* fusion or T-cell phenotype and the longer postnatal latency period suggest additional postnatal events are required for leukemic transformation in this subtype.
- Not all childhood cases develop *in utero*.

Postnatal Factors in Causation

- The observations of a peak age of development of childhood ALL of 2 to 5 years, an association of industrialization and modern or affluent societies with increased prevalence of ALL, and the occasional clustering of childhood leukemia cases have fueled two parallel infection-based hypotheses to account for postnatal events.
  — "Delayed-infection" suggests that some susceptible individuals with a prenatally acquired preleukemic clone had low or no exposure to common infections early in life because they lived in an affluent hygienic environment.
  — "Population-mixing" predicts that clusters of childhood ALL result from exposure of susceptible (nonimmune) individuals to common but fairly nonpathologic infections after population mixing with carriers.
  — t(1;19)/*E2A-PBX1* (also known as *TCF3-PBX1)* ALL appears to have a postnatal origin in most cases.

Acquired Genetic Changes

- More than three-fourths of all cases have recurring cytogenetic or molecular lesions with prognostic and therapeutic relevance (see **Table 55–1**).
- Hyperdiploidy (>50 chromosomes), which occurs in approximately one-third of pediatric cases and in 6 percent of adult cases, is associated with a more favorable prognosis.
- Hypodiploidy (<45 chromosomes) is associated with a poor prognosis.

TABLE 55–1	FREQUENCIES OF COMMON GENETIC ABERRATIONS IN CHILDHOOD AND ADULT ACUTE LYMPHOBLASTIC LEUKEMIA

Abnormality	Children (%)	Adults (%)
Hyperdiploidy (>50 chromosomes)	23–29	6–7
Hypodiploidy (<45 chromosomes)	1	2
t(1;19)(q23;p13.3) [*TCF3-PBX1*]	4 in white, 12 in black	2–3
t(9;22)(q34;q11.2) [*BCR-ABL1*]	2–3	25–30
t(4;11)(q21;q23) [*MLL-AF4*]	2	3–7
t(8;14)(q23;q32.3)	2	4
t(12;21)(p13;q22) [*ETV6-RUNX1*]	20–25	0–3
NOTCH1 mutations*	7	15
HOX11L2 overexpression*	20	13
LYL1 overexpression*	9	15
TAL1 overexpression*	15	3
HOX11 overexpression*	7	30
MLL-ENL fusion	2	3
Abnormal 9p	7–11	6–30
Abnormal 12p	7–9	4–6
del(7p)/del(7q)/monosomy 7	4	6–11
+8	2	10–12
Intrachromosomal amplification of chromosome 21 (iAMP21)	2	?

*Abnormalities found in T-cell ALL.
Source: *Williams Hematology*, 8th ed, Chap. 93, Table 93–1, p. 1411.

- The lymphoblasts from virtually all cases have acquired genetic changes that typically involve changes in chromosome number or structure.
- The most commonly recognized structural abnormalities result from translocations, followed by inversions, deletions, point mutations, and amplifications.
- Cooperative mutations are necessary for leukemic transformation and include genetic and epigenetic changes in key growth regulatory pathways.
- In one study, more than 40 percent of B-cell precursor ALL cases had mutations in genes encoding regulators of normal lymphoid development.
- The most frequent target was the lymphoid transcription factor *PAX5* (mutated in approximately 30% of cases), which encodes a paired-domain protein required for the pro-B-cell to pre-B-cell transition and B-lineage fidelity.
  — The second most frequently involved gene was *IKZF1* (mutated in almost 30% of the cases), encoding the IKAROS zinc finger DNA-binding protein that is required for the earliest lymphoid differentiation.
  — Approximately half of *BCR-ABL1* ALL cases had deletions of *CDKN2A/B* and *PAX5*.
- Overexpression of FLT3, a receptor tyrosine kinase important for development of hematopoietic stem cells, is a secondary event in almost all cases with either *MLL* rearrangements or hyperdiploidy.

CLINICAL FEATURES

- Symptoms may appear insidiously or acutely and presenting features generally reflect the degree of marrow failure and the extent of extramedullary spread (see Table 55–2).
- Patients typically present with signs or symptoms of anemia, e.g., pallor, fatigue, and lethargy, and in the older patient population, dyspnea, light-headedness, or angina.

TABLE 55–2   PRESENTING CLINICAL FEATURES IN CHILDREN AND ADULTS WITH ACUTE LYMPHOBLASTIC LEUKEMIA

Feature	Children	Adult
Age (years)		
<1	2	—
1–9	72–78	—
10–19	20–26	—
20–39	—	55
40–59	—	36
≥60	—	9
Male	56–57	62
Symptoms		
Fever	57	33–56
Fatigue	50	?
Bleeding	43	33
Bone or joint pain	25	25
Lymphadenopathy		
None	30	51
Marked (>3 cm)	15	11
Hepatomegaly		
None	34	65
Marked (below umbilicus)	17	?
Splenomegaly		
None	41	56
Marked (below umbilicus)	17	?
Mediastinal mass	8–10	15
CNS leukemia	3	8
Testicular leukemia	1	0.3

NOTE: Data are expressed as a percent of adult or childhood cases.
Source: *Williams Hematology,* 8th ed, Chap. 93, Table 93–2, p. 1412.

- Patients may have signs or symptoms of thrombocytopenia, e.g., petechiae, ecchymosis, and bleeding tendency, the degree of which can be enhanced by fever or infection.
- About half of the patients present with fever that is induced by pyrogenic cytokines (IL-1, IL-6, and TNF) released from leukemia cells; this typically resolves within 72 hours after the start of induction chemotherapy.
- About three-quarters of patients have hepatosplenomegaly and/or lymphadenopathy, the degree of which is more pronounced in pediatric cases.
- More than 8 to 10 percent of childhood cases and 15 percent of adult cases present with an anterior mediastinal mass that, in some cases, can compress the great vessels and trachea sufficiently to cause the superior mediastinal syndrome.
- More than 25 percent of pediatric cases present with bone or joint pain secondary to leukemia-cell infiltration or marrow necrosis.
- Infiltration of the testicle or lymphatic obstruction by leukemia cells can cause painless enlargement of the scrotum.
- Less common signs and symptoms include those resulting from leukemia-cell involvement of the CNS (e.g., headache, vomiting, alteration of mental function), renal collecting system (oliguria, anuria), eyes (diplopia, visual loss), salivary glands (Mikulicz syndrome), peripheral nerves (cranial nerve palsy), skin (leukemia cutis), or dorsal veins, and sacral nerves (priapism).
- In rare cases, the patient may present with spinal cord compression caused by epidural leukemia-cell mass.

LABORATORY FEATURES

- Anemia, neutropenia, and thrombocytopenia are common findings at presentation.
- Severity reflects the degree of marrow replacement by leukemic lymphoblasts (see Table 55–3).
- Twenty to forty percent present with blood neutrophil counts of less than ($<0.5 \times 10^9$/L).
- Patients can present with blood leukocyte counts ranging from 0.1 to 1500 $\times$ 10^9/L, and more than 10 percent will have leukocyte counts greater than ($>100 \times$ 10^9/L) with circulating blasts cells.
- As many as 16 percent of patients lack blasts in the blood film at the time of diagnosis, requiring a marrow biopsy for diagnosis.
- The leukemia blasts in over 70 percent of cases stain with the periodic acid–Schiff (PAS) reagent, are usually positive for terminal deoxynucleotidase (TdT) and typically negative for myeloperoxidase and nonspecific esterase.

TABLE 55–3 PRESENTING LABORATORY FEATURES IN CHILDREN AND ADULTS WITH ACUTE LYMPHOBLASTIC LEUKEMIA

	Percent of Total	
Feature	Children (White/Black)	Adults
Cell lineage		
T cell	15/24	
B-cell precursor	85/76	
Leukocyte count ($\times 10^9$/L)		
<10	47–49/34	41
10–49	28–31/29	31
50–99	8–12/14	12
>100	11–13/23	16
Hemoglobin concentration (g/dL)		
<8	48/58	28
8–10	24/22	26
>10	28/20	46
Platelet count ($\times 10^9$/L)		
<50	46/40	52
50–100	23/20	22
>100	31/40	26
CNS status*		
CNS1	67–79/60	92–95
CNS2	5–24/27	?
CNS3	3/3	5–8
Traumatic lumbar puncture with blasts	6–7/10	?
Leukemic blasts in marrow (%)		
<90	33/46	29
>90	67/54	71
Leukemic blasts in blood		
Present	87/90	92
Absent	13/10	8

*CNS-1: no blast cells in cerebrospinal fluid sample; CNS-2: <5 leukocytes/μL with blast cells in an atraumatic sample; CNS-3: ≥5 leukocytes/μL with blast cells in an atraumatic sample or the presence of a cranial nerve palsy; and traumatic lumbar puncture with blasts (≥10 erythrocytes/μL with blasts). Data on CNS2 and traumatic lumbar puncture with blasts not available in adults. Source: *Williams Hematology*, 8th ed, Chap. 93, Table 93–3, p. 1414.

- Findings that may precede the diagnosis of ALL by one to several months include:
  — Pancytopenia with an aplastic marrow (simulating aplastic anemia).
  — In rare cases, patients may present with a hypereosinophilic syndrome (e.g., pulmonary infiltration, cardiomegaly, and congestive heart failure), particularly males who have ALL cells with t(5;14)(q31;q32).
- Activation of the interleukin-5 gene on chromosome 5 by the enhancer element of the immunoglobulin heavy chain gene on chromosome 14 is thought to play a central role in leukemogenesis and the associated eosinophilia.
  — Occasional patients, principally male, present with thrombocytosis ($>400 \times 10^9$/L).
- Approximately 5 percent of patients, typically with T-cell ALL, may present with a mild coagulopathy.
- Serum immunoglobulin levels (particularly IgA and IgM) are decreased in about a third of childhood cases, particularly in association with B-cell ALL.
- Serum lactic acid dehydrogenase (LDH) is elevated in most patients and the level correlates with tumor burden and disease severity.
- Increased levels of serum uric acid are common in patients with large leukemic burden.
- Patients with massive renal involvement can have increased levels of creatinine, urea nitrogen, uric acid, and phosphorus.
- Less common laboratory abnormalities include hypercalcemia (caused by release of a parathyroid-like hormone from leukemia blasts), hyperuricemia (caused by an increased rate of cell turnover), elevated serum transaminases (caused by liver infiltration), or uremia (caused by renal failure secondary to kidney infiltration).
- Occasionally, patients with T-cell ALL may present with acute renal failure despite a relatively small degree of renal-cell infiltration by ALL cells.
- Liver dysfunction as a result of leukemic infiltration occurs in 10 to 20 percent of patients, usually is mild, and has no important clinical or prognostic consequences.
- Less common t(17;19)(q22;13.3) with *E2A-HLF* fusion, found in 0.5 percent of B-cell precursor ALL, is associated with:
  — Adolescent age.
  — Disseminated coagulopathy.
  — Hypercalcemia.
  — Dismal prognosis.
- Mediastinal mass and enlargement of the thymus may be seen on chest radiograph.
- About half of all pediatric cases present with periosteal reactions, osteolysis, osteosclerosis, or osteopenia, especially those with low leukocyte counts at presentation.
- A spinal radiograph may reveal vertebral collapse.

Evaluating CNS Disease

- It is essential to evaluate the cerebrospinal fluid (CSF) at diagnosis because of the high rate of CNS involvement.
  — CNS leukemia is defined by the presence of at least 5 leukocytes per microliter of CSF, or by the presence of cranial nerve palsies.
  — The presence of any leukemic blast cells in the CSF is associated with increased risk of CNS relapse.
- Contamination of the CSF by leukemic cells as a result of traumatic lumbar puncture at diagnosis is associated with an inferior treatment outcome in children with ALL.
  — Risk of traumatic lumbar puncture can be decreased by administering platelet transfusions to thrombocytopenic patients and by having the most experienced clinician perform the procedure after the patient is under deep sedation or general anesthesia.

Diagnosis and Cell Classification

- Examination of marrow aspirate is preferable for diagnosis of ALL.
- B-cell blasts in ALL are characterized by intensely basophilic cytoplasm, regular cellular features, prominent nucleoli, and cytoplasmic vacuolation.

- Analysis of a Wright-Giemsa stain (e.g., blood or marrow film) is insufficient to differentiate ALL from acute myeloid leukemia.
- Immunophenotyping of leukemia cells can help distinguish immunologic subtypes of ALL.
- A distinct subset of T-cell ALL that retain stem cell-like features, termed *early T-cell precursor ALL*, has been identified that is associated with a dire prognosis with conventional chemotherapy.
- Table 55–4 summarizes the salient presenting features of several recognized immunologic subtypes of ALL.
- Genetic classification
  — Approximately 75 percent of adult and childhood cases can be readily classified into prognostically or therapeutically relevant subgroups based on the modal chromosome number (or DNA content estimated by flow cytometry), specific chromosomal rearrangements, and molecular genetic changes.

TABLE 55–4   PRESENTING FEATURES OF ACUTE LYMPHOBLASTIC LEUKEMIA ACCORDING TO IMMUNOLOGIC SUBTYPE

Subtype	Typical Markers	Childhood (%)	Adult (%)	Associated Features
B-cell precursor	CD19+, CD22+, CD79a+, cIg±, sIg$^\mu$–, HLA-DR+			
Pro-B	CD10–	5	11	Infant or adult age group, high leukocyte count, initial CNS leukemia, pseudodiploidy, *MLL* rearrangement, unfavorable prognosis
Early pre-B	CD10+	63	52	Favorable age group (1–9 years), low leukocyte count, hyperdiploidy (>50 chromosomes)
Pre-B	CD10±, cIg+	16	9	High leukocyte count, black race, pseudodiploidy
B cell	CD19+, CD22+, CD79a+, cIg+, sIg$^\mu$+, sIgK↓, or sIg+	3	4	Male predominance, initial CNS leukemia, abdominal masses, often renal involvement
T lineage	CD7+, cCD3+			
T cell	CD2+, CD1±, CD4±, CD8±, HLA-DR–, TdT±	10	18	Male predominance, hyperleukocytosis, extramedullary disease
Pre-T	CD2–, CD1–, CD4–, CD8–, HLA-DR±, TdT+	1	6	Male predominance, hyperleukocytosis, extramedullary disease, unfavorable prognosis
Early T-cell precursor	CD1–, CD8–, CD5^{weak}, CD13+, CD33+, CD11b+, CD117+, CD65+, HLA-DR+	?	?	Male predominance, age >10 years, dismal prognosis

cCD3, cytoplasmic CD3; cIg, cytoplasmic immunoglobulin; CNS, central nervous system; sIg, surface immunoglobulin; TdT, terminal deoxynucleotidyl transferase.
Source: *Williams Hematology*, 8th ed, Chap. 93, Table 93–4, p. 1416.

— Two ploidy groups (hyperdiploidy >50 chromosomes and hypodiploidy <45 chromosomes) have clinical relevance. Hyperdiploidy, which is seen in approximately 25 percent of childhood cases and in 6 to 7 percent of adult cases, is associated with a favorable prognosis.
- Phenotype-specific reciprocal translocations are the most biologically and clinically significant karyotypic changes in ALL (see Table 55–5).

TABLE 55–5 CLINICAL AND BIOLOGIC FEATURES ASSOCIATED WITH THE MOST COMMON GENETIC SUBTYPES OF ACUTE LYMPHOBLASTIC LEUKEMIA

Subtype	Associated Features	Estimated Event-Free Survival (%)	
		Children	Adults
Hyperdiploidy (>50 chromosomes)	Predominant B-cell precursor phenotype; low leukocyte count; favorable age group (1–9 years) and prognosis in children	80–90 at 5 years	30–50 at 5 years
Hypodiploidy (<45 chromosomes)	Predominant B-cell precursor phenotype; increased leukocyte count; poor prognosis	30–40 at 3 years	10–20 at 3 years
t(12;21)(p13;q22) [*ETV6-RUNX1*]	CD13±/CD33± B-cell precursor phenotype; pseudodiploidy; age 1–9 years; favorable prognosis	90–95 at 5 years	Unknown
t(1;19)(q23;p13.3) [*TCF3-PBX1*]	CD10±/CD20–/CD34— pre-B phenotype; pseudodiploidy; increased leukocyte count; black race; CNS leukemia; prognosis depends on treatment	82–90 at 5 years	20–40 at 3 years
t(9;22)(q34;q11.2) [*BCR-ABL1*]	Predominant B-cell precursor phenotype; older age; increased leukocyte count; improved early outcome with tyrosine kinase inhibitor treatment	80–90 at 3 years	~60 at 1 year
t(4;11)(q21;23) with *MLL-AF4* fusion	CD10±/CD15±/CD33±/CD65± B-cell precursor phenotype; infant and older adult age groups; hyperleukocytosis; CNS leukemia; dismal outcome	32–40 at 5 years	10–20 at 3 years
t(8;14)(q24;q32.3)	B-cell phenotype; L3 morphology; male predominance; bulky extramedullary disease; favorable prognosis with short-term intensive chemotherapy including high-dose methotrexate, cytarabine, and cyclophosphamide	75–85 at 5 years	50–55 at 4 years
NOTCH 1 mutations	T-cell phenotype; favorable prognosis	90 at 5 years	50 at 4 years
HOX11 overexpression	CD10+ T-cell phenotype; favorable prognosis with chemotherapy alone	90 at 5 years	80 at 3 years
Intrachromosomal amplification of chromosome 21	B-cell precursor phenotype; low white blood cell count; intensified treatment required to avert a poor prognosis	30 at 5 years	?

Source: *Williams Hematology*, 8th ed, Chap. 93, Table 93–5, p. 1417.

DIFFERENTIAL DIAGNOSIS

- ALL should be considered in the differential diagnosis of patients with hypereosinophilia.
- ALL should be considered in the differential diagnosis of children and young adults with apparent aplastic anemia.
- Occasionally, hematogones in a regenerating marrow may mimic leukemic blast cells and require flow cytometry examination with optimal combinations of antibodies to distinguish these cells from residual leukemia cells.
- A major consideration in the differential diagnosis is whether the leukemic blasts represent of acute myelogenous leukemia (see Chap. 46).
- Marrow infiltration by small round-cell nonhematopoietic tumors, e.g., neuroblastoma, rhabdomyosarcoma, Ewing sarcoma, small cell lung cancer (see Chap. 12).
- Infectious diseases (e.g., mononucleosis especially those associated with thrombocytopenia) or hemolytic anemia (see Chap. 24 and Chap. 25) or pertussis (see Chap. 50).

THERAPY

Metabolic Complications

- Hyperuricemia can be treated with allopurinol (300 mg/d) or rasburicase (recombinant urate oxidase).
  - Allopurinol can decrease both the anabolism and catabolism of mercaptopurine by depleting intracellular phosphoribosyl pyrophosphate and by inhibiting xanthine oxidase.
  - If mercaptopurine and allopurinol are given together orally, the dosage of mercaptopurine generally must be reduced.
  - Rasburicase acts more rapidly than allopurinol and breaks down uric acid to allantoin, a readily excreted metabolite that is 5 to 10 times more soluble than uric acid. However, rasburicase is contraindicated in patients with glucose-6-dehydrogenase deficiency because hydrogen peroxide, a by-product of uric acid breakdown, can cause methemoglobinemia or hemolytic anemia.
- Hyperphosphatemia can be treated with a phosphate binder (e.g., aluminum hydroxide, calcium carbonate or acetate).

Hyperleukocytosis

- Hyperleukocytosis ($>100 \times 10^9$ white cells/L) is treated with
  - Either leukapheresis or exchange transfusions (in small children).
  - Preinduction therapy with low-dose glucocorticoids, with addition of vincristine and cyclophosphamide in cases of B-cell ALL, is a favored means of ameliorating hyperleukocytosis.
  - Hydration and alkalinization of urine through intravenous administration of sodium bicarbonate to reduce the risk of urate nephropathy during induction chemotherapy.

Infection Control

- Exercise precautions for immunocompromised persons (e.g., avoidance of overtly infected persons, uncooked vegetables, unpeeled fruits, fresh cut flowers).
- Broad-spectrum antibiotics for febrile patients with newly diagnosed ALL, especially in the setting of neutropenia.
- Trimethoprim-sulfamethoxazole, 2 to 3 days per week, for prophylaxis against pneumonia with *Pneumocystis*.
- Prophylaxis is started 2 weeks after remission induction and continues until 6 weeks after completion of all chemotherapy.

- Alternative treatments for patients who cannot tolerate trimethoprim sulfamethoxazole include aerosolized pentamidine and atovaquone (which should be taken with food or a milky drink).
- Live-virus vaccines should not be administered.

Antileukemic Therapy
- The aim of treatment is to achieve complete remission, in which there is no evidence of leukemia in the body and the marrow has been cleared of apparent lymphoblasts.

B-Cell ALL
- Aggressive cyclophosphamide-based regimens appear most effective for patients with B-cell ALL (L3 morphology, surface immunoglobulin-positive).
  — Effective CNS therapy is an essential component of successful regimens for B-cell ALL and generally consists of methotrexate and cytarabine administered both systematically and intrathecally.
  — B-cell ALL rarely, if ever, recurs after the first year; therefore, prolonged continuation therapy is not necessary.

Precursor B-cell ALL and T-cell ALL
- Cyclophosphamide and cytarabine for T-cell ALL.
- There are typically three standard phases of treatment for the average-risk patient, both children and adults:
  — Remission induction.
  — Consolidation.
  — Maintenance/continuation therapy.

Remission Induction
- Goal is to purge the body of leukemia cells to prevent further spread of the disease to the brain and spinal cord.
- Hospitalization is usually necessary at some point to help prevent infection and to administer blood products.
- Specific drugs vary and are different for adults and children.
- For induction, nearly everyone receives vincristine and a glucocorticoid (e.g., prednisone, prednisolone, or dexamethasone), and adults typically also receive an anthracycline, such as daunorubicin.
- Adding L-asparaginase to the induction regimen provides for response rates of approximately 98 percent in children and approaching 90 percent in adults with standard-risk disease.
- There are three forms of L-asparaginase, each with a different pharmacokinetic profile when given intravenously:
  — *Erwinia carotovora* L-asparaginase has a relatively short half-life and is generally given at 20,000 IU/m^2 three times per week for 6 to 12 doses.
  — *Escherichia coli* L-asparaginase is generally given at a dose ranging from 5000 to 10,000 IU/m^2 two to three times per week for 6 to 12 doses.
  — *Polyethylene glycol (PEG)* L-asparaginase (pegaspargase) has the longest half-life and usually is given every other week for two doses at 2,500 IU/m^2.
  — The dose intensity and duration of treatment are more important than the type of L-asparaginase used.
- Because of lower immunogenicity, improved efficacy, and less frequent administration, pegaspargase has replaced the native product as the first-line treatment for children in the United States.

Consolidation Therapy
- Defined as treatment given shortly after remission induction upon restoration of normal hematopoiesis.
- Regimens typically consist of high doses of multiple agents not used during induction therapy or readministration of the induction regimen.

- Consolidation therapy has improved outcome in pediatric patients, even in those with low-risk disease commonly used regimens in childhood cases include:
  — High-dose methotrexate (5 g/m^2) with or without 6-mercaptopurine.
  — High-dose L-asparaginase given for an extended period.
  — An epipodophyllotoxin plus cytarabine.
  — Combinations of dexamethasone, vincristine, L-asparaginase, doxorubicin, and thioguanine, with or without cyclophosphamide.
- Consolidation therapy for adult patients with ALL has become standard.
  — Consolidation regimens consisting of high-dose cytarabine and daunorubicin failed to improve outcome in randomized trials.
  — In adults, methotrexate dose probably should be limited to 1.5 to 2 g/m^2 because higher doses may lead to excessive toxicities.
- Prolonged (4-month) consolidation therapy with methotrexate, cytarabine, thioguanine, cyclophosphamide, and L-asparaginase yielded the same outcome as did short (1-month) consolidation therapy with cyclophosphamide and L-asparaginase alone.
- Some of the agents that appear to offer the greatest benefit in consolidation regimens are:
  — High-dose cytarabine for standard- and high-risk disease other than T-cell ALL.
  — High-dose cytarabine and mitoxantrone for very-high-risk ALL bearing the t(4;11) translocation or rearrangement involving the *MLL* gene (at 11q23).

Maintenance Therapy

- Maintenance, or continuation, therapy usually involves daily low-dose chemotherapy given for 2 to 3 years.
  — Because boys, but not girls, benefit from a third year of therapy, girls typically receive 2 years and boys 3 years of maintenance therapy.
  — In most adult trials, maintenance therapy is given for 2 years.
- Mature B-cell ALL rarely recurs after the first year, so prolonged maintenance therapy is not recommended.
- Maintenance therapy typically involves weekly administration of methotrexate (orally or intravenously) and daily doses of oral 6-mercaptopurine to patients who remain in remission.
- Intermittent pulses of vincristine and a glucocorticoid may improve the efficacy of such antimetabolite-based regimens.
- Studies show that maintenance therapy lowers the relapse rate in childhood ALL, except in cases of mature B-cell leukemia.
- Aggressive maintenance may be fatal for some children.
- One in 300 patients have an inherited deficiency of thiopurine *S*-methyltransferase, are highly sensitive to 6-mercaptopurine, and only can tolerate small amounts of drug.

Therapy of CNS

- Extra treatment measures typically are necessary for eradicating leukemia cells from sanctuary disease sites (e.g., brain, testes, and spinal cord) that do not achieve therapeutic drug concentrations during systemic chemotherapy.
- High rate of CNS relapse after successful systemic chemotherapy can be lowered to less than 2 percent with prophylactic therapy of the CNS.
- Intrathecal (IT) chemotherapy may be as effective as cranial irradiation:
  — IT methotrexate for low-risk and intermediate-risk ALL.
  — Combined IT methotrexate, hydrocortisone, and cytosine arabinoside for high-risk ALL.
- Low-dose radiation (e.g., 1,200 cGy) may provide adequate protection against CNS relapse if used in the setting of effective systemic chemotherapy.
- CNS relapse requires systemic therapy along with treatment of CNS (cranial irradiation 24 Gy plus combined triple IT therapy).
- The outcome after CNS relapse is poor, analogous to the outcome after marrow relapse.
- Survival after CNS relapse is usually less than 1 year in adults.

Allogeneic Hematopoietic Stem Cell Transplantation
- Controversial for patients during first remission.
- Typically considered for patients who have histocompatible donors and who:
  — Require extended (>4 weeks) of induction therapy because of refractory disease.
  — Are adults and have high leukocyte counts on presentation.
  — Develop hematologic relapse while on therapy or shortly thereafter.
  — High level of minimal residual disease after remission.

BCR-ABL-positive ALL
- The use of tyrosine kinase inhibitor imatinib in BCR-ABL–positive ALL.
- In combination with chemotherapy, tyrosine kinase inhibitor not only induced a higher complete remission rate but also a higher rate of molecular remission (~50%) in adults.

COURSE AND PROGNOSIS

Relapse
- Relapsed disease may occur at any site.
- Most relapses occur during treatment or within the first 2 years after its completion.
- In 25 percent of childhood ALL and in 65 percent of adult ALL, the disease will recur after consolidation and maintenance therapy.
- Factors that influence the likelihood of relapse include:
  — Age over 30 years.
  — A high white blood cell count at the time of diagnosis (e.g., $>50 \times 10^9$/L).
  — Disease that has spread beyond the marrow to other organs.
  — Certain genetic abnormalities, such as the presence of *MLL* gene rearrangements (at 11q23) or the Ph chromosome.
  — The need for extended (>4 weeks) induction therapy to attain complete remission.
- Poor prognosis:
  — Relapse while on therapy or after a short initial remission.
  — T-cell ALL immunophenotype.
  — The presence of the BCR-ABL translocation.
  — An isolated hematologic relapse.
  — Presence of minimal residual disease after reinduction treatment.
  — Adults with isolated CNS relapse.
- Marrow relapse is the most common site of relapse and portends a poor outcome.
- Typical signs or symptoms are anemia, leukocytosis, leukopenia, thrombocytopenia, bone pain, fever, or sudden decrease in tolerance to chemotherapy.
- Prolonged second remissions (>3 years) may be obtained with chemotherapy in about half of patients with a late relapse (e.g., >6 months after cessation of therapy), but only in about 10 percent of those with an early relapse.
- Testicular relapse:
  — One-third of patients with early testicular relapse and two-thirds of patients with late testicular recurrence became long-term survivors after salvage chemotherapy and testicular irradiation.
  — Late relapse after cessation of maintenance is compatible with subsequent long disease-free survival after treatment.
  — Treatment recommended is bilateral testicular irradiation with 20 Gy in 2-Gy fractions and systemic reinduction.
  — One-third of patients with isolated early testicular relapse and two-thirds with late relapse in this site survive long-term.
- CNS relapses:
  — Efficacy of salvage therapy depends on history of prior CNS irradiation.
  — Intensive chemotherapy and craniospinal irradiation can secure long-term remission in previously unirradiated patients.

Treatment Sequelae

- Currently, the induction mortality ranges between 2 percent and 11 percent in adult ALL.
- A major source of mortality is infection with bacteria or fungi.
- The death rate among elderly patients receiving remission induction therapy can be as high as 30 percent.
- Poor tolerance of chemotherapy and consequent reduction of dose intensity largely account for the generally poor clinical outcome in elderly patients.
- Table 55–6 lists the side effects associated with antileukemic therapy.

TABLE 55–6	SOME SIDE EFFECTS ASSOCIATED WITH ANTILEUKEMIC THERAPY	
Treatment	**Acute Complications**	**Delayed Complications**
Prednisone (or prednisolone)	Hyperglycemia, hypertension, changes in mood or behavior, acne, increased appetite, weight gain, peptic ulcer, hepatomegaly, myopathy	Avascular necrosis of bone, osteopenia, growth retardation
Dexamethasone	Same as prednisone, except for increased changes in mood or behavior and myopathy but less salt retention	Same as prednisone
Vincristine	Peripheral neuropathy, constipation, chemical cellulitis, seizures, hair loss	None
Daunorubicin, idarubicin, doxorubicin, or epirubicin	Nausea and vomiting, hair loss, mucositis, marrow suppression, chemical cellulitis, increased skin pigmentation	Cardiomyopathy (with high cumulative dose)
L-Asparaginase	Nausea and vomiting, allergic reactions (manifested as rashes, bronchospasm, severe pain at intramuscular injection site), hyperglycemia, pancreatitis, liver dysfunction, thrombosis, encephalopathy	None
Mercaptopurine	Nausea and vomiting, mucositis, marrow suppression, solar dermatitis, liver dysfunction: increased hematologic toxicity in persons lacking thiopurine methyltransferase	Osteoporosis (long-term use), acute myeloid leukemia in persons with thiopurine methyltransferase deficiency
Methotrexate	Nausea and vomiting, liver dysfunction, marrow suppression, mucositis (resulting from high-dose treatment), solar dermatitis	Leukoencephalopathy, osteopenia (resulting from long-term use)
Etoposide, teniposide	Nausea and vomiting, hair loss, mucositis, marrow suppression, allergic reactions (bronchospasm, urticaria, angioedema, hypotension)	Acute myeloid leukemia
Cytarabine	Nausea and vomiting, fever, skin rashes, mucositis, marrow suppression, liver dysfunction, conjunctivitis (resulting from high-dose treatment)	Decreased fertility (with high cumulative dose)

(continued)

TABLE 55-6	(CONTINUED)	
Treatment	Acute Complications	Delayed Complications
Cyclophosphamide	Nausea and vomiting, hemorrhagic cystitis, marrow suppression, syndrome of inappropriate secretion of antidiuretic hormone, hair loss	Bladder cancer or acute myeloid leukemia (rare), decreased fertility (with high cumulative dose)
Rituximab	Infusion reactions, mucocutaneous reactions, cardiac arrhythmias, lymphopenia	Reaction of virus infections, progressive multifocal leukoencephalopathy from JC virus infection
Intrathecal methotrexate	Headache, fever, seizure, marrow suppression, mucositis (in patients with renal dysfunction)	Encephalopathy or myelopathy (with high cumulative dose)
Brain irradiation	Hair loss, postirradiation somnolence syndrome (6–10 weeks after treatment)	Seizure, mineralizing microangiopathy, growth hormone deficiency, thyroid dysfunction, obesity, osteopenia, brain tumors, basal cell carcinoma, parotid gland carcinoma, hair loss, cataract (rare), dental abnormalities

Source: *Williams Hematology,* 8th ed, Chap. 93, Table 93–6, p. 1423.

- Potential acute side effects of therapy occurring during or shortly after induction therapy:
  — Hyperglycemia with glucocorticoid use in more than 10 percent of cases.
  — Pancreatitis in a subset of patients treated with L-asparaginase.
  — Mucositis with anthracycline or antimetabolite chemotherapy.
  — Tumor lysis syndrome.
  — Hypercoagulable state.
  — Complications of marrow suppression.
- Potential delayed side effects of therapy:
  — Neurologic impairment from CNS therapy.
  — Growth and development impairment.
  — Aseptic necrosis of the bone.
  — Obesity, which occurs in 30 percent of young adult survivors of ALL.
  — Testicular damage in boys.
- Risk of development of a second malignancy.
  — Brain tumors and acute myelogenous leukemia most common.
  — Median latency period is 9 to 20 years, depending on the type of second malignancy.

Prognostic Markers
- Of the many variables that influence prognosis, risk-categorization is the most important.
- Childhood ALL cases are divided into low-, standard-, or high-risk groups.

- Low risk:
  - B-cell-precursor phenotype.
  - Age 1 to 9 years.
  - Presenting leukocyte count less than 50×10^9/L.
  - Hyperdiploidy.
  - Absence of CNS or testicular involvement.
  - *ETV6-RUNX1* fusion.
  - Absence of hypodiploidy or other cytogenetic features of high-risk disease.
- Standard risk:
  - T-cell ALL and all cases of B-cell precursor ALL not meeting criteria for low- or high-risk disease.
- High risk:
  - Presenting leukocyte count greater than 50×10^9/L.
  - Presence of certain cytogenetic abnormalities, for example:
  - t(9;22)(q34;q11), resulting in *BCR-ABL* fusion gene.
  - ALL cells with t(8;14), t(2;8), or t(8;22) genetic translocations involving *c-MYC*.
  - Leukemia cells with t(1;19)(q23;p13.3) involving *E2A* and *PBX1*.
  - ALL cells with t(4;11) involving the *MLL-AF4* gene at 11q23 (dismal prognosis).
  - Most T-cell ALL.
  - Poor early response to therapy or induction failure.
- Adult ALL cases can be divided into standard- or high-risk groups (see Table 55–7).
- Standard risk:
  - Patients younger than 60 years of age.
  - Hyperdiploidy or absence of hypodiploidy.
  - Absence of adverse cytogenetic abnormalities.
- High risk:
  - Age greater than 60.
  - Presence of cytogenetic abnormalities noted for pediatric high-risk disease.
  - Presenting leukocyte count greater than 50×10^9/L.
  - Hypodiploidy.
  - Poor early response to therapy or induction failure.

TABLE 55–7	ADVERSE PROGNOSTIC FACTORS IN ADULT ALL	
Factors	B-Cell Precursor	T Cell
Age (years)*	>35	>35
Leukocyte count ($\times 10^9$/L)	>30	>100
Immunophenotype	Pro-B (CD10–)	Pre T
Genetics	t(9;22) [*BCR-ABL1*]	*HOX11L2* expression?
	t(4;11) [*MLL-AF4*]	*ERG* expression?
	Hypodiploidy?	
Treatment response	Delayed remission (>4 weeks)	Delayed remission (>4 weeks)
	Minimal residual disease >10^{-4} after induction	Minimal residual disease >10^4 after induction

*Continuous factor with increasing age associated with progressively worse outcome.
Source: *Williams Hematology*, 8th ed, Chap. 93, Table 93–7, p. 1424.

For a more detailed discussion, see Ching-Hon Pui: Acute Lymphoblastic Leukemia. Chap. 93, p. 1409 in *Williams Hematology*, 8th ed.

CHAPTER 56
The Chronic Lymphocytic Leukemias

DEFINITION

- Chronic lymphocytic leukemia (CLL) is a neoplastic disease characterized by accumulation of small, mature-appearing lymphocytes in blood, marrow, and lymphoid tissues.
- The most prevalent adult leukemia in western societies.
- The age-adjusted incidence rate for CLL in the United States is 4.2/100,000 persons according to the Surveillance Epidemiology and End-Result Program of the National Cancer Institute.
- The age-adjusted incidence rate of CLL worldwide is 2.5/100,000 persons as determined by the International Agency for Research on Cancer of the World Health Organization.
- In 98 percent of patients, the disease is of B-cell lineage; less than 2 percent of patients have T-cell lineage leukemia.
- Approximately 0.8 percent of all cancers and approximately 30 percent of all leukemias annually.
- CLL is very uncommon in Eastern Asia (e.g., Japan and Korea).

ETIOLOGY AND PATHOGENESIS

Environmental Factors

- There is no exogenous factor (e.g., chemical, solvent) that has been established to increase the risk of CLL.
- Radiation exposure both in the Japanese as a result of the atomic bomb detonations in World War II and in Western cultures in patients treated with radiation for spondylitis and uterine cancers did not show an increased risk of CLL, despite an increased incidence of the acute leukemias and chronic myelogenous leukemia.
- CLL B cells may have receptors for Epstein-Barr virus but are not subject to EBV infection.

Hereditary Factors

- Familial occurrence in some patients.
  - Multiple cases of this leukemia may be found within a single family.
  - May also be found in association with other indolent lymphoproliferative disorders.
  - First-degree relatives of patients with lymphoplasmacytic lymphoma or Waldenström macroglobulinemia (see Chap. 70) have a greater than three-fold risk of developing CLL.
- Genetic factors that contribute to increased incidence of CLL:
  - Early studies have associated the risk of developing aggressive CLL with polymorphisms in the gene encoding CD5 (located at 11q13), CD38 (located at 4p15), or tumor necrosis factor-α (TNF-α) and other genes mapping to 13q21.33-q22.2.
  - Disease-susceptibility associated with single nucleotide polymorphisms in or around genes encoding proteins involved in apoptosis or immune regulatory pathways, namely *CCNH* (located at 5q13.3), *APAF1* (located at 12q23), *IL16* (located at 15q26.3), *CASP8* (located at 2q33.1), *NOS2A* (located at 17q11.1), and *CCR7* (located at 17q21.2).

Immunoglobulin Expression

- The leukemic cells from over 90 percent of patients with CLL express low levels of monoclonal surface immunoglobulin.
- Sixty percent of patients cells express κ light chains and 40 percent with λ light chains.
- Evidence for selection in the immunoglobulin genes expressed by CLL argues that stimulation through the immunoglobulin receptor plays a role in leukemogenesis.
- CLL cells express IgM in 25 percent and both IgM and IgD in over 55 percent of cases and rarely express other immunoglobulin isotypes.

Monoclonal B-Cell Lymphocytosis

- Studies using flow cytometry have found populations of B cells with the phenotype of CLL cells in the blood of healthy individuals.
- These monoclonal B cells coexpress CD5 and CD19 and have low level expression CD20 and CD79b.
- Fourteen percent of healthy first-degree relatives with two or more family members with CLL have circulating monoclonal B cells of the CLL B-cell immunophenotype.
- Approximately 8 percent of healthy individuals over the age of 60 years of age have circulating monoclonal B cells of the CLL phenotype whether or not they have an absolute lymphocytosis.
- Patients with monoclonal B-cell lymphocytosis may develop frank CLL that eventually will require treatment at the rate of approximately one percent per year.

Cytogenetic Abnormalities

- Using Q-banding and/or G-banding techniques and improved methods for inducing leukemia cell proliferation *in vitro*, the leukemic cells from more than half of all CLL patients have clonal chromosomal abnormalities.

Chromosome 13 Anomalies

- The most common genetic abnormality and one found in about half of all patients is deletion on the long arm of chromosome 13, specifically at 13q14.-23.1 telomeric to the retinoblastoma gene (*RB-1*) and centromeric to and including the D12S25 region.
- Loss of microRNA *miR15* and/or *miR16-1* might contribute to leukemogenesis and account for the frequent deletions that are observed at 13q14.3.

Chromosome 12 Anomalies

- Trisomy 12 is the second common abnormality, found in about 20 percent of patients; half of these have trisomy 12 only.
- May not be a primary factor in leukemogenesis, but probably acquired during disease evolution.

Chromosome 11 Anomalies

- Approximately 20 percent of patients have a deletion(s) in the long arm of chromosome 11, termed 11q⁻, which is associated with relatively poor prognosis (11q22.3-q.23.1).
- Associated with younger age at diagnosis (< 55 years) and tend to have bulky cervical lymphadenopathy than patients without such genetic changes.
- Higher expression levels of CD38, FMC7, CD25, and surface immunoglobulin, and lower level expression of CD11a/CD18, CD11cd/CD18, CD31, CD48, and CD58.
- Distinct microRNA signatures and characteristic low-level expression of *miR-29* and *miR-18*.

Chromosome 6 Anomalies
- Involve deletions at 6q23 but can also involve deletions at 6q25–27 and/or 6q2.
- 6q21 and 6q24 generally have higher proportions of blood prolymphocytes, higher than average expression of CD38.
- Patients tend to have more aggressive disease than patients with normal cytogenetics or isolated deletions at 13q14.

Chromosome 17 Anomalies
- Deletions in the short arm of chromosome 17 at 17p13.1 are in approximately 10 percent of all patients. The critical gene in the region that typically is deleted is *TP5*.
- 17p– and/or *TP53* mutations generally have more advanced disease, a higher leukemia-cell proliferative rate, a shorter survival, and greater resistance to first-line therapy.
- Neoplastic cells from nearly half of the patients transform to an aggressive B-cell lymphoma (referred to as Richter syndrome or transformation) or B-cell prolymphocytic leukemia may have inactivating mutations in *TP53*.

Chromosome 14 Anomalies
- *t14;18* (or 2;18 and 22;18) translocations involving *BCL2* on chromosome 18 are uncommon. However, CLL cells from virtually all cases overexpress *BCL2* and this feature is characteristic of low-grade nodular B-cell lymphoma (see Chap. 62).

Chromosome 18 Anomalies
- Five percent have aberrant immunoglobulin gene arrangements with *BCL2* located on the long arm of chromosome 18, at 18q21.

Leukemia Cell Growth Kinetics
- In the spleen, proliferation of CLL cells occurs preferentially in the white pulp zones.
- Studies on patients who ingested heavy water to evaluate the growth kinetics of CLL cells *in vivo* revealed that the leukemic cells of each patient had birth rates ranging from 0.1 percent to greater than 1.0 percent of the entire clone per day.
  — This conflicts with the notion that CLL is principally an accumulative disease as a result of deficient apoptosis.
  — The study suggests that the blood lymphocyte count for any one patient is defined by a more dynamic process, in which leukemia cells are generated and die at appreciable rates.
- Expression of CXCL12 and CXCL13 by marrow stromal cells also could account for the accumulation of leukemia cells in the marrow, which invariably is infiltrated by leukemia cells in untreated patients with CLL.

Immunologic Defects
Immune Deficiency
- Combined immunoglobulin deficiency and impaired cellular immunity
  — Hypogammaglobulinemia is common in active disease.
  — T-cells although not intrinsically involved show impaired reactivity.
  — CLL B cells have little stimulatory activity in autologous or even allogeneic mixed lymphocyte culture and, thus, contribute to the immunodeficiency present in active disease.
- Increased incidence of common bacterial infections.
- Increased risk of opportunistic infections.
- High rate of opportunistic infections posttherapy requires use of prophylactic antibiotics and close monitoring for viral infections (e.g., cytomegalovirus).
- Higher risk of skin cancers.

Autoimmunity

- Autoimmune diseases frequently occur in CLL.
  - Autoimmune hemolytic anemia and immune thrombocytopenia are the most common.
  - Pure red cell aplasia and autoimmune neutropenia are less common.
  - Pathogenic autoantibodies are not produced by the neoplastic B-cell clone.

CLINICAL FEATURES

- Median age of patient at diagnosis is approximately 67 years.
- Male/female ratio is 2:1.
- Twenty-five percent of patients are asymptomatic, and the disease is detected because of lymphocytosis or lymph node enlargement.
- Many patients have fatigue, reduced exercise tolerance, or malaise.
- Some cases may present with chronic rhinitis secondary to nasal involvement of CLL cells.
- Patients with advanced disease may have weight loss, recurrent infections, bleeding, and/or symptomatic anemia.
  - Night sweats and fevers (the so-called B symptoms) are uncommon and should prompt evaluation for complicating infectious disease.
- Lymph nodes may become very large and coalescent.
- Eighty percent of patients have nontender lymphadenopathy at diagnosis.
- Approximately 50 percent have mild to moderate splenomegaly at presentation.
- Extranodal involvement is frequent but not commonly symptomatic.
  - CLL cell infiltrates all can develop in the scalp, subconjuctivae, prostate, gonads, or pharynx.
  - Occasionally, the leukemic cells infiltrate the lung parenchyma, producing nodular or miliary pulmonary infiltrates that can be detected on chest imaging.
  - Gastrointestinal tract also may be infiltrated with leukemic cells and may result in ulceration, gastrointestinal bleeding, or malabsorption.
  - Leukemic cell infiltration of the central nervous system is unusual but may produce headache, meningitis, cranial nerve palsy, obtundation, or coma.

LABORATORY FEATURES

Blood Findings

- The blood cell counts are characterized by an increase in the absolute lymphocyte count of greater than 5.0×10^9/L.
- The blood film has an increase in small, normal appearing lymphocytes to a degree related to lymphocyte count. Characteristically approximately one in six lymphocytes in the blood are CLL cells ruptured during preparation and are referred to as smudge cells.
- Fifteen percent of patients present with normocytic anemia.
- Twenty percent have a positive red cell antiglobulin (Coombs) test at some time in the disease.
- Thrombocytopenia caused by antiplatelet antibodies may develop at any time. In advanced disease, thrombocytopenia also may be a result of marrow replacement and/or splenic sequestration.

Marrow Findings

- Marrow is invariably infiltrated with small lymphocytes in one of four patterns:
  - Interstitial (or lacy): 30 percent. This is associated with a better prognosis and/or early stage disease.
  - Nodular: 10 percent.
  - Mixed interstitial/nodular: 25 percent.
  - Diffuse marrow replacement: 25 percent; associated with a poorer prognosis.

Lymph Node Findings

- Lymph nodes are affected by diffuse infiltrate of small lymphocytes that efface the node architecture and invade the subcapsular sinus.

Immunologic Studies

- Diagnosis of CLL requires sustained monoclonal lymphocytosis of greater than $5 \times 10^9/L$.
- The diagnosis of CLL rests on establishing the monoclonal nature of the lymphocytosis. For example, one usually determines if the light chain expression is either λ or κ (monoclonal) and not both (polyclonal).
- CLL cells typically express CD5+, CD10–, CD19+, CD20 (dull), CD23+, and CD103–; low expression of surface immunoglobulin; flow-level or absent expression of CD22 and CD79b.
- Cellular immune defects, possibly related to CLL cell expression of transforming growth factor (TGF)-β and the immune suppressive cell-surface phenotype of leukemia cells.
- FMC7, a monoclonal antibody that binds an epitope of CD20 formed when this surface antigen is present at high density, typically does not react with CLL cells.
- Higher content of cytoplasmic immunoglobulin.

Serum Protein Electrophoresis

- Most common finding is hypogammaglobulinemia.
- Reduction in the serum levels of IgM precedes that of IgG and IgA.
- Five percent of patients have a serum monoclonal protein.
- In some cases, there is defective and/or unbalanced immunoglobulin chain synthesis by the leukemic B-cell clone, resulting in μ heavy-chain disease and/or immunoglobulin light-chain proteinuria (see Chap. 71).

DIFFERENTIAL DIAGNOSIS

- See Table 56–1 for the immunophenotype of chronic B-cell leukemias/lymphomas.
- Monoclonal lymphocytosis versus causes of polyclonal lymphocytosis (see Chap. 50).
- Prolymphocytic leukemia (see discussion later in this chapter).
  - Fifty-five percent of circulating leukemic lymphocytes should have prolymphocytic morphology; larger size than CLL cells and a prominent nucleolus.
  - High levels of CD79b and surface immunoglobulin; low levels of CD5 (see Table 56–1).
- Hairy cell leukemia (see Chap. 57).
- Lymphomas with circulating neoplastic cells (see Chap. 59).
- Small lymphocytic lymphoma.
  - Low-grade small lymphocytic B-cell lymphoma is closely related to B-cell CLL in its biology and clinical features.
  - Associated with lymph node involvement.
- Mantle cell lymphoma (see Chap. 63).
  - Express many of the same surface antigens as CLL B cells.
  - Does not express CD23.
- Splenic marginal zone lymphoma (SMZL) (see Chap. 64).
  - Commonly is called splenic lymphoma with villous lymphocytes.
  - Mature B-cell phenotype and express IgM and IgD, but typically lack expression of CD23, CD43, CD10, BCL-6, and cyclin D.
  - Neoplastic B cells have weak or negative expression of CD5.
- Lymphomas of follicular center cell origin (see Chap. 62).
  - Small cleaved cell lymphomas express the CD10 (CALLA) antigen.

TABLE 56–1 IMMUNOPHENOTYPE OF CHRONIC B-CELL LEUKEMIAS/LYMPHOMAS

Disease Entity	sIg	CD5	CD10	CD11C	CD19	CD20	CD22	CD23	CD25	CD103
Chronic lymphocytic leukemia	+/–	++	–	–/+	+	+/–	–/+	++	–/+	–
Prolymphocytic leukemia	++	+	–	–/+	+	+/–	+	+/–	–	–
Hairy cell leukemia	+/–	–/+	–	++	+	+	++	–/–	+	++
Mantle cell lymphoma	+	++	–	–	+	+	+/–	–/+	–	–
Splenic margina zone lymphoma	+	–/+	–/+	+	+	+	+/–	–/+	–	–
Lymphoplasmacytoid lymphoma	+/–	–/+	–	–	+	+/–	+/–	–/+	+/–	–
Follicular center lymphoma	+	–	+	–	+	++	+	–/+	–	–

sIg, surface immunoglobulin.

– Leukemia cells do not express the surface antigen; + leukemia cells from most cases express the surface antigen; +/–, low-level expression; –/+, most cases either do not express the antigen or express it at very low levels; ++, high-level expression of the surface antigen in nearly all cases.

Source: *Williams Hematology*, 8th ed, Chap. 94, Table 94–1, p. 144C.

- Lymphoplasmacytic leukemias.
  — Express CD38, PCA-1, CD56, and CD85; low-level or lack of expression of CD19, CD20, CD24, CD72, and HLA-DR.
- Waldenström macroglobulinemia (see Chap. 70).
- Myeloma (see Chap. 69).
- T-cell lymphoproliferative disorders.
- T-cell CLL and T-cell prolymphocytic leukemia (see discussion later in this chapter).
- Large granular lymphocytic leukemia (see Chap. 58).
- Adult T-cell leukemia/lymphoma (see Chap. 67).
- Cutaneous T-cell lymphomas (see Chap. 66).

THERAPY, COURSE, AND PROGNOSIS

Clinical Staging

- Clinical staging is helpful in defining prognosis and deciding when to initiate therapy.
- Rai or Binet staging systems can be used (see Table 56–2 and Table 56–3).
  — Despite the advent of new prognostic markers, these staging systems still have independent prognostic value.

TABLE 56–2 **RAI CLINICAL STAGING SYSTEM**

Revised Staging System	Original Staging System	Clinical Features at Diagnosis	Median Survival, Years
Low risk	0	Blood and marrow lymphocytosis	12
	I	Lymphocytosis and enlarged lymph nodes	11
Intermediate risk	II	Lymphocytosis and enlarged spleen and/or liver	8
High risk	III	Lymphocytosis and anemia (hemoglobin below 11 g/dL)	5
	IV	Lymphocytosis and thrombocytopenia (platelets below 100,000/μL)	7

Source: *Williams Hematology,* 8th ed, Chap. 94, Table 94–2, p. 1442.

TABLE 56–3 **BINET CLINICAL STAGING SYSTEM**

Stage	Clinical Features at Diagnosis	Median Survival, Years
A	Blood and marrow lymphocytosis and less than 3 areas* of palpable lymphoid-tissue enlargement	12
B	Blood and marrow lymphocytosis and 3 or more areas of palpable lymphoid-tissue enlargement	9
C	Same as B with anemia (hemoglobin below 11 g/dL in men or 10 g/dL in women) or thrombocytopenia (platelets less than 1.0×10^{11}/L)	7

*An area is defined as the cervical, axillary, or inguinofemoral lymph nodes, or the liver and spleen. The liver and spleen together count as one area, as do the right and left cervical lymph nodes. However, bilateral enlargement of the axillary lymph nodes or the inguinofemoral lymph nodes each count as two areas. Thus, the number of enlarged lymphoid areas can range from one to five.
Source: *Williams Hematology,* 8th ed, Chap. 94, Table 56–3, p. 1443.

Other Prognostic Indicators
Leukemia Cell Doubling Time (LDT)
- The shorter the time it takes for the lymphocyte count to double, the worse the prognosis.
- If the lymphocyte count doubles in less than 1 year, median survival is about 5 years.

Immunoglobulin Gene Mutation Status
- Two groups are distinguished by the extent that their expressed immunoglobulin heavy chain variable region genes (IgHV) have undergone somatic mutation.
  — Half of all cases have leukemia cells that express nonmutated IgHV genes and have a greater tendency for disease progression.
  — The rest express IgHV genes with levels of base substitutions that distinguish them from their germ-line counterparts.
- One noted exception to this appears to be represented by patients who have leukemia cells that use a particular immunoglobulin gene, designated *IGHV3–21*.
  — Patients who have CLL cells that use a mutated *IGHV3–21* gene together with a λ immunoglobulin light chain encoded *IGHV3–21* apparently have a risk of aggressive disease similar to that of patients who have leukemia cells that express unmutated IgHV genes.

CD38
- High cell-surface expression of CD38 is associated with more aggressive disease and/or relatively poor prognosis.
- CD38-negative leukemia cells might later be found to have leukemia cells that express this surface antigen.

Zeta-Associated Protein of 70kDa (ZAP-70)
- CLL cases that use unmutated IGHV genes generally express levels of ZAP-70 comparable to normal T cells.
- CLL cases that use mutated IGHV genes generally do not express detectable levels of ZAP-70.
- CLL-cell expression of ZAP-70 appears to be a stronger prediction of need for early treatment than use of unmutated IGHV.

Serum Factors
- High-level in CLL cells of β_2-microglobulin (β_2M) is associated with adverse prognosis.

Indications for Treatment (See Table 56-4)
- Rai stage 0 to I, or Binet A should be monitored without therapy, unless they have evidence of progressive disease.
- Progressive disease:
  — An increase of 50 percent or more in blood lymphocyte count over a 2-month period or LDT of less than 6 months.

TABLE 56–4	INDICATIONS FOR THERAPY IN CLL
Anemia	
Thrombocytopenia	
Disease-related symptoms	
Markedly enlarged or painful spleen	
Symptomatic lymphadenopathy	
Blood lymphocyte count doubling time < 6 months	
Prolymphocytic transformation	
Richter transformation	

Source: *Williams Hematology*, 8th ed, Chap. 94, Table 94–4, p. 1446.

- — Transformation of CLL cells to a more aggressive histology causing worsening anemia and/or thrombocytopenia.
- — Increase of 50 percent or more in the size of the liver and/or spleen.
- — An increase of 50 percent or more on two consecutive exams performed about 2 weeks apart in the sum of the sizes of at least two lymph nodes, one of which must be greater than 6 cm.
- — Appearance of new palpable lymphadenopathy.
- Absolute lymphocyte count should not be used as the sole indicator for treatment.
- Stable disease:
  - — Patients who do not achieve a complete or partial response and who do not have progressive disease.

Response Criteria

- Response criteria for patients who have had prior therapy are the same as those used for initial therapy.
- Four major response criteria:
  - — Complete response.
  - — Partial response.
  - — Nonresponse.
  - — Progressive disease.
- Incomplete marrow recovery (CRi): patients who fulfill all criteria for complete response except for persistent anemia, thrombocytopenia, or neutropenia unrelated to CLL.
- A patient is defined as having a relapse if they achieved complete or partial response but experienced disease progression 12 or more months after completing therapy.

Complete Response

- Requires that the patient is free of clinical disease for at least 2 months after therapy.
- Normal complete blood counts, e.g., neutrophil count at least 1.5×10^9/L, lymphocyte count less than or equal to 4.0×10^9/L, platelets greater than or equal to 1.0×10^{11}/L, and hemoglobin greater than 11 g/dL without transfusion.
- Absence of fever, night sweats, weight loss, or other disease-related symptoms.
- Absence of hepatosplenomegaly or detectable adenopathy.
- Marrow with less than 30 percent lymphocytes and lacking pathologic lymphoid nodules.
- If the marrow is found to be hypocellular, a repeat marrow biopsy should be performed after 4 to 6 weeks, provided blood counts have recovered. A marrow biopsy should not exceed 6 months after the last treatment.

Partial Response

- For at least 2 months after therapy, the patient must have at least:
  - — A 50 percent reduction in the number of blood lymphocytes.
  - — A 50 percent reduction in lymphadenopathy or hepatosplenomegaly.
- Absolute neutrophil count of greater than or equal to 1.5×10^9/L or greater than 50 percent improvement over that noted prior to therapy.
- Blood platelets greater than 100×10^9/L.
- Hemoglobin greater than 11 g/dL.
- A 50 percent improvement in platelet or red cell counts over pretreatment values without transfusion.
- Patients who satisfy the criteria for a complete response but who have persistent lymphoid nodules in the marrow are classified as having a *nodular partial response*.

Progressive Disease

- Develop new lymphadenopathy; an increase in lymphadenopathy by greater than or equal to 50 percent.

- An increase in the liver or spleen size by greater than 50 percent or the appearance of hepatomegaly or splenomegaly while on therapy.
- An increase in the absolute lymphocyte count by greater than or equal to 50 percent.
- Transformation to a more aggressive histology (e.g., Richter syndrome), which should be established by lymph node biopsy.

Refractory Disease
- Patient who experiences disease progression within 6 months of completing therapy is considered to have disease that is refractory to such therapy.

Minimal Residual Disease (MRD)
- Improved leukemia-cell detection methods using flow cytometry or polymerase chain reaction (PCR) can reveal patients in complete response who have residual leukemia cells.
- Patients who experience eradication of MRD apparently have a longer treatment-free survival than do patients who have achieved a complete response but have persistent MRD.

Cytogenetics and Type of Therapy
- Del(17p) predicts resistance to standard chemotherapy and thus an inferior prognosis.
- Del(11q) has significantly lower response rates to single-agent chemotherapy (e.g., chlorambucil or fludarabine monophosphate).
  — Response of such patients to treatment with a combination drug regimen using an alkylating agent, such as cyclophosphamide, with a purine analogue, such as fludarabine monophosphate, did not differ significantly from that of patients who have CLL cells that lack this deletion.

Age and Type of Therapy
- Treatment regimens found safe and well tolerated in clinical trials might prove too toxic for older patients treated in the community.
- Cumulative Illness Rating Scale: evaluate the burden of comorbidity on elderly cancer patients:
  — "GO GO": Patients who are medically fit with no or just mild comorbidities and a normal life expectancy.
  — "SLOW GO": Patients who are medically less fit with multiple or severe comorbidities and an unknown life expectancy.
  — "NO GO": Patients who are frail and had fatal comorbidities and a very short life expectancy.

Therapeutic Agents
Deoxyadenosine Analogues
Fludarabine (9-β-D arabinofuranosyl-2-fl uoradenine, F-ara-A)
- Inhibits adenosine deaminase (ADA). (9-β-D arabinofuranosyl-2-fluoradenine, F-ara-A).
- Most widely used deoxyadenosine analogue in the treatment of CLL.
- Complete and partial responses achieved in 50 to 60 percent of previously treated patients, and in 70 to 80 percent of untreated patients, at a dose of 25 mg/m^2 intravenously per day for 5 consecutive days each 28-day cycle.
- An oral formulation of fludarabine has been approved for use in North America and Europe
  — The recommended adult dose in single-agent therapy is 40 mg/m^2 for 5 consecutive days each 28-day cycle, which is equivalent to the 25mg/m^2 intravenous dose.
- Patients who do not respond to two cycles of therapy are unlikely to respond to further cycles of fludarabine as single-agent therapy.
- Ability to prolong survival is not established.

- Major toxicities are hematologic (e.g., cytopenias) and immunologic (e.g., increased susceptibility to infection).
- Renal clearance represents approximately 40 percent of the total-body clearance, which can also be achieved via hemodialysis in patients who experience acute renal failure after drug therapy.
- Should not be administered to patients with a glomerular filtration rate of less than 17 mL/min per m^2.

Cladribine (2-chlorodeoxyadenosine)
- Resistant to ADA with similar activity spectrum as that of fludarabine.
- Forty to 60 percent of patients respond to monthly cycles of cladribine per oral (PO) at 0.12 mg/kg daily for 5 consecutive days.
- Patients resistant to fludarabine generally are also resistant to cladribine as single-agent therapy.
- Thrombocytopenia may be dose limiting.
- Myelotoxicity and impaired cellular immunity similar to that of fludarabine.
- Ability to prolong survival is not established.
- Median duration of partial remissions is 9 months; nonresponding patients have a short median survival of 4 months.

Pentostatin (2′-deoxycoformycin)
- Inhibits ADA.
- Generally is administered at a dose of 4 mg/m^2 weekly for 3 weeks followed by 4 mg/m^2 every other week for 6 weeks, followed by once a month for 6 months.
- More than 90 percent of the administered drug is excreted unchanged in the urine.

Alkylating Agents
Chlorambucil
- Daily oral dose, initially 2 to 4 mg, up to 6 to 8 mg/d; can be advanced to 6 to 8 mg if tolerated.
- Intermittent schedule, total dose 0.4 to 0.7 mg/kg given over 1 to 4 days every 2 to 4 weeks or on day 1. Cycle repeated every 2 to 4 weeks.

Bendamustine (Treanda)
- Administered at 70 to 100 mg/m^2 given intravenously on each of 2 consecutive days every 4 weeks demonstrated overall response rates of 50 to 90 percent and complete response 10 to 30 percent in patients with relapsed/refractory CLL.
- A phase III trial comparing the activity of chlorambucil versus bendamustine in the initial therapy of 319 patients with CLL demonstrated significantly higher response rates in patients treated with bendamustine.
- Myelosuppression is the major toxicity.
- For patients who experience grade 3 or greater hematologic toxicity following treatment, it is recommended that the dose be reduced to 50 mg/m^2 on days 1 and 2 of each cycle.
- If grade 3 hematologic toxicity recurs, then further reduction of the dose to 25 mg/m^2 on days 1 and 2 should be considered.
- In the event of grade 4 hematologic toxicity or clinically significant grade 2 or higher nonhematologic toxicity, then treatment should be delayed until such toxicity has resolved, or at the discretion of the treating physician.
- Not recommended for treatment of patients with a glomerular filtration rate of less than 23 mL/min per m^2.

Cyclophosphamide
- As active as chlorambucil.
- Daily oral dose, 50 to 100 mg.
- Intermittent schedule with 500 to 750 mg/m^2 given orally or intravenously every 3 to 4 weeks.

- Fluid intake of 2 to 3 L per day important while taking cyclophosphamide to decrease risk of hemorrhagic cystitis.

Alemtuzumab (Campath-1H)
- Also known as MabCampath or Campath.
- Humanized monoclonal antibody specific for CD52.

Relapse/Refractory CLL
- Approved for use in patients refractory to fludarabine as single-agent therapy.
- Patients typically are given successively increasing doses 1 mg, 3 mg, 10 mg, and then 30 mg per intravenous injection to mitigate the infusional reactions of fever, chills, and/or rash, which generally are more pronounced during the initial administrations of this antibody.
- Grade 4 neutropenia is not uncommon, but is not an indication to discontinue treatment.
- Overall response rate of approximately 30 percent and complete response rate of 2 percent.
- Acute toxicity with infusion includes rigors, hypotension, rash, and dyspnea.
- Generally not effective for reducing lymphadenopathy.
- Causes profound T-cell depletion and immunosuppression.
- Acute infusional toxicity can be mitigated by preinfusion hydrocortisone at a dose of 100 mg intravenously and by initiating therapy with smaller doses that are increased on subsequent treatment days, if the lower dose is well tolerated (c.g., 3 mg per dose, then 10 mg per dose, and then 30 mg per dose).
- Treated patients have an increased susceptibility to opportunistic infections (esp. cytomegalovirus), and should receive concomitant antimicrobial therapy in prophylaxis against infection.
- Patients with bulky lymphadenopathy (greater than 5 cm in diameter) appear unlikely to achieve a complete response to therapy with this agent.

Initial Therapy
- Yields a longer progression-free survival duration than does single-agent chlorambucil.
- Campath has a complete response rate of 24 percent, an overall response rate of 83 percent, and time-to-progression requiring alternative treatment of 23.3 months, which were significantly superior to the complete response rate of 2 percent, OR rate of 55 percent, and time-to-progression of 14.7 months observed in the patients treated with chlorambucil.
- The US Food and Drug Administration (FDA) approved intravenous alemtuzumab for use in the initial therapy of patients with CLL in September 2007.

Subcutaneous Administration
- Administered subcutaneously at 30 mg three times per week for 6 or more weeks.
- Blood concentrations of alemtuzumab achieved following subcutaneous administration were significantly lower than those observed following intravenous administration of the same amount of antibody.
- Requires longer treatment durations and/or greater amounts of alemtuzumab to achieve comparable clinical responses as intravenous alemtuzumab.
- Not FDA approved.
- Adverse events include grade 1 or 2 local bruising and discomfort at site of injection.

Rituximab (anti-CD20)
- Humanized monoclonal antibody specific for CD20.
- Studies using single-agent rituximab at a dose of 375 mg/m^2 intravenously each week for 4 weeks noted only partial responses and in a minority of CLL patients.
- Several clinical trials have demonstrated therapeutic benefit (see Table 56–5).
- Responses observed are generally partial, limited to lymph nodes with median time to progression of less than 8 months.

TABLE 56–5 **RITUXIMAB TREATMENT REGIMENS**

Rituximab Treatment	Prior Therapy	No. pts. Evaluable	% CR	% OR	Median TTP (mo.)
375 mg/m^2 IV qwk × 4	Yes	30	0	13	N/A
375 mg/m^2 IV qwk × 4	Yes	28	0	25	5
500-825 mg/m^2 IV qwk × 4	Yes	24	0	21	N/A
1.0-1.5 g/m^2 IV qwk × 4	Yes	7	0	43	N/A
2.25 g/m^2 IV qwk × 4	Yes	8	0	75	N/A
375 mg/m^2 IV TIW qwk × 4	Mixed	29	4	52	11
375 mg/m^2 IV qwk × 4 then q 6 mo. for 2 yr.	Yes	44	9	58	19

CR, complete remission; IV, intravenously; OR, overall response, TIW, three times per week; TTP, time to progression.
Source: *Williams Hematology,* 8th ed, Chap. 94, Table 94–5, p. 1452.

- Toxicity at high dose is extremely common but is generally at grade 1 or 2 (fevers and chills).
- The severity of and risk for infusion-related reactions abate with successive infusions.
- Problems related to the initial treatment can be mitigated by slowing the rate of infusion and by splitting the first dose, giving 100 mg rituximab on the first day and then the remainder of the 375 mg/m^2 dose on day 2.

Glucocorticoids

- For treatment of associated autoimmune diseases; 1 mg/kg daily, and then taper.
- Partial responses can be achieved with intravenous high-dose methylprednisolone at 1 g/m^2 per day for 5 days at monthly intervals.
- Prednisone, as a single agent, can control disease in approximately 10 percent of patients.

Other Agents

- *Cytosine arabinoside:* High-dose cytosine arabinoside has modest activity in advanced-stage CLL.
- *Etoposide:* Patients who do not respond to alkylating agents can achieve a partial remission.
- *Mitoxantrone* has apparent activity in CLL.

Combination Therapy
Chlorambucil and Prednisone

- The standard regimen when initiating treatment has been:
  — Chlorambucil 0.4 to 0.7 mg/kg orally on day 1.
  — Prednisone 80 mg orally days 1 to 5.
  — Repeat every 2 to 4 weeks.
- Eighty percent of patients may achieve partial or complete responses.

Fludarabine-Containing Regimens
Fludarabine and Cyclophosphamide (FC)

- Can induce responses in patients who appear resistant to single-agent fludarabine.
- Each 28-day cycle consists of fludarabine 20 mg/m^2 to 30 mg/m^2 intravenously daily (or 30-50mg/m^2 orally) for 3 days and cyclophosphamide intravenously or orally at 200 mg/m^2 to 300 mg/m^2 daily for 3 days.

- A response rate is seen in virtually all patients, but approximately 25 percent achieve complete remission.
- Higher degree of myelotoxicity than with either agent alone.

Fludarabine/Cyclophosphamide/Rituximab (FCR)

- Treatment with rituximab concomitant with fludarabine and cyclophosphamide (FCR) appears highly effective (Tables 56–6 and 56–7).
- When given at 375 mg/m^2 on day 1 of course 1 and then at 500 mg/m^2 on day 1 of courses 2 to 6, rituximab when used with fludarabine/cyclophosphamide induced complete response rate of 25 percent and overall response rate of 73 percent of previously treated patients.
- Thirty-two percent of the patients who achieved a complete response did not have evidence of MRD in the marrow by molecular testing.
- Large multicenter phase II trial established superiority of FCR over FC (see Table 56–6).
- Major toxicity of FCR is hematologic.

TABLE 56–6	CHEMOIMMUNOTHERAPY TREATMENT REGIMENS AS INITIAL THERAPY FOR PATIENTS WITH CHRONIC LYMPHOCYTIC LEUKEMIA				
Treatment Group/Regimen		No. Patients Evaluable	% CR	% OR	PFS at 24 Months
Sequential F – 25 mg/m^2 IV d 1–5, course 1–6; *after 2 mo. observation, then* R – 375 mg/m^2 IV weekly × 4		53	28	77	45%
Or					
Concurrent F – 25 mg/m^2 IV d 1–5, course 1–6; R – 375 mg/m^2 IV d 1, 4, course 1; d 1, course 2–6 *after 2 mo. observation, then* R – 375 mg/m^2 IV weekly × 4		51	47	90	67%
F – 25 mg/m^2 IV d 2–4, course 1; d 1–3, course 2–6 C – 250 mg/m^2 IV d 2–4, course 1; d 1–3, course 2–6 R – 375–500 mg/m^2 IV d 1, course 1–6		224	70	95	68%
P – 2 mg/m^2 IV d 1, course 1–6 C – 600 mg/m^2 IV d 1, course 1–6; R – 375 mg/m^2 IV d 1, course 2–6		64	41	91	61%
F – 25 mg/m^2 IV d 1–3; course 1–6 C – 250 mg/m^2 IV d 1–3; q28d; course 1–6 R – 375 mg/m^2 IV d 0, course 1; 500 mg/m^2 d 1, course 1–6		390	52	95	76%
Or					
F – 25 mg/m^2 IV d 1–3; q28d; course 1–6; C – 250 mg/m^2 IV d 1–3; q28d; course 1–6		391	27	88	62%

C, cyclophosphamide; CR, complete remission; d, day; IV, intravenously; F, fludarabine; No., number; OR, overall response; P, pentostatin; PD, progressive disease; PFS, progression free survival; R, rituximab.
Source: *Williams Hematology,* 8th ed, Chap. 94, Table 94–6, p. 1453.

TABLE 56–7	CHEMOIMMUNOTHERAPY TREATMENT REGIMENS FOR PATIENTS WITH CHRONIC LYMPHOCYTIC LEUKEMIA WHO HAVE BEEN PREVIOUSLY TREATED			

Treatment Group/Regimen	No. Patients Evaluable	% CR	% OR	Median TTP (mo.)
F – 25 mg/m^2 IV d 2–4, course 1; d 1–3, course 2–6	177	25	73	N/A
C – 250 mg/m^2 IV d 1, 4, course 1; d1, course 2–6				
R – 375 mg/m^2 d 1, course 1; 500 mg/m^2 d1, course 2–6				
P – 4 mg/m^2 IV d 1, course 1–6	32	25	75	N/A
C – 600 mg/m^2 IV d 1, course 1–6;				
R – 375 mg/m^2 IV d 1, course 2–6				
F – 25 mg/m^2 IV d 1–3, course 1–6	274	24	70	31
C – 250 mg/m^2 IV d 1–3; course 1–6				
R – 375 mg/m^2 IV, course 1; 500 mg/m^2 IV, course 2–6				
Or				
F – 25 mg/m^2 IV d 1–3, course 1–6	272	13	58	21
C – 250 mg/m^2 IV d 1–3; course 1–6				
C – 250 mg/m^2 IV d 3–5; course 1–6	28	4	46	16
F – 25 mg/m^2 IV d 3–5; course 1–6				
A – 30 mg/m^2 IV d 1, 3, 5; course 1–6				
R – 375–500 mg/m^2 IV d 2; course 1–6				
F – 30 mg/m^2 d 1–3; course 1–6	36	30	83	13
A – 30 mg/m^2 d 1–3; course 1–6				
F – 25 mg/m^2 IV d 1–3	6	17	83	N/A
A – 30 mg IV TIW × 12 wks				
A – 30 mg IV TIW × 24 wks. *then if there is PD or SD add* F – 40 mg/m^2 PO d 1–3; course 1; d 1–3, course 2–6	8	0	2	N/A

A, alemtuzumab; C, cyclophosphamide; CR, complete remission; d, day; IV, intravenously F, fludarabine; N/A, not applicable; No., number; OR, overall response; P, pentostatin; PD, progressive disease; PO, oral; R, rituximab; SD, stable disease; TIW, thrice weekly; TTP, time to tumor progression.
Source: *Williams Hematology*, 8th ed, Chap. 94, Table 94–7, p. 1454.

Fludarabine/Rituximab (FR)

- Appears well tolerated and more effective than treatment with single-agent fludarabine.
- Significantly better progression-free survival and overall survival than patients treated with fludarabine alone in long-term follow-up.

Fludarabine Regimens with Mitoxantrone

- Treatment with mitoxantrone, given at 10 mg/m^2 on the first day of each cycle, together with fludarabine, given at 30 mg/m^2 on days 1 through 3 of a 28-day cycle.
- Overall response rates of 80 percent in previously untreated patients and 60 percent in patients who were refractory to therapy with alkylating agents.
- The regimen of fludarabine at 25 mg/m^2 given on days 1 through 3 of a 28-day cycle together with cyclophosphamide at 200 mg/m^2 on days 1 through 3 and

mitoxantrone, given at 10 mg/m^2 on the first day of each cycle, yielded complete responses of 50 percent (and overall responses of 78%) after a median of 3 cycles in patients who had relapsed or who were resistant to standard therapy.

Fludarabine Regimens Containing Cisplatin or Oxaliplatin (OFAR Regimen)

- Cisplatin, administered at 100 mg/m^2 via continuous intravenous infusion over 4 days, has been used in combination with fludarabine given at 30 mg/m^2 via bolus intravenous infusion on days 3 and 4 of a 28-day cycle.
- Myelosuppression was the major dose limiting toxicity.
- The combination regimen involving use of oxaliplatin, fludarabine, cytarabine, and rituximab (OFAR) has activity in patients with relapsed/refractory CLL or Richter transformation.
- A phase I/II study determined the optimal dose of oxaliplatin at 25 mg/m^2 given intravenously on days 1 to 4 of each 28-day cycle.
- Intravenous fludarabine (at 30 mg/m^2) and cytarabine (1 g/m^2) are given on days 2 and 3 of each cycle along with rituximab, given at 375 mg/m^2 on day 3 of cycles 1 and then day 1 of each subsequent cycle.

Fludarabine/Prednisone

- Concomitant use of prednisone with fludarabine does not improve the response rate, but does increase the risk for opportunistic infection.

Fludarabine/Chlorambucil

- Treatment with this combination has not been shown to be significantly better than that with fludarabine alone.

Pentostatin-Containing Regimens

- Response frequencies similar to that of fludarabine-containing regimens that use otherwise similar agents.
- Treatment of previously treated patients with pentostatin at 4 mg/m^2 and cyclophosphamide at 600 mg/m^2 given on day 1 of each 21-day course.
  - Complete response rate is approximately 15 percent; overall response rate is approximately 75 percent in fludarabine-refractory patients.
- Pentostatin administered with cyclophosphamide and rituximab:
  - Effective for patients with relapsed CLL and in patients who have not received prior therapy.

Cladribine-Containing Regimens

- Response rates to 3 courses of cladribine at 4 mg/m^2 per day and cyclophosphamide 350 mg/m^2 per day for 3 days every 4 weeks in patients with refractory or recurrent CLL appeared inferior to those achieved in comparable patients treated with the combination of fludarabine and cyclophosphamide.
- Incorporation of rituximab into cladribine-containing regimens improves the effectiveness of therapy without substantially adding to treatment-related toxicity.

High-Dose Methylprednisolone and Rituximab

- The combination of high-dose methylprednisolone and rituximab (HDMP + R) appears highly active in the treatment of patients with refractory CLL, as well as in patients who had not received prior therapy.
- Does not employ agents that can cause significant myelosuppression.
- Fourteen patients with fludarabine-refractory CLL received 1 g/m^2 per day of intravenous methylprednisolone for 5 days on days 1 to 5 of each 28-day cycle together with rituximab at 375 mg/m^2 weekly for the 4 weeks of each cycle. Following three 4-week cycles of therapy, the treated patients

experienced a complete remission rate of 36 percent and an overall response
rate of 79 percent.
- HDMP reduced to 3 days per 28-day cycle, with the same dose of rituximab
yielded an overall response rates of 96 percent and a complete response rate of
32 percent after 3 cycles of therapy for patients who had not received prior
therapy.

Cyclophosphamide, Vincristine, and Prednisone (CVP)
- Effective in previously untreated patients and in some with refractory CLL.
- The dosages are cyclophosphamide 300 to 400 mg/m^2, orally, daily for 5 days,
vincristine 1 to 2 mg intravenously on day 1, and prednisone 40 mg/m^2 orally
per day for 5 days.

Cyclophosphamide, Doxorubicin, Vincristine, and Prednisone (CHOP)
- Has been evaluated in patients with advanced disease, but appears to have
a lower therapeutic index than purine-analog-containing chemotherapy
regimens.
- Mean survival of patients treated with CHOP was similar to that of patients who
received CVP over an 18-month period.
- Vincristine does not appear to add substantially to the CHOP regimen.

Splenectomy
- May ameliorate the cytopenias associated with advanced-stage CLL, particularly thrombocytopenia.
- May be effective in mitigating intractable or recurrent disease-associated autoimmune hemolytic anemia and/or thrombocytopenia, providing for sustained
improvement in the majority of patients who undergo this procedure.

Radiation Therapy
- Irradiation remains a useful technique for localized treatment to ameliorate
symptoms caused by nerve impingement, vital organ compromise, painful bone
lesions, or bulky disfigurement.
- Delivery of 200 Gy can result in rapid shrinkage of lymph nodes or masses.
- Splenic irradiation is useful in patients with painful splenomegaly.

Leukapheresis
- May reduce organomegaly and improve hemoglobin and platelet levels.
- Successful in ameliorating lymphocytosis and disease-related complications
in pregnant patients with CLL, obviating the use of other antileukemia
treatments until late pregnancy (when risk to the fetus is minimized) or after
delivery.

Supportive Measures
- Erythropoietin:
  — Used on patients who develop anemia as a disease-related complication.
  — May obviate or reduce the frequency of blood transfusions.
  — Can be associated with serious therapy-related complications, such as skin
  reactions, polycythemia, or thromboembolic disease.

Investigational Therapies
Hematopoietic Stem Cell Transplantation (HSCT)
Autologous HSCT
- Preparative regimen well tolerated.
- High risk for recurrent disease after transplant.
- May prolong disease-free survival.

Allogeneic HSCT

- May eradicate the leukemia cells to the levels that cannot be detected using sensitive molecular techniques to detect clonal immunoglobulin gene rearrangements.
- Patients who relapse following allogeneic HSCT may respond to infusions of donor leukocytes.
- Patients who had lymphadenopathy less than 5 cm and no comorbidities had a 5-year overall survival of 71 percent.

Nonmyeloablative Allogeneic HSCT

- Preparative regimen better tolerated than standard allogeneic HSCT.
- Complete chimerism, as well as best response, is not achieved immediately after transplantation but may take over 3 months to develop.
- Patients with refractory CLL can experience eradication of MRD several weeks following transplant, providing evidence of a graft-versus-leukemia effect.

Other Agents and Biologics

Flavopiridol (Alvocidib)

- Cyclin-dependent kinase inhibitor that has activity in CLL.

Lenalidomide (Revlimid)

- Patients with CLL appear more sensitive to lenalidomide than patients with other conditions.
  - Resulted in unacceptable toxicity when given at doses typically used in the treatment of myeloma.

Ofatumumab (Arzerra)

- Ofatumumab is a human monoclonal antibody (for the CD20 protein) that appears to inhibit early-stage B lymphocyte activation.
- Approved by the FDA in October of 2009 for use in treating patients with CLL refractory to fludarabine and alemtuzumab.

Active Immune Therapy and Gene Therapy

- Treatment of patients with autologous leukemia cells transduced with Ad-CD154 showed promising results in a phase I clinical study.

Disease Complications

Infection

- Major cause of morbidity/mortality.
- Susceptibility to infection correlates with hypogammaglobulinemia and/or T-cell lymphocytopenia.
  - Advanced-stage disease, hypogammaglobulinemia, and low levels of specific antibodies to pneumococcal capsular polysaccharide associated with greatest of severe or multiple infections.
- Monthly intravenous administration of pooled normal serum immunoglobulin (IVIG at 240 to 400 mg/kg every 3 to 4 weeks) can decrease frequency of infection.
- Autoimmune hemolytic anemia and immune thrombocytopenia.

Second Malignancies

- Most frequently melanoma, sarcoma, colorectal, lung, or myeloma.
- Higher recurrence rates of basal cell carcinoma after Mohs surgery (a surgical procedure used to treat common types of skin cancer) than the general population.
- Higher incidence of developing Merkel cell carcinoma (rare and highly aggressive cancer in which malignant cancer cells develop on or just beneath the skin and in hair follicles).

- Higher risk for developing more aggressive and/or metastatic squamous cell skin carcinomas than the general population.
- Multiple myeloma occurs at 10 times the expected rate in patients with CLL but evidently does not arise from the same malignant B-cell clone.
- Both untreated and treated CLL patients can develop acute myelogenous leukemia or myelodysplastic syndrome.
- Therapy-related acute myelogenous leukemia may develop after treatment with single-agent deoxyadenosine analogues, such as fludarabine or cladribine.

Pure Red Cell Aplasia

- Patients with CLL or ALL may develop pure red cell aplasia that is unrelated to therapy.
- For CLL patients, treatment with the combination of cyclosporine and prednisone appears to be superior to prednisone alone.

Richter Transformation

- Transformation to an aggressive, large cell, high-grade, B-cell lymphoma.
- Can occur at any time in the course of CLL.
- Occurs in approximately 3 percent of patients at a median of 2 years after diagnosis of CLL.
- Can develop in patients who had not received chemotherapy.
- Can arise from the original CLL clone.
- Chromosomal abnormalities are complex and include:
  — del 8p, del 9p, del 11q (11q23), 12(+), del 13q, 14q(+), del 17p, del 20 and/or translocations involving chromosome 12.
  — Trisomy 12 and chromosome 11 abnormalities are more frequent.
- Higher incidence of *P53* mutations at transformation.
- Three independent risk factors for transformation identified:
  — High-level expression of CD38 by leukemia B cells.
  — Absence of leukemia-cell deletion at 13q14.
  — Leukemia cell expression of certain IgHV genes, notably *IGHV4-39*.
- Clinical and laboratory features:
  — Increased serum lactic acid dehydrogenase activity in approximately 80 percent of patients.
  — Rapid lymph node enlargement in approximately 65 percent.
  — Fever and/or weight loss in approximately 60 percent.
  — Monoclonal gammopathy in approximately 45 percent.
  — Extranodal disease in approximately 40 percent.
- Not all patients with CLL that have rapid lymph node enlargement have Richter transformation.
- Infection with herpes simplex virus can cause acute lymphadenitis.
- Occasional cases of Richter transformation have histology resembling that of Hodgkin lymphoma (see Chap. 59), termed *Richter syndrome with Hodgkin lymphoma features*.
  — Richter syndrome with Hodgkin lymphoma features may respond favorably to therapy for Hodgkin lymphoma.
- Treatment similar to that of patients with high-grade lymphoma (see Chap. 61).
- Encouraging responses have been observed with OFAR regimen (see above).
- Median survival is 5 months after transformation.

CLL/PL and Prolymphocytic Transformation

- Fifteen percent of patients with CLL have a mixture of small lymphocytes and prolymphocytes (PL), the latter accounting for 10 to 50 percent of the lymphoid cells. These patients are considered to have CLL/PL.
- In eighty percent of CLL/PL cases, the proportion of PLs remains stable.

- Twenty percent of patients with CLL/PL undergo prolymphocytic transformation with greater than 55 percent of the leukemia cells having PL morphology (see below).
  — Progressive splenomegaly is characteristic.
  — Mean survival of 9 months after transformation.

Acute Lymphoblastic Leukemia
- Rare complication.
- Can arise from same cell clone as CLL.
- Associated with high levels of expression of *c-MYC* and surface immunoglobulin.

Prognosis
- No established cures for CLL.
- Spontaneous remissions are rare.
- Varies substantially between different patients depending on clinical stage and/or presence or absence of certain disease features associated with progression and/or adverse clinical outcomes.
- Female patients have longer survival.
- Male-to-female ratio is greater in patients diagnosed at younger ages (< 65 years).
- CLL relegated deaths occur more frequently in younger patients.
- Five-year relative survival is approximately 70 percent, 70 percent, 65 percent, and 40 percent for age groups younger than 40, 40 to 59, 60 to 79, and 80+ years, respectively, indicating that the 5-year survival does not vary significantly between the different age groups under the age of 80 years.
- Risk of CLL-unrelated deaths and secondary malignancies predominated older groups.

Prognostic Nomogram and Index for Overall Survival
- Can assist in predicting survival of untreated patients.
- Uses six independent covariates that were identified in a multivariate Cox proportional hazards assessment of outcomes data (see Table 56–8).
- Allows one to total the points identified on the top scale for each independent covariate (see Table 56–9).
- Total point score is then identified on a total point scale and based on the score the patients can then be stratified into low-risk, intermediate-risk, or high-risk categories (see Fig. 56–1).

TABLE 56–8	OVERALL SURVIVAL PROBABILITY AND RELATIVE RISK OF DEATH ACCORDING TO RISK GROUP (N = 1617)					
Risk Group	Index Score	No. of Patients	5-y OS (SE)	10-y OS (SE)	RR	95% CI
Low	1-3	194	0.97 (0.01)	0.80 (0.05)	1.00	Reference
Intermediate	4-7	1236	0.80 (0.01)	0.52 (0.03)	3.89	2.42-6.26
High	≥ 8	187	0.55 (0.04)	0.26 (0.06)	10.48	6.27-17.53

OS, overall survival; SE, standard error; RR, relative risk; CI, confidence interval.
Reproduced with permission from Wierda WG, O'Brien S, Wang X, et al: Prognostic nomogram and index for overall survival in previously untreated patients with chronic lymphocytic leukemia. *Blood* 109:4679, 2007. Copyright © the American Society of Hematology.
Source: *Williams Hematology*, 8th ed, Chap. 94, Table 94–8, p. 1462.

TABLE 56–9	PROGNOSTIC INDEX BASED ON PRESENCE OF RISK FACTORS			
	Point Contribution			
Characteristic	**0**	**1**	**2**	**3**
Age, y	—	<50	50-65	>65
β_2M, mg/L	<ULN	1-2 × ULN	>2 × ULN	N/A
ALC, × 10^9/L	<20	20-50	>50	N/A
Sex	Female	Male	N/A	N/A
Rai Stage	0-II	III-IV	N/A	N/A
No. of involved nodal groups	≤2	3	N/A	N/A

Index score is the sum total of the point for each of the 6 characteristics. An index score of 1–3 = low risk; 4–7 = intermediate risk; ≥ 8 = high risk. To convert β_2M from milligrams per liter to nanomoles per liter, multiply milligrams per liter by 85.

β_2M, β_2-microglobulin; LDH, lactic acid dehydrogenase; ALC, absolute lymphocyte count; ULN, upper limit of normal.

Reproduced with permission from Wierda WG, O'Brien S, Wang X, et al: Prognostic nomogram and index for overall survival in previously untreated patients with chronic lymphocytic leukemia. *Blood* 109:4679, 2007. Copyright © the American Society of Hematology.

Source: *Williams Hematology,* 8th ed, Chap. 94, Table 94–9, p. 1463.

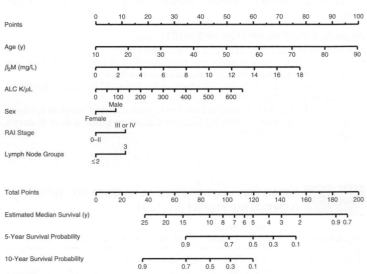

FIGURE 56-1 Nomogram for survival of untreated patients with CLL. The points identified on the top scale for each independent covariate in the top part of the figure are added together to determine the total prognosis score, which then is used on the total points scale (shown in the bottom part of the figure) to identify the estimated median survival time (years) and the probability of 5- and 10-year survival. (Reproduced with permission from Wierda WG, O'Brien S, Wang X, et al: Prognostic nomogram and index for overall survival in previously untreated patients with chronic lymphocytic leukemia. *Blood* 109:4679, 2007. Copyright © the American Society of Hematology.)

(Source: *Williams Hematology,* 8th ed, Chap. 94, Figure 94–4, p. 1462.)

B-CELL PROLYMPHOCYTIC LEUKEMIA

Definition

- Clinical and morphologic variant of CLL.
- Subacute lymphoid leukemia.
- Incidence: less than 10 percent that of CLL.
- Diagnosis of PLL requires that at least 55 percent of the circulating leukemic lymphocytes have prolymphocytic morphology.

Etiology and Pathogenesis

- Unknown etiology.

Cytogenetics

- Karyotype of the leukemia cells from many patients displays the 14q+ abnormality.
- Trisomy 12 is another recurrent abnormality.
- Deletions of the long arm of chromosome 6 (6q-) and rearrangement affecting chromosomes 1 and 12 are occasionally observed.
- Most common abnormalities:
  - 13q14 at 46 percent.
  - Trisomy 12 at 21 percent.
  - 14q32 at 21 percent.
- Loss of heterozygosity at 17p13.3 associated with inactivating mutations in the *TP53* gene is observed in as many as three quarters of the cases examined.

Cytogenesis

- Mature B-cell origin that have undergone immunoglobulin gene rearrangement.
  - IGHV4-34 genes.

Clinical Features

- Fifty percent of patients are older than 70 years.
- Often have advanced disease at presentation.
- Presenting symptoms include fatigue, weakness, weight loss, an acquired bleeding tendency, and early satiety because of splenomegaly.
- Massive splenomegaly occurs in about two-thirds of patients.
- Patients typically have relatively little palpable lymphadenopathy.
- In rare cases, patients may present with leukemic meningitis, leukemic pleural effusion, or malignant ascites.

Laboratory Features

- Frequently find normochromic, normocytic anemia with hemoglobin levels less than 11 g/dL.
- Platelet count is often less than 100×10^9/L.
- Lymphocyte count is greater than 100×10^9/L in 75 percent of patients.
- Hypogammaglobulinemia is common, and about one-third of patients have monoclonal gammopathy.
- Marrow is infiltrated diffusely with neoplastic lymphocytes.
- PLL cells typically express B-cell differentiation antigens and:
  - Variable levels of CD5 (only about half of all cases are CD5$^+$).
  - Generally express high levels of sIg, usually IgM or IgD and react strongly with antibody FMC7.
    High levels of CD22 and are often negative for CD23.

Therapy, Course, and Prognosis

- Indications for treatment:
  - Disease-related symptoms.
  - Symptomatic splenomegaly.
  - Progressive marrow failure.

— Blood prolymphocyte count greater than 20×10^9/L.
— Hemoglobin less than 10 g/dL in the absence of hemolysis.
— Platelet count less than 100×10^9/L.
- Treatment is with alkylating agents similar to those used for CLL, or combinations such as CHOP, yield response rates of 20 percent.
- Fludarabine or cladribine may be effective.
- Monoclonal antibodies (e.g., CAMPATH-1H, rituximab), alone or in combination with chemotherapy, may be effective.
- Splenic irradiation with 1000 to 1600 Gy delivered to the splenic bed, has been advocated as a palliative therapy for the disease.

T-CELL PROLYMPHOCYTIC LEUKEMIA

Definition

- Because of its relative aggressive clinical behavior, what formerly had been called T-cell CLL is categorized in the REAL classification as T-cell prolymphocytic leukemia (PLL) regardless of leukemia cell morphology (see Chap. 54).
- Incidence: less than 5 percent that of CLL.

Etiology and Pathogenesis

- Unknown etiology.
- There is a 3:2 male to female predominance.
- Incidence is five to six times higher in the southern islands of Japan than in Western societies.
- Infection with human T-lymphotropic virus type I (HTLV-1) may play a pathogenic role in a subset of patients.

Genetics

- Chromosomal regions most often overrepresented were:
  — 8q at 75 percent, 5p at 62 percent, and 14q at 37 percent, as well as 6p and 21 both at 25 percent.
- Chromosomal regions most often underrepresented were:
  — 8p and 11q at 75 percent, 13q at 37 percent, and 6q, 7q, 16q, 17p, and 17q at 25 percent.
- Less common cytogenetic rearrangements are:
  — del(6)t(X;6), (p14;q25), del(13)t(13;14)(q22;q11), t(5;13)(q34;p11), r(17)(p13q21), and t(17;20)(q21;q13).
- Alterations on chromosomes 5, 6, 8, 11, 13, 14, 17, and/or 21 apparently cluster into discrete regions that may contain genes that are deleted or amplified during leukemogenesis or disease progression.
- Strong association with mutations in the ataxia-telangiectasia–mutated (ATM) gene that maps to chromosome region 11q22.3–23.1.
- *MCP1* or *TCL1* on the short arms of chromosome 13 and 14, respectively, are implicated in the pathogenesis of T-PLL.

Clinical Features

- Presenting symptoms include fatigue, weakness, weight loss, and early satiety because of splenomegaly.
- About a third of patients have cutaneous involvement on the torso, arms, and face, which is usually present at diagnosis.
- Skin manifestations include diffuse infiltrated erythema and erythroderma, producing a nonscaling, papular, nonpruritic rash.
- Some cases present with central nervous system involvement.

Laboratory Features

- Blood lymphocyte counts often in excess of 10×10^9/L at presentation.
- T-lymphocyte infiltration of the marrow.

- Biopsy of erythematous skin lesions can reveal a perivascular or periappendiceal dermal infiltrate of lymphoid cells, often with prolymphocyte morphology.
- Leukemia cells typically express pan-T-cell differentiation antigens (e.g., CD2, CD3, CD5, and CD7), but not CD1, HLA-DR, or terminal transferase, reflecting a mature T-cell phenotype.
- In addition to pan-T-cell surface antigens, approximately:
  — Seventy-five percent of cases express CD4 (helper T-cell phenotype), but not CD8.
- Fifteen percent of cases express CD8 (suppressor/cytotoxic T-cell phenotype) but not CD4.
- Ten percent of cases express both CD4 and CD8 (less-mature T-cell phenotype).
- Leukemia cells have monoclonal T-cell receptor gene rearrangements.

Differential Diagnosis
Polyclonal T-Cell Lymphocytosis
- Cells typically are a mixture of CD4$^+$/CD8$^-$ and CD4$^-$/CD8$^+$ T cells and lack monoclonal T-cell receptor gene rearrangements.

T-Cell Large-Granular Lymphocytic Leukemia (see Chap. 58)
- Leukemia cells have large granular lymphocyte morphology.

Adult T-Cell Leukemia/Lymphoma (see Chap. 67)
- Endemic to the southwest of Japan and the Caribbean region.
- Patients have lymphadenopathy, hypercalcemia, and high white blood cell counts.
- Leukemia cells have polylobed or convoluted nuclei.
- Patients typically have antibodies to HTLV-I.

Mycosis Fungoides and Sézary Syndrome (see Chap. 66)
- Neoplastic cells have characteristic cerebriform nuclei.
- Shares many features with T-cell PLL.

Therapy, Course, and Prognosis
- Aggressive disease that is generally refractory to conventional alkylating agent chemotherapy.
- Treatment with deoxyadenosine analogues (e.g., 4 mg/m^2 each week for the first 4 weeks and then every other week or cladribine) is effective in inducing complete response or partial response in about half of patients.
- Topical glucocorticoids, mechlorethamine, carmustine, ultraviolet light B, PUVA, or total skin electron beam therapy is palliative for patients with extensive cutaneous involvement (see Chap. 66).
- Clinical trials have found that alemtuzumab induced responses in more than two-thirds of heavily pretreated relapsed/refractory patients with T-cell PLL.
- Systemic glucocorticoids may be palliative.
- High-dose chemoradiotherapy and allogeneic stem cell transplantation has had anecdotal success.
- Median survival is approximately 3 years for patients with PLL and 8 years for those with CLL.

For a more detailed discussion, see Thomas J. Kipps: Chronic Lymphocytic Leukemia and Related Diseases. Chap. 94, p. 1431 in *Williams Hematology,* 8th ed.

CHAPTER 57
Hairy Cell Leukemia

DEFINITION

- B-lymphocyte malignancy that principally involves the marrow and spleen.
- Reactive marrow fibrosis and blood cytopenias are frequent features.
- Irregular cytoplasmic projections on neoplastic B lymphocytes (which gives the disease its name), most striking when examined as a wet preparation by phase microscopy.

EPIDEMIOLOGY

- Estimated that about 700 cases per year occur in the United States (approximately 2% of all leukemias).
- Male:female ratio approximately 4:1.
- Median age at presentation approximately 50 to 55 years.

ETIOLOGY AND PATHOGENESIS

- No exogenous causes established.
- Disease is rare in persons of African or Asian descent.
- Hairy cells are B cells in a late (pre-plasma cell) stage of development.
- B cells have clonal immunoglobulin gene rearrangements.
- Express pan-B–cell markers (e.g., CD19, CD20, and CD22) and the plasma cell marker Prostate Cancer Antigen-1.
- Express additional surface antigens that are uncommon on B lymphocytes (e.g., CD11c, CD25, and CD103).
- Secrete cytokines that may impair normal hematopoiesis (e.g., tumor necrosis factor-α).

CLINICAL FEATURES

- Abdominal fullness/discomfort caused by massive splenomegaly (25%).
- Fatigue, weakness, weight loss (25%).
- Bleeding or infection (25%).
- Found incidentally to have abnormal blood count and/or splenomegaly (25%).
- Painful bony lesions (3%).
- Splenomegaly in 90 percent of patients (median splenic weight approximately 1300 g).
- Infections with common bacteria, viruses, fungi, *Mycobacterium kansasii, Pneumocystis jiroveci,* aspergillus, histoplasma, cryptococcus, *Toxoplasma gondii* or other opportunistic organisms, once common, are less frequent because of more effective initial therapy.
- Unusual findings include: cutaneous vasculitis, leukoclastic angiitis, erythema nodosum, polyarthritis, and Raynaud phenomenon.

LABORATORY FEATURES

- Eighty percent of patients have absolute neutropenia and monocytopenia.
- Severe neutropenia ($< 0.5 \times 10^9$/liter) in 30 percent of patients.
- Severe monocytopenia is hallmark of the disease.
- Anemia is present in three-quarters of patients.
- Moderate to severe pancytopenia found in 67 percent.

- Thrombocytopenia in about 75 percent of patients.
- Careful examination of the blood by light microscopy identifies hairy cells in 80 percent of patients (Fig. 57–1) and in > 90 percent of patients with flow cytometry.
- Liver function test abnormalities in 19 percent, azotemia in 27 percent, and hyperglobulinemia in 18 percent, which may be monoclonal.
- Occasionally leukocytosis is present as a result of circulating hairy cells. Extreme leukocytosis (>100 × 10⁹/L) can occur very infrequently, most often seen in the "hairy cell leukemia variant" (see below).
- Hairy cells comprise less than 20 percent of lymphocytes in patients with low white blood cell counts, but are the predominant cell in patients whose white blood cell count is greater than 10×10^9/L.
- Marrow biopsy shows focal or diffuse infiltrate of leukemic cells with characteristic surrounding halo of pale-staining cytoplasm (the "fried-egg" appearance) and a diffuse fine fibrillar network best appreciated with the periodic acid–Schiff stain (Fig. 57–1).
- Marrow is usually hypercellular, but occasionally hypocellular, mimicking aplastic anemia.
- Immunohistochemistry with CD22 and CD103 antibodies is more sensitive than morphology in detecting residual neoplastic cells in the marrow.
- Diffuse infiltration of splenic red pulp cords and sinuses by hairy cells.
- Irregular cytoplasmic projections can be found on light and electronic microscopy.
- Ribosomal-lamellar cytoplasmic complexes seen on electron microscopy in about 50 percent of patients.
- Cytoplasm stains strongly positive for tartrate-resistant acid phosphatase (TRAP) in approximately 95 percent of hairy cell cases. (This classic test has been replaced by flow cytometry for hairy cell markers.)
- Hairy cells most commonly coexpress high levels of CD11c, CD22, CD25, and CD103, but lack of expression of CD21 (Table 57–1).
- Cytogenetic abnormalities in hairy cell leukemia are very diverse and occur in about half the patients, often involving chromosome 5 (e.g., trisomy, interstitial deletions, pericentric inversions of chromosome 5).

DIFFERENTIAL DIAGNOSIS

- Hairy cell leukemia should be differentiated from nonlymphoid disorders that can present with pancytopenia, splenomegaly, and marrow fibrosis.
  — Primary myelofibrosis.
  — Mast cell disease.
- Hairy cell leukemia can be differentiated from other lymphoproliferative diseases via its clinical and laboratory features (Table 57–1).
- Hairy cell leukemia variant:
  — More often presents with high white blood cell counts (often > 100,000/μL).
  — Have a higher nucleus-to-cytoplasm ratio than do hairy cell leukemia cells.
  — TRAP staining is often negative or only weakly positive.
  — Not associated with neutropenia or monocytopenia.
  — Hairy cell variant cells are often negative for CD25 and CD103.
  — Lack ribosomal-lamellar complex on electron microscopy.
- Other B-cell lymphoproliferative disorders:
  — Chronic lymphocytic leukemia (see Chap. 56).
  — B-cell prolymphocytic leukemia (see Chap. 56).
  — Splenic lymphoma with circulating villous lymphocytes (see Chap. 64)
  — Lymphocytosis is more common.
  — Lymphocytes have more basophilic cytoplasm and generally do not express CD103.
  — TRAP staining is either negative or weakly positive.

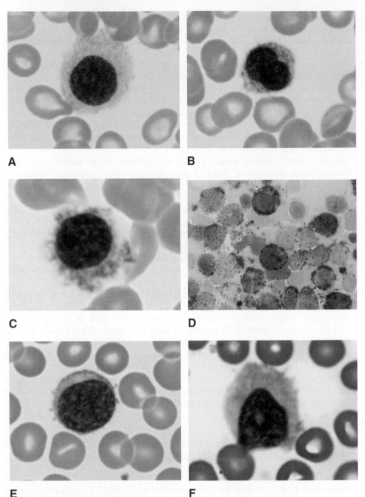

FIGURE 57-1 Cytologic findings in hairy cell leukemia. **A.** Typical hairy cell. The cytoplasmic margins are irregular with a frayed appearance. **B.** A common variation in the appearance of hairy cells is the nuclear contour that can be oval, reniform (as illustrated), or even lobated. The cell otherwise has features of hairy cell leukemia. **C.** Although rarely a dominant finding in the blood film, occasional cells are usually present that show prominent the hairy projections. **D.** The neoplastic cells of hairy cell leukemia consistently show bright positivity for acid phosphatase that is not extinguished by tartrate treatment (tartrate-resistant acid phosphatase). Acid phosphatase stain with tartrate. **E.** Splenic marginal zone lymphoma, also known as splenic lymphoma with villous lymphocytes. The neoplastic cells superficially resemble those in hairy cell leukemia, but rather than the frayed cytoplasmic margins typical of hairy cells, villous lymphocytes generally have a sparse number of irregularly distributed coarse cytoplasmic projections. Wright stain. **F.** Hairy cell leukemia variant. The cells in this rare disorder are generally larger than typical hairy cells and some cells have a single large nucleolus. The cytoplasm can closely resemble that seen in typical hairy cell leukemia. Table 57–1 indicates the CD-surface marker distinctions among the various morphologic cell types shown here with surface projections.
(Reproduced with permission from Robert W. Sharpe, MD, Department of Pathology, Scripps Clinic, LaJolla, CA.)
(Source: Williams Hematology, 8th ed, Chap. 95, Figure 95–1, p. XXX.)

TABLE 57–1   FEATURES OF HAIRY CELL LEUKEMIA AND SIMILAR DISORDERS

	Hairy-cell leukemia	Chronic lymphocytic leukemia	B-cell prolymphocytic leukemia	Splenic lymphoma with villous lymphocytes	Hairy cell leukemia variant
Male:female ratio	4:1	2:1	2:1	2:1	4:1
Palpable splenomegaly	75–95%	> 50%	> 90%	> 90%	> 90%
Palpable lymphadenopathy	5%	70%	30%	< 5%	< 5%
Pattern of splenic involvement	Red pulp	White pulp ± red pulp	White pulp ± red pulp	White pulp ± red pulp	Red pulp
Mean WBC($\times 10^9$/liter)	5	100	175	20	90
Tartrate-resistant acid-phosphatase	+	–	±	–	±
Immunophenotype					
sIg	+++*	+	+++	+++	+++
CD5	–†	+++	±	±	–
CD11c	+++++	+‡	±	±	±
CD19	+++	+	+++	+++	+++
CD20	+++++	+	+++	+++	+++
CD22	+++	±‡	+++	+++	+++
CD25	+++	+‡	±	±	–
CD103	++	–	–	±	±

* Symbols indicate intensity from very strong (+ + + + +) to weak (+) to negative (−). A (±) indicates that some cases are positive.
† A small percentage may express CD5.
‡ CD11c and CD25 are expressed weakly in the majority of B-cell CLL.

THERAPY

- Approximately 90 percent of patients require treatment at time of diagnosis. Indications include:
  - Symptomatic splenomegaly or lymphadenopathy.
  - Anemia (Hb level less than 10 g/dL).
  - Thrombocytopenia (platelet count $<100 \times 10^9$/L).
  - Granulocytopenia (neutrophil count $< 1.0 \times 10^9$/L) with recurrent bacterial or opportunistic infections.
  - Leukemic phase (white cell count $> 20 \times 10^9$/L).
  - Vasculitis.
  - Painful bony involvement.
- **Cladrabine** (2-Chlorodeoxyadenosine) is the treatment of choice for hairy cell leukemia.
  - A purine analogue given as a 7-day continuous intravenous infusion at 0.1 mg/kg per day. (Successful subcutaneous, oral, and weekly dosing has been reported.)
  - Can induce long-lasting complete responses in greater than 75 percent of patients. Initially, 91 percent have complete response and 7 percent a partial response.
  - Sixteen percent of complete responders have evidence of relapse at 48 months. Approximately 90 percent of patients initially treated with cladrabine who relapse will have a complete (62%) or partial response (26%) when retreated with the same drug.
  - In a subsequent study of 207 patients monitored for at least 7 years after cladrabine treatment, 95 percent had achieved a complete response and 5 percent a partial response after a single 7-day course. The overall survival at 108 months was 97 percent and the median disease-free duration for all responders was 98 months.
  - Notable toxicities of cladrabine:
    - Aseptic fever in setting of neutropenia.
    - T-cell depletion, particularly CD4$^+$ cells.
- **Pentostatin** (2′-deoxycoformycin):
  - A purine analogue that inhibits adenosine deaminase.
  - A good second choice drug for patients unresponsive or refractory to cladrabine.
  - Administered as an intravenous bolus of 4 mg/m^2 every other week for 3 to 6 months until maximum response as judged by decrease of blood and marrow hairy cells, reduced spleen size, and improvement in normal blood cell counts.
  - Complete response rates with pentostatin (~50%) are lower than that achieved with cladribine.
  - Pentostatin may not be effective in patients refractory to cladribine.
  - Notable toxicities:
    - Fever, rash, conjunctivitis.
    - Reversible renal dysfunction.
    - Mild hepatic toxicity.
    - Depletion of CD4$^+$ cells.
- **Interferon-α** (IFN-α):
  - Complete response rate is 8 percent; 74 percent achieve a partial response.
  - Not curative; 50 percent relapse less than 2 years after treatment.
  - Usual dosage schedule is 2×10^6 U IFN-α_{2b}/m^2 subcutaneously three times weekly for 12 months or 3×10^6 U IFN-α_{2a}/m^2 subcutaneously daily for 6 months and decreased to 3 times per week for an additional 6 months.
  - Not as effective as purine analogues.
  - Toxicity:
    - Flu-like symptoms (fever, myalgia, malaise).
    - Myelosuppression.

- **Rituximab**
  - Hairy cells express CD20 and thus an anti-CD20 monoclonal antibody is rational.
  - The responses have been modest but it should be considered in patient's refractory to cladribine and pentostatin.
  - 375 mg/m^2 intravenously weekly for 4 to 8 weeks.
  - A proportion (25 to 75%) of patients has a complete or partial remission, which may be sustained for several years in a proportion of responders. Others relapse and progress.
- **Anti-CD22 Immunotoxin BL22**
  - Anti-CD22 fused to a *Pseudomonas* exotoxin.
  - Can induce remissions in a high proportion of patients who are refractory to cladribine.
  - Associated with a reversible hemolytic uremic syndrome in a minority of patients.
- **Splenectomy**
  - Not curative.
  - Current indications:
    - Massive, painful, and/or ruptured spleen.
    - Pancytopenia and an active infection with opportunistic pathogen (e.g., *Mycobacterium*). Splenectomy usually results in marked increase in neutrophil and monocyte count and better response to antimicrobial treatment.
    - Failure of systemic chemotherapy.
- **Granulocyte colony-stimulating factor** (G-CSF):
  - May ameliorate neutropenia.
  - Adjunct to therapy in cases of infection.
- **Radiation**
  - Lytic bone lesions can be treated with low-dose irradiation.

CLINICAL COURSE

- With cladrabine treatment considered curable with overall survival rates in excess of 95 percent at 4 years.
- Remissions of over 10 years duration common.
- Minimal residual disease can be found in about 35 percent of long-term responders (median disease-free survival 16 years) but its presence does not necessarily predict for relapse since very long-term responders are as likely as not to have minimal residual disease by very sensitive techniques to identify marrow hairy cells.
- A plateau in relapse has not been reached at over 10 years of remission and, thus, a risk of late relapse exists.
- Relapsed patients after first treatment with cladrabine have a high response rate to retreatment with cladrabine or another agent.
- Infections, including by opportunistic organisms, the cause of death in over 50 percent of patients prior to the availability of cladrabine, are now uncommon.

For a more detailed discussion, see Darren Sigal and Alan Saven: Hairy Cell Leukemia. Chap. 95, p. 1483 in *Williams Hematology,* 8th ed.

CHAPTER 58
Large Granular Lymphocytic Leukemia

DEFINITION

- T-cell large-granular lymphocytic (T-LGL) leukemia results from the clonal expansion of large granular lymphocytes (LGL) with a T-cell (CD3+) phenotype and a clonal T-cell receptor gene rearrangement(s).
- Natural killer (NK)-LGL leukemia is a clonal expansion of LGL with a NK cell (CD3-) phenotype. It lacks convenient markers to determine clonality such as antigen receptor rearrangements.

T-LGL LEUKEMIA

Etiology and Pathogenesis

- Suggestive evidence of a role for human T lymphotropic virus (HTLV) retroviral infection in some patients.
- Most patients are not infected with either HTLV-I or HTLV-II.
- Cytomegalovirus implicated in rare cases of CD4+ T-LGL.
- Epstein-Barr virus implicated in some cases of NK-LGL.
- Leukemic cells have features of antigen-activated cytotoxic T lymphocytes (CTL), suggesting role for antigen in initial LGL expansion.
- Constitutive overexpression of the Fas ligand (CD178), which also is found at high levels in patients' sera, may be a factor in many disease manifestations (e.g., neutropenia, rheumatoid arthritis).

Clinical Features

- About half of patients have palpable splenomegaly.
- About one-third of patients have recurrent bacterial infections and/or "B symptoms" (e.g., low-grade fevers, night sweats, and/or weight loss) (aggressive variant) (see Table 58–1).
- About one-quarter of patients have rheumatoid arthritis, often with features of "Felty syndrome."
- Less than 10 percent of patients have lymphadenopathy.

Laboratory Features

- Immunophenotype of LGL cells in blood and marrow: CD3+CD8+CD16+ CD57+ CD4-CD56-, and, often, HLA-DR+.
- Patients have clonal T-cell–receptor gene rearrangement(s), usually involving α and β chains.
- Nearly 85 percent of patients have neutropenia, often less than 0.5×10^9/L.
- Approximately half of the patients have anemia, often caused by pure red cell aplasia and/or autoimmune hemolytic anemia.
- Approximately one-fifth of patients have thrombocytopenia.
- About one-quarter of patients do not have increased blood total lymphocyte counts.
- The median LGL count in patients is 4.0×10^9/L (normal mean 0.3×10^9/L) (Fig. 58–1).
- More than 90 percent of patients have LGL infiltration of the marrow and splenic red pulp.

TABLE 58–1   COMPARATIVE FEATURES OF LARGE GRANULAR LYMPHOCYTIC LEUKEMIA

Variable	T-cell LGL Leukemia (Indolent type)	T-cell LGL leukemia (Aggressive type)	NK-LGL leukemia (Aggressive type)	Chronic NK Lymphocytosis (Indolent type)
Median age (years)	60	40	40	60
Male:female ratio	1	2	1	7
Phenotype	CD3+CD16+CD57+ Clonal TCRαβ rearrangement	CD3+CD16+CD56+ Clonal TCRαβ rearrangement	CD3−CD16+CD56+	CD3−CD16+ CD56+
Clinical features	One-third asymptomatic Two-thirds symptomatic Cytopenias, splenomegaly, rheumatoid arthritis (~25% of patients).	Symptomatic, usually with B symptoms (fever, sweats, weight loss) Lymphadenopathy, hepatosplenomegaly.	Symptomatic, usually with B symptoms (fever, sweats, weight loss) Lymphadenopathy, hepatosplenomegaly	Most patients are asymptomatic; about 40% with signs (cytopenias, vasculitis, neuropathy, splenomegaly)
Treatment approach	Observation or immunosuppressive therapy, if required	Acute lymphoblastic leukemia –type therapy	Acute lymphoblastic leukemia –type therapy	Observation or immunosuppressive therapy if required
Prognosis	Relatively Good	Poor	Very Poor	Relatively Good

Source: *Williams Hematology*, 8th ed, Chap. 96, Table 96–3, p. 1495

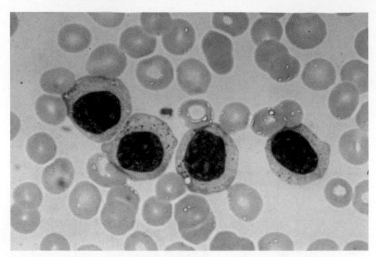

FIGURE 58-1 Blood film. Four large granular lymphocytes with azurophilic granules in cytoplasm. (Reproduced with permission from Bruce Cheson.)
(Source: *Williams Hematology,* 8th ed, Chap. 96, Fig. 96–1, p. 1494.)

- Marrow infiltration may be nodular or interstitial. If interstitial, it may be difficult to appreciate involvement without staining for neoplastic cells using immunocytochemistry.
- Patients commonly have elevated levels of certain autoantibodies and other serologic abnormalities (Table 58–2).

Differential Diagnosis

- T-LGL leukemia should be considered in patients with increased blood LGL counts and
    — Chronic or cyclic neutropenia.
    — Pure red cell aplasia.
    — Rheumatoid arthritis.
- T-LGL leukemia can be distinguished from NK-LGL leukemia by immunophenotype and clonal T-cell–receptor gene rearrangement (Table 58–1).

Therapy, Course, and Prognosis

- Chronic.
- Unusual cases that coexpress CD3 and CD56 may have a more aggressive clinical course.
- Significant morbidity/mortality from infections.
- Low-dose methotrexate 10 mg/m^2 orally once weekly or cyclophosphamide 100 mg PO daily, or cyclosporine may be effective in alleviating neutropenia/ anemia.
- Coexisting B-cell neoplasms (e.g., essential monoclonal gammopathy or chronic lymphocytic leukemia) occur in 25 percent of patients.

NK-LGL LEUKEMIA

Etiology and Pathogenesis

- Epstein-Barr virus infection implicated in the pathogenesis.

Clinical Features

- Fever, night sweats, weight loss are common (see Table 58–1).
- Massive hepatosplenomegaly typical.
- Lymphadenopathy and gastrointestinal tract involvement are common.
- Patients tend to be of younger age than those with CD3+ LGL leukemia.

Laboratory Features

- LGL lack expression of CD3 and clonal T-cell receptor rearrangements.
- NK-leukemic LGL is usually CD4+CD16+CD56+CD8−CD57-.
- LGL counts are generally high and may exceed 50×10^9/L.
- Severe neutropenia (e.g., $< 0.5 \times 10^9$/L) is observed in less than one-fifth of patients.
- Anemia and thrombocytopenia very common.
- Coagulopathy frequently occurs.
- Clonal cytogenetics may be present.
- Serologic abnormalities listed in Table 58–2 are uncommon in NK-LGL leukemia.

Therapy, Course, and Prognosis

- Acute presentation and aggressive course is common.
- Patients with chronic NK lymphocytosis may not require treatment.
- Effective combination chemotherapy has not been reported.
- Patients with NK-LGL usually die a few months after diagnosis despite aggressive multidrug chemotherapy.

TABLE 58–2 **SEROLOGIC FINDINGS IN CD3$^+$ LGL LEUKEMIA**

Feature	Percent of Patients
Rheumatoid factor	~60
Circulating immune complexes	~50
Antinuclear antibody	~40
Antineutrophil antibody	~40
Polyclonal hypergammaglobulinemia	~25
Positive antiglobulin (Coombs) test	~15
Monoclonal gammopathy	~8

Source: *Williams Hematology*, 8th ed, Chap. 96, Table 96–2, p. 1494.

For a more detailed discussion, see Thomas P. Loughran, Marshall E. Kadin: Large Granular Lymphocytic Leukemia. Chap. 96, p. 1493 in *Williams Hematology*, 8th ed.

CHAPTER 59
Hodgkin Lymphoma

DEFINITION

- Neoplasm of lymphoid tissue in most cases derived from germinal center B cells, defined by the presence of the Reed-Sternberg cells or its mononuclear variant Hodgkin cells with a characteristic immunophenotype and appropriate cellular background.
- The Reed-Sternberg and Hodgkin cell, the neoplastic cells defining Hodgkin disease, are considered of B-cell origin based on its clonal immunoglobulin gene rearrangements.
- Classic Hodgkin disease accounts for 95 percent of cases and contains four histologic subtypes that are distinguished on the basis of microscopic appearance and relative proportions of Reed-Sternberg cells, lymphocytes, and fibrosis: nodular sclerosis, mixed cellularity, lymphocyte-depleted, or lymphocyte-rich Hodgkin disease. A fifth subtype, nodular lymphocyte predominance has been added to the four classic histologic types (see Table 59–1).

EPIDEMIOLOGY

- In 2009 in the United Stated, there were 8510 cases of Hodgkin lymphoma.
- Incidence rate is influenced by socioeconomic and environmental factors.
- Bimodal age distribution: peak between ages 15 to 34 and in those older than age 60 years.
- Nodular sclerosis predominates in young adults.
- Mixed cellularity predominates in older ages.
- Presence of the Epstein-Barr virus (EBV) in Reed-Sternberg and Hodgkin cells is more common in less-developed countries and in pediatric and older adult cases.
- Role for EBV in etiology is suggested by evidence that serologically confirmed mononucleosis confers a threefold risk for Hodgkin disease in young adults.
- Increased risk among siblings and close relatives suggests genetic factors may contribute to disease susceptibility.

ETIOLOGY AND PATHOGENESIS

- Reed-Sternberg cells are relatively large cells that typically have bilobed nuclei with prominent eosinophilic nucleoli separated by a clear space from a thickened nuclear membrane (see Fig. 59–1).
- Reed-Sternberg cells represent monoclonal outgrowths of germinal center B cells that have incurred extensive somatic mutations, most likely in the course of the immune response to antigen.
- Mononuclear Reed-Sternberg cell variants, referred to as Hodgkin cells, have similar nuclear characteristics and may represent Reed-Sternberg cells cut in a plane that shows only one lobe of the nucleus.
- Nearly all Hodgkin and Reed-Sternberg cells have rearranged and somatically mutated immunoglobulin VH genes (IgHV).
- It is possible that Hodgkin and Reed-Sternberg cells originate from a preapoptotic germinal center B cell with unfavorable mutations that has escaped negative selection.
- Karyotypes are usually hyperdiploid with structural abnormalities but without pathognomonic chromosomal aberrations.

TABLE 59–1   CLASSIFICATION OF HODGKIN LYMPHOMA

Histologic Subtype	Immunophenotype
Nodular lymphocyte-predominant	CD20+ CD30− CD15− Ig+
Classic	CD20 −*CD30+ CD15+ Ig−
Nodular sclerosis	
Mixed cellularity	
Lymphocyte-rich	
Lymphocyte-depleted	

*Infrequently positive.
Source: *Williams Hematology,* 8th ed, Chap. 99, Table 99–1, p. 1528.

- Reed-Sternberg cells secrete a variety of cytokines and chemokines that may be responsible for the recruitment of nonmalignant cells that comprise the bulk of the cells in the tumor population.
- Hodgkin and Reed-Sternberg cells show a global loss of their B-cell phenotype, retaining only B-cell features associated with their interaction with T cells and their antigen-presenting function.
- The lack of expression of numerous B-cell genes is the result of loss of B-cell transcription factor expression (OCT2, BOB1, and PU.1) and epigenetic silencing.
- The main B-cell lineage commitment factor, PAX5, is typically expressed, but its target genes are downregulated.
- Because Hodgkin and Reed-Sternberg cells lack expression of functional B-cell surface receptors, rescue from apoptosis is probably an important mechanism of survival.
- Most prevalent genetic lesions in Hodgkin and Reed-Sternberg cells involve two signaling pathways:

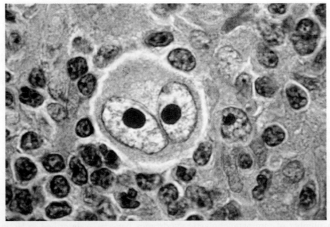

FIGURE 59–1 High magnification of lymph node section in a patient with Hodgkin lymphoma. A Reed-Sternberg cell is in the center of the field with the classic findings of giant size compared with background lymphocytes, binucleation, and prominent eosinophilic nucleoli. (Source: *Williams Hematology,* 8th ed, Figure 99–1, p. 1529.)

- — Janus kinase (JAK)-STAT: gains in JAK2 and inactivation of the negative regulator JAK-STAT signaling, suppressor of cytokine signaling 1, resulting in enhanced cytokine signaling.
- — Nuclear factor-κB (NF-κB): Genetic alterations include gains and amplifications of the NF-κB transcription factor REL in about half of all cases. Somatic mutations of the gene encoding the inhibitor of NF-κB (1κBα) occur in approximately 20 percent of cases. Inactivating mutations and deletions of the gene encoding A20, a negative regulator of NF-κB, have been found in approximately 40 percent of cases, nearly all of which were EBV-negative.
- Multiple-receptor tyrosine kinases are aberrantly expressed in Hodgkin and Reed-Sternberg, including platelet-derived growth factor receptor-α.
- Several factors point to the pathogenetic role of EBV in approximately 40 percent of classic Hodgkin lymphoma.
  - — The viral proteins latent membrane protein 1 (LMP1) and latent membrane protein 2 (LMP2), in particular, appear to have hijacked signaling pathways to promote the survival of EBV-infected Hodgkin and Reed-Sternberg cells.
  - — There is an inverse relationship between expression of multiple receptor tyrosine kinases and EBV expression.
  - — There is an ability of EBV to rescue crippled germinal center B cells in the laboratory.
  - — Mutations preventing any B-cell receptor expression are in EBV-positive Hodgkin and Reed-Sternberg cells.
  - — There is an inverse relationship between mutations reducing the expression of the NF- κB regulator A20 and EBV-positive Hodgkin and Reed-Sternberg cells.
- The different types of Hodgkin lymphoma have different types and quantities of cytokines, and these appear to provide for the distinctive histopathologic features and symptoms associated with each type; for example:
  - — CCL5, CCL17, CCL22 attract T-helper 2 (Th2) and T-regulatory cells.
  - — IL-8 attracts neutrophils.
  - — IL-10, TGF-β, galectin 1, and prostaglandin E_2 have immunosuppressive effects.

CLINICAL FEATURES

- Usual presentation is with painless lymph node enlargement.
- Constitutional symptoms may be present:
  - — "B" symptoms: fever above 38 °C, drenching night sweats, and weight loss of more than 10 percent of baseline body weight.
  - — Pel-Ebstein fever: high fevers for 1 to 2 weeks alternating with afebrile periods of similar length; virtually diagnostic of Hodgkin disease.
- Detection of an unusual mass or swelling in the superficial, supradiaphragmatic lymph nodes (60–70% cervical and supraclavicular, 15–20% axillary) is the most common presentation.
- Pruritus may be evident.
- Intrathoracic disease is present at diagnosis in 67 percent of patients.
- Mediastinal adenopathy is common.
- Immunologic dysfunction:
  - — All patients have multiple abnormalities of cellular immunity.
  - — Some defects persist even after successful treatment.
- Abnormalities in complete blood count are variable and nondiagnostic.
- A number of rare paraneoplastic syndromes have been described in Hodgkin lymphoma at the time of diagnosis.
  - — These include vanishing bile duct syndrome and idiopathic cholangitis with clinical jaundice, the nephrotic syndrome with anasarca, autoimmune

hematologic disorders (e.g., immune thrombocytopenia or hemolytic anemia), and neurologic signs and symptoms.

RADIOGRAPHIC FEATURES

- Intrathoracic disease detectable by computed tomography (CT) of the chest is present at diagnosis in two-thirds of patients.
- Whole-body F-F-fluorodeoxyglucose positron emission tomography (FDG-PET) and/or magnetic resonance imaging (MRI) correlate with CT evaluation and have resulted in few changes in stage or therapy.

CLINICAL AND PATHOLOGIC CORRELATION

There are five histologic subtypes of Hodgkin disease: nodular sclerosis, mixed cellularity, lymphocyte depletion, lymphocyte rich, and nodular lymphocyte predominance.

Nodular Sclerosis

- Approximately 40 to 70 percent of patients present with nodular sclerosis.
- Frequent involvement of the lower cervical, supraclavicular, and mediastinal lymph nodes in adolescents and young adults, particularly females.
  — In young females, frequent involvement in lower cervical, supraclavicular, and mediastinal lymph nodes.
  — Seventy percent have limited stage disease.
- Main distinguishing feature is the *lacunar cell,* a Reed-Sternberg cell variant that derives its appearance from retraction of its cytoplasm with immunophenotype CD30+ CD15+ CD20–.

Mixed Cellularity

- Affects both pediatric and older age groups.
- Strong association with prior EBV infection.
- Associated with advance stage disease.
- Mixed cellularity in 30 to 50 percent of patients.
- Classic Reed-Sternberg cells amid a cellular background of lymphocytes, eosinophils, plasma cells, and histiocytes.

Lymphocyte-Depletion

- Hodgkin and Reed-Sternberg cells are sparse.
- Present in older age groups.
- Systemic symptoms frequent.
- Widespread disease involving superficial and mediastinal lymph node groups, hepatosplenomegaly.
- May present with fever, jaundice, and pancytopenia.
- Associated with acquired immunodeficiency disorder (see Chap. 52).

Lymphocyte Rich

- Presenting features are very similar to the nodular lymphocyte-predominant subtype, although patients with the lymphocyte-rich subtype tend to be older.
- Classic CD30+ CD20
  — immunophenotype of Reed-Sternberg cells.

Nodular Lymphocyte Predominance

- Histologic pattern found in approximately 10 percent of patients.
- Patients typically present with disease in a localized lymph node area, especially the axilla.

- Male predominance, 4:1.
- The tumor is composed principally of benign lymphocytes with some histiocytes. Neutrophils and eosinophils are rare.
- CD20+CD15−CD30− lymphocytes with mononuclear but lobulated or folded nucleus referred to as popcorn cells. Unlike classic Hodgkin lymphoma, cells express B-lineage markers (e.g., CD20).

ANATOMIC DISTRIBUTION OF HODGKIN DISEASE

- Hodgkin lymphoma presents:
  — In the cervical nodes in 70 percent of patients.
  — In the axillary nodes in 12 percent of patients.
  — In the inguinal nodes in 9 percent of patients.
- The frequency of splenic involvement is approximately 35 percent.
  — Splenic involvement depends on histologic subtype; it is more frequent in mixed cellularity and lymphocyte depletion cases compared with lymphocyte predominant or nodular sclerosis.
- Disease distribution at presentation:
  — A minority of patients have exclusive subdiaphragmatic disease.
  — CT of the chest, abdomen, and pelvis and FDG-PET provide sensitive delineation of involved sites with the exception of the spleen and marrow.
- Staging (see Table 59–2).
- Use of chemotherapy in all stages of disease has reduced the critical nature of detecting subclinical disease.
- Marrow involvement occurs in approximately 10 to 15 percent of new patients and is more common in patients of older age, advanced stage, less favorable histology.

LABORATORY FEATURES

- There are no diagnostic laboratory features of Hodgkin lymphoma.
- A complete blood count may reveal one or another of neutrophilia, eosinophilia, lymphocytopenia, thrombocytosis, or anemia.

TABLE 59–2   ANN ARBOR STAGING CLASSIFICATION FOR HODGKIN LYMPHOMA

Stage

I   Involvement of a single lymph node region (I) or of a single extralymphatic organ or site (I_E)

II   Involvement of two or more lymph node regions on the same side of the diaphragm alone (II), or with involvement limited, contiguous extralymphatic organ tissue (II_E)

III Involvement of lymph node regions on both sides of the diaphragm (III), which may include the spleen (III_S), or limited, contiguous extralymphatic organ, or site (III_E), or both (III_{SE})

IV   Multiple or disseminated foci of involvement of one or more extralymphatic organs or tissues, with or without associated lymph node involvement

Modifying Features

A   Asymptomatic

B   Drenching night sweats; fever >38 °C; loss of more than 10% body weight in 6 months

X   Bulky disease: mass >10 cm; >0.33 mediastinal mass ratio

E   Involvement of a single, contiguous or proximal extranodal site

Mediastinal mass ratio is the ratio of the maximal width of a mediastinal mass relative to the maximal width of the mediastinum, as measured by CT imaging.
Source: *Williams Hematology*, 8th ed, Chap. 99, Table 99–2, p. 1533.

- Immune neutropenia can occur.
- Anemia: usually a result of chronic disease, but rarely may be caused by hemolysis secondary to high fever or associated with appositive direct antiglobulin (Coombs) test.
- Thrombocytopenia may occur as a result of marrow involvement, hypersplenism or an immune mechanism.
- Serum lactate dehydrogenase levels are elevated in 35 percent of patients at diagnosis.
- Elevated serum levels of β_2-microglobulin in the setting of normal renal function correlates with tumor burden and prognosis.
- Elevated serum levels of cytokines, including IL-6 and L-10, and soluble CD30 and CD2 may correlate with constitutional symptoms and/or advanced disease.
- Hypercalcemia is unusual in Hodgkin lymphoma and appears to be secondary to synthesis of increased levels of 1, 25-dihydroxyvitamin D by Hodgkin lymphoma cells.

DIFFERENTIAL DIAGNOSIS

- Biopsy of unexplained, persistent, or recurrent adenopathy should be reviewed by an experienced hematopathologist.
  — The most likely diagnosis is either Hodgkin or a non-Hodgkin lymphoma.
- Nonneoplastic conditions that simulate Hodgkin lymphoma include viral infections, particularly infectious mononucleosis.
- Cell depleted nodes of any histology may resemble the diffuse fibrosis variant of lymphocyte-depleted, including the depleted phase of lymph nodes from HIV-infected patients.

THERAPY

- Advances in radiotherapy technique deliver more precise dose distribution, sparing normal tissues.
- Radiotherapy.
  — Involved field: 3500 to 4400 Gy at 150 to 200 Gy per daily fraction (5 days per week).
  — Uninvolved fields (prophylactic) 3000 to 3500 Gy.
  — Therapy has been modified to reduce field size to areas of known or bulky disease. The dose also has been lowered particularly when used in combination with chemotherapy.
  — Initial disease reduction with chemotherapy results in less radiation exposure to the neck, female breast, heart, and lungs, all of which should result in fewer late complications.
- The first modern combination chemotherapy program was mechlorethamine (nitrogen mustard), Oncovin (vincristine), procarbazine, and prednisone (MOPP) regimen.
- Combination chemotherapy regimens for Hodgkin lymphoma (Table 59–3):
  — COPP: cyclophosphamide, vincristine, procarbazine, prednisone (Table 59–3).
  — ABVD: Adriamycin (doxorubicin), bleomycin, vinblastine, dacarbazine (Table 59–3):
    - Preferred primary regimen.
    - Used together with MOPP in alternating or "hybrid" regimens.
- Alternative regimens for advanced disease that incorporate G-CSF to mitigate neutropenia of high-dose chemotherapy (Table 59–3):
  — BEACOPP: bleomycin, etoposide, Adriamycin (doxorubicin), cyclophosphamide, vincristine, procarbazine, prednisone.
  — STANFORD V: bleomycin, etoposide, doxorubicin, nitrogen mustard, vincristine, vinblastine, prednisone ± G-CSF.

| TABLE 59–3 | COMBINATION CHEMOTHERAPY FOR HODGKIN LYMPHOMA |

Drug	Dose mg/m^2	Route	Schedule (days administered)	Cycle Length (days)
COPP				28
cyclophosphamide	650	IV	1,8	
vincristine	1.4*	IV	1,8	
procarbazine	100	PO	1–14	
prednisone	40	PO	1–14	
ABVD				28
doxorubicin	25	IV	1,15	
bleomycin	10	IV	1,15	
vinblastine	6	IV	1,15	
dacarbazine	375	IV	1,15	
COPP/ABVD				28
Alternate cycles of COPP with ABVD				
BEACOPP (Standard)				21
bleomycin	10	IV	8	
etoposide	100	IV	1–3	
doxorubicin	25	IV	1	
cyclophosphamide	650	IV	1	
vincristine	1.4*	IV	8	
procarbazine	100	PO	1–7	
prednisone	40	PO	1–14	
BEACOPP (Escalated)				21
bleomycin	10	IV	8	
etoposide	200	IV	1–3	
doxorubicin	35	IV	1	
cyclophosphamide	1250	IV	1	
vincristine	1.4*	IV	8	
procarbazine	100	PO	1–7	
prednisone	40	PO	1–14	
(G-CSF)	(+)	SQ	8+	
BEACOPP (14-day)				14
Standard BEACOPP given every 14 days with growth factor support.				
STANFORD V				12 weeks
nitrogen mustard	6	IV	day 1 on wk 1,5,9	
doxorubicin	25	IV	day 1 on wk 1,3,5,7,9,11	
vinblastine	6	IV	day 1 on wk 1,3,5,7,9,11	
vincristine	1.4*	IV	day 1 on wk 2,4,6,8,10,12	
bleomycin	5	IV	day 1 on wk 2,4,6,8,10,12	
etoposide	60 x 2	IV	day 1 & 2 on wk 3,7,11	
prednisone	40	PO	day 1 on wk 1–10, taper	
G-CSF for dose reduction, delay				

*Capped at 2 mg.
Source: *Williams Hematology,* 8th ed, Chap. 99, Table 99–3, p. 1535.

Favorable, Limited-Stage Disease

- Stage I or stage II supradiaphragmatic disease with no bulky sites and none or only one extranodal site.
- A more restrictive definition is used in Europe based on the number of Ann Arbor sites, erythrocyte sedimentation rate (ESR), age and extranodal sites, as well as bulky disease (see Table 59–4).
  - Approximately 35 percent of stages I and II patients meet this more limited definition of favorable disease.
- Management of stage II is controversial, but usually involves use of chemotherapy or combined chemoradiotherapy.
  - Trials demonstrated the superiority of involved field-radiotherapy plus anthracycline-containing chemotherapy compared with extended-field radiotherapy in early stage favorable Hodgkin lymphoma.
- With the goal of avoiding radiotherapy and its late effects, current studies are assessing interim FDG-PET scanning as a means of identifying patients (PET-negative) for whom radiotherapy can be omitted.
- Classic clinical stage I Hodgkin lymphoma patients presenting with inguinofemoral disease may be treated with shorter course of chemotherapy and involved-field radiotherapy.

Locally Extensive, Limited-Stage Disease

- Extensive mediastinal disease (greater than one-third of thoracic diameter) needs combined modality therapy (chemotherapy and radiation); 80 percent disease-free survival.

TABLE 59–4   PROGNOSTIC FACTORS FOR HODGKIN LYMPHOMA

Limited Stage		Advanced Stage
EORTC	GHSG	International Collaborative Study
Adverse Prognostic Factors		**Adverse Prognostic Factors**
MMR $\geq$ 0.35	MMR $\geq$ 0.35	Age $\geq$ 45 years
ESR >30 if symptomatic	ESR >30 if asymptomatic	Stage IV
ESR >50 if asymptomatic	ESR >50 if asymptomatic	Male sex
>3 Ann Arbor sites	>2 Ann Arbor sites	White blood count $\geq 15 \times 10^9$/L
Age $\geq$ 50	Extranodal disease	Lymphocyte count < 0.6 $\times$ 10^9/L or <8%
	Massive splenic disease	Albumin < 4 g/dL
		Hemoglobin < 10.5 g/dL
Presence of any factor is considered unfavorable.		Factors summed to yield the international prognostic score.
Two-thirds of limited stage patients have one or more adverse factors.		75% of patients have a score of 1–3.

EORTC, European Organization for the Research and Treatment of Cancer; GHSG, German Hodgkin Study Group; MMR, mediastinal mass ratio, which is the ratio of the maximal width of a mediastinal mass relative to the maximal width of the mediastinum, as measured by CT imaging; ESR, erythrocyte sedimentation rate.
Source: *Williams Hematology,* 8th ed, Chap. 99, Table 99–4, p. 1536.

Advanced Disease
- ABVD has become standard therapy.
- Interim analyses showed superior outcomes for BEACOPP.
  - Cure rates in excess of 80 percent for escalated BEACOPP, are the best ever recorded for a large phase III trial in advanced Hodgkin lymphoma.
  - BEACOPP has not been universally accepted as the new standard in advanced Hodgkin lymphoma because of concerns about the acute toxicity.
- The use of radiotherapy as a consolidation to combination chemotherapy in advanced Hodgkin lymphoma is controversial.
- Table 59–5 lists selected clinical trials for Hodgkin lymphoma.

Recurrent Disease
- Relapse after radiotherapy: chemotherapy results in an excellent rate of cure.
- High-dose therapy and autologous marrow or peripheral blood stem cell transplantation is the treatment of choice for patients who fail primary induction or who relapse after chemotherapy.
- Transplantation cure rates range from 40 to 60 percent.
- High-dose regimens include BEAM (carmustine, etoposide, cytarabine, melphalan), CBV (cyclophosphamide, carmustine, etoposide), and augmented CBV regimens.
- Second-line chemotherapy with ICE (ifosfamide, carboplatin, etoposide), DHAP (dexamethasone, cytarabine, cisplatin), or IGEV (ifosfamide, gemcitabine, vinorelbine) is used to achieve a minimal disease state prior to stem cell mobilization and transplantation.
- Treatment failures following autologous transplantation present a challenge, with longevity directly related to the time to relapse after transplant.
- Anti-CD20 antibody rituximab achieves high response rates in nodular lymphocyte-predominant Hodgkin lymphoma and can be used as retreatment or as an extended-treatment regimen.

COURSE AND PROGNOSIS
- Survival rate is 90 percent at 10 years up to age 44 years; 80 percent up to 54 years; 70 percent up to 64 years of age.

Clinical Prognostic Markers
- Prognostic markers for Hodgkin lymphoma are listed in Table 59–4.
- Adverse prognostic factors:
  - Male sex.
  - Age > 45 years.
  - Stage IV disease.
  - White blood count greater than or equal to 15×10^9/L.
  - Lymphocyte count less than 0.6×10^9/L or less than 8 percent of total leukocytes.
  - Hemoglobin concentration less than 10.5 g/dL.
  - Albumin concentration less than 4 g/dL.
- The European Organization for the Research and Treatment of Cancer (EORTC) defines four or more nodal sites, ESR greater than 50 mm/h in asymptomatic patients or ESR greater than 40 mm/h in symptomatic patients, and histology as indicators of intermediate disease (see Table 59–4).
- The presence of each factor reduced freedom from progression by about 7 percent.
- Patients in the worst prognostic group (five to seven factors) had a 42 percent freedom from progression at 5 years.
- FDG-PET imaging at the completion of treatment provides a high degree of negative predictive value, ranging from 81 to 100 percent.

TABLE 59–5	SELECTED RANDOMIZED CLINICAL THERAPEUTIC TRIALS IN HODGKIN LYMPHOMA			
Study (Number of patients)	Treatment	Failure-Free Survival (%)	Overall Survival (%)	Follow-up (years)
Limited stage, favorable and unfavorable				
Milan (140)	4 ABVD + IFRT	94	96	12
	4 ABVD + STLI	93	94	
		p = NS	p = NS	
NCIC-ECOG (399)	RT-containing	93	96	5
	4-6 ABVD	87	94	
		p = 0.006	p = NS	
Limited stage, favorable				
EORTC/GELA H9F(783)	6 EBVP + 20-IFRT	88	98	4
	6 EBVP + 30-IFRT	85	100	
	6 EBVP	69	98	
		p = 0.001	p = 0.241	
GHSG HD10 (1370)	2 ABVD + 30-IFRT	No difference to date*		4
	2 ABVD + 20-IFRT			
	4 ABVD + 30-IFRT			
	4 ABVD + 30-IFRT			
Limited stage, unfavorable				
EORTC/GELA H9U (808)	6 ABVD + 30-IFRT	91	95	4
	4 ABVD + 30-IFRT	87	94	
	4 BEACOPP + 30-IFRT	90	93	
		p = NS	p = NS	
GHSG HD11 (1422)	4 ABVD + 30-IFRT	No difference to date*		2.5
	4 ABVD + 20-IFRT			
	4 BEACOPP + 30-IFRT			
	4 BEACOPP+ 20-IFRT			
Advanced stage				
GHSG HD9 (1201)	8 COPP/ABVD + RT	69	83	5
	8 BEACOPP + RT	76	88	
	8 BEACOPPesc + RT	87	91	
		p <0.002	p <0.002	

ABVD, doxorubicin, bleomycin, vinblastine, dacarbazine; BEACOPP, bleomycin, etoposide, doxorubicin, cyclophosphamide, vincristine, procarbazine, prednisone; COPP, cyclophosphamide, vincristine, procarbazine, prednisone; EBVP, epirubicin, bleomycin, vinblastine, prednisone; ECOG, Eastern Cooperative Oncology Group; EORTC, European Organization for the Research and Treatment of Cancer; GELA, Groupe d'Etude des Lymphomes de l'Adulte; GHSG, German Hodgkin Study Group; IFRT, involved field radiotherapy; NCIC, National Cancer Institute of Canada; RT, radiotherapy; STLI, subtotal lymphoid irradiation.
*Interim analysis; **Interim analysis
Source: *Williams Hematology,* 8th ed, Chap. 99, Table 99–5, p. 1537.

- The positive predictive value of PET scanning at the end of chemotherapy is more variable and is related to disease extent and use of radiotherapy.
- Among patients referred for transplantation, sensitivity to standard-dose, second-line chemotherapy predicts for better survival: responding patients had an event-free survival of 60 percent versus 19 percent for those without a response.

Complications of Treatment

- The treatment of Hodgkin lymphoma is associated with important acute and chronic side effects.
- Late-treatment effects in the form second malignancy and cardiopulmonary disease can contribute to shortened longevity for cured patients. They increase with time and are currently the leading causes of death for Hodgkin lymphoma patients.
- Secondary malignancies:
  — Acute leukemia or myelodysplasia: the risk is proportional to cumulative dose of alkylating agents.
  — Increased risk of non-Hodgkin lymphoma, usually diffuse, aggressive, B-cell and are more frequent in nodular lymphocyte-predominant subtype.
  — Increased risk of development of solid cancer. Site is most often lung, stomach, bone, soft tissue. There is greater than threefold increased risk with radiation doses greater than 4 Gy and an eightfold risk for doses greater than 40 Gy. Elimination of routine axillary radiation, which is now standard, results in a 2.7-fold reduction in risk.
- Cardiac disease or breast cancer may occur in recipients of mediastinal irradiation.
- Radiation pneumonitis may occur depending on dose received by lung.
- Thyroid function abnormalities are common after neck irradiation, reaching a risk of 47 percent at 26 years.
- Current therapy programs use low-dose or no radiotherapy for all stages of disease.
- Vaccination against encapsulated organisms 10 to 14 days prior to the onset of treatment is advised.
- Early detection and prevention strategies for second cancers and cardiac disease should be considered in high-risk patients.
- Infertility frequent after MOPP chemotherapy. Banking sperm or eggs prior to therapy may be important in patients at risk for sterility.

For a more detailed discussion, see Sandra J. Horning: Hodgkin Lymphoma. Chap. 99, p. 1527 in *Williams Hematology*, 8th ed.

CHAPTER 60
General Considerations of Lymphoma: Epidemiology, Etiology, Heterogeneity, and Primary Extranodal Disease

EPIDEMIOLOGY

- Approximately 70,000 cases of non-Hodgkin lymphoma (NHL) will be diagnosed in 2010 and approximately 20,000 persons will die of the disease in the United States.
- NHL represents approximately 4.5 percent of cancers in the United States and 3.0 percent of cancer deaths, annually.
- The age-adjusted incidence rates for NHL in the United States are: 25.6 for white males, 18.4 for black males, 17.5 for white females, and 13.1 for black females.
- The risk of NHL in the United States is approximately three fold that of several underdeveloped countries and two fold that of several comparable industrialized country.
- There is a logarithmic increase in annual incidence in both men and women from late teenagers to octogenarians in the United States: males 15 to 19 years of age, 2.3 cases/100,000 persons; males 80 to 84 years of age, 140 cases/100,000 persons; females 15 to 19 years, 1.4 cases/100,000 persons; females 80 to 84 years, 100 cases per 100,000 persons.
- Follicular lymphoma represents approximately 25 to 30 percent of NHL cases in the United States but is uncommon in many developing countries and in Asia, especially China and Japan.
- Diffuse large B-cell lymphoma represents approximately 30 percent of NHL cases in the United States.
- The annual incidence of NHL, but not Hodgkin lymphoma, increased significantly between 1972 and 1995 in the United States and Western European countries. The increase probably started before 1972 but the United States National Cancer Institute did not track specific-site cancer incidence before that date.
- The rate is still increasing slightly for women and older men in the United States. Orbital adenexal lymphoma, and mantle cell lymphoma are increasing at a rate of 6 percent per year.
- There is no aggregate evidence sufficient to reach a level of medical or scientific certainty at this time that benzene, other solvents, pesticides, herbicides, dyes, various occupations, and other industrial exposures increase the relative risk of lymphoma as determined by the U.S. Public Health Service.
- There are instances of familial clustering and an increase in the relative risk of lymphoma in siblings of patients with lymphoma or related hematologic malignancies (e.g., myeloma). These so-called nonsyndromic examples of increased risk are likely explained by as yet undefined predisposition genes, akin to the Li-Fraumeni syndrome, which is the result of germ-line inheritance of p53.
- Several syndromic immunodeficiency states increase the relative risk of lymphoma in family members (see Table 60–2).

TABLE 60–1	**HISTOLOGIC SUBTYPES AND RELATIVE FREQUENCY OF THE NON-HODGKIN LYMPHOMAS (NHL)**

I. B-cell lymphomas (~88% of all NHL)
   A. 1. Diffuse large B-cell lymphomas (30%)
      2. T-cell rich large B-cell lymphoma
      3. Primary diffuse large B-cell lymphoma of the central nervous system
      4. Primary cutaneous diffuse large B-cell lymphoma
      5. Epstein-Barr virus (EBV)-positive diffuse large B-cell lymphoma of the elderly
      6. Diffuse large B-cell lymphoma arising in human herpesvirus (HHV)-8– associated multicentric Castleman disease
      Diffuse large B-cell lymphomas with features simulating Hodgkin lymphoma
   B. Follicular lymphoma (25%)
   C. Extranodal marginal zone lymphoma of mucosa-associated lymphatic tissue (MALT lymphoma) (7%)
   D. Small lymphocytic lymphoma-chronic lymphocytic leukemia (7%)
   E. Mantle cell lymphoma (5%)
   F. Primary mediastinal (thymic) large B-cell lymphoma (3%)
   G. Lymphoplasmacytic lymphoma-Waldenström macroglobulinemia (<2%)
   H. Nodal marginal zone B-cell lymphoma (<1.5%)
   I. Splenic marginal zone lymphoma (<1%)
   J. Extranodal marginal zone B-cell lymphoma (<1%)
   K. Intravascular large B-cell lymphoma (<1%)
   L. Primary effusion lymphoma (<1%)
   M. Primary cutaneous follicle center lymphoma (1%)
   N. Burkitt lymphoma–Burkitt leukemia (1.5%)
   O. Plasmablastic lymphoma <1.0%
   P. Lymphomatoid granulomatosis (<1%)

II. T-and NK-cell lymphomas (~12% of all NHL)
   A. Extranodal T or NK lymphoma
   B. Enteropathy-associated T-cell lymphoma
   C. Hepatosplenic T-cell lymphoma
   D. Subcutaneous panniculitis-like T-cell lymphoma
   E. Cutaneous T-cell lymphoma (Sézary syndrome and mycosis fungoides)
   F. Primary cutaneous gamma-delta T-cell lymphoma
   G. Anaplastic large-cell lymphoma
   H. Angioimmunoblastic T-cell lymphoma
   I. Primary T-cell lymphoma unspecified

III. Immunodeficiency-associated lymphoproliferative disorders (see **Table 60–2** for inherited diseases associated with immunodeficiencies and lymphoma)
   A. HIV-associated lymphoma
   B. Posttransplantation lymphoproliferative disorder
   C. Lymphoma associated with a primary immune disorder

Nosology based on the World Health Organization Classification of Tumors of Hematopoietic and Lymphoid Tissues. The parenthetical percentages are approximate but give a sense of the relative distribution of subtypes. The frequency of lymphoma type varies depending on the geographical area under consideration. The frequencies cited here are approximate and related to those observed in the United States, the United Kingdom, or Western Europe. Some very rare subtypes are not listed.
Source: *Williams Hematology,* 8th ed, Chap. 97, Table 97–1, p. 1500.

HISTOLOGIC HETEROGENEITY

- The World Health Organization has categorized over 30 unique histopathologic types of NHL and these are shown in Table 60–1 with their approximate relative frequency. Approximately 88 percent are B-cell lymphomas and approximately 12 percent are T-cell lymphomas. There are striking variations in the incidence of various subtypes of NHL in different geographic areas throughout the world.

EFFECT OF GENE POLYMORPHISMS

- Single nucleotide polymorphism base analysis has indicated that lymphomagenesis may be linked to polymorphic genes that are involved in apoptosis, cell cycle regulation, lymphocyte development, and inflammation. The polymorphisms could also be linked to individual susceptibility to certain environmental exposures.

INFECTIOUS AGENTS

- Adult T-cell leukemia-lymphoma is caused by human T-cell lymphocytotrophic virus- (HTLV)-1 (see Chap. 67).
- The Epstein-Barr virus genome has been found with a high prevalence in the neoplastic lymphocytes of African Burkitt lymphoma, posttransplantation lymphoma, human immunodeficiency virus (HIV)–related lymphoma, primary central nervous system lymphoma, primary effusion lymphoma, immunoblastic plasmacytoid B-cell lymphoma, oral cavity plasmablastic lymphoma, and extranodal NK/T-cell lymphoma. The precise role of this virus in lymphomagenesis has not been defined but it is likely to be an important facilitating factor in some of these lymphoma types.
- Human herpesvirus-8 is associated with Kaposi sarcoma, Castleman disease, and primary effusion lymphoma found most frequently in immunodeficiency associated with HIV infection.
- Hepatitis B and C virus have been implicated in the pathogenesis of lymphoma based on the seropositivity of cases compared with controls. Hepatitis C virus has a predilection for lymphocytes, and it has been specifically associated with diffuse large B-cell lymphoma, marginal zone lymphoma, and lymphoplasmacytic lymphoma but not follicular lymphoma. The etiologic role and pathogenetic mechanisms of these viruses have not been established.
- *Helicobacter pylori* can cause marginal zone B-cell lymphomas of mucosa-associated lymphatic tissue (MALT lymphoma), notably of the stomach. This organism is the first bacterium shown to be capable of inducing a human neoplasm (see Chap. 64).
- *Chlamydophila psittaci* has been associated with a majority of cases of a specific extranodal mucosa-associated lymphoid tissue lymphoma, ocular adnexal lymphoma.
- *Campylobacter jejuni* and *Borrelia burgdorferi* have been associated with immunoproliferative diseases of the small intestines and B-cell lymphoma of the skin.

IMMUNOSUPPRESSION AND AUTOIMMUNITY

- A number of inherited immunodeficiency syndromes listed in Table 60–2 are associated with a predisposition to lymphoma.
- Acquired immunodeficiency states including acquired immunodeficiency syndrome (AIDS)–related lymphoma and posttransplantation-related lymphoma usually have a B-cell lineage immunophenotype and often involve extranodal sites (e.g., skin or central nervous system), are aggressive in behavior, and often associated with Epstein-Barr virus infection of the neoplastic B lymphocytes.

TABLE 60–2 INHERITED SYNDROMES PREDISPOSING TO LYMPHOMA

Syndrome	Inheritance	Altered Genes Description	Mechanism	Leukemia Type
DNA repair defects				
Ataxia telangiectasia	R	ATM homozygotes Dominant-negative missense mutations	Genomic instability Increased translocations in T cells formed at the time of V(D)J recombination	T cell lymphoma, T-cell ALL, T-cell PLL, B-cell lymphoma
Bloom	R	BLM	Genomic instability	ALL, lymphoma
Nijmegen breakage	R	NBS1	Genomic instability Altered telomere maintenance	Lymphoid tumors, especially B-cell lymphoma
Tumor-suppressor gene defect				
Li-Fraumeni*	D	p53	Defect in tumor suppressor	CLL, ALL, Hodgkin and Burkitt lymphoma
Immunodeficiency states				
Common variable immunodeficiency	R and D	Defect in CD40 signaling	Failure of B-cell maturation	Burkitt, MALT, other B-cell lymphomas, Hodgkin lymphoma
Severe combined immunodeficiency disease (SCID)	R	ADA	Defective T- + B-cell function	B-cell lymphoma
Wiskott-Aldrich	X	WASP	Signaling and apoptosis	Hodgkin and non-Hodgkin lymphoma
X-linked immunodeficiency with normal or increased IgM	X	CD40L	CD40 ligand defect on T cell	Hodgkin and non-Hodgkin lymphoma
X-linked lymphoproliferative syndrome (XLP)	X	SAP	Defect in immune signaling	EBV-related B-cell lymphoma
Apoptotic defect				
Autoimmune lymphoproliferative syndrome (ALPS)	D	APT (FAS)	Germ-line heterozygous FAS mutations; defective apoptosis	Lymphoma

| | Altered Genes | | | |
Syndrome	Inheritance	Description	Mechanism	Leukemia Type
Unknown defect				
Dubowitz	R	Unknown	Unknown	ALL, lymphoma
Poland	D	May not be inherited	Unknown	ALL, lymphoma
WT	D	Unknown	Unknown	ALL, Castleman disease

ALL, acute lymphocytic leukemia; CLL, chronic lymphocytic leukemia; D, dominant; EBV, Epstein-Barr virus; MALT, mucosa-associated lymphatic tissue lymphoma; R, recessive; T-PLL, T prolymphocytic leukemia; X, X-linked.
*Li-Fraumeni or Li-Fraumeni–like syndrome has been described in which a gene other than p53 is mutated. hCHK2 in particular has been described as etiologic. We have not included these variants in the table because we are uncertain if lymphoma is one of the cancers for which susceptibility is increased.
Source: *Williams Hematology*, 8th ed, Chap. 97, Table 97–2, p.1502.

- The occurrence of Ig (V) mutations in acquired immunodeficiency-related lymphoma strongly suggests a germinal center B lymphocyte transformation.
- The incidence and severity of immunodeficiency-related lymphoma have increased in relationship to the use of more powerful immunosuppressive agents, such as cyclosporine and in the setting of mismatched T-cell depleted allogeneic hematopoietic stem cell grafts.
- Several autoimmune disorders are associated with an increased relative risk of lymphoma. These include systemic lupus erythematosus, Sjögren syndrome, autoimmune thyroid disease, and, perhaps, rheumatoid arthritis. For example, NHL is increased 6.5-fold and MALT lymphoma of the parotid gland 1000-fold in Sjögren syndrome.

SPECIFIC CHROMOSOME ABNORMALITIES AND HISTOLOGIC SUBTYPE

- Chromosome abnormalities involving all 22 autosomes and the sex chromosomes can occur with lymphoma.
- Lymphomas have a high frequency of fusion genes usually one of two types: oncogenes activated by juxtaposing with immunoglobulin or T cell receptor genes or by forming chimeric genes that activate mutant kinases or transcription factors.
- Approximately 85 percent of cases of follicular lymphoma have a t(14;18) (q32;q21)(*IgH;BCL-2*) in the lymphoma cells. Presumably the overexpression of BCL-2 contributes to an anti-apoptotic effect favoring an accumulation of long-lived centrocytes (see Chap. 62).
- In Burkitt lymphoma cells t(8;14)(q24;q32), principally, or t(2;8)(p13;q24) or t(8;22)(q24;q11) is present in the Burkitt cell. The common feature is the formation of a fusion gene involving the *MYC* gene at band q24 on chromosome 8 with either the *IgH* or *Igκ* or *Igλ* genes (see Chap. 65).
- The t(2;5)(p23;q35) in the cells of anaplastic large cell lymphoma (ALCL) involves the *NPM* gene at 5p35 and the ALCL tyrosine kinase (*ALK*) gene at 2p23, resulting in a novel oncoprotein, p80. The translocation occurs in about 50 percent of cases in adults and a higher proportion of children.
- Four translocations, t(11;18)(*API2;MALT1*), t(1;14)(*IgH-BCL10*), t(14;18)(*IgH; Malt1*), and t(3;14)(*IgH;FOXP1*) have been associated with marginal zone

lymphomas of the MALT type at different sites. In the first three translocations shown, the oncogenic product targets the nuclear factor-κB pathway (see Chap. 64).

- Most cases of mantle cell lymphoma have t(11;14)(q13;q32) in the lymphoma cells. This translocation juxtaposes CCND1 and the IgH genes and results in upregulation of cyclin D1, used as a marker in the diagnosis of this disease (see Chap. 63).

GENERAL APPROACHES TO LYMPHOMA MANAGEMENT

- Complete history and physical examination to determine extent of superficial lymphadenopathy, evidence of extranodal involvement, and presence of B symptoms (fever, >38 °C, night sweats, weight loss >10% body weight in last 6 months).
- Staging should be carried out to determine extent of disease as shown in Table 60–3.
- Although the Ann Arbor Staging System was developed for Hodgkin lymphoma, it is used for NHL staging as well (see Table 60–4).

PRIMARY EXTRANODAL LYMPHOMA

- Lymphomas involving extranodal sites most commonly occur simultaneously with nodal involvement at time of diagnosis or during course of the disease.
- Lymphoma only found in extranodal sites after staging procedures (see Table 60–3) is called *primary extranodal lymphoma*.
- Solitary extranodal lymphoma can occur in any organ. Lymphoma should be considered in the differential diagnosis of any solitary mass.
- The histology of primary extranodal lymphoma is usually marginal zone lymphoma of mucosa associated lymphoid tissue or diffuse large B-cell lymphoma. Other lymphoma types may occasionally be the histologic diagnosis.
- Therapy is usually a combination of excision, radiotherapy, multidrug chemotherapy, and a lymphocyte-directed monoclonal antibody. Rituximab, cyclophosphamide, hydroxydoxorubicin (Adriamycin), vincristine (Oncovin) and

---

TABLE 60–3　STAGING PROCEDURES FOR LYMPHOMA

I. Initial studies
   A. History and physical examination
   B. Biopsy specimen
   C. Pathologic diagnosis
   D. Flow cytometry
   E. Immunohistochemistry
   F. Cytogenetic analysis
   G. CT/PET scans of neck, chest, abdomen, and pelvis
II. Additional studies
   A. Immunoglobulin and T-cell-receptor gene rearrangement studies
   B. Polymerase chain reaction for *BCL-1* and *BCL-2*
   C. Ultrasonography and MRI to clarify abnormalities
   D. CT scan or MRI of brain if neurologic signs or symptoms
   E. Analysis of cerebrospinal fluid if neurologic signs or symptoms
   F. Gastrointestinal studies (imaging and or endoscopy) if Waldeyer ring involvement

---

CT, computed tomography; MRI, magnetic resonance imaging; PET, positron emission tomography.
Source: *Williams Hematology*, 8th ed, Chap. 97, Table 97–3, p.1504.

TABLE 60–4	ANN ARBOR STAGING SYSTEM

Stage I*	Restricted to one lymph node-bearing area
Stage II*	Two or more areas of nodal involvement on one side of the diaphragm
Stage III*	Lymphatic involvement on both sides of the diaphragm
Stage IV	Liver, marrow involvement, or extensive extranodal disease

- Status "A": Absence of fevers, sweats, or weight loss.
- Status "B": Unexplained fevers >38 °C (100.4 °F), drenching night sweats, weight loss of >10% of body weight in the preceding 6 months represent
- Clinical Stage: Assigned stage based only on history, physical findings, and laboratory and imaging studies.
- Pathologic Stage: Assigned stage based only on areas of biopsy-proven involvement
- Substage E: Localized, extranodal disease

*The spleen is considered a single nodal area.
Source: *Williams Hematology*, 8th ed, Chap. 97, Table 97–4, p. 1504.

prednisone (R-CHOP) is one commonly used regimen for extranodal B-cell malignancies.
- The pathobiology underlying a propensity of primary extranodal lymphoma to arise simultaneously in paired organs (kidneys, ovaries, breasts, eyes, adrenals, and others) is unknown.
- Specific types include:
  — *Bone.* Primary lymphoma may affect any bone but usually the long bones are involved. If the skull is involved, central nervous system invasion may occur.
  — *Breast.* Primary lymphoma of the female breast mimics carcinoma. Staging finds lymph node, marrow, or other extranodal sites of involvement in half the cases.
  — *Central nervous system.* Involvement of the leptomeninges may produce headache, stiff neck, and cranial nerve impairment; brain involvement can result in headache, lethargy, papilledema, focal neurologic signs, or seizures; spinal cord involvement can result in back pain, extremity weakness, paresis, and paralysis. Usually aggressive type of diffuse large B-cell lymphoma. Intracerebral lymphoma is a feature of acquired immunodeficiency syndrome.
  — *Chest and lung.* Primary pulmonary lymphoma may present as a solitary mass in the lung and require lung biopsy for diagnosis. Primary chest wall lymphoma can be accompanied by fever, sweating, and dyspnea and require excisional biopsy for diagnosis. Primary endobronchial lymphoma may follow lung transplantation and cause airway obstruction.
  — *Endocrine glands.* Primary adrenal lymphoma usually presents bilaterally and may lead to adrenal insufficiency. Primary thyroid lymphoma often develops on the background of autoimmune (Hashimoto) thyroiditis. Primary pituitary lymphoma can result in pituitary insufficiency, including diabetes insipidus.
  — *Eye.* Ophthalmic lymphoma is the most common orbital malignancy and includes lymphoma involving the eyelids, conjunctiva, lacrimal sac, lacrimal gland, orbit, or intraocular space. Ophthalmic lymphoma accounts for approximately 7 percent of primary extranodal lymphoma cases.
  — *Gastrointestinal tract.* This is the most common form of primary extranodal lymphoma, accounting for approximately one-third of cases. The most common site of involvement is the stomach, followed by the ileum, cecum, colon, and rectum. The liver, pancreas, and gallbladder may also be the site of extranodal lymphoma. Symptoms are related to the site involved (e.g., nausea, vomiting, diarrhea, bleeding).

— *Genitourinary tract.* Primary lymphoma of the testes presents as painless enlargement and may be bilateral. Primary lymphoma of the ovary is often bilateral and presents as abdominal masses sometimes felt on abdominal or pelvic examination. Cases limited to the uterus, uterine cervix, vagina, or vulva may occur. Lymphomatous involvement of both kidneys usually presents with renal failure. Bilateral ureteral involvement presents with obstructive renal failure. Primary lymphoma of the bladder or of the prostate may occur.

— *Heart.* Primary cardiac lymphoma may involve the heart or pericardium. Patients may present with dyspnea, edema, arrhythmia, or pericardial effusion with tamponade. Masses may occur in the right atrium (most common), pericardium, right ventricle, left atrium, or left ventricle.

— *Paranasal sinuses.* May present with local pain, upper airway obstruction, rhinorrhea, facial swelling, or epistaxis. Usually diffuse large B-cell lymphoma in the United States and Western Europe and T-cell and NK cell lymphoma in Asia.

— *Skin.* The three main types of cutaneous B-cell lymphoma are: primary cutaneous marginal zone B-cell lymphoma, primary cutaneous follicular center B-cell lymphoma, and primary cutaneous large B-cell lymphoma (leg type). The first two are indolent lymphomas and the last type is an aggressive lymphoma. These lymphomas may present as soft tissue masses, mimicking sarcoma, until a biopsy and histopathologic diagnosis is obtained.

— *Spleen.* Primary splenic lymphoma is rare since concomitant marrow involvement is present in most cases. The issue of whether splenic lymphoma is extranodal arises but since lymphoma is usually confined to the red pulp and not the white pulp, it can be considered extranodal.

 For a more detailed discussion, see Kenneth A. Foon and Marshall A. Lichtman: General Considerations of Lymphoma: Epidemiology, Etiology, Heterogeneity, and Primary Extranodal Disease. Chap. 97, p. 1497 in *Williams Hematology*, 8th ed.

CHAPTER 61
Diffuse Large B-Cell Lymphoma

DEFINITION

- Diffuse large B-cell lymphomas (DLBCLs) are a heterogeneous group of aggressive lymphomas of large, transformed B cells.
- DLBCLs can arise *de novo* or may transform from a low-grade lymphoma, such as small lymphocytic lymphoma or follicular lymphoma.
- Table 61–1 lists the variants and subtypes of DLBCL.

EPIDEMIOLOGY

- Most common B-cell lymphoid neoplasm in the United States and Europe and accounts for approximately 28 percent of all mature B-cell lymphomas.
- The most common presentation is in late middle-aged and older persons.
- Median age at diagnosis is approximately 65 years.

ETIOLOGY AND PATHOGENESIS

- Molecularly heterogeneous disease with multiple complex chromosomal translocations and genetic abnormalities as identified by cytogenetics and gene expression profiling.
- Disease is derived from B cells that have undergone somatic mutation in the immunoglobulin (Ig) genes.
- *BCL6* gene rearrangements may be specific for DLBCL.
  - Approximately 40 percent of cases in immunocompetent persons and approximately 20 percent of HIV-related cases display *BCL6* rearrangements.
  - BCL6 protein mediates the specific binding of several transcription factors to DNA.
- Approximately 30 percent of patients have the t(14;18) translocation involving *BCL2* and the Ig-heavy-chain gene.
  - The presence of *p53* mutation in combination with *BCL2* denotes that the tumor is derived from a transformation of a prior follicular lymphoma.
- Aberrant somatic mutation occurs in more than 50 percent of cases and targets multiple loci (e.g., *IGH*, *PIM1*, *MYC*, *RhoH/TTF* (ARHH), *PAX5*, *c-MYC*).
- Three molecular subtypes have been identified determined by gene expression profiling:
  - Germinal center B-like (GCB): arise from normal germinal center B cells.
  - Activated B-cell-like (ABC): may arise from postgerminal center B cells that are arrested during plasmacytic differentiation.
  - Primary mediastinal B-cell lymphoma: might arise from thymic B cells.

CLINICAL FEATURES

- Lymph nodes are enlarged, nontender, firm but rubbery and are typically found in the neck or abdominal mass.
- Systemic "B" symptoms of fatigue, fever, night sweats, and weight loss occur in 30 percent of patients at presentation.
- Approximately 50 to 60 percent of patients have disseminated DLBCL (stage III or IV) upon presentation.

TABLE 61-1	DIFFUSE LARGE B-CELL LYMPHOMA: VARIANTS AND SUBTYPES

I. Diffuse large B-cell lymphoma, not otherwise specified (NOS)
   A. Common morphologic variants
      1. Centroblastic
      2. Immunoblastic
      3. Anaplastic
   B. Rare morphologic variants
   C. Molecular subgroups
      1. Germinal center B-cell–like
      2. Activated B-cell–like
   D. Immunohistochemical subgroups
      1. CD5-positive DLBCL
      2. Germinal center B-cell–like
      3. Nongerminal center B-cell–like
II. Diffuse large B-cell lymphoma subtypes
   A. T-cell/histiocyte-rich large B-cell lymphoma
   B. Primary DLBCL of the CNS
   C. Primary cutaneous DLBCL, leg type
   D. EBV-positive DLBCL of the elderly
III. Other lymphomas of large B cells
   A. Primary mediastinal (thymic) large B-cell lymphoma
   B. Intravascular large B-cell lymphoma
   C. DLBCL associated with chronic inflammation
   D. Lymphomatoid granulomatosis
   E. ALK-positive DLBCL
   F. Plasmablastic lymphoma
   G. Large B-cell lymphoma arising in HHV8-associated multicentric
      Castleman disease
   H. Primary effusion lymphoma
IV. Borderline cases
   A. B-cell lymphoma, unclassifiable, with features intermediate between
      diffuse large B-cell lymphoma and Burkitt lymphoma
   B. B-cell lymphoma, unclassifiable, with features intermediate between
      diffuse large B-cell lymphoma and classic Hodgkin lymphoma

ALK, anaplastic lymphoma kinase; DLBCL, diffuse large B-cell lymphoma; EBV, Epstein-Barr virus; HHV, human herpes virus.
Source: *Williams Hematology*, 8th ed, Chap. 100, Table 100–1, p. 1548.

- Other sites that may be affected include testis, bone, thyroid, salivary glands, skin, liver, breast, nasal cavity, paranasal sinuses, pleural cavity, and central nervous system (CNS).
- Marrow involvement occurs in 15 percent of patients.
- CNS involvement may occur after testicular or paranasal sinuses involvement.
- Some patients might have discordant disease in which the lymph nodes are involved with DLBCL but the marrow histopathology may be that of a low-grade lymphoma.
- Patients with lymphoma in the Waldeyer ring have an increased risk of gastrointestinal lymphoma.

LABORATORY FEATURES

Blood and Marrow

- Lymphoma involvement of the marrow occurs in approximately 15 percent of cases.

Cell Immunophenotype

- The malignant cells have surface monoclonal Ig of either κ or λ light-chain type.
  — The most commonly expressed surface Ig is IgM.
- Lymphoma cells generally express the pan-B cell antigens: CD19, CD20, CD22, PAX5, and CD79a.
  — The cells also express CD45 and less commonly CD10 or CD5.
- CD5+ DLBCL may be more aggressive with worse prognosis.

Histopathology

- Lymph nodes are usually effaced by a diffuse infiltrate of large lymphocytes.
- Other rare morphologic variants occur, for example, with a myxoid or fibrillary appearance.

PROGNOSTIC FACTORS

- In 1993, a model was proposed to assign a prognosis to patients with aggressive lymphoma undergoing treatment with doxorubicin-containing chemotherapeutic regimens termed the *international prognostic index* (IPI) (see Table 61–2).
  — The 5-year survival rates for patients age 60 years or younger with IPI scores of 0, 1, 2, and 3 were 83, 69, 46, and 32 percent, respectively (see Table 61–3).
- Gene-expression profiling has also been used to delineate groups of patients with DLBCL who may differ in their response to therapy and prognosis.
- The relative expression of six genes can identify three prognostic groups:
  — High-level expression of *LMO2*, *BCL6*, and *FNI* correlated with prolonged survival.
  — High-level expression of *BCL2*, *CCND2*, and *SCYA3* correlated with short survival.
- Patients with an elevated β_2-microglobulin level and high serum lactic acid dehydrogenase (LDH) have a poor prognosis.
- Approximately 70 percent of DLBCL cases are of germinal center origin, as demonstrated by BCL6 protein and have a more favorable prognosis.
- Survivin, a member of the inhibitor of apoptosis family of proteins, is expressed in 60 percent of patients with DLBCL and is associated with a poor prognosis.
- High number of infiltrating CD4+ T cells in lymph nodes involved with DLBCL is associated with a better prognosis.
- High-level expression of cyclin D3, serum vascular endothelial growth factor, plasma cytokines such as interleukin (IL)-2, IL-10, and IL-6, or *p53* gene mutation are associated with a poor prognosis.

TABLE 61–2	INTERNATIONAL PROGNOSTIC FACTOR INDEX FOR NON-HODGKIN LYMPHOMA

Risk Factors

Age >60 years

Serum lactic acid dehydrogenase greater than twice normal

Performance status ≥2

Stage III or IV

Extranodal involvement at >1 site

Each factor accounts for 1 point, for a total score that ranges from 0 to 3 for patients <61 years of age. The latter age-adjusted index includes all variables except for age and extranodal sites. For patients ≥61 years of age, a total score ranges from 0 to 5 and includes each variable shown in this table.

Source: *Williams Hematology,* 8th ed, Chap. 100, Table 100–2, p. 1549.

TABLE 61–3 **OUTCOME ACCORDING TO RISK GROUP DEFINED BY THE INTERNATIONAL PROGNOSTIC INDEX**

International Index	No. of Risk Factors	Complete Response Rate (%)	Relapse-Free Survival (%)		Survival (%)	
Age-Adjusted International Prognostic Index, Patients >60 Years of Age						
			2-Year	5-Year	2-Year	5-Year
Low	0 or 1	87	79	70	84	73
Low-intermediate	2	67	66	50	66	51
High-intermediate	3	55	59	49	54	43
High	4 or 5	44	58	40	34	26
Age-Adjusted International Index, Patients <61 Years of Age						
			2-Year	5-Year	2-Year	5-Year
Low	0	92	88	86	90	83
Low-intermediate	1	78	74	66	79	69
High-intermediate	2	57	62	53	59	46
High	3	46	61	58	37	32

Source: *Williams Hematology,* 8th ed, Chap. 100, Table 100–3, p. 1549.

- Fluorine-18-fluorodeoxyglucose-positron emission tomography (FDG-PET) is used for staging and monitoring patients.

THERAPY

- DLBCL is potentially curable with combination chemotherapy.
- The dose intensity administered during the first 12 weeks of therapy determines survival.

Early Stage DLBCL (Stages I and II)
- Localized disease occurs in approximately 25 percent of patients.
- Combining chemotherapy with radiation therapy improved outcome (see Table 61–4).
  - Patients in a study received eight cycles of cyclophosphamide, hydroxy-daunorubicin, Oncovin (vincristine), and prednisone (CHOP) chemotherapy or three cycles of CHOP plus involved-field radiotherapy and had a 5-year overall response rate of 82 percent and a progression-free survival rate of 72 percent compared with patients who received chemotherapy alone.
  - Patients with poor risk factors had a worse overall survival.
  - The treatment advantage of CHOP plus involved-field radiation for the first 7 years diminished as a result of lymphoma recurrence between 5 and 10 years.
- Systemic chemotherapy has improved the outcome of patients with localized aggressive lymphoma.
- Rituximab has changed the therapeutic paradigm in advanced DLBCL and is incorporated in most treatment regimens.

Advances Stages of DLBCL (Bulky Stages I and II or III and IV)
- Table 61–5 lists different chemotherapy regimens for intermediate- and high-grade lymphoma.
- The results of the Monoclonal Antibody Therapeutic International Trial (MInT) suggest that six cycles of rituximab with a CHOP-like regimen is the best therapy for young patients with good-prognosis DLBCL.
  - R-CHOP now is the standard of care for younger patients with DLBCL.
  - Adding etoposide to R-CHOP or intensifying the doses of drugs in CHOP therapy is under study.

TABLE 61–4 **TREATMENT OF LIMITED-STAGE AGGRESSIVE LYMPHOMA**

Patient Population	Number of Patients	Treatment	5-Year OS (p value) (%)
Stages I and II, nonbulky	401	8 cycles CHOP vs. 3 cycles CHOP + IFRT	72 (p = 0.05) 82
Bulky stages I, IE, II, and IIE	399	8 cycles CHOP vs. 8 cycles CHOP + IFRT	73* 87 (p = 0.24)
Age >60 years, IPI O	576	4 cycles CHOP vs. 4 cycles CHOP + IFRT	72 68 (p = 0.5)
Age <61 years, localized stages I and II, IPI O	647	ACVBP vs. 3 cycles CHOP + IFRT	90 87 (p <0.001)
Age >60 years with IPI >O	60	R-CHOP + IFRT	92

CHOP, cyclophosphamide, doxorubicin, vincristine, prednisone; IFRT, involved-field radiation therapy; IPI, international prognostic index; OS, overall survival; R-CHOP, rituximab, cyclophosphamide, doxorubicin, vincristine, prednisone.
*OS for 172 complete remission patients randomized to observation versus involved-field radiation therapy.
Source: *Williams Hematology*, 8th ed, Chap. 100, Table 100–4, p. 1552.

TABLE 61–5 **COMBINATION CHEMOTHERAPY FOR INTERMEDIATE- AND HIGH-GRADE LYMPHOMA**

Regimen	Dose	Route	Days of Treatment	Interval between Treatment Cycles (Days)	Cycles
R-CHOP-21					
Rituximab	375 mg/m^2	IV	1	21	6–8
Cyclophosphamide	750 mg/m^2	IV	1		
Doxorubicin	50 mg/m^2	IV	1		
Vincristine	1.4 mg/m^2	IV	1		
Prednisone	100 mg/day	PO	1–5		
CHOP-14					
Cyclophosphamide	750 mg/m^2	IV	1	14	6–8
Doxorubicin	50 mg/m^2	IV	1		
Vincristine	1.4 mg/m^2	IV	1		
Prednisone	100 mg/day	PO	1–5		
I-CHOP					
Cyclophosphamide	1000 mg/m^2	IV	1	14	6
Doxorubicin	70 mg/m^2	IV			
Vincristine	2 mg	IV	1		
Prednisone	100 mg	PO	1–5		
CHOPE-21					
Cyclophosphamide	750 mg/m^2	IV	1	21	6–8
Doxorubicin	50 mg/m^2	IV	1		
Vincristine	2 mg/m^2	IV	1		
Etoposide	100 mg/m^2	IV	1–3		
Prednisone	100 mg/day	PO	1–5		

(continued)

TABLE 61–5 **COMBINATION CHEMOTHERAPY FOR INTERMEDIATE- AND HIGH-GRADE LYMPHOMA (CONTINUED)**

Regimen	Dose	Route	Days of Treatment	Interval between Treatment Cycles (Days)	Cycles
Dose-Adjusted R-EPOCH*					
Rituximab	375 mg/m^2	IV	1	21	6–8
Etoposide	50 mg/m^2/day	CIV	1–4 (96 hours)		
Doxorubicin	10 mg/m^2/day	CIV	1–4 (96 hours)		
Vincristine	0.4 mg/day	CIV	1–4 (96 hours)		
Cyclophosphamide	750 mg/m^2/ day	IV	5		
Prednisone	60 mg/m^2/day	PO	1–5		
ESHAP (for relapsed lymphoma)					
Etoposide	40 mg/m^2	IV	1–4	21	
Methylprednisone	500 mg/m^2	IV	1–5		
Cytarabine	2 mg/m^2	IV	5		
Cisplatin	25 mg/m^2	CIV	1–4		
DHAP (for relapsed l lymphoma)					
Dexamethasone	40 mg/m^2	PO or IV	1–4	21	
Cisplatin	100 mg/m^2	CIV	1		
Cytarabine	2 mg/m2	IVq12h x 2 doses	2		
R±ICE (for relapsed lymphoma)					
Rituximab	375 mg/m^2	IV	1	14	
Mesna	5000 mg/m^2	IV	l (day 2)		
Carboplatin	AUC = 5 (maximum 800 mg)	IV	1 (day 2)		
Etoposide	100 mg/m^2	IV	1–3		
Neulasta	6 mg	SQ	1 (day 4)		

AUC, area under the curve; CIV, continuous intravenous infusion; I-CHOP, intensified-CHOP; IV, intravenously; PO, by mouth; SQ, subcutaneously.

*Doses of etoposide, doxorubicin, and cyclophosphamide are increased 20% over the dose in the previous cycle if the nadir of the absolute neutrophil count in the previous cycle was ≥ 0.5 × 109/L.

The reader is advised to verify drugs, doses, and administration schedules of these regimens.

Source: *Williams Hematology,* 8th ed, Chap. 100, Table 100–5, p. 1554.

Chemotherapy in Patients Older than Age 60 Years

- Patients older than age 60 years with a low or low-intermediate IPI have a lower relapse-free and overall survival rate than younger patients.
- The best therapy based on recent studies for patients over the age of 60 years is six cycles of R-CHOP.

Role of High-Dose Chemotherapy and Autologous Hematopoietic Stem Cell Transplantation (Auto-HSCT) in Initial Therapy

- High-dose chemotherapy and auto-HSCT is not recommended for most patients with diagnosed DLBCL.

- A subgroup of patients with poor prognostic features may benefit from such aggressive therapy and should be considered for auto-HSCT in the context of a clinical trial.
- Abbreviated courses of chemotherapy prior to transplantation are not beneficial, and patients should receive a full course of standard chemotherapy and achieve a maximum response prior to transplantation.

Recurrent and Refractory DLCBL

Chemotherapy

- A substantial proportion of patients are either refractory or will relapse after chemotherapy.
- Relapse usually occurs within the first 2 to 3 years after diagnosis but is uncommon after 4 years of diagnosis.
- Cure of relapsed or refractory patients may first require response to a differently configured regimen followed by auto-HSCT.
- Responses to monotherapy are generally not long-lasting.
- The addition of rituximab to the ifosfamide-carboplatin-etoposide (ICE) chemotherapy regimen (R-ICE) increased the complete response rate of patients with relapsed or primary refractory DLBCL under consideration for auto-HSCT.

Autologous Stem Cell Transplantation (Auto-HSCT)

- Patients with relapsed or primary refractory DLBCL who achieve complete response before auto-HSCT generally have better outcomes than those who achieve only partial response.
- Disease sensitivity at the time of auto-HSCT has remained the most significant prognostic variable for predicting treatment outcome.
- Patients who undergo auto-HSCT when the disease is resistant to the initial induction therapy have less than a 20 percent probability of disease-free survival.

Allogeneic Hematopoietic Stem Cell Transplantation (Allo-HSCT)

- The overall relapse and progression rate for the allo-HSCT patients at 5 years was 23 percent compared with 38 percent in the auto-HSCT patients.
- Allo-HSCT cannot be recommended before auto-HSCT except in the context of a clinical trial.
- Radioimmunotherapy as monotherapy: not recommended for DLBCL.
- Patients with relapsed disease should receive multidrug chemotherapy.
- Auto-HSCT should be performed if chemosensitivity is demonstrated and no contraindications are present.
- If patients are elderly or have comorbid conditions, the goal should be palliation.
- Radiotherapy can be used to alleviate symptoms at a particular site of involvement.

Therapy for Specific Subtypes and Clinical Presentations

Primary Testicular Lymphoma

- Represents 1 to 2 percent of all lymphomas, with an estimated incidence of 0.26 per 100,000 males per year.
- Represents the most common testicular tumor in men older than 50 years of age.
- Eighty to 90 percent of primary testicular lymphomas are DLBCL, with a mean age at diagnosis of 68 years.
- Most patients present with stage I-II with isolated involvement of the right or left testis equal in frequency.
- Six percent of testicular lymphoma cases have bilateral involvement.
- Primary testicular lymphoma tends to disseminate to several extranodal sites, including the contralateral testis, CNS, skin, Waldeyer ring, lung, pleura, and soft tissues.
- Treatment using radiation therapy alone provides suboptimal disease control, even for patients with stage I disease.

- Chemotherapy with anthracycline-containing regimens (e.g., R-CHOP) is recommended after orchiectomy.

Lymphoma during Pregnancy
- Fourth most frequent malignancy diagnosed during pregnancy, occurring in approximately 1 in 6000 deliveries.
- The risks to the fetus of treatment are greatest during the first trimester.
- Patients with supradiaphragmatic stage I disease may be considered for localized radiotherapy as a temporary measure until the second trimester, when chemotherapy holds less risk for the fetus.
- Patients close to delivery should be treated with full-dose chemotherapy as soon after pregnancy as possible.

PRIMARY MEDIASTINAL LARGE B-CELL LYMPHOMA

- Arises in the mediastinal lymphatic structures, probably from a thymic B-cell precursor.
- Variant type of DLBCL accounts for approximately 3 percent of lymphomas, and is most commonly seen in young and middle-aged adults, with about two-thirds of cases in females.

Clinical Features
- The clinical presentation is typically an anterior mediastinal mass that is locally invasive of neighboring tissues that may lead to airway obstruction and superior vena cava syndrome in approximately 40 percent of patients.
- Distant nodal involvement at presentation is more suggestive of typical DLBCL with mediastinal involvement.
- Relapses tend to be extranodal, including the liver, gastrointestinal tract, kidneys, ovaries, and CNS.
- Marrow involvement is very unusual.

Histopathologic Findings
- Primary mediastinal B-cell lymphoma and Hodgkin lymphoma share gene-expression profiles, raising questions about biologic relationships.
- Rarely, multinucleated cells may sometimes mimic Reed-Sternberg cells along with other morphologic similarities to Hodgkin lymphoma.
- Fibrotic bands may intersperse with the tumor cells, sometimes referred to as primary B-cell mediastinal lymphoma with sclerosis.
- Primary mediastinal lymphoma lacks the CD30 and CD15 antigens characteristic of Hodgkin lymphoma, and it expresses the B-cell–associated antigens CD19, CD20, CD22, and CD79a.

Treatment
- Incorporation of rituximab in dose-adjusted EPOCH resulted in 100 percent overall survival and 91 percent event-free survival, compared with 78 percent overall survival and 67 percent event-free survival observed with dose-adjusted EPOCH without rituximab.
  - Although outcomes appear to be superior for more intensive therapies over CHOP-type regimens in retrospective studies, they have not been compared in prospective randomized trials with R-CHOP.

LYMPHOMATOID GRANULOMATOSIS

- Rare lymphoproliferative disorder characterized by angiocentric and angiodestructive Epstein-Barr virus (EBV)-positive B-cell proliferation associated with extensive reactive T-cell infiltration.
  - Approximately two-thirds of cases occur in males.

— The median age of presentation is in the fifth decade of life, although pediatric cases occur.

Clinical Findings

- Most common sites of involvement are the lungs (90%). Other common sites of involvement include the skin (25–50%), kidney (30–40%), liver (29%), and the CNS (26%).
- The spleen and lymph nodes are often less involved.
- The distribution of disease leads to cough, dyspnea, and sometimes chest pain.
- Fever, weight loss, and joint pain are very frequent.
- Abdominal pain and diarrhea as a result of gastrointestinal involvement and various neurologic signs, including diplopia, ataxia, mental status changes, and others may be evident.
- Skin involvement can be morphologically diverse (e.g., ulcerations, plaques, maculopapules) but are usually accompanied by subcutaneous nodules.
- The pulmonary lesions are usually bilateral, nodules in the lower half of the lung. They may cavitate. Nodules may also be found in the brain and kidney and sometimes other locales.

Histopathologic Findings

- The grading of lymphomatoid granulomatosis relates to the proportion of EBV-positive B cells relative to the reactive lymphocytes in the background.
- Grade 1 lesions contain a polymorphous lymphoid infiltrate without cytologic atypia.
- Grade 2 lesions contain occasional large lymphoid cells or immunoblasts in a polymorphous background.

Treatment and Prognosis

- The clinical prognosis is variable in lymphomatoid granulomatosis with a median survival of 2 years.
- Poor prognostic findings include neurologic involvement and higher pathologic grade.
- Treatment consists of combination chemotherapy containing a glucocorticoid.

INTRAVASCULAR LARGE B-CELL LYMPHOMA

- A rare type of extranodal large B-cell lymphoma characterized by selective growth of lymphoma cells within the lumina of vessels, sparing the large arteries and veins.
- This tumor usually occurs in adults in the sixth and seventh decade.
- It occurs equally in men and women.
- The clinical manifestations of this lymphoma are extremely variable.
- Symptoms are related to the organs affected.
- Two types of clinical patterns have been recognized:
  — European countries: patients develop brain and skin involvement.
  — Asian countries: patients present with multiorgan failure, hepatosplenomegaly, pancytopenia, and hemophagocytic syndrome.
  — B symptoms (fever, drenching sweats, and weight loss) are common in both types.
- Skin lesions range from single to striking clusters of nodules and tumors.
  — They may be painful and appear as violaceous plaques, erythematous nodules, or tumors that may ulcerate.
  — These lesions commonly appear on the arms and legs, abdomen and breasts but may occur anywhere.
- Increased LDH levels and β_2-microglobulin levels are observed in the serum of most patients.

- Elevated erythrocyte sedimentation rate and abnormalities in hepatic, renal, and thyroid function are common.
- Tumor cells express B-cell–associated antigens and occasionally express CD5.
- Anthracycline-based chemotherapy has been used for treatment. The addition of rituximab to chemotherapy regimens has improved clinical outcomes.
  — Progression-free survival (PFS) and overall survival (OS) rates at 2 years after diagnosis were 56 and 66 percent, respectively, in the rituximab-chemotherapy group, compared with 27 and 46 percent for patients in the chemotherapy group ($p = 0.001$ for PFS and $p = 0.01$ for OS).
- For patients with CNS involvement, more intensive chemotherapy with drugs such as methotrexate and cytarabine that reach the CNS is required.

POSTTRANSPLANT LYMPHOPROLIFERATIVE DISORDERS (PTLD)

- PTLD results from lymphoid or plasmacytic proliferations that develop in the setting of immunosuppressive therapy for solid organ or marrow transplantation.
- Occurs in approximately 1 to 2 percent of solid-organ transplant recipients.
  — There is a clear association between PTLD and the type of organ transplanted.
- Cardiac-lung and intestinal transplantation have the highest incidence of PTLD.
- The highest incidence occurs in the first years of transplantation.
- The incidence of PTLD after HSCT ranges from 0.5 to 1 percent.
- The onset of posttransplant lymphoma in most patients is related to B-cell proliferation induced by infection with EBV in the setting of chronic immunosuppression.
- Involvement of the grafted organ occurs in approximately 30 percent of patients and may lead to organ damage and fatal complications.
- Management of PTLD is not uniform.
- Reduction of immunosuppression is the first step in the treatment of these patients.
- Many cases of polyclonal PTLD may resolve completely with a reduction in immunosuppressive therapy.
- Patients with late PTLD and more aggressive monoclonal PTLD are less likely to respond.
- Rituximab has shown promising results when incorporated into treatment regimens.
- The only baseline factor predicting response was a normal level of serum LDH at day 80 of treatment.
- The following sequence is generally recommended:
  — If possible, the first step is reduction in immunosuppression, followed by four weekly cycles of rituximab if reduction of the immunosuppression is ineffective.
  — If both steps are ineffective, then six cycles of R-CHOP are recommended.

T-CELL-HISTIOCYTE-RICH LARGE B-CELL LYMPHOMA

- Characterized by effacement of the architecture of the lymph node by a lymphohistiocytic infiltrate with a diffuse or vaguely nodular growth pattern.
- Accounts for less than 5 percent of all cases of DLBCL and occurs at a younger age on average.
- The median age of onset is in the fourth decade.
- A male predominance is noted.
- This subtype more often presents with advanced stage disease, and often in multiple extranodal sites, and with an elevated serum LDH.
- The lymphoma infiltrates the spleen, liver, and marrow with greater frequency than does DLBCL.

- Marrow involvement occurs in approximately one-third of the cases, a frequency considerably higher than in DLBCL and patients are more likely to develop "B" symptoms than patients with DLBCL.
- When treated with CHOP-like regimens, most series suggest that the outcome for these patients is similar to patients with typical DLBCL.
- Six cycles of R-CHOP for advanced disease would be a reasonable initial approach to therapy.

PRIMARY CUTANEOUS DLBCL, LEG TYPE

- Composed solely of large transformed B cells with a predilection for the skin of the leg.
- Primary cutaneous DLBCL, leg type constitutes approximately 4 percent of all primary cutaneous B-cell lymphomas.
- The median age at the time of presentation is 60 to 70 years.
- Lymphomatous tumors affect the skin of the legs in most cases, but approximately 10 percent arise at other sites.
- The B cells are usually positive for CD20 and usually express *BCL2* and *FOX-P1*.
- Lymphoma cells often find translocations involving *MYC*, *BCL6*, or *IGH* genes.
- The gene-expression profile of these lymphoma cells is often the same as activated B-cell like DLBCL.
- Anthracycline-containing chemotherapy with rituximab should be considered as initial therapy. The incorporation of rituximab improves the response rates and overall survival.

ANAPLASTIC LYMPHOMA KINASE-POSITIVE LARGE B-CELL LYMPHOMA

- An uncommon neoplasm of large immunoblast-like B cells that stain for nuclear and or cytoplasmic anaplastic lymphoma kinase (ALK) protein.
- The lymphoma cells may undergo plasmablastic differentiation.
- The average age of presentation is in the fourth decade with a male predilection.
- Most patients present with advanced stage disease.
- The most common affected nodal areas are in the neck and mediastinum.
- Common extranodal involvement include the liver, spleen, bone, and gastrointestinal tract.
- The lymphoma cells are large immunoblasts with a large central nucleolus.
- The lymphoma cells stain for the ALK protein, usually with a granular cytoplasmic appearance but nuclear staining may also occur. These cells are usually CD3, CD20, CD30, CD79a negative.
- Occasional cases may have a t(2;17)(p23;q23) that results in a clathrin-ALK fusion protein.
- The clinical course of ALK-positive large B-cell lymphoma is aggressive with a median survival time of 24 months.
- Tumors are usually all negative for CD20, making the utility of rituximab uncertain.

 For a more detailed discussion, see Michael Boyiadzis and Kenneth A. Foon: Diffuse Large B-Cell Lymphoma. Chap. 100, p. 1547 in *Williams Hematology*, 8th ed.

CHAPTER 62
Follicular Lymphomas

- Follicular lymphoma (FL) is an indolent lymphoid neoplasm that is derived from mutated germinal center B cells and exhibits a nodular or follicular histologic pattern. It is typically composed of a mixture of small, cleaved follicle center cells referred to as centrocytes and large noncleaved follicular center cells referred to as centroblasts. The disease has masqueraded under multiple previous monikers, including "nodular lymphoma" in the Rappaport classification and "follicle center cell lymphoma" in the Working Formulation.
- FL accounts for approximately 20 to 25 percent of adult non-Hodgkin lymphomas (NHL) in the United States, with an annual incidence of approximately 14,000 new cases per year.
- The disease is uncommon in persons younger than age 20 years, and pediatric cases appear to represent a separate disease entity that is typically localized, lacks the translocation 14;18 and BCL-2 expression, and has a very good prognosis.

CLINICAL FEATURES

Symptoms and Signs
- Patients with FL usually present with painless diffuse lymphadenopathy.
- Less frequently, patients may have vague abdominal complaints, including pain, early satiety, and increasing girth, which are caused by a large abdominal mass.
- Approximately 10 percent of patients present with B symptoms (fever, drenching night sweats, or loss of 10% of their body weight).

Staging the Disease
- Evaluation involves performance of a medical history, physical examination (with attention to the lymph nodes in Waldeyer ring and size and involvement of liver and spleen); laboratory testing (including a complete blood count, examination of the blood film and a differential white cell count, lactic acid dehydrogenase [LDH], β_2-microglobulin, comprehensive metabolic panel, serum uric acid level); lymph node biopsy; marrow aspiration and biopsy; flow cytometric analysis of blood, marrow, and lymph node cells; and computed tomography (CT) of the chest, abdomen, and pelvis.
- Excisional lymph node biopsies are strongly preferred for the initial histologic diagnosis, although in cases in which nodal masses are inaccessible, generous needle core biopsies may suffice.
- The diagnosis should not be established solely on the basis of flow cytometry of the blood or marrow, or on cytologic examination of aspiration needle biopsies of lymph node or other tissue.
- In selected circumstances, additional CT scans of the neck, positron emission tomography (PET)/CT imaging, measurement of the cardiac ejection fraction, serum protein electrophoresis, quantitative immunoglobulins, and hepatitis C testing may be useful.

LABORATORY FEATURES

Lymph Node Morphology
- Exhibits a predominantly nodular lymph node pattern; however, the neoplastic follicles are distorted and as the disease progresses, the malignant follicles efface the nodal architecture.

- The World Health Organization has developed a three grade classification system according to the proportion of centroblasts detected microscopically.
- Nearly all authorities now agree, however, that grade 3B FL behaves aggressively and should be treated with anthracycline-containing regimens (e.g., rituximab, cyclophosphamide, doxorubicin, vincristine, prednisone [R-CHOP]) similar to diffuse large B-cell lymphoma.

Cytogenetics

- The classic cytogenetic finding is the t(14;18)(q32;q21) translocation that juxtaposes the *BCL-2* gene on band q21 of chromosome 18 with the immunoglobulin (Ig) heavy-chain gene on band 32 of chromosome 14 . This alteration occurs in 85 to 90 percent of cases and virtually all cases with a grade 1 histopathology (> 95% centrocytes).
- The Ig enhancer element results in amplified expression of the translocated gene product and, thus, overexpression of BCL-2 protein leading to inhibition of apoptosis of affected B cells.
- However, detection of the t(14;18) translocation in lymphoid cells is neither necessary nor sufficient for the diagnosis of FL.
- Additional cytogenetics abnormalities are found in 90 percent of patients, most commonly, loss of 1p, 6q, 10q, and 17p, and gains of 1, 6p, 7, 8, 12q, X, and 18q/dup.

PROGNOSTIC FACTORS

Clinical and Laboratory Values

- There are five adverse prognostic factors: age (>60 years vs. ≤60 years), Ann Arbor stage (III–IV vs. I–II), hemoglobin level (<120 g/L vs. ≥120 g/L), number of nodal areas (>4 vs. ≤, and serum LDH level (high vs. normal).
- Three risk groups are defined: low risk (0–1 adverse factors, 36% of patients), intermediate risk (2 factors, 37% of patients, hazard ratio [HR] of 2.3), and poor risk (≥ 3 adverse factors, 27% of patients, HR = 4.3). See **Fig. 62–1** for outcomes following chemotherapy with and without rituximab.

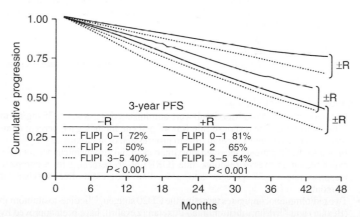

FIGURE 62-1 Progression-free survival of 827 patients with FL stratified by the Follicular Lymphoma International Prognostic Index (FLIPI) into low risk (0–1 risk factors, 40% of patients, *black lines*), intermediate risk (2 risk factors, 33% of patients, *blue lines*), or high risk (3–5 risk factors, 27% of patients, *red lines*). Of the 827 patients, 267 were treated with chemotherapy regimens without rituximab (*dotted lines*) and 560 were treated with rituximab-containing regimens (*solid lines*). (*Reproduced with permission from Federico M, Bellei M, Pro B, et al: J Clin Oncol June 20;25(185):8008, 2007.*)

(Source: *Williams Hematology,* 8th ed, Chap. 101, Fig. 101–3, p.1567.)

Gene Expression Profiling

- Two gene-expression signatures allow construction of a survival predictor that enables segregation of patients into four quartiles with disparate median lengths of survival (13.6, 11.1, 10.8, and 3.9 years), independent of clinical prognostic variables.
- One signature (immune-response 1) is associated with a good prognosis and includes genes encoding T-cell markers (e.g., *CD7*, *CD8B1*, *ITK*, *LEF1*, and *STAT4*) as well as genes that are highly expressed in macrophages (e.g., *ACTN1* and *TNFSF13B*).
- The immune-response-2 signature is associated with a poor prognosis and includes genes preferentially expressed in macrophages, dendritic cells, or both (e.g., *TLR5*, *FCGR1A*, *SEPT10*, *LGMN*, and *C3AR1*).

THERAPY

Radiotherapy

- Patients with stage I or II FL represent only 10 to 30 percent of all cases in most series.
- Standard management for stage I or limited contiguous stage II disease involves the administration of involved field radiotherapy (35 to 40 Gy).
- Adjuvant chemotherapy does not appear to improve survival in this setting.

Observation (Watch and Wait)

- Excellent survival has also been observed in patients with early stage disease who received no initial therapy.
- In a group of 43 selected patients, 56 percent were free from the requirement for treatment for at least 10 years and 86 percent were alive 10 years after diagnosis.
- Based on this study, many authorities have concluded that "watchful waiting" is an acceptable alternative to radiotherapy for stage I or II FL.
- Because there is no conclusive evidence that survival of FL patients is improved by immediate institution of therapy, or that conventional management (other than allogeneic hematopoietic stem cell transplantation) can cure the disease, a "watch-and wait" approach is also recommended for patients with extensive stage II or stage III or IV FL.

Single Agent Chemotherapy

- Patients can be palliated effectively with a variety of single chemotherapy agents (Table 62–1).

Monoclonal Antibody Therapy

- Four weekly infusions of rituximab were administered at a dose of 375 mg/m^2 to patients with FL. The response rate was 48 percent, including a 6 percent complete response rate and a median time to progression of approximately 1 year.
- In one study, 38 patients received rituximab as initial and maintenance therapy, experiencing an overall response rate (ORR) of 76 percent, with a complete response rate of 37 percent and a median progression-free survival of 34 months.
- Two radioimmunoconjugates targeting the CD20 antigen, [131]iodine-tositumomab (Bexxar) and [90]yttrium-ibritumomab tiuxetan (Zevalin), have been approved by the U.S. Food and Drug Administration for relapsed, refractory, and transformed indolent lymphomas.
- In a randomized study comparing treatment of patients with relapsed FL with either ^{90}Y-ibritumomab tiuxetan or rituximab, the ORR (86 vs. 55%) and the complete response (CR) rate (30 vs. 15%) were both statistically superior in the group treated with the radioimmunoconjugate. Similarly, ^{131}I-tositumomab was compared with unlabeled tositumomab in a randomized trial of relapsed

TABLE 62–1	THERAPEUTIC REGIMENS FOR FOLLICULAR LYMPHOMA

Agent(s)	Dose	Route	Day(s) of Treatment	Repeat Cycle at Day
Single agents				
Chlorambucil	0.08–0.12 mg/kg	PO	Daily	
	or 0.4–1.0 mg/kg	PO	1	28
Cyclophosphamide	50–100 mg/m^2	PO	Daily	
	or 300 mg/m^2	PO	1–5	28
Fludarabine	25 mg/m^2/day	IV	1–5	28
Pentostatin	4 mg/m^2	IV	1	14
Cladribine	0.1 mg/kg/day	IV (continuous)	1–7	28
	or 0.14 mg/kg/day	IV (2 h)	1–5	28
Bendamustine	100–120 mg/ m^2/day	IV	1, 2	21 or 28
Rituximab	375 mg/m^2/day	IV	1, 8, 15, 22	
Combination therapy				
Stanford CVP				
Cyclophosphamide	400 mg/m^2	PO	1–5	21
Vincristine	1.4 mg/m^2 (maximum 2 mg)	IV	1	21
Prednisone	100 mg/m^2	PO	1–5	21
R-CVP				
Rituximab	375 mg/m^2	IV	1	21
Cyclophosphamide	1000 mg/m^2	IV	1	21
Vincristine	1.4 mg/m^2 (maximum 2 mg)	IV	1	21
Prednisone	100 mg	PO	1–5	21
R-CHOP				
Rituximab	375 mg/m^2	IV	1	21
Cyclophosphamide	750 mg/m^2	IV	1	21
Doxorubicin	50 mg/m^2	IV	1	
Vincristine	1.4 mg/m^2	IV	1	
Prednisone	100 mg	PO	1–5	
FND				
Fludarabine	25 mg/m^2	IV	1–3	28
Mitoxantrone	10 mg/m^2	IV	1	
Dexamethasone	20 mg	IV or PO	1–5	
CF				
Cyclophosphamide	600–1000 mg/m^2	IV	1	
Fludarabine	20 mg/m^2	IV	1–5	21–28

Source: *Williams Hematology*, 8th ed, Chap. 101, Table 101–1, p. 1568.

indolent lymphoma and both the ORR (55 vs. 19% and the CR rate (33 vs. 8%) were higher in patients receiving the radiolabeled antibody.

- The major toxicity of radioimmunotherapy is delayed myelosuppression. Growth factor administration and transfusions are required in approximately 20 percent of patients. A potential long-term concern with both radiolabeled antibody formulations is the potential development of myelodysplasia and acute leukemia as late complications. Hypothyroidism may also occur as a delayed toxicity of ^{131}I-labeled tositumomab in approximately 10 percent of patients.

Combination Chemotherapy

- In one study, induction therapy consisting of eight cycles of rituximab/cyclophosphamide/vincristine/prednisone (R-CVP) was compared with eight cycles of CVP without rituximab in 321 patients with newly diagnosed disease. R-CVP was superior to CVP alone in terms of ORR (81 vs. 57%), CR rate (41 vs. 10%), time to progression (32 months vs. 15 months), time to treatment failure (27 months vs. 7 months), and overall survival (OS; 83 vs. 77% at 4 years, p = 0.029).
- Similarly, R-CHOP was compared with CHOP for first-line treatment of 428 patients with advanced stage FL. R-CHOP exhibited a superior ORR (96 vs. 90%), time to treatment failure (p < 0.001), duration of response (p = 0.001), and OS (p = 0.016) compared with CHOP alone.

Hematopoietic Stem Cell Transplantation

- The role of high-dose chemoradiotherapy and allogeneic hematopoietic stem cell transplantation in the management of patients remains highly controversial.
- A randomized trial of 89 patients with relapsed disease showed that transplanted patients experience a marginal OS advantage compared with patients randomized to continued conventional salvage chemotherapy without transplantation. When used as part of initial therapy for high-risk patients, randomized studies demonstrate no improvement in OS.
- Adverse outcomes associated with autologous hematopoietic stem cell transplantation include treatment-related mortality (3–5%) and a substantial increase in the incidence of secondary myelodysplasia and acute myelogenous leukemia, occurring in 7 to 19 percent.
- Although allogeneic hematopoietic transplantation affords long-term progression free survival for approximately 40 to 50 percent of patients with relapsed disease, transplant-related mortality rates range from 20 to 40 percent because of the usual advanced age of patients.

For a more detailed discussion, see Oliver W. Press: Follicular Lymphoma. Chap. 101, p. 1565 in *Williams Hematology*, 8th ed.

CHAPTER 63
Mantle Cell Lymphomas

- Mantle cell lymphoma (MCL) cells display an immunophenotype similar to lymphocytes in the mantle zone of normal germinal follicles, surface immuno-globulin (sIg) M+, sIgD+, CD5+, CD20+, CD10–, CD43+. In contrast to chronic lymphocytic leukemia (CLL) or small lymphocytic lymphoma (SLL), MCL cells typically do not express CD23.
- MCL had been previously classified as an intermediate-grade lymphoma and called "intermediate lymphocytic lymphoma." It also had been termed *centro-cytic lymphoma* and previously confused with other types of lymphoma or leu-kemia, such as SLL, CLL, or marginal zone lymphoma.

PATHOPHYSIOLOGY

- Insight into the pathophysiology of MCL was realized with discovery of the cytogenetic abnormality t(11;14) (q13;q32) in the tumor cells, a translocation resulting in the over expression of the cell cycle regulator cyclin D1.
- However, it is almost certain that additional genetic events are involved in devel-opment of the fully transformed state as low numbers of cells carrying the t(11;14) translocation have been found in the blood of some healthy individuals without any evidence of disease.
- The *ATM* (ataxia-telangiectasia mutant) gene is mutated in approximately 40 percent of patients. *ATM* inactivation facilitates genomic instability in lym-phoma cells through impaired response to DNA damage.
- Additional genetic anomalies that could contribute to the disease include losses in chromosomes 1p13-p31, 2q13, 6q23-27, 8p21, 9p21, 10p14-15, 11q22-23, 13q11-13, 13q14-34, 17p13, and 22q12; gains in chromosomes 3q25, 4p12-13, 7p21-22, 8q21, 9q22, 10p11-12, 12q13, and 18q11q23; and high copy-number amplifications of certain chromosomal regions.

CLINICAL FEATURES

- The typical presentation is that of an older patient with lymphadenopathy in sev-eral sites (e.g., cervical, axillary, inguinal).
- The patient may be asymptomatic but a significant proportion may have fever, night sweats, or weight loss.
- The liver may be enlarged and the spleen is enlarged in 40 percent of patients at the time of diagnosis. In 25 percent of the cases, there is symptomatic gastroin-testinal involvement.
- A number of adverse prognostic features of MCL have been identified, includ-ing the expression of the Ki67 proliferation antigen in a high proportion of lym-phoma cells, high serum level of β_2-microglobulin in the absence of renal dys-function, high serum levels of lactic acid dehydrogenase (LDH), presence of blastoid cytology, advanced patient age, late Ann Arbor stage, extranodal pre-sentation, constitutional symptoms, among others.
- A prognostic model called the Mantle Cell International Prognostic Index (MIPI) has been introduced, which uses four independent prognostic factors: age, performance status, LDH, and leukocyte count.
- There is no consensus on the risk of central nervous system (CNS) disease in patients with MCL or the need to give CNS prophylaxis. Studies have reported an incidence of CNS of 4 percent and a 5-year actuarial risk of 26 percent.

LABORATORY FEATURES

- Approximately 50 percent of patients present with blood and marrow involvement, sometimes with an overt leukemic phase, but more often with subtle involvement as detection of the malignant lymphocyte immunophenotype by flow cytometry of blood or marrow cells.
- Almost all cases of MCL show overexpression of cyclin D1 mRNA. The rare cases that are negative for cyclin D1 usually overexpress cyclin D2 or D3.
- MCL cells stain strongly for the antiapoptotic molecule BCL-2 and are negative for the germinal center markers CD10 and BCL-6.

DIAGNOSIS

- The immunophenotype of MCL has some similarities to that of CLL or SLL.
- In contrast to CLL or SLL, MCL cells react strongly with FMC7, a weak anti-CD20 mAb, and typically do not express CD23.
- All cases of MCL express cyclin D1, typically at levels that are much higher than that of other lymphomas.

THERAPY

- MCL is currently considered incurable but long-term remissions occur depending on the Mantle Cell International Prognostic Index (Fig. 63–1).

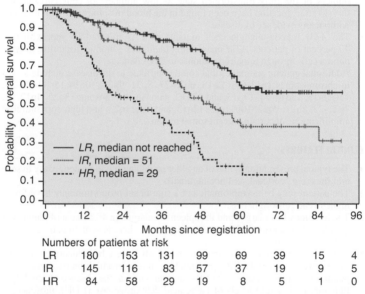

FIGURE 63-1 Overall survival according to the Mantle Cell International Prognostic Index (MIPI). *LR* indicates low risk, prognostic score less than 5.7; *IR* indicates intermediate risk, prognostic score 5.7 or more but less than 6.2; and *HR* indicates high risk, prognostic score 6.2 or more. The prognostic score is calculated as $[0.03535 \times \text{age (years)}] + 0.6978$ (if ECOG >1) + $[1.367 \times \log_{10}(\text{LDH/ULN})] + [0.9393 \times \log_{10}(\text{WBC count})]$. ECOG, Eastern Cooperative Oncology Group performance status score; LDH, lactic acid dehydrogenase; ULN, upper limits of normal; WBC, white blood cell. (Reproduced with permission from Hoster E, Dreyling M, Klapper W, et al: *Blood* Jan 15;111(2):558-565, 2008.)

(Source: *Williams Hematology*, 8th ed, Chap. 102, Fig. 102–3, p. 1580.)

- Localized disease is rare. Because of the presence of advanced disease at presentation, most patients require systemic therapy.
- MCL is responsive to doxorubicin-containing chemotherapy, but the complete remission rates are approximately 35 percent, the duration of response is 10 to 12 months, and the median survival 3 to 4 years, all of which are lower when compared with other lymphoma subtypes.
- Fludarabine has been tested in a small number of untreated MCL patients and has achieved an overall response rate of approximately 40 percent with a complete remission rate of approximately 30 percent. The median overall survival (OS) in this study was 2 years.
- The anti-CD20 monoclonal antibody rituximab is the most important recent addition to the therapy of lymphomas, including MCL. Rituximab alone produces an approximate 40 percent response in patients with untreated MCL. However, the lymphoma cells of some patients can lose expression of CD20 after repeated therapy.
- In patients with blood involvement, the first dose of rituximab should be infused slowly and with close monitoring during initial therapy because of the risk of tumor lysis syndrome or cytokine-release syndrome.
- Several studies suggest that cytarabine adds significantly to the response, as demonstrated by the difference in response between patients treated with essentially similar chemotherapeutic regimens without cytarabine (e.g., cyclophosphamide/adriamycin/vincristine/prednisone (CHOP) vs. dexamethasone/high-dose cytosine arabinoside/cisplatin (DHAP).
- Based on all these findings, chemotherapy for MCL is characterized by increasingly intensive combinations of therapy, including CHOP-R (plus rituximab), EPOCH-R, R modified hyper CVAD, and several others, with and without autologous hematopoietic stem cell transplantation as consolidation.
- The inherent resistance of MCL to conventional doses of chemotherapy is evident at relapse. Among the studied salvage therapies, the proteasome inhibitor bortezomib has shown a 31 percent response rate as single-agent therapy. Temsirolimus is a promising mTOR inhibitor that has also shown a 38 percent overall response rate in relapsed MCL. Lenalidomide has shown a 53 percent overall response rate with 13 percent complete remissions.
- Based on the radiation sensitivity of MCL, radioimmunoconjugates of anti-CD20 antibodies have shown substantial response rates in patients given the agents as initial therapy and in those with relapsed disease. However, such therapy should be considered primarily for patients who do not have extensive marrow involvement (e.g., < 15%) to avoid excessive myelotoxicity.
- A reduced intensity allograft can achieve progression free survival and event-free survival rates of 40 to 80 percent and overall survival rates of 55 to 86 percent after a median follow-up of 2 to 3 years, with 5 to 30 percent acute graft-versus-host disease and 0 to 24 percent treatment-related mortality. Some experts believe that hematopoietic stem cell transplantation offers the best option for long-term remission in this disease.

For a more detailed discussion, see Jorge E. Romaguera and Peter W. McLaughlin: Mantle Cell Lymphoma. Chap. 102, p. 1575 in *Williams Hematology*, 8th ed.

CHAPTER 64
Marginal Zone B-Cell Lymphoma

- The marginal zone lymphomas (MZLs) are derived from memory-type or antigen-experienced B cells that reside in regions contiguous to the outer part of the mantle zones of B-cell follicles.
- The World Health Organization (WHO) defines three separate MZL entities, namely, the extranodal marginal zone B-cell lymphoma of mucosa-associated lymphoid tissue (currently known as MALT lymphoma), the nodal marginal zone B-cell lymphoma (previously termed *monocytoid lymphoma*), and the splenic marginal zone B-cell lymphoma (with or without circulating villous lymphocytes).
- Gastric MALT lymphoma is one of the best examples of a microbiologic (*Helicobacter pylori*) cause of a human malignancy.

PATHOPHYSIOLOGY

- MALT lymphomas arise from mucosa-associated lymphoid tissues in the context of chronic inflammation.
- Other bacterial infections are possibly implicated in the pathogenesis of MZLs arising in the skin (*Borrelia burgdorferi*), in the ocular adnexa (*Chlamydophila psittaci*), and in the small intestine (*Campylobacter jejuni*).
- Hepatitis C virus (HCV) appears involved in the pathogenesis of splenic MZL through antigen-driven stimulation of the lymphoma clone.
- There is, however, a great and incompletely explained geographic variation in the strength of these associations.
- An increased risk of developing MALT lymphoma has been also reported in individuals affected by autoimmune disorders, especially Sjögren syndrome and systemic lupus erythematosus.
- Several recurrent chromosomal translocations have been described in extranodal MZLs. Three of them [t(11;18)(q21;q21), t(1;14)(p22;q32), and t(14;18) (q32;q21)] are the most characterized, and, interestingly, they all appear to affect the same signaling pathway, activating nuclear factor-kappa B (NF-κB), a transcription factor that plays a major role in immunity, inflammation, and apoptosis.

CLINICAL FEATURES

- The most common site of MALT lymphoma is the stomach, encompassing at least one-third of all cases.
- Extranodal MZLs may also arise at many other sites, including the salivary gland, the thyroid, the upper airways, the lung, the ocular adnexa (lacrimal gland, conjunctiva, eyelid, orbital soft tissue), the breast, the liver, the urogenital system, the skin and other soft tissues, and even the dura.
- As a general rule, the presenting symptoms of extranodal MZLs are related to the primary location.
- Elevated serum lactic acid dehydrogenase (LDH) or serum β_2-microglobulin levels, as well as constitutional B symptoms, are extremely rare at presentation.
- MALT lymphoma can remain localized for a prolonged period within the tissue of origin, but regional lymph nodes can sometimes be infiltrated and dissemination at multiple sites is not uncommon, occurring in up to one-fourth of cases.

DIAGNOSIS

- The presence *H. pylori* must be determined by histochemistry or, alternatively, urea breath test.
- The B cells of MZLs show the immunophenotype of the normal marginal zone B cells present in spleen, Peyer patches, and in lymph nodes. Therefore, the tumor B cells express surface immunoglobulins and pan-B antigens (CD19, CD20, and CD79a), express the marginal zone-associated antigens CD35 and CD21, and lack expression of CD5, CD10, CD23, or high-level expression of cyclin D1.
- The tumor cells of extranodal MZL typically express immunoglobulin (Ig) M, less often IgA, or IgG, whereas splenic zone lymphoma is typically IgD-positive.
- In addition to routine histology and immunohistochemistry, fluorescence *in situ* hybridization analysis or use of polymerase chain reaction for detection of t(11;18) may be useful for identifying patients who are unlikely to respond to antibiotic therapy for *H. pylori*.
- The very rare splenic MZL comprises less than 1 percent of all lymphomas. More than half of the cases present circulating villous lymphocytes with characteristic fine, short cytoplasm polar projections. When these are more than 20 percent of the lymphocyte count, the term *splenic lymphoma with villous lymphocytes* is commonly used.

STAGING

- The initial staging procedures should include a gastroduodenal endoscopy with multiple biopsies taken from each region of the stomach, duodenum, gastroesophageal junction, and from any abnormal-appearing site.
- Endoscopic ultrasound is recommended to evaluate the regional lymph nodes and gastric wall infiltration.
- Other recommended laboratory and radiologic studies include measurement of serum LDH and β_2-microglobulin; computed tomography of the chest, abdomen, and pelvis; and marrow aspirate and biopsy (see Table 64–1).
- Multiorgan involvement is not uncommon and complete staging procedures are recommended for patients with non-gastric mantle zone B-cell lymphoma.

THERAPY

- Eradication of *H. pylori* with antibiotics plus proton-pump inhibitor regimens should be the sole initial treatment of localized (i.e., confined to the stomach) *H. pylori*-positive gastric MALT lymphoma. *H. pylori* eradication results in complete regression of gastric MALT lymphoma in approximately 50 to 75 percent of cases.
- Histologic evaluation of repeat biopsies remains an essential follow-up procedure, with multiple biopsies taken 2 to 3 months after treatment to document that the lymphoma is not progressing and that *H. pylori* eradication has been achieved.
- Treatment of *H. pylori* is based on triple or quadruple therapy, including a proton-pump inhibitor, clarithromycin and amoxicillin or metronidazole for 14 days, or a proton-pump inhibitor, metronidazole, tetracycline, and bismuth subcitrate for 14 days (Table 64–2).
- Patients who do not respond or have only a partial response to antibiotic therapy should be considered for surgery or radiotherapy.
- Because gastric MALT lymphoma is multifocal, the surgical procedure is a total gastrectomy with its associated complications.Surgery has not been shown to achieve superior results in comparison with organ-preserving strategies.
- On the contrary, excellent disease control can be achieved with involved field radiotherapy alone for stages I and II MALT lymphoma of the stomach without evidence of *H. pylori* infection or with persistent lymphoma after antibiotic eradication.

TABLE 64–1	RECOMMENDED MINIMUM STAGING PROCEDURES FOR EXTRANODAL MARGINAL ZONE LYMPHOMA

- History (duration and presence of local or systemic symptoms)
- Physical examination (careful evaluation of all lymph node regions, inspection of the upper airways and tonsils, clinical evaluation of the size of liver and spleen, detection of any palpable mass)
- Laboratory tests, including complete blood cell counts and examination of a blood film, lactic acid dehydrogenase, evaluation of renal and liver function
- Standard posteroanterior and lateral chest radiographs
- Abdominal and pelvic computed tomography
- Search for *Helicobacter pylori* infection (biopsy histology or breath test) is needed in gastric lymphoma. Other chronic infections that may have a pathogenetic role should also be investigated when lymphoma presents at certain sites (i.e., *Borrelia burgdorferi* in cutaneous localizations, *Chlamydophila psittaci* in the ocular adnexa, and *Campylobacter jejuni* in the small bowel).
- Marrow biopsy
- Additional investigations may include:
  1. *For gastric lymphoma:* gastroduodenal endoscopy with multiple gastric biopsies from all the visible lesions and the noninvolved areas and gastric endoscopic ultrasound
  2. *For intestinal presentation:* esophagogastroduodenoscopy, small-bowel studies and colonoscopy
  3. *For pulmonary lesions:* bronchoscopy and bronchoalveolar lavage

Source: *Williams Hematology,* 8th ed, Chap. 103, Table 103–1, p. 1585.

TABLE 64–2	STANDARD ANTI-*HELICOBACTER* TREATMENTS BASED ON CONSENSUS GUIDELINES

Triple therapy
- Proton-pump inhibitor (standard dose, twice daily)
- Clarithromycin (500 mg twice daily)
- Amoxicillin (1000 mg twice daily) or metronidazole (500 mg twice daily) for 14 days

Quadruple therapy
- Proton-pump inhibitor (standard dose twice daily)
- Metronidazole (500 mg three times daily)
- Tetracycline (500 mg four times daily)
- Bismuth subcitrate (120 mg four times daily for 14 days)

Quadruple therapy is an alternative first choice treatment in areas with a high prevalence (>15–20%) of clarithromycin resistance, or in patients who have previously received a macrolide antibiotic. Bismuth-containing quadruple therapy is the best second-choice treatment. Proton-pump inhibitor plus amoxicillin or tetracycline and metronidazole are recommended if bismuth is not available.
Source: *Williams Hematology,* 8th ed, Chap. 103, Table 103–2, p. 1585.

- The optimal management of nongastric disease is not clearly established and should be "patient-tailored," taking into account the site, the stage, and the clinical characteristics of the individual patient.
- In general, the treatment used for *H. pylori*-negative cases can be applied to nongastric MALT lymphoma. Radiation therapy is considered the treatment of choice for localized lesions. MALT lymphomas at different sites have been successfully eradicated with involved field radiation therapy encompassing the involved organ alone with doses of approximately 30 to 36 Gy.
- Patients with systemic disease should be considered for systemic chemotherapy and/or immunotherapy with anti-CD20 monoclonal antibodies.
- Patients with splenic marginal zone lymphoma usually have widespread disease. Nevertheless, a watch and wait approach is probably sufficient following splenectomy since most patients display an indolent course.

For a more detailed discussion, see Emanuele Zucca: Marginal Zone B-cell Lymphomas. Chap. 103, p. 1583 in *Williams Hematology*, 8th ed.

CHAPTER 65
Burkitt Lymphoma

- Burkitt lymphoma (BL) may present in three distinct forms: endemic (African), sporadic, and immunodeficiency-associated.
- Evidence for involvement of the c-*MYC* gene came from studies on the recurrent translocations in BL involving the long arm of chromosome 8, which involved the c-*MYC* locus.

EPIDEMIOLOGY

- The endemic form is found in eastern equatorial Africa, with a peak age incidence at 4 to 7 years, and is nearly twice as frequent in boys as in girls.
- Sporadic BL, defined as cases outside of endemic African regions, accounts for 1 to 2 percent of all patients with non-Hodgkin lymphoma (NHL).
- The incidence is higher in males than in females, and the median age of onset is 30 years.
- Immunosuppression-related Burkitt lymphoma increased in incidence during the AIDS epidemic.

PATHOPHYSIOLOGY

- The unifying feature of all three types of BL is activation of the c-*MYC* gene, typically resulting from translocations involving the long arm of chromosome 8, which carries c-*MYC*. Such translocations commonly involve also the long arm of chromosome 14, which carries the immunoglobulin heavy chain gene complex, but might instead involve chromosome 2 or 22, which carries the immunoglobulin kappa or lambda light chain gene complex, respectively. The constitutive activation of c-*MYC* increases the expression of a number of genes encoding proteins involved in cell proliferation.
- Translocations are thought to occur via double-strand breaks that occur during the normal B-cell class-switch reaction and somatic hypermutation.
- A distinctive feature of BL is the translocations involving the long arm of chromosome 8 and chromosomes 14, 2, or 22. Up to one-third of cases also might have alterations involving the short arm of chromosome 17 at 17p13.1, involving the *TP53* gene encoding p53. Loss of p53 function might be selected in BL cells that otherwise would be induced to undergo apoptosis in response to overexpression of c-*MYC*.
- The incidence of Epstein-Barr virus (EBV) positivity in the various forms of BL: it is found in essentially all patients with African BL, 30 to 40 percent of patients with immunosuppression associated BL, and in 20 percent of patients with nonendemic form of disease.

CLINICAL FEATURES

- The endemic (African) form often presents as a jaw or facial bone tumor. It may spread to extranodal sites, especially to the marrow and meninges. Almost all cases are EBV positive.
- The nonendemic or American form presents as an abdominal mass in approximately 65 percent of cases, often with ascites. Extranodal sites, such as the kidneys, gonads, breast, marrow, and central nervous system (CNS) may be involved. Involvement of the marrow and CNS is much more common in the nonendemic form.

- Tumor lysis syndrome is very common following induction chemotherapy but also can occur spontaneously prior to therapy, especially in patients with a high tumor burden. Spontaneous tumor lysis is a poor prognostic indicator.
- The syndrome results in some or all of the following: hyperuricemia and hyperuricosuria, hyperkalemia, hyperphosphatemia, hypocalcemia, metabolic acidosis, and uric acid nephropathy with renal failure.

LABORATORY FEATURES

- Patients with bulky disease may have Burkitt cells in marrow and blood with accompanying suppression of normal blood counts.
- Rare cases, often males, may present principally with marrow and blood involvement, so-called Burkitt cell leukemia.
- The serum lactic acid dehydrogenase is often elevated as a reflection of the high cell turnover, especially in patients with bulky disease.
- BL cells are mature B cells that typically express CD19, CD20, CD22, CD79a, and surface IgM. BL cells lack expression of CD5 or CD23.

DIAGNOSIS

- All cases of BL have a translocation between the long arm of chromosome 8, the site of the c-*MYC* protooncogene (8q24), and one of three translocation partners: the Ig heavy-chain region on chromosome 14; the κ light-chain locus on chromosome 2; or the λ light-chain locus on chromosome 22.
- The translocations involving *c-MYC* can be detected by fluorescence *in situ* hybridization (FISH).

STAGING

- Although virtually all lymphoma is staged with a uniform set of parameters, staging in BL employs a very distinct system (Table 65–1).

THERAPY

- BL is a highly aggressive tumor; however, therapy with multi-agent chemotherapeutic programs results in excellent long-term remission rates and long-term survival of up to 85 percent of children.

TABLE 65–1   MURPHY STAGING SYSTEM FOR BURKITT LYMPHOMA

Stage I: Single nodal or extranodal site excluding mediastinum or abdomen
Stage II: Single extranodal tumor with regional nodal involvement
    Two extranodal tumors on one side of diaphragm
    Primary gastrointestinal tumor with or without associated mesenteric nodes
    Two or more nodal areas on one side of diaphragm
Stage IIR: Completely resected intraabdominal disease
Stage III: Two single extranodal tumors on opposite sides of diaphragm
    All primary intrathoracic tumors
    All paraspinal or epidural tumors
    All extensive primary intraabdominal disease
    Two or more nodal areas on opposite sides of diaphragm
Stage IIIA: Localized, nonresectable abdominal disease
Stage IIIB: Widespread multiorgan abdominal disease
Stage IV: Initial CNS or marrow involvement (< 25%)

Adapted with permission from Perkins AS, Friedberg JW: *Hematology Am Soc Hematol Educ Program* 341–348, 2008.
Source: *Williams Hematology,* 8th ed, Chap. 104, Table 104–1, p. 1590.

- Risk stratification allows patients with limited disease to be treated with less intensive therapy than more advanced cases and still achieve very high responses.
- The specific regimens that have been developed to treat BL are generally adapted from pediatric experience.
- There are no studies directly comparing regimens, with most employing cyclophosphamide, doxorubicin, vincristine, methotrexate, ifosfamide, etoposide, high-dose cytarabine, rituximab, but always with intrathecal chemotherapy.
- In general, shorter durations of chemotherapy (i.e., 6 months) are as good as longer (18 months) periods of treatment.
- BL has a high proliferative rate, so subsequent chemotherapy cycles should be started as soon as hematologic recovery occurs. Waiting for a fixed period between cycles may lead to regrowth of resistant tumor cells between cycles.
- Given the high proliferative rate of the tumor, and the effect of chemotherapy, upfront treatment for tumor lysis syndrome should occur, especially in patients with a high lactic acid dehydrogenase level or bulky disease. Carefully monitored hydration (~3 liters of saline per day), allopurinol or rasburicase, the latter especially useful in high risk or spontaneous cases because of rapid onset of action. Continuous venovenous hemofiltration has been very useful in permitting concomitant full-dose chemotherapy, while preventing lysis syndrome and renal failure.
- In the highly active antiretroviral therapy (HAART) era, HIV-positive patients with BL should be treated similarly to immunocompetent patients.

 For a more detailed discussion, see Jonathan W. Friedberg and Archibald S. Perkins: Burkitt Lymphoma. Chap. 104, p. 1589 in *Williams Hematology,* 8th ed.

CHAPTER 66
Cutaneous T-Cell Lymphoma (Mycosis Fungoides and Sézary Syndrome)

DEFINITION

- Mycosis fungoides (and its variant Sézary syndrome) are malignant proliferations of mature memory T lymphocytes of the phenotype CD4+CD45RO+ (memory T cells). They invariably involve the skin and are the principal forms of cutaneous T-cell lymphoma.
- Other types of lymphoma may also have prominent skin involvement (see Table 66–1).

EPIDEMIOLOGY

- Cutaneous T-cell lymphoma are two-fold more common in males than females.
- Median age at diagnosis is 55 years.
- In the United States, there are approximately 1000 cases per year representing about 1.5 percent of lymphomas.

CLINICAL FINDINGS

- Patients usually present with nonspecific skin lesions (chronic dermatitis) occurring years before diagnosis.
- Early in disease, patients are often diagnosed with eczema (spongiotic dermatitis), psoriatic-like dermatitis, or other nonspecific dermatoses associated with pruritus.
- Histologic diagnosis may be difficult in early stages. Neoplastic infiltrates may be minimal, masked by normal inflammatory cells, and the neoplastic mature CD4+ phenotype may be misinterpreted as normal inflammatory cells.
- Mycosis fungoides may be divided into patch stage (patch-only disease), plaque stage (both patches and plaques) and tumor stage (more than one tumor along with patches and plaques).
- A *patch* is defined as a flat lesion with varying degrees of erythema with fine scaling; a *plaque* is defined as a demarcated, erythematous, brownish lesion, with variable scaling of at least 1 mm elevation above the skin surface; a *tumor* extends at least 5 mm above the surface (tumors are usually in a setting of patches and plaques) (see Fig. 66–1).
- Mycosis fungoides d'emblée is an aggressive form with a poor prognosis characterized by tumors arising *de novo* in the absence of patches or plaques.
- Lesions have a predisposition for skin folds and non–sun exposed areas (bathing-trunk distribution) but in later stages they can be generalized and involve the face, palms, soles, and other areas.
- Progression through stages usually occurs over years but some cases may present with late stage lesions.
- Pruritus may be mild or severe and is one of the principal quality of life issues for patients. It can lead to insomnia, depression, and suicidal ideation.
- Erythrodermic skin involvement occurs in about 5 percent of patients and can be slight to severe. It can be associated with scaling, keratoderma, painful fissures in the hands and feet, nail dystrophy and loss. Severely inflamed skin can lead to bacterial infection, fever, chills, and septicemia.

TABLE 66–1	**WORLD HEALTH ORGANIZATION–EUROPEAN ORGANIZATION FOR RESEARCH AND TREATMENT OF CANCER CLASSIFICATION OF PRIMARY CUTANEOUS T-CELL AND NATURAL KILLER CELL LYMPHOMAS**

I. Mycosis Fungoides
  A. Mycosis fungoides variants and subtypes
    1. Folliculotropic mycosis fungoides
    2. Pagetoid reticulosis
    3. Granulomatous slack skin

II. Sézary Syndrome

III. Adult T-Cell Leukemia/Lymphoma

IV. Primary Cutaneous CD30+ Lymphoproliferative Disorders
  A. Primary cutaneous anaplastic large cell lymphoma
  B. Lymphomatoid papulosis

V. Subcutaneous Panniculitis-Like T-Cell Lymphoma

VI. Extranodal Natural Killer/T-Cell Lymphoma, Nasal Type

VII. Primary Cutaneous Peripheral T-Cell Lymphoma, Unspecified
  A. Primary cutaneous aggressive epidermotropic CD8+ T-cell lymphoma (provisional)
  B. Cutaneous γδT-cell lymphoma (provisional)
  C. Primary cutaneous CD4+ small/medium-sized pleomorphic T-cell lymphoma (provisional)

VIII. Precursor Hematologic Neoplasm
  A. CD4+/CD56+ hematodermic neoplasm (blastic NK-cell lymphoma)

Source: *Williams Hematology,* 8th ed, Chap. 105, Table 105–1, p. 1596.

- Sézary syndrome describes patients with pruritus, generalized exfoliative erythroderma, lymphadenopathy, and CD4+ lymphocytes with hyperconvoluted nuclei in the blood (see **Figs. 66–1** and **66–2**). It has the worst prognosis of the various types of mycosis fungoides.
- Depending on stage of presentation, lymphadenopathy and other organ involvement may occur.
- Lymphadenopathy is usually evident in 50 percent of patients at diagnosis and increases as disease progresses.

LABORATORY FINDINGS

Skin Biopsy
- Skin biopsy may be compatible with several benign dermatoses early in the disease.
- Classic mycosis fungoides lesions show a superficial lymphocytic infiltrate: lymphocytes may be large or small but have characteristic cerebriform nuclear convolutions. Epidermotropism with clusters of lymphocytes in the epidermis around Langerhans cells referred to as Pautrier abscesses. Later in the disease large lymphocytes may extend into the dermis.

Immunophenotype
- The neoplastic cells are mature helper-inducer T-cells expressing CD3,CD4, and CD45RO but not CD8. CD7, expressed on normal blood T cells, may be absent on mycosis fungoides lymphocytes in the skin and blood and on Sézary cells. Loss of CD26 expression is a hallmark of the neoplastic lymphocytes.

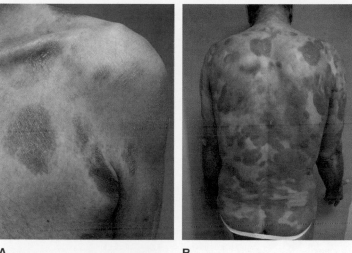

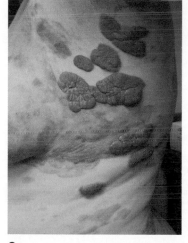

FIGURE 66-1 Mycosis fungoides. **A.** Erythematous atrophic patches with fine scale. **B.** Extensive patches and thicker plaques. **C.** Tumors on the background of preexisting patches and plaques. (Source: *Williams Hematology,* 8th ed, Chap. 105, Fig. 105–1, p.1596.)

Cytochemistry

- Mycosis fungoides cells stain for acid phosphatase, α-naphthyl acetate esterase, and β-glucuronidase; but generally are negative for CD25, peroxidase, alkaline phosphatase, and esterase.

Blood and Marrow

- Mycosis fungoides cells may be found in the blood in advanced disease, and in this setting, the marrow also contains mycosis fungoides cells. In Sézary

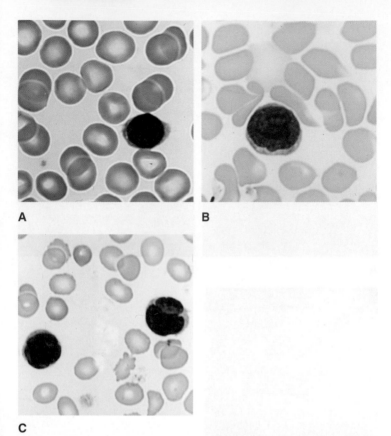

FIGURE 66–2 Blood lymphocytes. **A.** Normal small lymphocyte. **B.** Sézary cell. Note the nuclear swirls and the light microscopic appearance of the Sézary cell nucleus. Without careful inspection in cases of lymphocytosis, Sézary cells can be mistaken for small lymphocytes seen in chronic lymphocytic leukemia. **C.** Blood lymphocytes from a patient with mycosis fungoides and disseminated disease involving marrow and blood. Note clefted appearance of the nucleus. *(Reproduced with permission from Lichtman's Atlas of Hematology www.accessmedicine.com.)* (Source: *Williams Hematology,* 8th ed, Chap. 105. Fig. 105–5, p.1598.)

syndrome, blood and marrow involvement with neoplastic lymphocytes is the rule (see Figs. 66–2 and 66–3).

Lymph Node Biopsy
- Enlarged lymph nodes should have an excisional biopsy regardless of the T stage.
- Most early cases do not show effacement of node, but atypical lymphocytes in the paracortical T-cell zone are present.
- Later, lymph nodes may show partial or complete effacement and a monomorphic infiltrate of mycosis fungoides cells.

Chromosomal and Genic Findings
- The neoplastic lymphocytes have *TCRVβ* gene rearrangement.

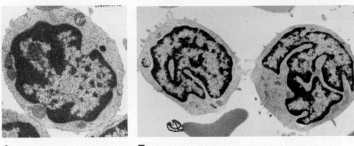

FIGURE 66-3 Transmission electron micrographs of lymphocytes. **A.** Normal lymphocyte. **B.** Two lymphocytes from a patient with Sézary cells in the blood. The latter have the striking cerebriform nuclear abnormalities characteristic of Sézary cells. *(Reproduced with permission from Lichtman's Atlas of Hematology, www.accessmedicine.com.)*
(Source: *Williams Hematology,* 8th ed, Chap. 105. Fig. 105–6, p.1599.)

- Cytogenetic findings are not seen consistently. Loss of 10q heterozygosity and microsatellite instability are present in advanced disease. Microsatellite instability is a condition in which damaged DNA results from defects in normal DNA repair. Microsatellites (sections of DNA), which consist of a sequence of repeating units of 1 to 6 base pairs in length, when unstable either shorten or lengthen.
- Homozygous deletions of tumor suppressor genes *PTEN* and *CDKN2A* on chromosomes 9p and 10p is associated with progressive disease.

STAGING

- Mycosis fungoides is stratified according to the *tumor, node, metastasis, blood (TNMB) classification* (see Table 66–2).
- Staging is of importance because it determines the therapeutic approach.
- Cutaneous lesions are stratified using the *T staging system* (see Table 66–2).
- The presence of tumors (T3) may indicate a worse prognosis than erythroderma (T4).
- Lymph nodes are assigned the *N category* in the classification (Table 66–2).
- Superficial adenopathy, although present in many patients, is usually not prominent early in the disease but progresses with progressive skin involvement.
- Magnetic resonance imaging is used to identify intraabdominal adenopathy.
- The M stage (metastatic disease) is the most significant prognostic indicator (Table 66–2).
- Patients with liver, spleen, pleural, and lung involvement have a median survival less than 1 year.
- Blood involvement is categorized in the *B* category in the classification system (Table 66–2).
- The percentage of neoplastic T cells in blood increases with progressive disease but sensitive techniques can find small concentrations of neoplastic T cells in the blood at diagnosis in many patients.

DIFFERENTIAL DIAGNOSIS

- Several benign dermatoses can mimic mycosis fungoides and may even have *TCR* gene rearrangements. Examples are psoriasis and psoriasiform dermatoses (eczema, pityriasis rubra pilaris, drug eruptions, and others).
- Adult T-cell leukemia lymphoma may have skin lesions simulating mycosis fungoides. May have other distinctive clinical features and serum HTLV1 antibodies (see Chap. 67).

TABLE 66–2	**TNMB CLASSIFICATION OF MYCOSIS FUNGOIDES**

T: Skin

   T1: Limited patches, papules, or plaques covering < 10% of the skin surface
      (T1a = patch only; T1b = plaques ± patches)
   T2: Generalized patches, papules, or plaques covering 10% of the skin
      surface (T2a = patch only; T2b = plaques ± patches)
   T3: At least one tumor (≥1 cm in diameter)
   T4: Generalized erythroderma over at least 80% body surface area

N: Lymph nodes

   N0: No clinically abnormal peripheral lymph nodes; biopsy not required
   N1: Clinically abnormal peripheral lymph nodes; histopathology Dutch
      grade 1 or NCI LN0 to 2
   N2: Clinically abnormal peripheral lymph nodes; histopathology Dutch
      grade 2 or NCI LN3
   N3: Clinically abnormal peripheral lymph nodes; histopathology Dutch
      grades 3–4 or NCI LN4
   NX: Clinically abnormal peripheral lymph nodes; no histologic confirmation

M: Visceral organs

   M0: No visceral organ involvement
   M1: Visceral organ involvement; requires histologic confirmation and specify
      organ

B: Blood

   B0: Atypical circulating cells not present (< 5%); specify "a" if flow cytometry is
      negative for clonal T lymphocytes or "b" if positive for clonal T lympho-
      cytes
   B1: Atypical circulating cells present (> 5%, minimal blood involvement);
      specify "a" if flow cytometry is negative for clonal T lymphocytes or "b" if
      positive for clonal T lymphocytes
   B2: Leukemia (≥ 1.0×10^9 cells/L, CD4 to CD8 ratio of 10 or higher, evidence
      of a T-cell clone in the blood)

CTCL, cutaneous T-cell lymphoma.
NOTE: T indicates the size of the tumor and whether it has invaded nearby tissue. N indicates the regional lymph nodes that are involved. M indicates distant metastasis. B indicates whether there are tumor cells in the blood.
Source: *Williams Hematology,* 8th ed, Chap. 105, Table 105–2, p. 1599.

- Pagetoid reticulosis consists of cutaneous plaques. It affects young males and has a benign course.
- Primary cutaneous CD30-positive lymphomas may have tumors that mimic mycosis fungoides. This is an indolent disease and may regress spontaneously. It should be distinguished from CD30+ transformation of mycosis fungoides and secondary skin involvement of CD30+ nodal lymphoma.
- Lymphoid papulosis is a benign skin disorder. Crops of pruritic, painful erythematous papules or nodules that ulcerate and heal spontaneously.
- The clinical findings, results of skin and node biopsy, blood T cell analysis, immunophenotype of T cells, TCR studies, and observation often can distinguish these diseases from mycosis fungoides.

TREATMENT

- Treatment is divided into skin-directed and systemic therapy.
- Skin-directed therapy is the mainstay in early phases of disease and as an adjunct for systemic disease.

TABLE 66–3	THERAPEUTIC OPTION FOR MYCOSIS FUNGOIDES AND SÉZARY SYNDROME

Skin-Directed Therapy	Systemic Therapy

Topical therapy
  Topical glucocorticoids
  Nitrogen mustard (mechlorethamine)
  Carmustine (BCNU, nitrosourea)
  Retinoids (bexarotene, tretinoin)
  Topical tacrolimus (Protopic)
  Imiquimod (Aldara)
	Immunomodulators
	  Interferon-α
	  Extracorporeal photopheresis
	  (ECP)
	  Antibodies/fusion proteins
	    Denileukin diftitox (ONTAK,
	    DAB$_{389}$–IL-2)
	  Alemtuzumab (Campath)

Light therapy
  UVB and PUVA
  Photodynamic therapy
  Electron beam
  Localized
  Total-skin
	Retinoids
	  Oral bexarotene (Targretin)
	  Acitretin (Soriatane)
	  Isotretinoin (Accutane)
	Histone deacetylase inhibitors
	  Vorinostat (Zolinza)
	  Romidepsin (Istodax)
	Chemotherapy (alone or in
	  combinations)
	  Oral prednisone, methotrexate,
	  doxorubicin, cyclophosphamide;
	  chlorambucil; pentostatin,
	  cladribine, fludarabine,
	  pralatrexate, several others

PUVA, psoralen and ultraviolet radiation of the A spectrum; UVB, ultraviolet radiation of the B spectrum.
Source: *Williams Hematology*, 8th ed, Chap. 105, Table 105–5, p. 1601.

- Therapeutic options for mycosis fungoides are listed in Table 66–3 and in Figure 66–4. Details of their use are described in *Williams Hematology*, 8th edition, Chap. 105, p.1601.
- Therapeutic modalities produce remission in most patients, but cure is uncommon.
- Topical glucocorticoids may be useful for pruritus, but they should not be used for long periods because they inhibit collagen synthesis and predispose to cutaneous infection. They should not be used on face, neck, or intertriginous areas. They can foster acne, glaucoma, and cataracts.
- Topical nitrogen mustard for early cutaneous disease has low toxicity but is not curative. It is also inconvenient to use as it must be applied daily to large areas of skin and frequent allergic responses occur. In responders, treatment should be continued for a year (or until lesions disappear) and then can be decreased in frequency for an additional year or two.
- Topical retinoids (e.g., bexarotene) can induce complete responses in 20 percent and improvement in an additional 40 percent. Approved for use in patients refractory to another topical therapy. Must not be used in pregnant women.
- Phototherapy with ultraviolet (UV) radiation in the form of UVA or UVB spectrum can be useful in early disease, patches, and very thin plaques. Given at least three times per week for 4 to 8 weeks to achieve maximal response. May result in complete clearing of lesions. Acute cutaneous burning can occur and slight increase in long-term risk of other skin cancers.
- Psoralen with ultraviolet A light (PUVA): Psoralen dose of 0.6 mg/kg, orally, 2 hours before ultraviolet A light therapy, three times per week, followed by maintenance therapy given every 2 to 4 weeks indefinitely.

Therapies for Cutaneous T-Cell Lymphomas

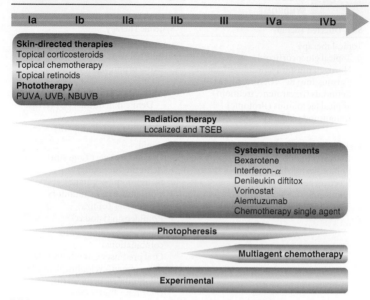

FIGURE 66-4 Cutaneous T-cell lymphoma treatment algorithm. NBUVB, narrowband ultraviolet B; PUVA, psoralen ultraviolet A; TSEB, total-skin electron beam; UVB, ultraviolet B. (Source: *Williams Hematology,* 8th ed, Chap. 105. Fig. 105–7, p.1600.)

- PUVA results in 60 percent complete remission rate for patients with cutaneous plaques. Lower response rates for patients with generalized erythroderma or tumors. Adverse effects include mild nausea, pruritus, and sunburn-like changes.
- PUVA is not curative.
- Electron-beam therapy: 80 percent complete remission rate; 20 percent disease-free at 3 years; 4 Gy/week (total dose 36 Gy in 8 to 9 weeks). Can be given to specific lesions or to total skin surface.
- Oral retinoids (e.g., bexarotene) 300mg/m^2 per day induces overall response in about 50 percent of patients and a complete response in about 1 in 50 patients. Virtually all patients develop central hypothyroidism and hypertriglyceridemia. Requires treatment with thyroid replacement and lipid lowering agents. Headaches, leukopenia, pruritus may occur. Usually used in more advanced stages. Must not be given to pregnant women or those considering pregnancy.
- Histone deacetylase inhibitors (e.g., vorinostat and romidepsin), interferon-α, a variety of single agent chemotherapy (e.g., pralatrexate, cyclophosphamide, fludarabine, doxorubicin), and combined agent chemotherapy have been used. Single agent therapy is occasionally effective but duration of response has been short, usually. Combined agent therapy is more toxic, about 25 percent of patients have a good response but long-term disease-free survival is extremely uncommon (see *Williams Hematology,* 8th ed, Chap. 105, p. 1603).
- Several other therapies are under study.

COURSE

- Median survival after diagnosis is about 12 years.
- Prognosis is dependent on the stage.
- Lymph node involvement signifies a poorer prognosis, and visceral involvement indicates poorest prognosis with median survival of less than 1 year.
- Fifty percent of deaths in patients with mycosis fungoides result from infection.
- Septicemia and bacterial pneumonia are common. *Pseudomonas* sp. and *Staphylococcus* sp. are particularly common and originate in skin.
- Herpes virus infection occurs in 10 percent of patients.
- Widespread organ involvement in late stages contributes to mortality.

PRIMARY CUTANEOUS ANAPLASTIC LARGE CELL LYMPHOMA

- CD30+ cutaneous lymphoproliferative disease is the second most common cutaneous T-cell lymphoma after mycosis fungoides and represents about 25 percent of cutaneous T-cell disorders.
- Represents a spectrum from lymphomatoid papulosis, a benign self-limited form, to cutaneous anaplastic large cell lymphoma (ALCL), a more progressive form.
- CD30+ primary cutaneous ALCL presents with skin involvement without evidence of extracutaneous disease for at least 6 months after presentation (Fig. 66–5).

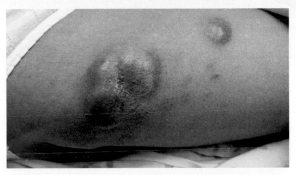

A

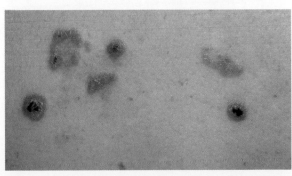

B

FIGURE 66-5 CD30+ lymphoproliferative disorders. **A.** Primary cutaneous anaplastic large cells lymphoma. Large cutaneous tumors on the anterior thigh. **B.** Lymphomatoid papulosis. Numerous small erythematous papules and small nodules. Some with necrotic centers in crops. Some lesions show spontaneous regression.
(Source: *Williams Hematology*, 8th ed, Chap. 105. Fig. 105–8, p.1604.)

- CD30+ primary cutaneous ALCL can occur at any age; median incidence is about 65 years and males are affected slightly more than females.
- The lesions are brownish to violaceous nodules or tumors, solitary (often) but can be numerous and widely distributed, and may regress spontaneously.
- On biopsy, at least 75 percent of the cells should express CD30 and usually CD4 but are negative for CD15, do not express ALK-1, or have the t(2;5), unlike systemic ALCL.

LYMPHOID PAPULOSIS

- Lymphoid papulosis is a clonal, usually self-limited disease characterized by crops of erythematous, dome-shaped papules or nodules that may ulcerate. They regress over a few months with minor residuals of scarring or atrophy.
- Lymphoid papulosis, rarely, can evolve into a more aggressive cutaneous lymphoma. It is also associated with a higher incidence of lymphoid and non-lymphoid malignancies than unaffected persons.

For a more detailed discussion, see Larisa J. Geskin: Cutaneous T-Cell Lymphoma (Mycosis Fungoides and Sézary Syndrome). Chap. 105, p. 1595 in *Williams Hematology,* 8th ed.

CHAPTER 67
Mature T-Cell and Natural Killer Cell Lymphomas

CLASSIFICATION

- The lymphomas of mature T cells and natural killer (NK) cells are shown in Table 67–1. The cutaneous forms are discussed in Chap. 66.

T-CELL LEUKEMIAS

T-Cell Prolymphocytic Leukemia

- Prolymphocytes (large [T] lymphocytes usually with prominent nucleoli) represent at least 50 percent of lymphocytes in the blood. They often have nuclear convolutions.
- T-prolymphocytes characteristically express pan-T-cell markers: CD2, CD3, CD5, and CD7.
- In the majority of cases, prolymphocytes express CD4 but not CD8 (i.e., malignant cell of T-helper cell origin). In occasional morphologically identical cases, CD4 may be weakly expressed or absent and CD8 may be weakly positive. CD52 is highly expressed and can be a target of therapy.
- Inversion of chromosome 14 is the most common cytogenetic abnormality and is found in 80 percent of patients. The t(14;14) occurs in 10 percent of patients. Associated abnormalities of chromosome 8 (e.g., t(8;8)) are common as well. Several other chromosomes (e.g., 6, 11, 17) may also be abnormal.
- Represents 20 percent of prolymphocytic leukemias; the remainder have a B-cell phenotype.
- The male:female ratio is 1.5:1.
- The tissue (e.g., lymphatic tissue) involvement and blood involvement coexist and are striking in both locations.
- Most patients have generalized lymphadenopathy and hepatosplenomegaly with marrow replacement and lymphoma cells dominating the white cell count (usually >100 × 10⁹/L).
- Anemia and thrombocytopenia are nearly always evident at diagnosis.
- Skin involvement occurs in approximately 20 percent of patients.
- Serology for the human lymphocytotropic virus-1 is negative.
- The clinical course is usually rapid. Median survival is less than 1 year.
- No standard chemotherapeutic treatment program has been developed. For example, cyclophosphamide, hydroxydaunorubicin (doxorubicin), vincristine (Oncovin), prednisone (CHOP) therapy does not produced long-term remissions.
- Pentostatin and cladribine can induce responses in approximately 40 percent of patients; but, complete remissions are infrequent (~10%) and long-term responses (>1 year) are uncommon.
- Alemtuzamab, a humanized monoclonal antibody against CD52, given three times weekly, has induced good responses in over 50 percent of patients.
- Allogeneic hematopoietic stem cell transplantation can induce a long-term remission of the disease.
- Occasional patients may have a chronic course of a few years but then evolve to a rapidly progressive phase.

TABLE 67-1	WORLD HEALTH ORGANIZATION CLASSIFICATION OF MATURE T-CELL AND NATURAL KILLER CELL NEOPLASMS

Leukemic neoplasms:
    T-cell prolymphocytic leukemia
    T-cell large granular lymphocytic leukemia
    Aggressive NK-cell leukemia
Nodal neoplasms:
    Adult T-cell leukemia/lymphoma
    Anaplastic large cell lymphoma
    Peripheral T-cell lymphoma, unspecified
    Angioimmunoblastic T-cell lymphoma
Extranodal neoplasms:
    Hepatosplenic T-cell lymphoma
    Nasal NK/T-cell lymphoma
    Enteropathy-type T-cell lymphoma
    Subcutaneous panniculitis T-cell lymphoma
Cutaneous neoplasms
    Mycosis fungoides
    Sézary syndrome
    Primary cutaneous CD-30 positive T-cell lymphoproliferative disorders

CD, cluster of differentiation; NK, natural killer.
Source: *Williams Hematology*, 8th ed, Chap.106, Table 106–1, p. 1609.

T-Cell Large Granular Lymphocytic Leukemia (see also Chap. 58)

Demographic Features

- Accounts for approximately 3 percent of all T cell/NK cell neoplasms.
- Median age of onset is 60 years.
- Approximately 85 percent of cases in Western countries are indolent.
- An aggressive variant (15% of cases) occurring in younger patients is most prevalent in Asia and South America.

Clinical Findings

- Persistence of elevated numbers of large granular lymphocytes in the blood (usually $> 0.2 \times 10^9$/L). The absolute large granular lymphocyte count may be lower and a clonal proliferation still be present based on T-cell receptor chain gene rearrangement studies.
- Marrow may show prominent infiltrate of large granular lymphocytes.
- Anemia occurs in 50 percent and neutropenia in 80 percent of patients. Severe neutropenia ($< 0.5 \times 10^9$/L) occurs in half the patients. Mild thrombocytopenia occurs in 20 percent of patients.
- Recurrent bacterial infections are notable in patients with severe neutropenia.
- Splenomegaly in about 35 percent at diagnosis, principally from massive accumulation of neoplastic cells in the spleen.
- Pure red cell aplasia occurs in approximately 15 percent of cases.
- One-third of cases associated with clinical evidence of rheumatoid arthritis (thought to reflect immune system dysregulation).
- In patients in which evidence of rheumatoid arthritis is present, the clinical features are indistinguishable from Felty syndrome.
- Circulating immune complexes, autoantibodies to various tissues, and polyclonal hypergammaglobulinemia also highlight the immune dysregulation.
- T-cell receptor chain gene rearrangement is a diagnostic hallmark along with clinical features.
- The large granular lymphocyte immunophenotype is CD3+CD8+CD57+.

Treatment

- Treatment may not be necessary initially. Severe neutropenia with recurrent infections, severe anemia or thrombocytopenia, or symptomatic splenomegaly may require therapy. No standard approach has been set in phase III clinical trials.
- Methotrexate, 10 mg/m^2 orally weekly, combined with prednisone, 1 mg/kg per day orally for 1 month and then tapered is one approach. A majority so treated have marked improvement.
- Cyclosporine, 7.0 mg/kg per day orally, or cyclophosphamide, 100 mg per day orally, may be used. Taper and use minimum required, once cell counts reach acceptable levels.
- Several early trials of various agents (e.g., tipifarnib, an oral farnesyltransferase inhibitor) and monoclonal antibodies (e.g., siplizumab, an anti-CD2) are under way.
- Although infrequent cases with an aggressive course may occur, most cases are indolent and the clonal abnormality remains relatively stable. The median survival is approximately 13 years.

Aggressive NK Cell Leukemia

- Represents less than 1 percent of all T-cell lymphomas.
- The Epstein-Barr virus implicated in its pathogenesis.
- Compared with most lymphomas, affects younger patients; median age at diagnosis 40 years.
- Most common among Asians or those of Asian ancestry.
- Usually fulminant presentation with fever, night sweats, cytopenias, hepatosplenomegaly.
- Disseminated intravascular coagulation (see Chap. 86), hemophagocytic syndrome (see Chap. 37), and multiorgan failure may be evident.
- Lymphadenopathy is often evident.
- Cutaneous involvement is not a feature.
- Lymphocytosis is present in the blood and marrow, but percent of neoplastic lymphocytes in the blood is quite variable from low to markedly elevated.
- Immunophenotype of lymphocytes by flow cytometry is CD2+CD3+CD8+ CD56+CD57−.
- Deletions of 17p13 and 6q21-25 most common cytogenetic abnormalities. Isochromosome 7 also occurs. 17p13 is site of the p53 gene.
- Serum lactic acid dehydrogenase markedly elevated.
- Standard multidrug chemotherapy is ineffective for this aggressive disease.
- Multidrug therapy (as used for poor-risk acute lymphocytic leukemia for initial therapy, including central nervous system prophylaxis, followed by high-dose consolidation therapy, in anticipation of allogeneic hematopoietic stem cell transplantation) is an intensive approach that can lead to a prolonged response.
- Anti-CD2 antibody, siplizumab, has been effective in only 1 of 16 patients in a phase I trial.
- An indolent form of NK cell leukemia, not separately classified as yet, exists. It presents as a chronic lymphocytosis with NK cell markers and no other signs or symptoms; easily distinguished clinically from the fulminant, prevalent form described above.

NODAL MATURE T-CELL NEOPLASMS

Adult T-Cell Leukemia/Lymphoma

Epidemiology and Pathogenesis

- Viral-induced lymphoproliferative disease with foci of occurrence in areas of Japan, South America, the Caribbean Basin, and equatorial Africa.
- Caused by a retrovirus, human lymphocytotropic virus (HTLV)-1, prevalent in the same regions as the clinical disease.

- Among HTLV-1 carriers, the lifetime risk of the disease is about 4 percent.
- Male:female ratio of disease 1.2:1 and median age of onset is approximately 60 years.
- Virus can be transmitted by blood-borne routes (e.g., transfusion), breast milk (mother to infant), and sexual intercourse.

Clinical Findings

- The presentation is variable: (a) smoldering disease, (b) chronic process with leukemic phase, (c) an aggressive lymphoma without overt blood involvement, (d) an aggressive leukemia with extensive marrow and blood lymphocytosis, or (e) a leukemic and lymphomatous presentation simultaneously.
- Lymphadenopathy, splenomegaly without overt leukemic involvement of blood and marrow may be evident in the lymphomatous presentation, although blood and marrow involvement frequently develops later.
- Lymph node enlargement occurs in virtually all patients although the nodes may be small, initially. Generalized lymphadenopathy is the rule and most have ret-roperitoneal adenopathy but mediastinal lymphadenopathy is very infrequent.
- The lymph node histopathology may mimic (a) diffuse large-cell lymphoma, (b) mixed large and small cell lymphoma, (c) large-cell immunoblastic lymphoma but no correlation exists with these different patterns of node effacement and clinical course.
- Blood lymphocytosis and marrow infiltration marks the leukemic phenotype. The lymphocyte count at diagnosis may range from 5×10^9/L to >100 $\times 10^9$/L.
- The lymphoid cells have characteristic clefted and lobulated nuclear shapes (Fig. 67–1) and express a mature T-helper cell phenotype, CD2+CD3+CD4+ and often CD25. Clonal rearrangement of the T-cell receptor β-chain is characteristic.

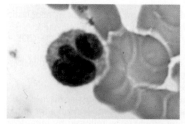
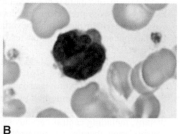

A   **B**

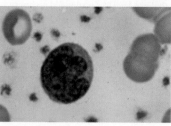

C

FIGURE 67-1 Blood film from a patient from the Caribbean region with adult T-cell leukemia-lymphoma. **A–C.** Note highly lobulated and clefted nuclei in lymphocytes, findings characteristic of this disease.
(Reproduced with permission from Lichtman's Atlas of Hematology, www.accessmedicine.com.)
(Source: *Williams Hematology,* 8th ed, Chap. 106, Fig. 106–1, p. 1612.)

- Anemia and thrombocytopenia are not prominent features at the time of diagnosis.
- Extranodal sites of involvement include the skin; lungs; gastrointestinal tract, especially the liver; and central nervous system.
- Skin involvement occurs in two-thirds of patients. Erythematous patches, plaques, papules, erythroderma, nodules or tumors alone or in combination may develop. Epidermal T-cell infiltration and lesions mimicking Pautrier microabscesses are found on histologic examination.
- The skin lesions may be indistinguishable from mycosis fungoides on inspection or even histologic examination but usually can be distinguished by serology for HTLV-1.
- Meningeal involvement may be evident by lymphocytosis in the cerebrospinal fluid.
- Spinal cord myelopathy and spastic paraparesis are two neurologic syndromes associated with this disorder.
- Decrease in B-cell function occurs through induction of suppressor cells; opportunistic infections are common even in the indolent forms.
- Hypercalcemia is often a feature and results from paraneoplastic production of parathyroid hormone-related proteins by osteoclasts. The osteoclastogenesis is mediated by the neoplastic T cells.
- The hypercalcemia is associated with polydipsia, polyuria, weakness, lethargy, and confusion.
- Radionuclide bone scans show a diffuse uptake throughout the skeleton, findings not usually seen in other lymphomas.
- Isolated osteolytic lesions may also occur.

Treatment

- Anthracycline-containing, multidrug therapy can induce a complete remission in approximately 30 percent of patients; however, it does not confer an increase in survival.
- Several other multidrug regimens (up to eight drugs) have been tried with complete remission rates of approximately 35 percent but the median survival with several different combinations has not exceeded 1 year.
- Allogeneic hematopoietic stem cell transplantation has had a high fatality rate (40%). The median survival of patients treated was less than 2 years.
- Interferon-α and zidovudine have resulted in partial remissions, some lasting several years.
- Monoclonal antibodies to CD25 with or without attached radionuclides have shown promising results.
- Denileukin diftitox (interleukin 2 coupled with diphtheria toxin) has induced complete remissions in pretreated patients.
- There is as yet no standardized approach that can be used as a basis for providing the treatment most likely to lead to long-term, disease-free survival.

Course

- Median survival for the lymphomatous or leukemic form of the disease is about 1 year.
- The "indolent" form, which is largely expressed in the skin, with little organ, marrow, or blood involvement, has a median survival of 2 years. (This form can be confused with cutaneous T-cell lymphoma described in Chap. 66)

Anaplastic Large Cell Lymphoma
Epidemiology and Pathogenesis
- Accounts for 5 percent of T-cell lymphomas.
- Has a bimodal age distribution: children and adolescents and older persons.
- Cells react with anti-CD30 and sometime referred to as CD30+ lymphomas.

- The cells in 65 percent of cases are positive for anaplastic lymphoma kinase (ALK).
- ALK-positive anaplastic large cell lymphoma cells contain a t(2;5)(p23;q35) fusing the *NPM* and *ALK* genes. The resultant *NPM-ALK* fusion gene encodes a p80 fusion oncoprotein. A small proportion of cases have translocations of *ALK* with other partners.
- Genomic and protein expression patterns indicate that the ALK-positive and ALK-negative anaplastic large cell lymphoma are two different diseases, although similar histopathologically.

Clinical and Laboratory Findings

- The cells of T-cell variants of anaplastic large-cell lymphoma are CD2+CD3+ CD4+CD5+CD7+.
- The cells of T-cell variants of anaplastic large cell lymphoma express granzyme B and perforin but have T-cell receptor gene rearrangements indicating its T-cell origin.
- Cutaneous CD30+ anaplastic large-cell lymphoma is a distinct entity and is discussed in Chap. 66.
- This type of lymphoma is usually an aggressive disease presenting with systemic symptoms of fever, chills, and weight loss, and nodal and extranodal involvement.
- The T-cell variant has a greater predilection for skin involvement and less predilection for marrow (and blood) and extranodal sites than does the null-cell variant.
- There are some distinctions between the ALK-positive and ALK-negative type. The former has a better prognosis.
- Ninety percent of children have the ALK-positive cell type.
- Marrow involvement is overt in about 30 percent of cases but if marrow is stained for CD30-positive or ALK-positive cells, approximately 60 percent of cases have marrow involvement.
- The histopathology is made up of large pleomorphic lymphoma cells in approximately 85 percent of cases, small to medium sized cells in 7 percent and a mixed small and large cell-sized variant with frequent macrophages in 7 percent. In each case, the cells stain for CD30.

Treatment

- Usually behaves as an aggressive lymphoma but is among the most responsive T-cell lymphomas to multidrug therapy containing an anthracycline antibiotic.
- Doxorubicin, bleomycin, vinblastine, and dacarbazine (ABVD) or high-dose methotrexate, doxorubicin, cyclophosphamide, vincristine, prednisone, and bleomycin (MACOP-B) each result in a 70 percent complete remission rate and a 5-year overall survival rate of 60 percent.
- There has not been a large experience with allogeneic hematopoietic stem cell transplantation but it can be very effective, even in patients with refractory or relapsed disease after multiagent chemotherapy.

Peripheral T-Cell Lymphoma (Unspecified)

- These T-cell lymphomas do not fit into a specified World Health Organization category of T-cell lymphoma.
- They represent about 30 percent of all T-cell lymphomas in Western countries.
- They are uncommon in children. Males are two-fold more likely than females to be affected.
- They are considered more aggressive than diffuse large B-cell lymphoma.
- Usually present with prominent (bulky) lymphadenopathy and widespread disease.
- Extranodal sites and marrow may be involved but blood involvement at presentation is uncommon.
- Patients have a high frequency of fever, night sweats, and weight loss.

- Pruritus, eosinophilia, or the hemophagocytic syndrome (see Chap. 37) may be present.
- Neoplastic cells express a CD4 or CD8 αβ T-cell phenotype but deletion of any of the pan-T cell antigens is common.
- Rearrangement of the T-cell receptor β chain gene is present in the neoplastic T cells.
- Elevated serum lactic acid dehydrogenase is very frequent.
- Use of multidrug lymphoma regimens that include an anthracycline antibiotic results in very few long-term survivors. These lymphoma cells are chemotherapy-resistant with current regimens that contain alkylating agents, anthracycline antibiotics, or topoisomerase II inhibitors.
- Use of high-dose consolidation therapy with autologous stem cell rescue for patients who have entered a remission on multidrug chemotherapy has increased 5-year overall survival for that subset of patients.
- There is little experience with allogeneic hematopoietic stem cell transplantation but transplantation-related mortality is considerable.

Angioimmunoblastic T-Cell Lymphoma

- Represents approximately 20 percent of T-cell lymphomas and 1 percent of all lymphomas.
- Median age of onset approximately 65 years. Males are affected slightly more often than females.
- Two types can occur: one evolving from angioimmunoblastic lymphadenopathy with dysproteinemia and the other arising *de novo*.
- Lymph node histopathology is characterized by nodal effacement and loss of germinal centers with a pleomorphic cellular infiltrate that in addition to neoplastic T cells has a background of plasma cells, immunoblasts, eosinophils, and macrophages. Small arborizing blood vessels are an important and prominent feature in the node.
- The neoplastic cells are CD4+ αβ T cells with β or γ T-cell receptor rearrangement (CD4+ follicular helper T cells). Pan T-cell markers are evident (e.g., CD2, CD3, CD5).
- The neoplastic T cells express CD10 in about 90 percent of cases, a marker characteristic of this type of lymphoma.
- CD8 cellular staining is present, but on reactive T cells in the background.
- Immunoglobulin gene rearrangements may be found in 20 percent of cases; but, they represent expanded clones of Epstein Barr virus-carrying B cells.
- Epstein-Barr virus-positive B cells are frequently present scattered throughout the node and is thought to be a secondary infection related to immunodeficiency.
- Patients present with widespread lymphadenopathy and splenomegaly with frequent involvement of marrow, liver, and skin. Pruritus may accompany the rash.
- Fever, night sweats, weight loss are very common at diagnosis.
- Pleural and peritoneal effusions (ascites) and arthritic manifestations may be present.
- Laboratory abnormalities include polyclonal hypergammaglobulinemia, immune complexes, cold agglutinins, rheumatoid factor, and other anti-tissue antibodies.
- The most frequent cytogenetic abnormalities are trisomy 3, trisomy 5, and involvement of the X chromosome. Complex karyotypes are a poor prognostic sign.
- Most patients are treated with anthracycline antibiotic-containing multidrug regimens. As in most other T-cell lymphomas, the initial response rate is about 40 percent, but survival is not extended significantly by such treatment.
- The course is usually aggressive and median survival is approximately 3 years.
- Poor prognostic signs are male sex, mediastinal lymphadenopathy, anemia, and complex cytogenetic patterns at the time of diagnosis.
- Large B-cell lymphoma may supervene, often Epstein Barr virus-positive.

EXTRANODAL NK CELL AND T-CELL LYMPHOMAS

Extranodal NK/T-cell Lymphoma

- Although most cases are NK cell malignancies, the cells in some cases have a cytotoxic T cell phenotype. Hence, the double nomenclature of NK/T cell.
- Nasal type (formerly called midline granuloma) always associated with Epstein-Barr virus infection and the blood titer of viral DNA is positively correlated with extent of the disease and a poor prognosis.
- More prevalent in Native Americans, Mexicans, and in Central and South Americans than those of European descent. Cases are more common in males than females and more prevalent at middle age (median age 50 years). Children can be affected.
- Nasal form 5-fold more common than extranasal form.
- Nasal form involves midline facial structures. The tumor induces vascular damage and necrosis.
- The neoplastic cellular histopathology is quite varied but the cells usually are CD2+CD56+CD3− but with CD3ε+ cytoplasmic staining. Cytotoxic molecules such as granzyme and perforin are positive. *In situ* hybridization for Epstein-Barr virus encoded RNA (EBER) is positive in all tumor cells and a negative reaction should result in consideration of other possible diagnoses.
- Patients present with symptoms of nasal obstruction or with epistaxis. Nasal examination shows a mass lesion and destruction of midline structures (e.g., nasal septum), but the tumor can extend to paranasal sinuses, orbit, palate, and oropharynx.
- Although typically localized to the nasopharynx and neighboring structures at presentation, the disease can spread to cervical lymph nodes, skin, gastrointestinal tract, and testes.
- Extranodal NK/T-cell lymphomas may also occur without initial confinement to the nasopharynx.
- These extranodal and extrapharyngeal lymphoma presentations are variable. Nodular ulcerating skin lesions are frequent. Intestinal involvement with perforation is common. Numerous other extranodal sites may be involved. Lymph node involvement may be present. Marrow and blood involvement can occur and can overlap with NK cell leukemia.
- The hemophagocytic syndrome may develop in the setting of this T-cell lymphoma.
- Local radiation and multidrug chemotherapy, including an anthracycline antibiotic, is usually used. One example of a useful intensive regimen is prednisone, methotrexate, doxorubicin, cyclophosphamide, and etoposide (ProMace) coupled with cytarabine, bleomycin, vincristine, methotrexate with leucovorin rescue (CytaBOM) with or without local radiation.
- Approximately 50 percent of patients may have a complete remission. The median overall survival is approximately 12 months but the 5-year free-survival was as high as 25 percent in some studies.
- High-dose chemotherapy with autologous stem cell rescue has been useful, occasionally.
- There is limited experience with allogeneic hematopoietic stem cell transplantation.

Enteropathic-Associated T-cell Lymphoma

- Accounts for less than 1 percent of lymphomas but for 25 percent of all intestinal lymphomas.
- Often preceded by gluten-sensitive enteropathy (celiac disease). Therefore, prevalent in geographic regions in which celiac disease is prevalent (Northern Europe) but can occur, sporadically, worldwide.
- A disease of adults. Median age at diagnosis 55 years. Male:female ratio is 3:1.
- Relapse while on a gluten-free diet may precede onset of lymphoma in patients with preceding celiac disease.

- Lymphoma is confined to the jejunum and ileum with invasion of the mucosa by interepithelial neoplastic T cells. Macroscopically, lesions appear as raised mucosal masses with ulcerations. May appear as a solitary mass.
- A preceding history of celiac disease may be described but is not invariable. Weight loss, small bowel diarrhea (steatorrhea), nausea and vomiting are usual, either as a result of the relapse of celiac disease or the malabsorptive effects of the infiltrating small bowel lymphoma.
- The diagnosis is usually made by histologic examination of the resected or biopsied portion of small bowel.
- Therapy is difficult because of the associated enteropathy. Many patients put on a multidrug lymphoma regimen cannot complete therapy.
- Complications while on therapy are common. These include gastrointestinal bleeding, small bowel perforation, and enterocolonic fistulae.
- Some patients may require enteral or parenteral feeding during therapy.
- A very good response in some studies has occurred in 35 percent of patients; but, relapse occurs at a median interval of 6 months and the 5-year relapse-free survival is under 20 percent.
- Most patients die either of complications of therapy or disease progression.

Hepatosplenic T-Cell Lymphoma

- Represents less than 1 percent of lymphomas.
- One-fifth of cases arise on background of immunodeficiency (e.g., immunosuppressive therapy for solid organ transplantation).
- The neoplastic cells are CD3+CD56+CD4−CD8− T-cells.
- T cells express γδ receptor chains and clonal rearrangement of the T-cell receptor δ-chain is present. Granzyme M is expressed but usually not granzyme B or perforin.
- The typical patient is a young male (median age 35 years) who presents with prominent splenomegaly and hepatomegaly without lymphadenopathy.
- Fever, night sweats, weight loss, and cytopenias (marked thrombocytopenia, leukopenia, anemia) as a result of marrow involvement are very common.
- An elevated serum lactic acid dehydrogenase is common.
- The most common cytogenetic abnormality in the lymphoma cells is isochromosome 7 (i(7)(q10) with trisomy 8. The i(7) is so common it may be a marker for this disease and the genetic effects responsible for the phenotype.
- Intensive multidrug therapy fails in most cases. Complete remissions occur in approximately 5 percent of patients with anthracycline antibiotic–containing regimens. Responses are usually short-lived. The median survival is 8 months.
- Allogeneic hematopoietic stem cell transplantation has been used uncommonly but some success has been reported.

Subcutaneous Panniculitis-Like T-Cell Lymphoma

- A very uncommon form of lymphoma occurring in less than 1 percent of cases.
- The median age of presentation is 30 years and 20 percent of cases are under age 20 years.
- About one-fifth of patients have an associated autoimmune disease, usually disseminated lupus erythematosus.
- Most common presentation is that of multiple, painful subcutaneous nodules on the trunk and extremities without other apparent sites of involvement. The nodules may range from 0.5 to several centimeters in diameter and may become necrotic.
- The lesions may regress, only to reappear later.
- Fever, night sweats, and weight loss is present in 50 percent of patients. Cytopenias may be present at diagnosis.
- The hemophagocytic syndrome may accompany this lymphoma in as many as 20 percent of patients.

- The cells have a mature $\alpha\beta$ T-cell phenotype and usually are CD8+ and express granzyme B, and perforin.
- Dissemination to lymph nodes is very unusual.
- The 5-year survival is approximately 80 percent. However, onset of the hemophagocytic syndrome is a very bad prognostic sign.
- Multidrug lymphoma therapy has been the mainstay of treatment but studies indicate less intensive regimens (e.g., chlorambucil, prednisone, cyclosporine) may be as useful.
- A distinction from cutaneous $\gamma\delta$ T-cell lymphoma is important because the latter does not have as favorable a prognosis.

HYPEREOSINOPHILIA AND T-CELL LYMPHOMAS

- Blood eosinophilia of $>1 \times 10^9$/L occurs in approximately 20 percent of T-cell lymphomas and about 20 percent of patients with the hypereosinophilic syndrome have a clonal T-cell expansion as the underlying cause.
- The neoplastic T-cells secrete IL-5, the principal eosinophilopoietin. Intratumoral IL-5 elaboration is closely correlated with blood eosinophilia.
- The clonal expansion of T cells, manifest principally by blood hypereosinophilia progress to overt and progressive T-cell lymphoma in >25 percent of patients over 10 years of observation.

 For a more detailed discussion see Oscar B. Goodman Jr and Nam H. Dang: Mature T-Cell and Natural Killer Cell Lymphomas. Chap. 106, p. 1609 in *Williams Hematology*, 8th ed.

CHAPTER 68
Essential Monoclonal Gammopathy

DEFINITION

- The presence of a serum monoclonal immunoglobulin (Ig) or a serum and urine monoclonal immunoglobulin light chain in the absence of evidence for a B-cell tumor (e.g., B-cell lymphoma, macroglobulinemia, myeloma, plasmacytoma, amyloidosis) over a period of observation.
- The monoclonal immunoglobulin may be of any isotype and may occasionally be of multiple isotypes (see Table 68–1).
- Synonyms for essential monoclonal gammopathy include (a) monoclonal gammopathy, (b) benign monoclonal gammopathy, (c) monoclonal gammopathy of unknown significance, with the acronym MGUS. The latter seems less appropriate now that the significance of this diagnosis is precisely known, and it is one of many examples of nonprogressive, clonal disorders with a predisposition to undergo clonal evolution to a malignant disorder (e.g., adenomatous colonic polyp).

EPIDEMIOLOGY

- May occur at any age but very unusual before puberty and increases in frequency with age. Frequency approximately 1 percent in those over 25 years, 3 percent in those over 70 years, and 10 percent in those over 80 years of age based on zonal electropheresis studies.
- Frequency higher with more sensitive immunologic techniques (e.g., isoelectric focusing or immunoblotting).
- Frequency significantly greater among Americans of African descent than those of European descent in comparative age-groups.
- Frequency greater in males than females.
- Familial aggregation of persons with essential monoclonal gammopathy occurs.
- Essential monoclonal gammopathy may harbinger the future development of a B-cell neoplasm, notably myeloma. A large proportion of patients with myeloma evolve from a preceding essential monoclonal gammopathy.

ETIOLOGY AND PATHOGENESIS

- Result from the growth of single B-lymphocyte into a clone of cells that elaborate a monoclonal immunoglobulin and or monoclonal light chains. Cessation of expansion of the clone occurs and the size of the clone remains stable, at a steady-state of approximately 1 to 5×10^{10} cells, indefinitely.
- At this clone size, organ pathology such as osteolysis, hypercalcemia, renal disease, or hematopoietic suppression does not occur. Polyclonal immunoglobulin synthesis is usually normal and, thus, increased frequency of infections is not a feature.
- IgA or IgG monoclonal gammopathy arise from a somatically mutated post-switch pre plasma cell, and IgM monoclonal gammopathy arises from a mutated germinal center B lymphocyte without evidence of isotype switching. This feature influences the result of clonal progression: IgA and IgG monoclonal gammopathy tends to evolve into myeloma or amyloidosis and IgM monoclonal gammopathy tends to progress to lymphoma or macroglobulinemia.
- The monoclonal immunoglobulin may react against self-antigen(s), resulting in symptomatic disease (e.g., neuropathy) that depends on the self-antigen involved and its blood or tissue distribution (see Table 68–2).

TABLE 68–1	**TYPES OF MONOCLONAL IMMUNOGLOBULIN SYNTHESIZED BY ABNORMAL B-CELL CLONE**

IgG, IgA, IgM, IgE, IgD
IgG + IgA, IgG + IgM, IgG + IgA + IgM
Monoclonal κ or λ light chain (Bence Jones proteinuria)

Source: *Williams Hematology*, 8th ed, Chap. 108, Table 108–1, p.1636.

CLINICAL FEATURES

- Persons with essential monoclonal gammopathy do not have symptoms or signs of myeloma or another B-cell lymphoproliferative disease (e.g., anemia, marrow plasmacytosis, lymph node enlargement, plasmacytoma, bone lesions, or amyloid deposits).
- Individuals usually are detected by the unexpected identification of a monoclonal protein in plasma or urine by zonal protein electrophoresis or another technique (see "Laboratory Detection," below).
- Patients occasionally have features of diseases that may result from the interaction of the monoclonal protein with antibody specificity for a plasma or cell protein (e.g., acquired von Willebrand disease, neuropathy, others). Table 68–2 lists the diseases that can occur as a result of this effect of the monoclonal protein.

LABORATORY DETECTION

Zonal Electrophoresis and Serum Light Chain Assay

- Serum protein electrophoresis and serum light chain assays to determine κ:λ light chain ratio.
- Molecules of each monoclonal protein have identical size and charge and thus migrate as a narrow band.
- Electrophoresis also can be done on concentrated samples of urine or cerebrospinal fluid (CSF).
- Immunoelectrophoresis and immunofixation electrophoresis are used to identify the heavy-chain class and light-chain type of monoclonal proteins.

TABLE 68–2	**FUNCTIONAL ABNORMALITIES ASSOCIATED WITH ESSENTIAL MONOCLONAL GAMMOPATHY**

Plasma protein disturbances
Antierythrocyte antibodies, acquired von Willebrand disease, immune neutropenia, cryoglobulinemia, cryofibrinogenemia, acquired C1 esterase inhibitor deficiency (angioedema), acquired antithrombin, insulin antibodies, antiacetylcholine receptor antibodies, "antiphospholipid" antibodies, dysfibrinogenemia
Renal disease
Neuropathies
Deep venous thrombosis

Source: *Williams Hematology*, 8th ed, Chap. 108, Table 108–2, p.1637.

LABORATORY FEATURES

- The monoclonal protein is usually IgG, but may be IgM, IgA, IgD, IgE, serum and urine-free light chains, or bi- or triclonal gammopathy (see Table 68–1).
- IgG in 70 percent, IgM in 15 percent and IgA in 10 percent of cases. A few percent have biclonal or triclonal Ig proteins or solely light chains in the urine (Bence Jones proteinuria).
- In IgG monoclonal gammopathy, the concentration of M protein is usually less than 3.0 g/dL and in IgA and IgM, less than 2.5 g/dL, but there are significant exceptions to this rule.
- Features of a B-cell malignancy are absent.
- Patients with monoclonal gammopathy usually have normal polyclonal immunoglobulin levels as opposed to patients with myeloma or macroglobulinemia who do not.
- Blood cell counts and marrow examination are normal. The proportion of plasma cells in marrow is usually <5 percent.
- Plasma cell labeling index is low (<1 percent).
- Blood T-lymphocyte subsets are normal.
- Serum β_2-microglobulin level is not elevated.
- Marrow microvessel density is three times that of normal individuals but less than that of marrow vasculature in patients with myeloma (although some overlap occurs).
- Interphase fluorescence *in situ* hybridization frequently uncovers numerical abnormalities (monosomy or trisomy) of chromosomes but progression to a symptomatic B-cell disease is not correlated with presence or absence of hyperdiploidy or hypodiploidy.

OLIGOCLONAL IMMUNOGLOBULINS

- Detected by high-resolution electrophoresis in patients with acute-phase reactants or polyclonal hyperglobulinemia.
- Oligoclonal immunoglobulins are frequent in the CSF of patients with neurologic conditions, e.g., multiple sclerosis.
- Serum oligoclonal or monoclonal immunoglobulins occur in patients with AIDS.

NEUROPATHIES AND MONOCLONAL GAMMOPATHY

Occurrence, Clinical, Laboratory, and Pathologic Findings

- Approximately 4 percent of patients with monoclonal gammopathy have neuropathy.
- IgM monoclonal gammopathy more strongly associated with neuropathy than patients with IgG or IgA.
- Approximately 10 percent of patients with idiopathic neuropathy have a monoclonal protein, a frequency about eight times that of age-matched comparison groups.
- Pathogenesis unclear (see *Williams Hematology,* 8th ed, Chap. 108, p. 1637 for discussion).
- Dysesthesias of hands and feet, loss of vibration and position sense, ataxia, intention tremor, and atrophy of distal muscle groups can occur, especially in association with IgM gammopathy.
- Patients with IgG or IgA gammopathy usually have chronic inflammatory demyelinating neuropathy. A minority have sensory axonal or mixed neuropathy.
- Severity of neuropathy can range from (a) mild with minor motor and/or sensory signs with or without mild functional impairment, (b) moderately disabling but with full range of activities, or (c) severely disabling interfering with walking, dressing, eating.

- The course may be remitting or progressive.
- IgA gammopathy may be associated with dysautonomia.
- Decreased nerve conduction velocity indicates demyelinization; decreased sensory potentials indicates axonal loss; electromyography may indicate denervation of muscles.
- Nerve biopsies may detect demyelinization of nerve fibers or axonal degeneration.

Management

- At least seven approaches have been used to improve the neuropathic findings: (a) intravenous IgG; (b) glucocorticoids; (c) immunoabsorption of perfused blood with staphylococcal protein A; (d) plasma exchange or plasmapheresis; (e) immunosuppressive cytotoxic chemotherapy with cyclophosphamide, fludarabine or chlorambucil with or without glucocorticoids; (f) rituximab; (g) high-dose cytotoxic therapy with autologous hematopoietic stem cell rescue.
- Plasma exchange (acute benefit) followed by immunosuppressive chemotherapy (chronic benefit) is a sequence sometime used.
- In patients with IgM and neuropathy, therapists may start with intravenous IgG as a less toxic initial approach.
- Response rates to each type of therapy are low and the duration of response unpredictable.
- Mild symptoms may not be an indication for therapy because of the low response rate and the noxious effects of therapy.

COINCIDENTAL DISORDERS

- Essential monoclonal gammopathy has been reported coincidental to a large number of conditions (see Table 68–3).
- Since the incidence of essential monoclonal gammopathy increases with age, other disorders that increase with age may be expected to co-associate without having any pathogenetic relationship and few studies have examined formally whether a causal relationship exists.
- Gaucher disease is one disorder in which a pathogenetic relationship may exist.

THERAPY, COURSE, AND PROGNOSIS

- Patterns of outcome in patients with essential monoclonal gammopathy:
  - Twenty-five percent of patients progress to develop myeloma, amyloidosis, macroglobulinemia, lymphoma, chronic lymphocytic leukemia over a 25-year period of observation. (Approximately 1% per year progress to some form of B-cell malignancy.)
  - Twenty-five percent of patients have a modest increase in Ig protein levels over time but do not progress to a B-cell malignancy.
  - Fifty percent of patients die of unrelated causes.
  - Although studies have shown some variables at diagnosis that may predict for earlier progression in groups of patients (e.g., higher marrow plasma cell concentrations, higher monoclonal Ig levels, lower levels of polyclonal Ig, abnormal serum light chin ratio), they are not sufficiently predictive in a single patient. In addition, there is no evidence, as yet, that early treatment is worthwhile.
  - Currently, neither gene expression analysis nor cytogenetic findings are sufficient to predict time of progression.
  - Rarely, the monoclonal protein disappears spontaneously.
  - Periodic reevaluation is required to determine the stability of the clinical course after diagnosis and to identify evidence of progression during long periods of observation.
- Therapy is generally not required for essential monoclonal gammopathy unless the monoclonal protein impairs the function of a normal plasma (e.g., acquired antithrombin) or tissue constituent (e.g., neuropathy) (see Table 68–2).

TABLE 68–3	DISORDERS REPORTED IN COINCIDENCE WITH MONOCLONAL GAMMOPATHY

Axial bone fracture

Connective tissue diseases and autoimmune diseases: Crohn disease, cryoglobulinemia, Hashimoto thyroiditis, lupus erythematosus, myasthenia gravis, pernicious anemia, polymyalgia rheumatica, psoriatic arthritis, rheumatoid arthritis, scleroderma, Sjögren disease

Corneal diseases: pseudo–Kayser-Fleischer ring, corneal gammopathy

Cutaneous diseases: Schnitzler syndrome, urticaria, hyperkeratotic spicules, pyoderma gangrenosum (neutrophilic dermatoses), psoriasis, scleromyxedema

Diffuse idiopathic skeletal hyperostosis

Endocrine diseases: hyperparathyroidism

Gaucher disease, type I

Hepatic disease: cirrhosis, hepatitis

Hereditary spherocytosis

Infectious diseases: bacterial endocarditis, *Corynebacterium* species, cytomegalovirus, human immunodeficiency virus, *Mycobacterium tuberculosis*, purpura fulminans

Metabolic disease: hyperlipidemia

Neutropenia, chronic

Osteoporosis

Pituitary macroadenoma

Pregnancy

Pseudomyeloma (severe osteoporosis)

Carcinomas: colon, lung, prostate, other

Myeloproliferative diseases: acute and chronic myelogenous leukemia, chronic neutrophilic leukemia, polycythemia vera

T-cell lymphomas, Hodgkin lymphoma

After chemotherapy, radiotherapy, or marrow, kidney, or liver transplantation

Transient, monoclonal, or oligoclonal gammopathies

Factitious hyperferremia

Factitious increase in C-reactive protein

Vitamin B_{12} deficiency

Source: *Williams Hematology,* 8th ed, Chap. 108, Table 108–3, p. 1638.

For a more detailed discussion, see Marshall A. Lichtman: Essential Monoclonal Gammopathy. Chap. 108, p. 1635 in *Williams Hematology,* 8th ed.

CHAPTER 69
Myeloma

DEFINITION

- Myeloma is a malignancy of terminally differentiated B cells (plasma cells) that produces a complete and/or partial (light chain) monoclonal immunoglobulin protein.
- Clinical and laboratory manifestations are heterogeneous, but typically include:
  - A monoclonal immunoglobulin in plasma and/or monoclonal light chains in plasma and urine. In rare cases, the cells do not secrete a monoclonal protein in the plasma.
  - Decreased polyclonal immunoglobulin secretion by residual normal plasma cells, which predispose to infections.
  - Myeloma cell proliferation in marrow leading to impaired hematopoiesis.
  - Osteolytic bone disease.
  - Often hypercalcemia as a result of osteolysis.
  - Sometimes renal dysfunction as a result light chain casts or hypercalcemia.
- Nearly 85 percent of newly diagnosed myeloma patients who have gene-expression-defined good-risk disease fare so well with therapy that the prospect of cure now appears tenable.

EPIDEMIOLOGY

- Myeloma accounts for more than 1 percent of all malignancies and for 10 percent of hematologic neoplasms.
- The age-adjusted incidence of myeloma is affected by gender and ethnicity: White men 6.6/100,000 persons, white females 4.2/100,000, black men 13.7/100,000 and black females 9.9/100,000.
  - The incidence of myeloma increases with age exponentially from age 40 years onward. Occasional cases occur in individuals in the third and fourth decade of life.
- Analysis of the aggregate of studies does not support a role for chemical agents, such as benzene or other solvents, pesticides, herbicides, or others as causative factors.
- Radiation, once thought to be a cause, appears not to be after reanalysis of the data in the Japanese population surviving the atomic bomb blasts.
- Several studies indicate an increased risk of myeloma in overweight and obese individuals. This relationship might be mediated by elevated IL-6 secreted by fat cells and fatty tissue stroma.

ETIOLOGY AND PATHOGENESIS

- Myeloma may result from errors in the process of immunoglobulin class switching, somatic hypermutation, or antigen receptor gene rearrangement of variable (V), diversity (D) and joining (J) gene segments (VDJ recombination) leading to mutational errors (double-strand DNA breaks) and, for example, translocations involving the *IgH* gene, fusing it to genes involved in cell proliferation or cell survival, and a resultant neoplastic change in late B-cell progenitor.
- Among patients with essential monoclonal gammopathy, progression to a progressive B-cell neoplasm (e.g., lymphoma, myeloma, AL amyloidosis) is 1 percent per year.
  - Many patients with myeloma have a preceding period of essential monoclonal gammopathy.

- Genetic abnormalities by standard cytogenetic and fluorescence *in situ* hybridization (FISH) are evident in two-thirds of patients with myeloma.
- DNA hyperdiploidy is present in about three-quarters of all patients.
- Typically, there are multiple abnormalities in each karyotype.
- Hyperdiploid myeloma typically has multiple trisomies of odd numbered chromosomes 3, 5, 7, 9, 11, 15, 19, and 21.
- Nonhyperdiploid myeloma usually is associated with *immunoglobulin heavy chain (IgH)* gene translocations located at chromosome 14q32 observed in about two-thirds of patients by FISH and in some patients translocations involving the λ light chain locus on chromosome 22. Translocations involving the κ locus on chromosome 2 are rare.
- There are five principal recurrent chromosomal rearrangements involving the *IgH* gene (14q32) and a gene(s) located on another chromosome that account for approximately 40 percent of all genetic abnormalities seen in myeloma.
  — 11q13, *cyclin D1* gene.
  — 4p16.3, fibroblast growth factor gene, *FGF-R3*, and multiple myeloma SET domain gene *MMSET*.
  — 6p21, *cyclin D3* gene.
  — 16q23, musculoaponeurotic fibrosarcoma gene (*MAF*).
  — 20q11, *MAFB* gene.
- Alterations in gene copy number detectable by FISH and comparative genomic hybridization are important for disease progression.
  — Alterations include gain of chromosome 1q, loss of chromosome 1p, deletion 13p, and deletion 17p.
  — Gain of the gene *AGO2*, important in microRNA regulation and expression, located at 8q24, is related to a poor prognosis.
  — Mutational activation of the *NRAS* or *KRAS* oncogenes and inactivation of *CDKN2A*, *CDKN2C*, *CDKN1B*, and/or *PTEN* tumor-suppressor genes are related to disease progression.
  — Late events involve inactivation of *TP53* and secondary translocations of *c-MYC*.
- The interaction of myeloma cell with the marrow microenvironment plays a role in disease progression and drug resistance.
- Osteolytic bone lesions are a hallmark of advanced myeloma, eventually developing in 70 to 80 percent of patients.

CLINICAL AND LABORATORY FEATURES

- Table 69–1 summarizes the commonly accepted diagnostic criteria for myeloma.
- The International Myeloma Working Group has issued simplified criteria (see Table 69–2).
- The most critical criterion of symptomatic disease and, hence, initiation of therapy, is evidence of organ or tissue impairment (end-organ damage) manifested by anemia, hypercalcemia, lytic bone lesions, renal insufficiency, hyperviscosity, amyloidosis, or recurrent infections, referred to as "CRAB" for hypercalcemia, *r*enal failure, *a*nemia, and *b*one lesions (see Table 69–3).
- The principal diagnostically important findings are an increase in marrow plasma cells in the presence of a serum or urine monoclonal protein.
  — The extent of the neoplastic plasma cell infiltrate may range from just above the normal upper limit of 8 to 10 percent of marrow cells to a virtual complete replacement of marrow with myeloma cells.
- Myelomatous involvement of the marrow typically causes anemia, but when advanced may also contribute to neutropenia and thrombocytopenia.
- Overproduction of interleukin (IL)-6 by marrow stroma, normal accessory cells, and/or myeloma cells may contribute to the anemia by upregulating hepatic production of hepcidin, which blocks release of iron from macrophages and inhibits iron absorption from the intestine.

TABLE 69–1	**CRITERIA FOR DIAGNOSIS OF MYELOMA***

Major criteria
   Plasmacytomas on tissue biopsy
   Marrow plasmacytosis with >30% plasma cells
   Monoclonal globulin spike on serum electrophoresis >3.5 g/dL for
   immunoglobulin (Ig) G or >2.0 g/dL for IgA; 1.0 g/24 h of κ or λ light-chain
   excretion on urine electrophoresis in the absence of amyloidosis
Minor criteria
   Marrow plasmacytosis 10–30%
   Monoclonal globulin spike present, but less than the levels defined above
   Lytic bone lesions
   Normal IgM < 0.05 g/dL, IgA < 0.1 g/dL, or IgG < 0.6 g/dL

*The diagnosis of plasma cell myeloma is confirmed when at least one major and one minor criterion or at least *three minor criteria* are documented in *symptomatic* patients with *progressive* disease. The presence of features not specific for the disease, such as the following, supports the diagnosis, particularly if of recent onset: anemia, hypercalcemia, azotemia, bone demineralization, or hypoalbuminemia.
Source: *Williams Hematology,* 8th ed, Chap. 109, Table 109–1, p. 1650.

TABLE 69–2	**SIMPLIFIED CRITERIA FOR THE CLASSIFICATION OF MYELOMA***

M-protein in serum and/or urine
Marrow (clonal) plasma cells* or plasmacytoma
Related organ or tissue impairment (ROTI), end-organ damage, including bone
   lesions

*If flow cytometry is performed, most plasma cells (>90%) will show a "neoplastic" phenotype.
NOTE: Some patients may have no symptoms but have related organ or tissue impairment.
Source: *Williams Hematology,* 8th ed, Chap. 109, Table 109–2, p. 1650.

TABLE 69–3	**DIAGNOSTIC CRITERIA FOR MYELOMA REQUIRING THERAPY**

Presence of an monoclonal immunoglobulin* in serum and/or urine plus clonal
   plasma cells in the marrow and /or a documented clonal plasmacytoma
PLUS one or more of the following:[†]
   Calcium elevation (>11.5 mg/dL) [>2.65 mmol/L]
Renal insufficiency (creatinine >2 mg/dL) [177 μmol/L or more]
Anemia (hemoglobin <10 g/dL or 2 g/dL [‡] or 1.25 μmol/L <NORMAL)
   Bone disease (lytic lesions or osteopenia)

*In patients with no detectable monoclonal immunoglobulin, an abnormal serum free-light chain (FLC) ratio on the serum FLC assay can substitute and satisfy this criterion. For patients, with no serum or urine monoclonal immunoglobulin and normal serum FLC ratio, the baseline marrow must have >10% clonal plasma cells; these patients are referred to as having "nonsecretory myeloma." Patients with biopsy-proven amyloidosis and/or systemic light-chain deposition disease (LCDD) should be classified as "myeloma with documented amyloidosis" or "myeloma with documented LCDD," respectively, if they have >30% plasma cells and/or myeloma-related bone disease.
[†]Must be attributable to the underlying plasma cell disorder.
[‡]Hemoglobin of 10 g/dL is 12.5 mmol/L [or 100 g/L].
Source: *Williams Hematology,* 8th ed, Chap. 109, Table 109–3, p. 1651.

- Thrombocytopenia is uncommon in early phases of myeloma, even with extensive marrow myeloma cell replacement.
- Most patients have an inappropriate erythropoietin response for the level of their anemia.
- Bleeding occurs in 15 percent of patients with IgG myeloma and in 30 percent of patients with IgA myeloma.
- Thrombocytosis should alert one to the possibility of hyposplenism because of amyloid deposition in the spleen.
- Hypercoagulable states may result from defective fibrin structure and fibrinolysis because of increased immunoglobulin levels, increased acquired protein C resistance, and increased synthesis of proinflammatory cytokines, such as IL-6.
- Lupus anticoagulants also have been reported in association with myeloma.

Immunoglobulin Abnormalities

- Virtually all patients with myeloma secrete a monoclonal immunoglobulin that can be detected by immunofixation analysis.
  — Approximately 60 percent of myeloma patients have detectable monoclonal IgG (usually >3.5 g/dL), 20 percent have monoclonal IgA (typically >2 g/dL), and 20 percent have only monoclonal immunoglobulin light chains. Excess light-chain proteinuria, however, can accompany IgG, IgA, and, especially, IgD myeloma.
- As a result of the advent of highly sensitive assays for serum light chains, an extremely small proportion of patients may have nonsecretory myeloma (no apparent extracellular monoclonal protein).
- Myelomas producing monoclonal IgD, IgE, IgM, or more than one immunoglobulin class are rare.
- The presence of a low concentration of serum monoclonal immunoglobulin by zonal electrophoresis should alert to the possibility of IgD myeloma, especially when associated with excess λ light chains in the serum and light-chain proteinuria, as 80 percent of IgD myeloma are of the λ light-chain variety.
  — Even patients with light-chain type myeloma, nonsecretory myeloma, or IgD or IgE myeloma often have depressed levels of normal, polyclonal serum IgG, IgA, and IgM.
- The half-life of free light chains is 2 to 4 hours, providing a means to assess the effects of therapy on the myeloma cell mass more quickly than by following plasma immunoglobulin.
- Intact immunoglobulins have a half-life of 17 to 21 days, and responses in immunoglobulin levels to therapy are much slower to become apparent.
- Reestablishment of a normal serum κ and λ light chain ratio (0.3–1.6) is now also included in the definition of stringent complete response by the Uniform International Response Criteria.
- IgA isotype adversely affects outcome in multivariate analysis.

Marrow Findings

- The marrow can be diffusely infiltrated but commonly displays considerable site-to-site variation in myeloma cell density in a given patient (focal or nodular involvement). Mixed patterns may also occur.
- Cytologically, myeloma cells resemble plasma cells, exhibiting varying degrees of maturity.
- More aggressive forms of myeloma may have larger cells with a centrally located nucleus, which has open chromatin and punched nucleoli, indicating increased transcriptional activity.
- Osteoclasts are often increased and osteoblasts decreased. Amyloid deposition, recognized on Congo red stain, may be diffuse or focal and sometimes only perivascular.

- Secondary myelodysplasia (dysmorphic red cells, granulocytes, and megakaryocytes) can develop after prolonged treatment with alkylating agents.
  — Pancytopenia in the context of a hypercellular marrow should prompt cytogenetic and interphase FISH studies to detect the most commonly encountered genetic changes associated with therapy-related myelodysplastic syndromes. (See Chap. 42)
- In flow cytometric phenotypic studies to identify mature plasma cells, they coexpress CD56.
- In less than 20 percent of cases, the plasma cells express CD20 or CD117 (KIT).
- Metaphase cytogenetic studies should be performed to identify the one-third of newly diagnosed patients harboring cytogenetic abnormalities associated with poor prognosis, especially hypodiploidy or chromosome 1 abnormalities.
- Plasma cell labeling index, as determined by tritiated thymidine or bromodeoxyuridine techniques, that exceed 0.5 percent is associated with a relatively short survival.

Renal Disease

- Some form of renal impairment occurs in 30 to 50 percent of myeloma patients at diagnosis, with up to 10 percent of patients requiring hemodialysis during their course of management.
- Myeloma cast nephropathy is the most common cause of renal impairment and is also referred to as myeloma kidney.
  — Myeloma kidney is caused by the formation of tubular casts in the distal nephron formed by the binding of light chains to uromodulin (Tamm-Horsfall protein).
  — Myeloma kidney obstructs the distal nephron and parts of the ascending loop of Henle and contributes to development of interstitial nephritis.
  — There is considerable variation in the nephrotoxic proclivity of light chains (e.g., λ light chains are more nephrotoxic than the κ type).
  — The second most common cause of nephropathy is hypercalcemia.
- AL amyloidosis associated with light-chain immunoglobulin proteinuria usually presents as the nephrotic syndrome, with very little light-chain secretion in the urine, but can lead, over time, to renal failure (see Chap. 72).
  — Amyloid deposits can be detected by Congo red staining.
  — AL amyloidosis is more common in patients with λ light-chain myeloma proteins than in patients with κ light-chain myeloma, especially those with λ light-chain proteins that have immunoglobulin variable regions belonging to the λ VI light-chain subgroup.
- The differential diagnosis of nephrotic syndrome in the myeloma patient should include renal vein thrombosis.
- Acquired adult Fanconi renal syndrome is also caused by κ light chains.
- Tumor cell involvement of the kidneys is uncommon.
  — Kidney biopsy can be helpful in accurately diagnosing the type of renal disease.
- A new dialysis filter has been developed that removes light chains with great efficiency.
- In general, cast nephropathy-induced renal impairment is (partially) reversible in approximately 50 percent of patients.

Pain

- Pain suffered by persons with myeloma frequently results from vertebral compression fractures.
- Localized pain can also be induced by regional tumor growth.

Infections

- Infection is a leading cause of morbidity and mortality in myeloma patients.
- Hypogammaglobulinemia reflecting suppression of CD19+ B lymphocytes results in susceptibility to encapsulated organisms.
- Deficiencies in cellular immune function account for the recurrent infections commonly seen.
- Abnormalities in T-cell function include reversed CD4+/CD8+ T-cell ratios, severe disruptions in the T-cell repertoire, and abnormal intracellular signal transduction impairing T-cell activation.
- In patients with persistently low CD4+ counts, *Pneumocystis jiroveci* prophylaxis should be considered.

Neuropathy

- Neurologic abnormalities generally are caused by regional myeloma cell growth compressing the spinal cord or cranial nerves.
- Polyneuropathies are observed with perineuronal or perivascular (*vasa nervorum*) amyloid deposition.

Hyperviscosity

- Hyperviscosity occurs in less than 10 percent of patients with myeloma.
  - Symptoms of hyperviscosity result from circulatory problems, leading to cerebral, pulmonary, renal, and other organ dysfunction (see Chap. 70).
  - Patients with IgA myeloma have hyperviscosity more frequently than do patients with IgG myeloma.
  - Among patients with IgG myeloma, those with tumors expressing immunoglobulins of the IgG_3 subclass are the most susceptible.

Extramedullary Disease

- Plasma cell leukemia ($\geq 2.0 \times 10^9$/L of blood) is rare at presentation, but can develop in approximately 5 percent of patients as a terminal disease manifestation.
- Visceral organ involvement of liver, lymph nodes, spleen, kidneys, breasts, pleura, meninges, and cutaneous sites should be suspected in the presence of elevated serum levels of lactic acid dehydrogenase (LDH).

Spinal Cord Compression

- Spinal cord compression has traditionally been treated with local radiotherapy and/or decompressive laminectomy.
- In patients suffering from systemic disease, chemotherapy that includes high-dose dexamethasone pulsing, as part of the combination oral dexamethasone, daily thalidomide, and 4 days of continuous-infusion cisplatin, doxorubicin, cyclophosphamide, and etoposide (DT PACE).
  - DT PACE has been shown to provide effective treatment. In the absence of symptom relief and lack of tumor shrinkage on MRI within 1 week, local radiation should be added.
  - If cord compression results from vertebral collapse without identifiable plasmacytoma on MRI, radiation may not be beneficial, and decompressive laminectomy may be the treatment of choice.
  - The local doses of radiotherapy to the spinal cord should not exceed 30 Gy, and liberal use of local radiation for the management of rib fractures is discouraged because it reduces marrow tolerance to chemotherapy.

INITIAL EVALUATION OF THE PATIENT WITH MYELOMA

- Minimal evaluation requirements include evaluation of the complete blood count; myeloma protein studies; examination of the blood film for the presence of rouleaux or circulating myeloma cells; a multichemical scan for the detection

of hypercalcemia, azotemia, serum β_2-microglobulin, C-reactive protein, and elevation of LDH (see Table 69–4).
- Myeloma protein studies should include:
  — Serum protein electrophoresis.
  — Serum-free light-chain assay, and a 24-hour urine collection to quantify 24-hour total urinary protein and measure quantity of light chains.
  — Urinary light chains are also referred to as "Bence Jones protein."
  — Immunofixation of serum and urine is needed for the immunoglobulin heavy- and light-chain isotype determination.
- Marrow aspiration and biopsy should include genetic studies (e.g., FISH and cytogenetics) and flow cytometry.
- Radiographic examination usually comprises a metastatic bone survey.
- MRI and CT-PET are more sensitive than the bone survey, and better capture early bone disease, the extent of bone disease, and extramedullary disease.
- Assessment of the heart by echocardiogram and electrocardiogram is useful to detect cardiac amyloidosis.
- Measurement of brain natriuretic peptide and N-terminal prohormone B-type natriuretic peptide are useful screening tests to detect cardiac dysfunction caused by amyloidosis or light chain deposition disease (LCDD).

Staging
- The Salmon-Durie staging system has been in use for more than 30 years but is being replaced by newer staging systems (see Table 69–5).
- The Southwest Oncology Group introduced an international staging system (ISS) based on two widely available parameters, serum β_2-microglobulin and albumin, and recognizes three stages (see Table 69–6).
  — Stage I is defined by β_2-microglobulin < 3.5 mg/L and albumin ≥ 3.5 g/100 mL.
  — The intermediate stage II has neither features of stage I or III.
  — Stage III is characterized by a β_2-microglobulin of ≥ 5.5 mg/L.
  — A weakness of the ISS is that it does not take cytogenetics into account.

Imaging Studies
- Radiographic studies should include a chest radiograph to determine cardiopulmonary status as well as a metastatic bone survey, including a rib series and long bone images.

TABLE 69–4 ASSESSMENT OF MULTIPLE MYELOMA

Complete blood count and differential count; examination of blood film

Chemistry screen, including calcium, creatinine, lactic acid dehydrogenase, BNP, proBNP

β_2-microglobulin, C-reactive protein

Serum protein electrophoresis, immunofixation, quantification of immunoglobulins, serum-free light chains

24-h urine collection for protein electrophoresis, immunofixation, quantification of immunoglobulins including light chains

Marrow aspirate and trephine biopsy with metaphase cytogenetics, FISH, immunophenotyping; gene array, and plasma cell labeling index (if available)

Bone survey and MRI; CT-PET (if available)

Echocardiogram with assessment of diastolic function and measurement of interventricular septal thickness; ECG

BNP, brain natriuretic peptide; CT, computed tomography; ECG, electrocardiogram; FISH, fluorescence *in situ* hybridization; MRI, magnetic resonance imaging; PET, positron-emission tomography; proBNP, prohormone B-type natriuretic peptide.
Source: *Williams Hematology,* 8th ed, Chap. 109, Table 109–5, p. 1657.

TABLE 69–5	ASSESSMENT OF MYELOMA TUMOR MASS (SALMON-DURIE)

I. High tumor mass (stage III) ($>1.2 \times 10^{12}$ myeloma cells/m^2)*
   One of the following abnormalities must be present:
   A. Hemoglobin <8.5 g/dL, hematocrit $<25\%$
   B. Serum calcium >12 mg/dL
   C. Very high serum or urine myeloma protein production rates:
      1. IgG peak >7 g/dL
      2. IgA peak >5 g/dL
      3. Urine light chains >12 g/24 h
   D. >3 lytic bone lesions on bone survey (bone scan not acceptable)
II. Low tumor mass (stage I) ($<0.6 \times 10^{12}$ myeloma cells/m^2)*
   All of the following must be present:
   A. Hemoglobin >10.5 g/dL or hematocrit $>32\%$
   B. Serum calcium normal
   C. Low serum myeloma protein production rates:
      1. IgG peak <5 g/dL
      2. IgA peak <3 g/dL
      3. Urine light chains <4 g/24 h
   D. No bone lesions or osteoporosis
III. Intermediate tumor mass (stage II) (0.6–1.2 $\times$ 10^{12} myeloma cells/m^2)*
   All patients who do not qualify for high or low tumor mass categories are
      considered to have intermediate tumor mass.
   A. No renal failure (creatinine ≤ 2 mg/dL)
   B. Renal failure (creatinine >2 mg/dL)

*Estimated number of neoplastic plasma cells.
Source: *Williams Hematology,* 8th ed, Chap. 109, Table 109–6, p. 1657.

- Roentgenographically detectable osteolytic lesions require at least 50 to 70 percent loss of bone mass, and represent advanced bone destruction.
- MRI has allowed detection and characterization of focal intramedullary disease in two-thirds of patients at time of diagnosis, even before the onset of bone destruction.
- Fluoro-2-deoxyglucose (FDG)-PET scanning is a convenient tool of whole-body imaging when performed in the context of CT scanning.
  — Because PET imaging is dependent upon metabolic uptake, active disease is often identified before bony destruction.
- Bone densimetric analysis is advised to establish the need for bisphosphonate therapy and should be performed annually.

TABLE 69–6	INTERNATIONAL STAGING SYSTEM (ISS)	
Stage I:	28%	β_2M <3.5
		ALB ≥3.5
Stage II:	39%	β_2M <3.5
		ALB <3.5
		or
		β_2M 3.5–5.5
Stage III:	33%	β_2M >5.5

%, percent of all patients with myeloma; ALB, serum albumin in g/dL; β_2M, serum β_2-microglobulin in mg/L.
Source: *Williams Hematology,* 8th ed, Chap. 109, Table 109–7, p. 1657.

DIFFERENTIAL DIAGNOSIS

- Table 69–7 presents diagnostic criteria for myeloma.

TREATMENT AND PROGNOSIS

Management of Newly Diagnosed Myeloma

- The goal of myeloma therapy has changed from achieving disease control to achieving long-term disease-free survival, if not cure.
- Four prospective randomized European studies found that auto-hematopoietic stem cell transplantation (HSCT) confers superior event-free and/or overall survival when compared with standard chemotherapy therapy.
- Vincristine, doxorubicin (Adriamycin), and dexamethasone (VAD) has long been used as the standard induction chemotherapy, but has been replaced by the advent of novel drugs.
- Combinations that include alkylating agents should be avoided, since these drugs could damage normal hematopoietic stem cells and make stem cell harvesting for subsequent autologous transplantation more difficult.
- An International Myeloma Working Group panel recommends collecting stem cells within the first six cycles of treatment with regimens containing thalidomide, lenalidomide, or bortezomib.
- The concept of two sequential (tandem) auto-HSCT was based on the notion that in adult acute leukemia, cures were not observed unless a complete remission rate of 40 percent was achieved. Because a single transplantation yields a rate of 20 percent, it was hypothesized that a tandem auto-HSCT would yield a complete remission rate of 40 percent.
  — Studies reported that patients who benefitted most from a second transplantation were those who did not achieve at least a very good partial remission after the first transplantation.
- Combination therapy with novel drugs achieve complete remission rates comparable to those obtained with auto-HSCT.
- Novel agents overcome the adverse prognostic implications of certain cytogenetic changes such as del 13, t(4;14), or del 17p.
- Complete remission rates as a surrogate marker for eventual outcome may prove to be inadequate.
  — A complete remission for 3 years rather than mere achievement of the remission is critical for long-term survival.

TABLE 69–7　SYMPTOMATIC MYELOMA	
Symptoms and Laboratory Features	Frequency (%)
Bone pain (spine, chest, less common in long bones)	65
Weakness and fatigue	50
Anemia	65
Renal insufficiency	20
Hypercalcemia	20
Serum monoclonal immunoglobulin (Ig) peak on standard electrophoresis	80
Monoclonal Ig peak on immunofixation of serum or urine	97
Monoclonal IgG	50
Monoclonal IgA	20
Monoclonal light chains only	20
Urinary monoclonal light chains	75
Marrow plasmacytosis >10%	90

Source: *Williams Hematology*, 8th ed, Chap. 109, Table 109–4, p. 1651.

— Patients who achieved complete remission and subsequently relapsed had an inferior outcome to patients who never attained complete remission.
• In another study, bortezomib was combined with 4-days of oral dexamethasone, daily thalidomide, and 4 days of continuous-infusion cisplatin, doxorubicin, cyclophosphamide, and etoposide (DT PACE).
— Unprecedented high overall survival, event-free survival, and duration of complete remission when compared with other studies.
— An anticipated cure fraction in the order of 50 percent in the 85 percent of patients who have a low-risk gene-expression profile.
— Del 17p was the only adverse cytogenetic feature for patients with this regimen.

Therapy for the Transplantation-Ineligible Patient
• The traditional age limit for autotransplantation is 65 years, although elderly patients should be considered for transplantation provided they have good organ function.
• The standard of care for elderly patients is melphalan and prednisone (MP).
• Four randomized controlled trials suggest that melphalan, prednisone, and thalidomide (MPT) provide significant benefit compared with MP alone.
— The combination of bortezomib (Velcade), melphalan, and prednisone (VMP) may be an alternative initial regimen in elderly patients.
— The trial showed a complete remission of approximately 30 percent and partial remission of approximately 90 percent with an overall survival at approximately 15 months reaching 90 percent, which was significantly better than MP-treated historical controls (66%).
• Lenalidomide, bortezomib, and dexamethasone combination therapy in patients with newly diagnosed myeloma provided a partial response rate of 100 percent with approximately 75 percent achieving a very good partial response rate or better in one study.
— With a median follow-up of 21 months, the estimated 18-month progression-free and overall survival for the combination treatment with or without stem cell transplantation was 75 percent and 97 percent, respectively.
• Bortezomib can cause peripheral neuropathy, transient cytopenias, or herpes zoster reactivation. The latter necessitates antiviral prophylaxis.
• The combination of melphalan, prednisone, and lenalidomide may also be useful as initial management of elderly patient.
— A study reported a complete response rate of approximately 25 percent with an event-free survival at 1 year at approximately 90 percent.
• In patients with preexistent polyneuropathy, it is probably wise to avoid bortezomib and thalidomide, whereas lenalidomide may be less suitable for patients with renal impairment.
• In patients with preexisting thromboembolism, thalidomide and lenalidomide are best avoided. The presence of cytogenetic abnormalities would favor the use of VMP or perhaps melphalan, lenalidomide, and prednisone.
• The combination of thalidomide and dexamethasone was superior to dexamethasone alone.
• Patients who have had prior thalidomide exposure should probably best be treated with one of the other novel agents.
• The combination of lenalidomide and dexamethasone had activity in both bortezomib-naïve and previously treated patients.
• The randomized phase III APEX study found a median overall survival of 30 months in the bortezomib group versus 24 months in the dexamethasone group.
• The choice of therapy for relapsed or refractory patients depends on a number of factors, including time since last therapy; prior exposure to novel agents, alone or in combination; and drug-induced comorbidities, for example, neuropathy, renal malfunction, and loss of patient physiologic reserve.
— The most important predictor of outcome at the time of relapse was the 70-gene risk score.

- High-risk relapse, usually characterized by rapid if not explosive myeloma growth, has a poor prognosis, requiring immediate reinduction with a potent combination regimen, such as VTD-PACE, followed by salvage transplantation, especially in patients who have obtained more than 3 years benefit from their initial transplants.

Allogeneic Hematopoietic Stem Cell Transplantation (Allo-HSCT)

- Early experience with myeloablative allogeneic transplantation has not been encouraging because of a high mortality, varying from 30 to 50 percent.
- In order to combine the cytoreductive effect of high-dose therapy with the benefit of the graft-versus-myeloma (GVM) effect, a single auto-HSCT was used initially, followed approximately 3 months later with a reduced intensity allograft, a concept also referred to as a tandem auto-"mini"-allograft.
  — There are no studies comparing tandem auto-HSCT prospectively with tandem auto-"mini"-allografting.
- Significant morbidity and mortality with a posttransplantation mortality of 11 to 18 percent with chronic graft-versus-host disease (GVHD) occurring in 43 to 74 percent of patients.
- GVHD did not protect from relapse.
- Nearly two-thirds of patients who had normal metaphase cytogenetics, implying good-risk disease, were alive at 7 years.
- Tandem auto-"mini"-allografting should be limited to patients with high-risk disease in whom higher initial morbidity and mortality may be more acceptable.
- Chromosomal alterations del 13 or del 17p are associated with poor outcome for patients receiving an allograft.
- Good-risk patients will do exceeding well with current auto-HSCT approaches, especially when combined with novel drugs, making it difficult to justify subjecting such patients to allografting.
- Routine allografting for myeloma cannot be recommended for high-risk patients.

Monitoring Disease Markers for Documentation of Response and Relapse

- The criteria for assessing response developed by the European Bone Marrow Transplant Registry have been supplanted by a new system for evaluating response, the International Uniform Response Criteria proposed by the International Myeloma Working Group (see Table 69–8).
- Survival endpoints include progression-free survival, event-free survival, and disease-free survival.
- Stable disease is no longer used as a measure of treatment efficacy.
- Duration of a response is calculated from the onset of response and only counts the subgroup of responding patients.
- Disease features can change with successive relapses: clonal evolution occurs, resulting in loss of previously secreted complete immunoglobulin and switch to only light-chain secretion ("Bence Jones escape") or entire loss of immunoglobulin-secretory capacity, often associated with extramedullary spread, best signified by increased LDH levels and lesions found on CT-PET examination.
  — Occasionally, unexplained anemia or pancytopenia accompanies disappearing myeloma protein markers, necessitating prompt marrow examination to detect fulminant relapse.
- Monthly determinations of myeloma protein should be performed during induction therapy.
- After two to four induction cycles and prior to high-dose melphalan-based auto-HSCT, the disease should be restaged, including marrow examination with cytogenetics and MRI and/or CT-PET of indicator lesions.

TABLE 69–8	UNIFORM RESPONSE CRITERIA FROM THE INTERNATIONAL MYELOMA WORKING GROUP

Response Subcategory*	Response Criteria
CR	Negative immunofixation of the serum and urine and disappearance of any soft-tissue plasmacytomas and <5% plasma cells in marrow.†
sCR	CR as defined above plus Normal FLC ratio and Absence of clonal cells in marrow† by immunohistochemistry or immunofluorescence.‡
VGPR	Serum and urine M-component detectable by immunofixation but not on electrophoresis or 90 or greater reduction in serum M-component plus urine M-component <100 mg per 24 h.
PR	>50% reduction of serum M-protein and reduction in 24-h urinary M-protein by >90% or to <200 mg per 24 h. If the serum and urine M-protein are unmeasurable, >50% decrease in the difference between involved and uninvolved FLC levels is required in place of the monoclonal Ig criteria. If serum and urine monoclonal Ig are unmeasurable, and serum-free light assay is also unmeasurable, >50% reduction in plasma cells is required in place of M-protein, provided baseline marrow plasma cell percentage was >30%. In addition to the above listed criteria, if present at baseline, a >50% reduction in the size of soft-tissue plasmacytomas is also required. Not meeting criteria for CR, VGPR, PR, or progressive disease.

CR, complete response; FLC, free light chain; PR, partial response; sCR, stringent complete response; SD, stable disease; VGPR, very good partial response.

*All response categories require two consecutive assessments made at any time before the institution of any new therapy; CR and PR and SD categories also require no known evidence of progressive or new bone lesions if radiographic studies were performed. Radiographic studies are not required to satisfy these response requirements.

†Confirmation with repeat marrow biopsy not needed.

‡Presence/absence of clonal cells is based upon the κ/λ of >4:1 or <1:2. Alternatively, the absence of clonal plasma cells can be defined based on the investigation of phenotypically aberrant plasma cells. The sensitivity level is 10^3 (less than on phenotypically aberrant plasma within a total of 1000 plasma cells). Examples of aberrant phenotypes include (1) CD38+^{dim} and CD56+^{strong}, CD19−, and CD45−; (2) CD38+^{dim}, CD138+, CD56++, and CD28+; (3) CD138+, CD19−, CD56++, and CD117+.

NOTE: SD is not recommended for use as an indicator of response; stability of disease is best described by providing the time-to-progression estimates.

Source: *Williams Hematology*, 8th ed, Chap. 109, Table 109–8, p. 1670.

— Such restaging should determine whether intramedullary or extramedullary disease has been reduced.

• Disease monitoring should be performed at least every month for the first year and at a minimum every other month thereafter.

Prognosis

• The prognosis of myeloma is determined by three factors:
  — Patient factors (e.g., age, comorbid conditions).
  — Tumor biology and disease burden (e.g., intrinsic cell drug sensitivity).
  — Type of therapy applied (e.g., newer thalidomide derivatives and proteasome inhibitors).

• Cytogenetic findings associated with poor outcome include:
  — Hypodiploidy and deletions 13q and 17p13.
  — Mutations at locus of the tumor-suppressor gene *TP53*.

— Gains and translocations of chromosome 1 are associated with more aggressive and more advanced myeloma.
— Gain of the 1q21 region (amp1q21) increases from approximately 40 percent at diagnosis to 70 percent at relapse.
  • Both the proportion of cells with 1q21 and the copy number increases at relapse, suggesting the existence of a gene-dosage effect involved in drug resistance.
  • The gene *CKS1B* located at 1q21 controls the G1 to S transition of the cell cycle and has been linked to shorter progression-free survival after auto-HSCT.
• Hyperdiploidy, which accounts for almost half of the patients with abnormal cytogenetics and involves nonrandom gains of chromosomes 3, 5, 7, 9, 11, 15, 19, and 21, is associated with chemosensitive disease and better overall survival.
• Translocation t(11;14) also confers a better outcome.
• Interphase FISH does not depend on cycling cells and can detect abnormal cells in as many as 80 to 90 percent of cases.
— FISH can also detect cytogenetically silent translocations.
• In the Eastern Cooperative Oncology Group, three distinct prognostic groups were recognized in patients treated with conventional chemotherapy:
— A poor prognosis was typified by t(4;14) and/or t(14;16) and/or del 17p.
— An intermediate prognosis by del 13q, but without t(4;14),t(14;16) or del 17p.
— A good prognosis group who have t(11;14) or no abnormalities.
• Del 13q, t(4;14), and del 17p all are associated with short event-free and overall survival.
• On multivariate analysis, only del 17p and t(4;14) independently predicted for event-free survival and overall survival.

SPECIAL DISEASE MANIFESTATIONS

IgM Myeloma
• IgM myeloma is distinct from Waldenström macroglobulinemia (see Chap. 70).
• Plasma cells, rather than the lymphoplasmacytic infiltrate, are seen to dominate the marrow of myeloma.
• DNA-aneuploidy and the presence of lytic bone lesions support a diagnosis of myeloma.

Solitary Plasmacytoma
• Solitary plasmacytoma of bone or soft tissue requires the absence of indicators of systemic disease, such as marrow plasmacytosis, anemia, or other lytic or soft-tissue lesions.
• Radiation therapy at doses of 40 to 50 Gy to the plasmacytoma.
— Approximately 50 percent of patients with solitary plasmacytoma have low monoclonal immunoglobulin levels in serum or urine and these typically disappear with radiation treatment.
• CT is recommended for evaluation of early bone disease.
• The detection of a solitary MRI lesion (cytologically proven) in the setting of essential monoclonal gammopathy changes the diagnosis to solitary plasmacytoma.
• In contrast to most patients with plasma cell myeloma, patients with solitary plasmacytoma or essential monoclonal gammopathy have normal serum immunoglobulin levels.
• Multiple solitary plasmacytomas may be seen at the outset as a result of advanced imaging by MRI and PET, or these may develop over time in approximately 5 percent of patients with apparently solitary plasmacytoma (see Table 69–9).
• Random marrow examinations should be negative.
• Patients with soft-tissue solitary plasmacytomas can often be cured with appropriate local radiation (dose of at least 4.5 Gy).

TABLE 69–9	MULTIPLE SOLITARY PLASMACYTOMAS (± RECURRENT)

No monoclonal immunoglobulin in serum and/or urine*

More than one localized area of bone destruction or extramedullary tumor of clonal plasma cells which may be recurrent

Normal marrow

Normal skeletal survey and magnetic resonance image of spine and pelvis if done

No related organ or tissue impairment (no end organ damage other than the localized bone lesions)

*A small monoclonal immunoglobulin may sometimes be present.
Reproduced with permission from The International Myeloma Working Group. Criteria for the classification of monoclonal gammopathies, multiple myeloma and related disorders: a report of the International Myeloma Working Group. *Br J Haematol* 121:749, 2003 (Table IX). Source: *Williams Hematology*, 8th ed, Chap. 109, Table 109–9, p. 1671.

- By contrast, this local treatment approach fails in the majority of patients with solitary plasmacytomas of bone.
- Local radiation, typically administered with high-dose dexamethasone, also has a palliative role for the treatment of focal lesions.

AL Amyloidosis

- When clinical features of congestive heart failure, nephrotic syndrome, malabsorption, coagulopathy, skin rash (oral mucosal rash, "raccoon's eyes") or neuropathy are present, a careful search for primary amyloidosis should be carried out (see Chap. 72).

Smoldering Myeloma

- Smoldering myeloma is a form of myeloma in which there is no evidence of end-organ damage at diagnosis.
- Smoldering disease progresses to active myeloma in over 80 percent of patients followed for 25 years.
- The risk of progression to myeloma is correlated with the proportion of plasma cells in the marrow (greater or less than 10%) and the height of the monoclonal immunoglobulin (greater than or less than 3.0 g/dL)
- Whereas the progression of essential monoclonal gammopathy to a progressive disease B-cell neoplasm is linear over 25 years of observation (1%/year), the risk of progression of smoldering myeloma decreases with time: 10 percent/year in the first 5 years, 3 percent/year in the next 5 years, and 1 percent/year in the next 5 years.
- Patients with smoldering myeloma have historically been monitored without therapy until evidence of progression.
- Once the diagnosis is established, through careful monitoring of disease markers over the duration of 2 to 3 months, these patients have been treated with thalidomide plus bisphosphonate therapy at some institutions.

EMERGENT COMPLICATIONS OF NEW MYELOMA THERAPY

- Patients with myeloma are at an increased risk for deep venous thrombosis and pulmonary embolism.
  — Particularly when known risk factors are present: history of prior venous thromboembolism (VTE), immobilization, and/or dehydration.
- The incidence of VTE is highest during the first 3 to 4 months following diagnosis and occurs in approximately 3 to 4 percent of patients receiving either dexamethasone alone or MP, but is much higher when newer agents are combined with dexamethasone and melphalan.

— A number of procoagulant abnormalities have been described in myeloma, including endothelial damage, paraprotein interference with fibrin structure, elevated von Willebrand multimers, elevated factor VIII, decreased protein S, and acquired activated protein C resistance.

- The incidence of VTE with single-agent thalidomide is approximately 2 to 4 percent in newly diagnosed and in relapsed patients, comparable to that observed with dexamethasone alone or MP, implying that thalidomide alone does not increase the risk of VTE.
  — However, the risk for VTE increases significantly when thalidomide is combined with either dexamethasone, melphalan, doxorubicin, or cyclophosphamide, or with other multiagent chemotherapy.
  — Most VTEs occur within the first 60 days of therapy.
- Single-agent lenalidomide does not appear to increase VTE, at least not in the setting of myeloma relapse, but is associated with a marked increased in VTE risk when lenalidomide is combined with dexamethasone.
- Bortezomib did not seem to increase the risk of VTE.
- Prevention of VTE is based on the assessment for known risk factors for VTE:
  — Myeloma-related (hyperviscosity, newly diagnosed status).
  — Therapy-related (high-dose dexamethasone [≥480 mg/month], doxorubicin, multiagent chemotherapy).
  — Individual factors (age, history of VTE, inherited thrombophilia, obesity, immobilization, central venous line, infections, surgery, administration of erythropoietin).
  — Factors related to comorbidities (acute infection, diabetes mellitus, cardiac or renal dysfunction).
- Therapy-related risks factor most in the risk-equation of VTE.
- The following thromboprophylaxis is recommended:
  — Acetylsalicylic acid (aspirin) in either a standard dose of 325 mg/day or in a low-dose of 81 mg/day for patients with one or no risk factor.
  — Low-molecular-weight heparin (LMWH) once a day, or full-dose warfarin for patients if two or more risk factors or therapy-related risks are present.
- The recommended duration of prophylaxis in general is 6 to 12 months.
- Long-term prophylaxis may be indicated in some patients.

Peripheral Neuropathy

- Bortezomib and thalidomide-induced peripheral neuropathy should be distinguished from other causes, such as paraneoplastic neuropathies, antecedent chemotherapy with neurotoxic agents (vincristine or cisplatinum), diabetes mellitus, or AL amyloidosis.
- If significant weakness or asymmetry of signs is present, a neurologic consultation must be obtained along with electromyography and nerve conduction studies.
- Second-generation, more selective proteasome inhibitors such as carfilzomib may have reduced neurotoxicity.
- Lenalidomide when combined with bortezomib may have a neuroprotective effect.
- Symptomatic treatment for thalidomide- and bortezomib-induced neuropathy usually comprises gabapentin, pregabalin, or tricyclic antidepressants.

Bisphosphonates

- Bisphosphonates are synthetic, stable analogues of inorganic pyrophosphate.
- The most commonly used bisphosphonates in myeloma are pamidronate and zoledronic acid.
- Most experts currently recommend 2 years of bisphosphonate therapy with extended therapy for selected patients with active bone disease.

Osteonecrosis of the Jaw

- Osteonecrosis of the jaw (ONJ) is a severe "bone" disease, associated with bisphosphonate therapy that affects the jaws and typically presents as infection with necrotic bone in the mandible or maxilla.
- ONJ usually presents as pain and/or numbness in the affected area, soft-tissue swelling, drainage, and tooth mobility.
- Risk of developing ONJ increases with duration of bisphosphonate exposure and is 5 to 15 percent at 4 years.
- A further predisposing factor for ONJ is invasive dental procedures such as extractions.
- Approximately 50 percent of affected patients had dental work prior to developing ONJ.
- To prevent ONJ, patients should be referred for dental evaluation prior to commencing intravenous bisphosphonates and should be advised to maintain excellent oral hygiene and avoid dental procedures while receiving these agents.
- Antibiotic prophylaxis before dental procedures may reduce the incidence of ONJ in patients receiving bisphosphonate therapy.
- Patients who had developed spontaneous ONJ have a significantly higher risk of nonhealing and ONJ recurrence.

For a more detailed discussion, see Frits van Rhee, Elias Anaissie, Edgardo Angtuaco, Twyla Bartel, Joshua Epstein, Bijay Nair, John Shaughnessy, Shmuel Yaccoby, Bart Barlogie: Myeloma. Chap. 109, p. 1645 in *Williams Hematology*, 8th ed.

CHAPTER 70
Macroglobulinemia

DEFINITION

- Waldenström macroglobulinemia (WM) is a lymphoid neoplasm resulting from the accumulation, predominantly in the marrow, of a clonal population of lymphocytes, lymphoplasmacytic cells, and plasma cells, which secrete a monoclonal immunoglobulin (Ig) M.
- WM corresponds to lymphoplasmacytic lymphoma (LPL) as defined in the Revised European-American Lymphoma (REAL) and World Health Organization classification systems.
- Most cases of LPL are WM; less than 5 percent of cases are IgA-secreting, IgG-secreting, or nonsecreting LPL.

EPIDEMIOLOGY

- The age-adjusted incidence rate of WM is 3.4 per 1 million among males and 1.7 per 1 million among females in the United States.
- The incidence rate is higher among Americans of European descent. Americans of African descent represent approximately 5 percent of all patients.
- Approximately 20 percent of patients are of Eastern European descent, specifically of Ashkenazi-Jewish ethnic background.
- Approximately 20 percent of 257 sequential patients with WM presenting to a tertiary referral center had a first-degree relative with either WM or another B-cell disorder.

PATHOGENESIS

Cytogenetic Findings

- Loss of all or part of chromosomes 17, 18, 19, 20, 21, 22, X, and Y have been commonly observed, and gains in chromosomes 3, 4, and 12 also occur.
- Chromosome 6q deletions encompassing 6q21–25 have been observed in up to half of WM patients.

Nature of the Tumor Cell

- The marrow B-cells in WM undergo maturation from small lymphocytes with large focal deposits of surface immunoglobulins, to lymphoplasmacytic cells or to plasma cells that contain intracytoplasmic immunoglobulins.

CLINICAL FEATURES

- Table 70–1 lists clinical and laboratory features at the time of diagnosis for 356 patients in a large study.
- Presenting symptoms most commonly are fatigue, weakness, weight loss, episodic bleeding, and manifestations of the hyperviscosity syndrome.
- Physical findings include:
    — Lymphadenopathy.
    — Hepatosplenomegaly.
    — Dependent purpura and mucosal bleeding.
    — Dilated tortuous retinal veins.
    — Multiple flesh-colored papules on extensor surfaces (deposits of IgM reacting to epidermal basement membrane antigens).

TABLE 70–1	CLINICAL AND LABORATORY FINDINGS FOR 356 CONSECUTIVE NEWLY DIAGNOSED PATIENTS WITH WALDENSTRÖM MACROGLOBULINEMIA

	Median	Range	Normal Reference Range
Age (years)	58	32–91	NA
Gender (male/female)	215/141		NA
Marrow involvement (% of area on slide)	30	5–95	NA
Adenopathy (% of patients)	15		NA
Splenomegaly (% of patients)	10		NA
IgM (mg/dL)	2620	270–12,400	40–230
igG (mg/dL)	674	80–2770	700–1600
IgA (mg/dL)	58	6–438	70–400
Serum viscosity (cp)	2.0	1.1–7.2	1.4–1.9
Hematocrit (%)	35	17–45	35–44
Platelet count ($\times 10^9$/L)	275	42–675	155–410
White cell count ($\times 10^9$/L)	6.4	1.7–22	3.8–9.2
β_2M (mg/dL)	2.5	0.9–13.7	0–2.7
LDH (U/mL)	313	61–1701	313–618

β_2M, β_2-microglobulin; cp, centipoise; LDH, lactic acid dehydrogenase; NA, not applicable.
Source: *Williams Hematology*, 8th ed, Chap. 111, Table 111–1, p. 1697.

— Peripheral sensory neuropathy.
— Raynaud phenomenon, especially upon exposure to cold.
— Splenomegaly and lymphadenopathy are uncommon.

Morbidity Mediated by the Effects of IgM
- Table 70–2 lists the physiochemical and immunologic properties of the monoclonal IgM Protein.

The Hyperviscosity Syndrome
- Symptoms usually occur when the monoclonal IgM concentration exceeds 50 g/L or when serum viscosity is >4.0 centipoises (cp) but can occur at lower serum concentrations of IgM.
- Presence of cryoglobulins contributes to increasing blood viscosity, as well as to the tendency to induce erythrocyte aggregation.
- Frequent symptoms are headache; impaired vision; mental status changes, such as confusion or dementia; altered consciousness that may progress to coma; ataxia; or nystagmus.
- Ophthalmoscopic changes include link-sausage appearance of retinal veins, retinal hemorrhages, and papilledema and/or distended and tortuous retinal veins, hemorrhages, and papilledema.
- Congestive heart failure may develop, particularly in the elderly.

TABLE 70–2   **PHYSICOCHEMICAL AND IMMUNOLOGIC PROPERTIES OF THE MONOCLONAL IGM PROTEIN IN WALDENSTRÖM MACROGLOBULINEMIA**

Properties of IgM Monoclonal Protein	Diagnostic Condition	Clinical Manifestations
Pentameric structure	Hyperviscosity	Headaches, blurred vision, epistaxis, retinal hemorrhages, leg cramps, impaired mentation, intracranial hemorrhage
Precipitation on cooling	Cryoglobulinemia (type I)	Raynaud phenomenon, acrocyanosis, ulcers, purpura, cold urticaria
Autoantibody activity to myelin-associated glycoprotein, ganglioside M_1, sulfatide moieties on peripheral nerve sheaths	Peripheral neuropathies	Sensorimotor neuropathies, painful neuropathies, ataxic gait, bilateral foot drop
Autoantibody activity to IgG	Cryoglobulinemia (type II)	Purpura, arthralgia, renal failure, sensorimotor neuropathies
Autoantibody activity to red blood cell antigens	Cold agglutinins	Hemolytic anemia, Raynaud phenomenon, acrocyanosis, livedo reticularis
Tissue deposition as amorphous aggregates	Organ dysfunction	Skin: bullous skin disease, papules, Schnitzler syndrome Gastrointestinal: diarrhea, malabsorption, bleeding Kidney: proteinuria, renal failure (light-chain component)
Tissue deposition as amyloid fibrils (light-chain component most commonly)	Organ dysfunction	Fatigue, weight loss, edema, hepatomegaly, macroglossia, organ dysfunction of involved organs (heart, kidney, liver, peripheral sensory and autonomic nerves)

Source: *Williams Hematology,* 8th ed, Chap. 111, Table 111–2, p. 1697.

- Inappropriate red cell transfusion can exacerbate hyperviscosity and may precipitate cardiac failure.

Cryoglobulinemia

- The monoclonal IgM can behave as a cryoglobulin (type I) in up to 20 percent of patients.
- Symptoms result from impaired blood flow in small vessels and include Raynaud phenomenon, acrocyanosis, and necrosis of the regions most exposed to cold, such as the tip of the nose, ears, fingers, and toes.

IgM-Related Neuropathy

- Peripheral neuropathy occurs in up to 40 percent of cases.
- The nerve damage is mediated by diverse pathogenetic mechanisms:
  — IgM antibody activity toward nerve constituents causing demyelinating polyneuropathies.
  — Endoneurial granulofibrillar deposits of IgM without antibody activity, associated with axonal polyneuropathy.
  — Tubular deposits in the endoneurium associated with IgM cryoglobulin.
  — Amyloid deposits or neoplastic cell infiltration of nerve structures is less common.
- Half of patients with IgM neuropathy may have a distinctive clinical syndrome that is associated with antibodies against a minor 100-kDa glycoprotein component of nerve, myelin-associated glycoprotein (MAG).
  — The anti–MAG related neuropathy is typically distal and symmetrical, affecting both motor and sensory functions; it is slowly progressive with a long period of stability.
  — Most patients present with sensory complaints; imbalance and gait ataxia, owing to lack of proprioception; and leg muscles atrophy in advanced stages.
- Patients with monoclonal IgM to gangliosides may have a demyelinating sensory neuropathy with chronic ataxic neuropathy sometimes presenting with ophthalmoplegia.
  — Monoclonal IgM proteins that bind to gangliosides with a terminal trisaccharide moiety, including ganglioside M_2 (GM_2) and GalNac-GD1A, are associated with chronic demyelinating neuropathy and severe sensory ataxia, unresponsive to glucocorticoids.
- Anti-sulfatide monoclonal IgM proteins are associated with sensory-motor neuropathy.
- The POEMS syndrome (polyneuropathy, organomegaly, endocrinopathy, M protein, and skin changes) is rare in patients with WM.

Cold Agglutinin Hemolytic Anemia (see Chap. 25)

- Monoclonal IgM may be cold agglutinins with binding activity for cell antigens at temperatures below 37 °C, producing chronic hemolytic anemia (see Chap. 25).
  — This disorder occurs in <10 percent of WM patients.
  — It is associated with cold agglutinin titers greater than 1:1000 in most cases.
  — Mild to moderate chronic hemolytic anemia can be exacerbated after cold exposure.
  — The agglutination of red cells in the skin circulation also causes Raynaud syndrome, acrocyanosis, and livedo reticularis.

IgM Tissue Deposition

- The monoclonal protein can deposit in several tissues as amorphous aggregates.
- Amorphous deposits in the dermis are referred to as macroglobulinemia cutis.
- Deposition of monoclonal IgM in the lamina propria and/or submucosa of the intestine may be associated with diarrhea, malabsorption, and gastrointestinal bleeding.
- The incidence of cardiac and pulmonary involvement is higher in patients with monoclonal IgM than with other immunoglobulin isotypes.

Manifestations Related to Tissue Infiltration by Neoplastic Cells

- Pulmonary involvement in the form of masses, nodules, diffuse infiltrate, or pleural effusions is uncommon; the overall incidence of pulmonary and pleural findings is approximately 4 percent.

- Malabsorption, diarrhea, bleeding, or gastrointestinal obstruction may indicate involvement of the gastrointestinal tract at the level of the stomach, duodenum, or small intestine.
- Skin
  — Can be the site of dense lymphoplasmacytic infiltrates, similar to that seen in the liver, spleen, and lymph nodes, forming cutaneous plaques and, rarely, nodules.
  — Chronic urticaria and IgM gammopathy are the two cardinal features of the Schnitzler syndrome, which is not usually associated initially with clinical features of WM although evolution to WM is not uncommon.

LABORATORY FINDINGS

- Anemia is the most common finding.
- Normocytic and normochromic anemia is present and rouleaux formation is often pronounced.
- Hemoglobin estimate can be inaccurate.
- Leukocyte and platelet counts are usually within the reference range at presentation.
- A raised erythrocyte sedimentation rate is almost always present.
- Thrombin time is often prolonged, and the prothrombin time and activated partial thromboplastin time may be prolonged.
- Serum levels of IgG and IgA are normal or low.

Marrow Findings

- Hypercellular, with diffuse infiltration of lymphocytes, plasmacytoid lymphocytes, and plasma cells (see **Fig. 70–1**).
- Contains lymphoid cells with monoclonal surface membrane and/or cytoplasmic immunoglobulin.

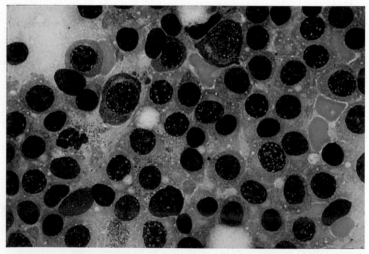

FIGURE 70–1 A Marrow film from a patient with Waldenström macroglobulinemia. Note infiltrate of mature lymphocytes, lymphoplasmacytic cells, and plasma cells.
(Reproduced with permission from Marvin J. Stone, MD.)
(Source: *Williams Hematology,* 8th ed, Chap. 111, Fig. 111–4, p. 1700.)

- Increased numbers of mast cells admixed with aggregates of malignant lymphocytes.
- A solely paratrabecular pattern of lymphocyte infiltration is unusual and should raise the possibility of follicular lymphoma.
- The lymphocyte immunoprofile is sIg+CD19+CD20+CD22+CD79+.
- In up to 20 percent of cases, the lymphocytes may also express CD5, CD10, or CD23.

Immunologic Abnormalities

- High-resolution electrophoresis combined with immunofixation of serum and urine is recommended for identification and characterization of the IgM monoclonal protein.
- Testing for cold agglutinins and cryoglobulins should be performed at diagnosis.
  - If present, subsequent serum samples should be analyzed at 37 °C for determination of serum monoclonal IgM level.
  - Although Bence Jones proteinuria is frequently present, it exceeds 1 g/24 h in only 3 percent of cases. Whereas IgM levels are elevated in WM patients, IgA and IgG levels are most often depressed and do not recover after successful treatment.

Serum Viscosity

- Serum viscosity should be measured if the patient has signs or symptoms of hyperviscosity syndrome.
- Among the first clinical signs of hyperviscosity are the appearance of peripheral and midperipheral dot and blot-like hemorrhages in the retina.
- In more severe cases of hyperviscosity, dot, blot, and flame-shaped hemorrhages can appear in the macular area along with markedly dilated and tortuous veins with focal constrictions resulting in "venous sausaging," as well as papilledema.

RADIOLOGIC FINDINGS

- Marrow involvement can be documented by MRI studies of the spine in more than 90 percent of patients.
- CT of the abdomen and pelvis demonstrates enlarged nodes in approximately 40 percent of WM patients.

RESPONSE CRITERIA IN WM (See Table 70-3)

- Major response: >50 percent decrease in serum Ig level.
- Minor response: based on ≥25 to <50 percent decrease in serum IgM level.
- An important concern with the use of IgM as a surrogate marker of disease is that it can fluctuate, independent of extent of tumor cell killing, particularly with newer biologically targeted agents such as rituximab and bortezomib.

TREATMENT

- Initiation of therapy should not be based on the IgM level *per se*, as this may not correlate with the clinical manifestations of WM.
- Initiation of therapy is appropriate for patients with constitutional symptoms, such as recurrent fever, night sweats, fatigue as a consequence of anemia, or weight loss.
  - Progressive symptomatic lymphadenopathy or splenomegaly provide additional reasons to begin therapy.
  - Anemia with a hemoglobin value of ≤10 g/dL or a platelet count of ≤100 × 10^9/L owing to marrow infiltration, also justifies treatment.
- Plasmapheresis is used to help manage the hyperviscosity syndrome.

TABLE 70–3	SUMMARY OF UPDATED RESPONSE CRITERIA FROM THE 3RD INTERNATIONAL WORKSHOP ON WALDENSTRÖM MACROGLOBULINEMIA
Complete response (CR)	Disappearance of monoclonal protein by immunofixation; no histologic evidence of marrow involvement, and resolution of any adenopathy/organomegaly (confirmed by CT scan), along with no signs or symptoms attributable to WM. Reconfirmation of the CR status is required at least 6 weeks apart with a second immunofixation.
Partial response (PR)	A ≥50% reduction of serum monoclonal IgM concentration on protein electrophoresis and a decrease in adenopathy/organomegaly on physical examination or on CT scan. No new symptoms or signs of active disease.
Minor response (MR)	A ≥25% but <50% reduction of serum monoclonal IgM by protein electrophoresis. No new symptoms or signs of active disease.
Stable disease (SD)	A <25% reduction and <25% increase of serum monoclonal IgM by electrophoresis without progression of adenopathy/organomegaly, cytopenias, or clinically significant symptoms because of disease and/or signs of WM.
Progressive disease (PD)	A ≥25% increase in serum monoclonal IgM by protein electrophoresis confirmed by a second measurement or progression of clinically significant findings because of disease (i.e., anemia, thrombocytopenia, leukopenia, bulky adenopathy/organomegaly) or symptoms (unexplained recurrent fever ≥38.4°C, drenching night sweats, ≥10mL/kg loss, or hyperviscosity, neuropathy, symptomatic cryoglobulinemia or amyloidosis) attributable to WM.

Source: *Williams Hematology,* 8th ed, Chap. 111, Table 111–3, p. 1704.

Initial Therapy

- Alkylating agents (e.g., chlorambucil), nucleoside analogues (cladribine or fludarabine), the monoclonal antibody rituximab, as well as combinations are considered reasonable choices for the initial therapy of WM.
- Exposure to alkylating agents or nucleoside analogues should be minimized in patients who are candidates for autologous stem cell transplantation, which typically is reserved for those younger than 70 years of age.

Alkylating Agents Therapy

- Chlorambucil has been administered on both a continuous (i.e., daily dose schedule) and an intermittent schedule.
  — Oral chlorambucil on a continuous schedule: Orally 0.1 mg/kg per day, every 6 weeks.

— Oral chlorambucil on an intermittent schedule: Orally 0.3 mg/kg per day for 7 days once every 6 weeks.
- Median response duration was greater for patients receiving intermittent- versus continuous-dose chlorambucil (46 vs. 26 months).
- Chlorambucil (8 mg/m^2) plus prednisone (40 mg/m^2) given orally for 10 days, every 6 weeks, resulted in a major response (i.e., reduction of IgM by more than 50%) in 72 percent of patients.
- Pretreatment factors associated with shorter survival in the entire population of patients receiving single-agent chlorambucil are:
  — Patients older than 60 years, male sex, hemoglobin less than 10 g/dL, leukocytes less than 4×10^9/L, and platelets less than 150×10^9/L.

Nucleoside Analogue Therapy

- Cladribine, administered as a single agent by continuous intravenous infusion, by 2-hour daily infusion, or by subcutaneous bolus injections for 5 to 7 days result in major responses in 40 to 90 percent of patients who received primary therapy, whereas in the previously treated patients, responses ranged from 38 to 54 percent.
- Fludarabine (25 mg/m^2 for 5 days) administered every 28 days to previously untreated or treated patients, resulted in an overall response rate of 38 to 100 percent or 30 to 40 percent, respectively.
- Major toxicities of nucleoside analogue therapy are myelosuppression and T-cell depletion, resulting in increased risk for opportunistic infections.
- Factors predicting a better response to nucleoside analogues:
  — Younger age at the start of treatment (<70 years).
  — Higher pretreatment hemoglobin (>9.5 g/dL).
  — Higher platelet count (>75 × 10^9/L).
  — Disease that does not relapse while on therapy.
  — A long interval between first-line therapy and initiation of a nucleoside analogue in for relapsed disease.
- Harvesting autologous blood stem cells succeeds on the first attempt in most patients who did not receive nucleoside analogue therapy, compared with as few as one-third of patients who received a nucleoside analogue.

CD20-Directed Antibody Therapy

- Rituximab is a chimeric monoclonal antibody that targets CD20, a widely expressed antigen on lymphoplasmacytic cells in WM.
- Standard doses of rituximab (i.e., four once-weekly infusions of 375 mg/m^2) induced major responses in approximately 30 percent of previously treated or untreated patients.
- The median time to treatment failure with rituximab ranged from 8 to over 27 months.
- A transient increase of serum IgM may be noted immediately following initiation of treatment with rituximab in many WM patients.
  — The increase in IgM following initiation of therapy with rituximab does not portend treatment failure and most patients return to their baseline IgM level by 12 weeks.
  — Plasmapheresis should be considered in these patients in advance of rituximab therapy.
- Rituximab should not be used as sole therapy for the treatment of patients at risk for hyperviscosity symptoms.
- Time to response to rituximab therapy exceeds 3 months on the average.
- Patients with baseline serum IgM levels of <60 g/L are more likely to respond.
- The objective response rate was significantly lower in patients who had either low serum albumin (<35 g/L) or a serum monoclonal protein greater than 40 g/L.

- Patients who had normal serum albumin and relatively low serum monoclonal protein levels derived a substantial benefit from rituximab with a time to progression exceeding 40 months.

Combination Therapies

- A regimen of rituximab, cladribine, and cyclophosphamide used in previously untreated patients resulted in a partial response in approximately 95 percent of WM patients.
- The combination of rituximab and fludarabine led to an overall response rate of 95 percent, with 83 percent of patients achieving a major response.
  — The median time to progression was 51 months.
- The combination of rituximab, dexamethasone, and cyclophosphamide achieved a major response in 74 percent of patients on this study, and the 2-year progression-free survival was 67 percent.
- A study using cyclophosphamide, doxorubicin, vincristine, prednisone (CHOP) in combination with rituximab (R-CHOP) achieved a major response in 77 percent of patients with relapsed or refractory disease.
- One study using two cycles of oral cyclophosphamide with subcutaneous cladribine as initial therapy reported a partial response in 84 percent of patients and the median duration of response of 36 months.
- A study evaluating fludarabine plus cyclophosphamide reported a response in 78 percent of patients and median time to treatment failure of 27 months.
- Various combination therapy regimens:
  — Nucleoside analogues and alkylating agents.
  — Rituximab in combination with nucleoside analogues.
  — Rituximab, nucleoside analogues, plus alkylating agents.
  — Rituximab and cyclophosphamide-based therapy.

Therapy for Relapsed or Refractory Patients
Proteasome Inhibitor

- Bortezomib is a proteasome inhibitor that induces apoptosis of primary WM lymphoplasmacytic cells.
  — All but 1 of 27 patients with relapsed or refractory disease, who received up to eight cycles of bortezomib at 1.3 mg/m^2 on days 1, 4, 8, and 11, had a response.
  — The overall response rate was 85 percent, with 10 and 13 patients achieving a minor ($<25\%$) and major ($<50\%$) decrease in IgM level.
  — Responses occurred at median of 1.4 months.
  — The median time to progression for all responding patients in this study was 7.9 (range: 3–21.4+) months.
  — The most common grade III/IV toxicities were sensory neuropathies (22.2%), leukopenia (18.5%), neutropenia (14.8%), dizziness (11.1%), and thrombocytopenia (7.4%).
  — Major responses occurred in 6 out of 10 (60%) previously treated patients.
- The combination of bortezomib, dexamethasone, and rituximab as primary therapy in patients with WM resulted in an overall response rate of 96 percent, and a major response rate of 83 percent.
  — The incidence of grade 3 neuropathy was approximately 30 percent but was reversible in most patients following discontinuation of therapy.

CD52-Directed Antibody Therapy

- Alemtuzumab is a humanized monoclonal antibody that targets CD52, an antigen expressed on marrow lymphoplasmacytic cells in WM patients, as well as on mast cells, which are increased in the marrow of patients with WM.

- Patients received three daily test doses of alemtuzumab (3, 10, and 30 mg intravenously) followed by 30 mg alemtuzumab intravenously three times a week for up to 12 weeks.
  — Among 25 patients evaluable for response, the overall response rate was 76 percent, which included 8 (32%) major responders and 11 (44%) minor responders.
- High rates of response to alemtuzumab as salvage therapy have also been reported.

Thalidomide and Lenalidomide

- Thalidomide as a single agent, and in combination with dexamethasone and clarithromycin, was examined in patients with WM.
  — Dose escalation from the thalidomide start dose of 200 mg daily was hindered by development of side effects.
  — A higher thalidomide dose (200 mg orally daily) along with dexamethasone (40 g orally once a week) and clarithromycin (500 mg orally twice a day) achieved a response in only 2 of 10 previously treated patients.
- In a study of lenalidomide and rituximab in WM, patients were started on lenalidomide at 25 mg daily on a syncopated schedule in which therapy was administered for 3 weeks, followed by a 1-week pause for an intended duration of 48 weeks.
  — Patients received 1 week of therapy with lenalidomide, after which rituximab (375 mg/m^2) was administered once weekly on weeks 2 to 5, and again on weeks 13 to 16.
  — The overall and major response rates in this study were 50 and 25 percent, respectively, and the median time to progression for responders was 18.9 months.
  — Most patients continued to have anemia despite treatment with lenalidomide.

High-Dose Therapy and Autologous Hematopoietic Stem Cell Transplantation

- High-dose chemotherapy followed by autologous stem cell transplantation in WM patients, previously treated with a median of three (range: 1–5) prior regimens, was well tolerated with an improvement in response status observed for seven patients.
- WM patients who received autologous transplantation, which included primarily relapsed or refractory patients, the 5-year progression-free and overall survival rate was 61 and 33 percent, respectively.
- Chemosensitive disease at time of the autologous transplantation was the most important prognostic factor for nonrelapse mortality, response rate, and progression-free and overall survival.

COURSE AND PROGNOSIS

- Table 70–4 lists several scoring systems that have been proposed for WM.
- Median duration of survival is 5 to 10 years.
- Major negative prognostic factors:
  — Age older than 65 years.
  — Anemia.
  — Thrombocytopenia (platelet count of < 100 to 150 × 10^9/L) or neutropenia (< 1.5 × 10^9/L) as adverse prognostic factors.
  — Elevated serum β_2-microglobulin levels (> 30 g/L).
  — Level of monoclonal IgM protein.
  — The presence of cyroglobulins.

TABLE 70–4 **PROGNOSTIC SCORING SYSTEMS IN WALDENSTRÖM MACROGLOBULINEMIA**

Study*	Adverse Prognostic Factors	Number of Groups	Survival
Gobbi et al.	Hgb <9 g/dL	0–1 prognostic factors	Median: 48 months
	Age >70 years	2–4 prognostic factors	Median: 80 months
	Weight loss		
	Cryoglobulinemia		
Morel et al.	Age ≥65 years	0–1 prognostic factors	5-year: 87% of patients
	Albumin <4 g/dL	2 prognostic factors	5-year: 62%
	Number of cytopenias:	3–4 prognostic factors	5-year: 25%
	Hgb <12 g/dL		
	Platelets <150 × 10^9/L		
	WBC <4 × 10^9/L		
Dhodapkar et al.	β_2M ≥3 g/dL	β_2M <3 mg/dL + Hgb ≥12 g/dL	5-year: 87% of patients
	Hgb <12 g/dL	β_2M <3 mg/dL + Hgb <12 g/dL	5-year: 63%
	IgM <4 g/dL	β_2M ≥3 mg/dL + IgM ≥4 g/dL	5-year: 53%
		β_2M ≥3 mg/dL + IgM <4 g/dL	5-year: 21%
Application of International Staging System Criteria for Myeloma to WM Dimopoulos et al.	Albumin ≤3.5 g/dL	Albumin ≥3.5 g/dL + β_2M <3.5 mg/dL	Median: NR
	β_2M ≥3.5 mg/L	Albumin ≤3.5 g/dL + β_2M <3.5 or β_2M 3.5–5.5 mg/dL	Median: 116 months
		β_2M >5.5 mg/dL	Median: 54 months
International Prognostic Scoring System for WM Morel et al.	Age >65 year	0–1 prognostic factors (excluding age)	5 year: 87% of patients
	Hgb <11.5 g/dL	2 prognostic factors (or age >65 years)	5 year: 68%
	Platelets <100 × 10^9/L	3–5 prognostic factors	5 year: 36%
	b_2M >3 mg/L		
	IgM >7 g/dL		

β_2M, β_2-microbloulin; Hgb, hemoglobulin; NR, not reported; WBC, white blood cell count.
*Gobbi PG et al. *Blood* 83:2939, 1994. Morel P et al. *Blood* 96:852, 2000. Dhodapkar MV et al. *Blood* 98:41, 2001. Dimopoulos M et al. *Leuk Lymphoma* 45:1809, 2004. Anagnostopoulos A et al. *Clin Lymphoma Myeloma* 7:205, 2006. Morel P et al. *Blood* 113:4163, 2009.
Source: *Williams Hematology*, 8th ed, Chap. 111, Table 111–4, p. 1705.

For a more detailed discussion, see Steven P. Treon and Giampaolo Merlini: Macroglobulinemia. Chap. 111, p. 1695 in *Williams Hematology*, 8th ed.

CHAPTER 71
Heavy-Chain Diseases

DEFINITION

- The heavy-chain diseases (HCDs) are neoplastic disorders of B cells that produce monoclonal immunoglobulins (Ig) consisting of truncated heavy chains without attached light chains.
- The diagnosis is established from immunofixation of serum, urine, or secretory fluids in the case of α-HCD or from immunohistologic analysis of the proliferating lymphoplasmacytic cells in nonsecretory disease.
- In decreasing order of incidence, HCD involves synthesis of defective α, γ, or μ heavy chains.
- There is a high frequency of autoimmune disorders preceding or concurrent with the diagnosis of HCD, particularly γ HCD.
- Table 71–1 summarizes the clinical features of the three types of HCD.

ETIOLOGY AND PATHOGENESIS

- The etiology of γ-HCD and μ-HCD is unknown.
- In α-HCD, the lymphoplasmacytic infiltration of the intestinal mucosa is thought to be a response of the alimentary tract immune system to protracted luminal antigenic stimulation.

CLINICAL AND LABORATORY FEATURES

γ-HCD

- Median age at presentation is in the late sixties.
- Clinical features different from those of myeloma because renal disease and osteolytic lesions rarely occur.
- Has various clinical and pathologic features that can be divided into three broad categories:
  — Disseminated lymphoproliferative disease.
  — Localized proliferative disease: Approximately 25 percent of patients.
  — No apparent proliferative disease: Approximately 15 percent of patients.
- Most γ-HCD proteins are dimers of truncated heavy chains without associated light chains.
- The serum protein electrophoretic pattern is extremely variable, but a monoclonal peak is detected in over two-thirds of patients.
- The median value of the monoclonal spike at diagnosis in one study of 19 patients was 1.6 g/dL.
- The amount of HCD protein in the urine usually is small (<1 g/24 h), but may reach 20 g/24 h.
- Patients commonly have moderate, normochromic, normocytic anemia.
- Autoimmune hemolytic anemia has been reported.
- Bone lesions are rare.

α-HCD

- Defined by the recognition of truncated monoclonal α chains without associated light chains.
- Characteristic sharp spike of monoclonal gammopathy is not found on serum protein electrophoresis.

TABLE 71–1   SUMMARY OF FEATURES OF THE HEAVY-CHAIN DISEASES

Feature	Type of Heavy-Chain Disease		
	α	γ	μ
Year described	1968	1964	1969
Incidence	Rare	Very rare	Very rare
Age at diagnosis	Young adult (<30 years)	Older adult (60–70 years)	Older adult (50–60 years)
Demographics	Mediterranean region	Worldwide	Worldwide
Structurally abnormal monoclonal protein	IgA	IgG	IgM
MGUS phase	No	Rarely	Rarely
Urine monoclonal light chain	No	No	Yes
Urine abnormal heavy chain	Small amounts	Often present	Infrequent
Sites involved	Small intestine, mesenteric lymph nodes	Lymph nodes, marrow, spleen	Lymph nodes, marrow, liver, spleen
Pathology	Extranodal marginal zone lymphoma (MALT or IPSID)	Lymphoplasma-cytoid lymphoma	Small lymphocytic lymphoma, CLL
Associated diseases	Infection, malabsorption	Autoimmune diseases	None
Therapy	Antibiotics, chemotherapy	Chemotherapy	Chemotherapy

CLL, chronic lymphocytic leukemia; Ig, immunoglobulin; IPSID, immunoproliferative small intestinal disease; MALT, mucosa-associated lymphoid tissue; MGUS, monoclonal gammopathy of undetermined significance.

Adapted with permission from Witzig TE, Wahner-Roedler DL: Heavy chain disease. *Curr Treat Options Oncol* 3:247, 2002.

Source: *Williams Hematology*, 8th ed, Chap. 112, Table 112–1, p. 1710.

- Identification of the α-HCD protein depends on immunoselection or immuno-fixation.
- Majority of cases have been reported in northern Africa, Israel, and surrounding Middle Eastern countries.
- At presentation, the patients commonly are in their teens or early twenties.
- Common clinical features on presentation include recurrent or chronic diarrhea, weight loss, fevers, and/or growth retardation.
- Digital clubbing is a frequent finding.
- Moderate hepatomegaly occurs in about 25 percent of patients.
- Mesenteric lymphadenopathy is common, sometimes presenting as an abdominal mass, whereas extraabdominal lymphadenopathy is rare.
- In many cases, the abnormal heavy chain only can be found in the intestinal secretions.
- The jejunum is the usual site of involvement, with dense plasma-cell infiltration of the mucosa appearing during early stage disease (stage A). Infiltration of

more blastic-appearing plasma cells is found extending beyond the lamina propria into the muscularis layer during later stages (stages B and C).

- Spread of neoplastic lymphoplasmacytic cell infiltration to mesenteric lymph nodes is characteristic of stage C disease.
- *Immunoproliferative small intestinal disease* (IPSID) is applied to small intestinal lesions which pathologic features are identical to those of α-HCD regardless of the type of immunoglobulin synthesized.

μ-HCD

- Median age at presentation is in the late fifties.
- Infiltration of marrow with lymphocytes and plasma cells is common.
- Patients may have osteolytic lesions or pathologic fractures.
- Anemia is frequent.
- Lymphocytosis and thrombocytopenia are uncommon.
- Two-thirds of patients have monoclonal Ig light chains in the urine.
- Patients present symptoms of a lymphoproliferative malignancy (e.g., chronic lymphocytic leukemia, B-cell lymphoma, Waldenström macroglobulinemia, or multiple myeloma).
- Diagnosis typically requires a combination or electrophoretic, immunoelectrophoretic, immunofixation, and immunophenotypic techniques.
- In a minority of cases, the Ig heavy chain can be identified by electrophoresis of serum or urine samples as a discrete homogenous band of β mobility.
- Immunoelectrophoresis and/or immunofixation are required to detect an Ig heavy-chain protein that does not react with either anti-κ or anti-λ antisera.
- Immunophenotypic analyses of biopsy material can reveal lymphoplasmacytic cells that stain positive for cytoplasmic Ig heavy chain, but not for Ig light chain.
- Bence Jones proteinuria is found in over half the cases of μ-HCD.
- Cases of nonsecretory μ-HCD have been reported.
- The presence of vacuolated plasma cells in the marrow of a patient with a lymphoplasmacytic proliferative disorder should always suggest the possibility of μ-HCD.

DIFFERENTIAL DIAGNOSIS

- All patients presenting with a lymphoplasma cell proliferative disorder should be evaluated for γ-HCD and μ-HCD.
- The digestive form of α-HCD should be differentiated from other B-cell lymphomas.

THERAPY, COURSE, AND PROGNOSIS

γ-HCD

- Clinical course is variable and, thus, depends on the clinical features.
- Survival ranges from 1 month to over 20 years.
- Patients with lymphadenopathy on presentation have a more aggressive course than do patients with little evidence of lymphoproliferative disease.
- The amount of serum γ-HCD protein usually parallels the severity of the associated malignant disease.
- Disappearance of the monoclonal component from serum and urine associated with apparent complete response has been induced by chemotherapy, radiotherapy, or surgical removal of a localized lymphatic mass.
- In an asymptomatic patient, therapy is usually not necessary.
- In symptomatic patients with a low-grade lymphoplasmacytic malignancy, a trial of chlorambucil may be beneficial.
- Melphalan and prednisone can be used if the proliferation is predominantly plasmacytic.

- A trial of cyclophosphamide, vincristine, and prednisone with or without doxo-rubicin is reasonable for patients with evidence of a progressive lymphoplasma cell proliferative process or high-grade B-cell lymphoma.
- Rituximab monotherapy was given in two cases, resulting in clinical responses in both.

α-HCD

- Clinical course is variable but generally progressive in the absence of therapy.
- Antibiotic therapy with tetracycline, metronidazole, or ampicillin is indicated for stage A disease patients who do not have parasitic infection.
  — Antibiotic therapy can result in complete response in 70 percent of patients.
- Patients with stage B or C disease or stage A lesions without improvement after a 60-month course of antibiotic treatment should be given chemotherapy. The treatment regimens are those commonly used to treat B-cell lymphoma (e.g., R-CHOP).
- Surgical resection should be considered for focal or bulky transmural lym-phomatous tumors in the gastrointestinal tract and extramedullary plasmacy-toma.
- Autologous hematopoietic stem cell transplantation has been recommended for patients with advanced or refractory disease.

μ-HCD

- There is no specific therapy for μ-HCD.
- Chemotherapy is similar to that used in chronic lymphocytic leukemia (see Chap. 56) or in myeloma (see Chap. 69).
- Clinical course is variable, with survival ranging from 1 month to 11 years after appearance of symptoms.

 For a detailed discussion, see Dietlind L. Wahner-Roedler and Robert A. Kyle: Heavy-Chain Disease. Chap. 112, p. 1709 in *Williams Hematology*, 8th ed.

CHAPTER 72
Amyloidosis

DEFINITION

- Amyloidosis is a clinical syndrome resulting from disorders of secondary protein structure, in which a precursor protein is secreted from the cell in a soluble form, only to become insoluble at some tissue site, ultimately compromising organ function.
- The term *amyloid* is used to describe a substance with a homogeneous eosinophilic appearance by light microscopy, a green birefringence on polarizing electron microscopy, and a characteristic β-pleated sheet appearance by x-ray diffraction.
- Terms such as *primary, secondary, senile, dialysis-associated*, and *myeloma-associated* have been abandoned in favor of the etiologically based, chemical terminology (Table 72–1) (e.g., immunoglobulin light chain amyloidosis is termed *AL amyloidosis*).
- The incidence of AL amyloidosis is approximately 4.5 per 100,000 persons in the United States.
- Amyloid A (AA) amyloidosis is increasingly rare, occurring in less than 1 percent of persons with chronic inflammatory diseases in the United States and Europe.
- AA amyloidosis is more common in Turkey and the Middle East, where it occurs in association with familial Mediterranean fever.
- AA is the only type of amyloidosis that occurs in children.
- Amyloid β_2-microglobulin ($A\beta_2M$) amyloidosis usually manifests as deposits in the joint synovial and occurs in patients on long-term dialysis.
  — $A\beta_2M$ amyloidosis is also declining in incidence with changes in dialysis techniques.
- The inherited amyloidoses are rare in the United States, with an estimated incidence of less than approximately 1 per 100,000 persons.
- Amyloidogenic transthyretin (ATTR) amyloidosis is the most common form of familial amyloidosis and is associated with mutations of the gene encoding transthyretin (TTR).

ETIOLOGY AND PATHOGENESIS

- The exact mechanism of fibril formation is unknown and may be different among the various types of amyloid.
- Amyloid precursor proteins typically consist of long fibrils composed of relatively small precursor proteins with molecular weights between 4,000 and 25,000 daltons.
- Each amyloid fibril protein has a precursor molecule in the serum.
  — The secondary structures of many of the proteins have substantial β-pleated sheet structure. The known exceptions include serum amyloid A (SAA) and cellular prion protein (PrP^c), which contain little or no β folding in the precursor protein despite extensive β-sheet in the deposited fibrils.
- Amyloid formation involves:
  — Stimulus-generated change in the serum concentration or primary structure of amyloid precursor proteins.
  — Conversion of the precursor protein to amyloid fibrils.
- In some cases, the aberrant secondary structure seen in amyloid formation reflects a hereditary alteration in amino acid sequence that predisposes to fibril formation.

TABLE 72–1	THE MODERN (CHEMICAL) CLASSIFICATION OF HUMAN AMYLOIDOSIS

Amyloid Protein	Precursor Protein	Clinical Syndrome(s)
AL	Immunoglobulin light chains or light-chain fragments	Plasma cell disorders
AH	Immunoglobulin heavy chain	Systemic amyloidosis
ATTR	Transthyretin (TTR)	Familial amyloidotic polyneuropathy, familial amyloid cardiomyopathy, senile systemic amyloidosis, isolated vitreous amyloidosis
AA	Apo-SAA	Inflammation-associated, acquired, or inherited (tumor necrosis factor receptor-associated periodic syndrome, TRAPS, and familial Mediterranean fever)
$A\beta_2M$	β_2-Microglobulin	Dialysis-associated amyloid
AApoAI	Apolipoprotein A-I	Familial amyloidosis involving various organs
AApoAII	Apolipoprotein A-II	Familial renal amyloidosis
AFib	Fibrinogen α chain	Familial renal amyloidosis
ALys	Lysozyme	Familial systemic amyloidosis
ACys	Cystatin C	Hereditary cerebral hemorrhage with amyloidosis, Icelandic type
$A\beta$	β-Protein precursor	Alzheimer disease, Down syndrome, hereditary cerebral hemorrhage with amyloidosis, Dutch type
AprP	Prion protein	Creutzfeldt-Jakob and Gerstmann-Sträussler-Scheinker diseases
AGel	Gelsolin	Hereditary corneal amyloidosis
AKer	Keratoepithelin	Hereditary corneal amyloidosis
ALac	Lactoferrin	Hereditary corneal amyloidosis
ACal	Calcitonin	Medullary carcinoma of the thyroid (in multiple endocrine neoplasia)
AIAPP	Amylin (islet amyloid polypeptide)	Insulinoma, type II diabetes mellitus
AANF	Atrial natriuretic factor	Isolated atrial amyloidosis
APro	Prolactin	Pituitary amyloid
ACytokeratin	Keratin	Cutaneous amyloidosis
Abri/ADan	Bri/Dan	Familial British and Danish dementia
AIns	Insulin	Iatrogenic
AMed	Lactadherin	Senile aortic
APin	To be named	Pindborg tumor-associated protein

Source: *Williams Hematology,* 8th ed, Chap. 110, Table 110–1, p. 1684.

- — Examples include TTR, lysozyme, fibrinogen, cystatin c, gelsolin, amyloid-β protein precursor (AβPP), or apolipoprotein A-I (ApoA1).
- In other cases, wild-type molecules are the fibril precursor.
  - — Examples include immunoglobulin light chain, β$_2$-microglobulin, ApoA1, and others.
- Several major proteins can form amyloid fibrils.
- AL protein (immunoglobulin light chain):
  - — AL amyloidosis is usually caused by a plasma cell neoplasm in the marrow and can occur in isolation or along with myeloma (see Chap. 69).
  - — Myeloid fibril deposits are composed of intact 23-kDa monoclonal immunoglobulin light chains.
  - — Although all kappa (κ) and lambda (λ) light-chain subtypes have been identified in amyloid fibrils, λ subtypes predominate.
  - — λ VI subtype appears to have unique structural properties that predispose it to fibril formation, often in the kidney.
- AL amyloidosis can be seen in other B lymphoproliferative disorders, including macroglobulinemia and lymphoma.
- AL amyloidosis should be distinguished from nonamyloid monoclonal immunoglobulin deposition disease (MIDD), in which the deposited immunoglobulin consists of both heavy and light chains, of which κ chains predominate.
- AA proteins (amyloid A proteins):
  - — AA amyloidosis occurs in response to inflammation and as a familial syndrome.
  - — The AA amyloid fibrils are usually composed of an 8-kDa, 76-amino-acid amino-terminal portion of the 12-kDa precursor, SAA.
  - — SAA is a polymorphic protein encoded by a family of active serum amyloid A (SAA) genes, which are acute phase apoproteins synthesized in the liver and transported by high-density lipoprotein (HDL3) in the plasma.
  - — Years of an underlying inflammatory disease causing an elevated SAA usually precedes fibril formation.
- ATTR proteins (transthyretin):
  - — Occurs in several familial syndromes and in senile amyloid.
  - — ATTR amyloidosis also is known as familial amyloidotic polyneuropathy or cardiomyopathy.
  - — Variant TTR molecules are prone to dissociation from stable tetramers and to unfolding, leading to misfolding, polymerization, and fibril formation.
  - — Evidence of an age-related "trigger" is that senile cardiac amyloidosis, caused by the deposition of fibrils derived from normal wild-type TTR, is exclusively a disease of older people.
- Aβ$_2$M (β$_2$-microglobulin):
  - — Occurs in chronic hemodialysis patients.
  - — Carpal tunnel and joint synovial membrane involvement is common.
- AP protein (P component):
  - — A minor protein component of amyloid deposits.
  - — Intravenously injected purified P component preferentially binds to amyloid deposits.
  - — This property has been exploited clinically, using radiolabeled P component, to localize and quantify the total body burden of amyloid in the so-called serum amyloid P (SAP) scan.
  - — Has structural homology with C-reactive protein.
- Apo E allele (Apo E4):
  - — Strongly associated with Alzheimer disease.
- In some instances, the amyloid precursors undergo proteolysis, which may enhance the kinetics of folding into a prefibrillar structural intermediate.
- In some of the amyloidoses (e.g., Aβ or AA), a normal proteolytic process may be disturbed, yielding a higher than normal concentration of a prefibrillar molecule.

DIAGNOSIS

- It is important to determine the type of amyloid because different types of amyloidosis may require different therapies.
- A tissue biopsy demonstrating amyloid fibrils is necessary for the diagnosis of amyloidosis.
  - Amyloidosis is diagnosed by demonstration of Congo red–binding material with characteristic apple-green fluorescence under polarized light microscopy in a biopsy specimen.
  - Subcutaneous fat aspiration and rectal biopsy will identify 80 to 90 percent of patients later found to have amyloid elsewhere.
  - Biopsy of an organ with impaired function is a high-yield procedure.
- Identification of a plasma cell neoplasm distinguishes AL amyloidosis from other types of amyloidosis.
  - There is often an increased percentage of plasma cells in the marrow.
  - Monoclonal light chain can be detected in serum or concentrated urine of approximately 90 percent of patients.
  - A monoclonal serum protein by itself is not diagnostic of amyloidosis, since essential monoclonal gammopathy is common in older patients.
- Consider the diagnosis in patients with:
  - Unexplained kidney disease with nephrotic syndrome.
  - Unexplained neuromuscular disease, congestive heart failure, or malabsorption.
- The cardinal finding in AL amyloidosis is monoclonal immunoglobulin light chain.
- AA amyloidosis should be suspected in patients with renal amyloidosis and a chronic inflammatory condition or infection.

CLINICAL FEATURES

- The clinical manifestations of amyloidosis vary widely and arise because of amyloid deposition and interference with normal organ function.
- Most common presenting symptoms and signs are:
  - Weakness and weight loss.
  - Purpura, particularly in loose facial tissue.
  - Symptoms and physical findings that reflect the extent of organ dysfunction because of amyloid involvement.
- AL amyloidosis affects the following organs:
  - Kidney:
    - Nephrotic syndrome, renal insufficiency.
  - In a small proportion of patients (~10%), amyloid deposition occurs in the renal vasculature or tubulointerstitium, causing renal dysfunction without significant proteinuria.
  - Liver and spleen:
  - Organ enlargement, hepatic cholestasis, and/or traumatic rupture of enlarged spleen.
  - Profound elevation of alkaline phosphatase with only mild elevation of transaminases is characteristic of hepatic amyloidosis.
  - Gastrointestinal tract:
  - Macroglossia, obstruction, ulceration, hemorrhage, malabsorption, and/or diarrhea.
  - Heart:
  - Congestive heart failure, cardiomegaly, and/or arrhythmias.
  - Low voltage R waves in the echocardiogram.
  - Restrictive cardiomyopathy.
  - Skin:
  - Lesions ranging from papules to large nodules, purpura.
  - Nervous system:

- — Peripheral neuropathies, postural hypotension (autonomic neuropathy).
- — Respiratory tract.
- — Blood:
  - • Coagulopathy because of depletion of fibrinogen, factor IX, and/or factor X.
- — Soft tissues:
- — Macroglossia, carpal tunnel syndrome, skin nodules, arthropathy, alopecia, nail dystrophy, submandibular gland enlargement, periorbital purpura, and hoarseness of voice.
- • AA Amyloidosis:
  - — Can occur at any age.
  - — Primary clinical manifestation is proteinuria and/or renal insufficiency.
  - — Hepatosplenomegaly in association with chronic inflammatory disorders.
  - — Cardiomyopathy rarely occurs.
  - — With chronic inflammatory diseases, amyloid progression is slow and survival is often more than 10 years, particularly with treatment for end-stage renal disease.
- • $A\beta_2M$ Amyloidosis:
  - — Several distinct rheumatologic conditions are observed in $A\beta_2M$ amyloidosis, including carpal tunnel syndrome, persistent joint effusions, spondyloarthropathy, and cystic bone lesions.
  - — Carpal tunnel syndrome usually produces the first symptom of disease.
  - — Persistent joint effusions accompanied by mild discomfort occur in up to 50 percent of patients on dialysis for more than 12 years.
- • ATTR Familial Amyloidosis: clinical features are similar to AL amyloidosis.
  - — The TTR variant, Val-122-Ile, is a common allele in the African American population and is associated with cardiomyopathy.

OTHER FORMS OF AMYLOIDOSIS

- • The hereditary renal amyloidoses (amyloidosis ApoA-I [AApoAI], ApoA-II [AApoAII], amyloidosis fibrinogen α-chain [AFib], amyloidosis lysozyme [ALys]) can resemble AL amyloidosis with renal involvement.
- • The clinical differentiation is suggested by the family history and immunohistologic staining of biopsy material with antibodies specific for candidate amyloid precursor proteins.

Amyloidoses Localized to the Central Nervous System

- • AL amyloidosis deposits are rarely found in the central nervous system, although they may be found in the cerebral vessels.
- • The primary central nervous system amyloidoses include amyloidosis cystatin C (ACys); hereditary cerebral hemorrhage with amyloidosis-Icelandic type, in which the precursor is the protease inhibitor cystatin c.

Localized Light Chain Amyloidosis

- • The tracheobronchial tree is the most common site of localized AL amyloidosis; it does not progress to systematic disease.

Other Localized Amyloidosis

- • Atrial natriuretic factor amyloidosis (AANF) affects older persons, often with congestive heart failure.
- • In calcitonin amyloid (ACal), the precursor protein is calcitonin.
- • In pancreatic islet cell amyloid polypeptide amyloidosis (AIAPP), the precursor protein is a polypeptide (IAPP), also known as amylin.
- • In prolactin amyloid (Apro), prolactin or its fragments are found in the pituitary amyloid.

- Three proteins (gelsolin, keratoepithelin, and lactoferrin) have been found in fibrils from patients with autosomal dominant corneal amyloidosis.
  - Medin, an integral fragment of lactadherin, which is produced in aortic smooth muscle cell, forms the amyloid seen in the aorta of all older humans.
  - Insulin has been found in fibrils at the site of insulin injection.
  - Cytokeratin has been found in amyloidosis localized to the skin.

TREATMENT AND PROGNOSIS

- Potential treatments of the amyloidoses can be directed at interfering with any of several pathogenetic processes.
- No specific treatment is available for amyloid disorders other than that caused by AL amyloidosis.

AL Amyloidosis

- Assessment of treatment response: Complete hematologic response is defined as absence of monoclonal protein in serum and urine by immunofixation electrophoresis, normal serum-free light-chain ratio and marrow biopsy with less than 5 percent plasma cells with no clonal predominance by immunohistochemistry.
- Rate of disease progression is variable.
- Clinically apparent cardiac involvement is an important determinant of outcome.
- Serum concentration of N-terminal probrain natriuretic peptide (NT-proBNP) is a sensitive biomarker of AL amyloidosis-associated cardiac dysfunction and a strong predictor of survival following aggressive treatment.
- High circulating levels of free light chains are associated with poor outcome.
  - Improved organ function may be evident 3 to 6 months following treatment.
  - The rate of clinical response is higher in patients with a complete hematologic response.
- High-dose intravenous melphalan chemotherapy (HDM) followed by autologous blood stem cell transplantation (autoSCT) is presently considered the most effective treatment for AL amyloidosis.
  - Amyloid deposition in the gastrointestinal tract predisposes to gastrointestinal bleeding that can be exacerbated by amyloid-associated coagulopathies, such as factor X deficiency.
  - Anasarca is common in patients with nephrotic syndrome and is exacerbated by granulocyte colony-stimulating factor administration.
  - Hypotension from cardiac disease or autonomic nervous system involvement; atrial and ventricular arrhythmias in patients with amyloid cardiomyopathy; difficulties with endotracheal intubation as a consequence of macroglossia; and spontaneous splenic, hepatic, and esophageal rupture can arise during treatment.
- Patients with severe systolic or diastolic heart failure because of amyloid cardiomyopathy are intolerant of chemotherapy and glucocorticoid-containing regimens. Thus, orthotopic heart transplantation may be required as a life-saving procedure.
- There is a small experience with allogeneic and syngeneic marrow transplantation for AL amyloidosis. This approach deserves further investigation in the context of clinical trials.
- The conventional treatment is low-dose oral melphalan with prednisone.
  - Median patient survival is approximately 18 months.
  - Many patients are unable to tolerate the fluid retention and worsening congestive heart failure associated with glucocortioid treatment.
- The use of oral melphalan as a single agent achieved a partial hematologic response in patients who received doses of melphalan greater than 300 mg administered continuously.

- Experience with myeloma has indicated that dexamethasone accounted for most (80%) of the plasma cell reduction achieved with infusional vincristine, doxorubicin (Adriamycin), and dexamethasone (VAD) and avoided the potential toxicity of vincristine and doxorubicin (Adriamycin).
  — Pulsed high-dose dexamethasone has been reported to benefit AL amyloidosis patients.
  — The toxicity of dexamethasone used with the same schedule of the VAD regimen in AL amyloidosis patients is substantial. A less toxic schedule (40 mg/day for 4 days every 21 days) induced organ response in 35 percent of patients in a median time of 4 months, without significant toxicity.
  — Dexamethasone 1 day a week is less toxic than 4-day pulses in patients with myeloma.
- Thalidomide itself can induce responses in up to half of patients treated with it alone or in combination with dexamethasone, but it is poorly tolerated in patients with AL amyloidosis.
  — Side effects prevent dose escalation above 200 to 300 mg/day.
  — Thalidomide combined with cyclophosphamide and dexamethasone (CTD regimen) in an oral regimen has been shown to be effective in inducing hematologic responses in approximately 75 percent (complete response: approximately 20%; partial response: approximately 55%) of patients with low treatment-related mortality of approximately 4 percent and median overall survival of 40 months.
- Lenalidomide with dexamethasone produced hematologic responses in approximately 70 percent of patients with significant organ responses.
  — Lenalidomide can exacerbate azotemia in patients with renal amyloidosis.
- Bortezomib in combination with dexamethasone reduces the concentration of the circulating monoclonal protein.
  — The median time to hematologic response is on the order of a month, and hematologic responses of 50 to 88 percent are being seen.
- Supportive care to decrease symptoms and support organ function plays an important role in the management of this disease.
- Achieving a balance between heart failure and intravascular volume depletion is particularly important especially in patients with autonomic nervous system involvement or nephrotic syndrome.
- Digoxin and calcium channel blockers should be avoided in AL amyloidosis and TTR cardiac amyloidosis because these drugs may bind to amyloid fibrils and exacerbate the cardiomyopathy.
- Patients with recurrent syncope may require permanent pacemaker implantation and ventricular arrhythmias can be treated with amiodarone and, in some patients, implantable defibrillators.
- Orthostatic hypotension can be severe and difficult to manage.
- Supportive treatment for amyloid-associated kidney disease, as for other causes of nephrotic syndrome includes salt restriction, diuretics, and treatment of secondary hyperlipidemia.
- Adequate protein intake should be maintained.
- Both hemodialysis and peritoneal dialysis are used for amyloidosis-associated end-stage renal disease.
- Diarrhea is a common and an incapacitating problem.
- Duloxetine may be effective in controlling pain of neuropathy.
- Nonnephrotoxic analgesics may be used as adjuvant agents.
- Bleeding in AL amyloidosis is frequent and multifactorial because capillary fragility (amyloid deposition in vessel walls) and coagulopathy (adsorption of clotting factor X by amyloid deposits).
  — Factor X is difficult to replace with plasma and patients with life-threatening bleeding caused by factor X deficiency should be treated with recombinant factor VII.
- In patients with massive macroglossia, surgical resection has not been effective.

AA Amyloidosis

- The major therapy in AA amyloidosis is treatment of the underlying inflammatory or infectious disease.
- For familial Mediterranean fever, colchicine in a dose of 1.2 to 1.8 mg per day orally is the appropriate treatment.
  — Colchicine has not been helpful for AA amyloidosis of other causes.
- Eprodisate interferes with the interaction of AA amyloid protein and glycosaminoglycans in tissues and thus prevents fibril formation and deposition.

Aβ_2M Amyloidosis

- The treatment for Aβ_2M amyloidosis is difficult because the 12 kDa β_2-microglobulin molecule is too large to pass through a dialysis membrane.
- Patients on chronic ambulatory peritoneal dialysis usually have lower plasma levels of β_2-microglobulin than those on hemodialysis.
- Patients who have received kidney transplants after developing Aβ_2M have an improvement in symptoms.

ATTR Familial Amyloidosis

- Without intervention, survival after ATTR disease onset is 5 to 15 years.
- Orthotopic liver transplantation, which removes the major source of variant TTR production and replaces it with normal TTR, is the major treatment for ATTR amyloidosis.
- Cardiomyopathy may worsen after liver transplantation.

Monoclonal Immunoglobulin Deposition Diseases (MIDD)

- In some patients with clonal plasma cell disorders, nonfibrillar aggregation and deposition of Ig light or heavy chains can occur.
  — Kidney and heart are the most frequent sites for MIDD.
  — Once the diagnosis of MIDD is established, determination of whether the patient has myeloma (e.g., serum and urine evaluation for monoclonal protein, marrow aspiration and biopsy, skeletal survey) should be made.

For a more detailed discussion, see Vaishali Sanchorawala, Daniel R. Jacobson, David C. Seldin, and Joel N. Buxbaum: The Amyloidoses. Chap. 110, p. 1683 in *Williams Hematology*, 8th ed.

PART IX

DISORDERS OF PLATELETS AND HEMOSTASIS

CHAPTER 73
Clinical Manifestations, Evaluation, and Classification of Disorders of Hemostasis

EVALUATION OF A SUSPECTED BLEEDING DISORDER

History

- A systematic approach is required to elicit and interpret all relevant information. Extensive, direct discussion between physician and patient is necessary to uncover the sometimes subtle details pertinent to a history of bleeding.
- Many otherwise healthy individuals, more often women than men, will report easy bruising and/or excessive bleeding.
- Patients with severe hemorrhagic disorders invariably have significantly abnormal histories of bleeding, either spontaneous or after trauma and/or interventions (e.g., biopsies or surgical procedures).
- Typical clinical manifestations occur with specific hemostatic disorders, as outlined in Table 73–1.
- When evaluating the absence of prior bleeding, it is important to determine whether or not the patient has been exposed to significant hemostatic challenges, such as dental extraction, surgery, trauma, or childbirth.
- It is also important to attempt to obtain objective confirmation of the bleeding event and the severity, such as the need for blood transfusions, the development of anemia requiring iron replacement, hospitalization because of bleeding, ambulatory evaluation of a bleeding tendency, and the results of any laboratory studies done previously.
- A medication history is essential, with particular attention to nonprescription drugs (e.g., aspirin or nonsteroidal antiinflammatory drugs [NSAIDs]) and other drugs taken regularly and therefore easily forgotten, including herbal and other alternative medicines.
- A nutritional history is necessary to evaluate intake of vitamin K, vitamin C, and the adequacy of general nutrition.

TABLE 73–1   CLINICAL MANIFESTATIONS TYPICALLY ASSOCIATED WITH SPECIFIC HEMOSTATIC DISORDERS

Clinical Manifestations	Hemostatic Disorders
Mucocutaneous bleeding	Thrombocytopenias, platelet dysfunction, von Willebrand disease
Cephalhematomas in newborns, hemarthroses, hematuria, and intramuscular, intracerebral, and retroperitoneal hemorrhages	Severe hemophilias A and B; severe deficiencies of factor VII, factor X, or factor XIII; severe type 3 von Willebrand disease; and afibrinogenemia
Injury-related bleeding and mild spontaneous bleeding	Mild and moderate hemophilias A and B; severe factor XI deficiency; moderate deficiencies of fibrinogen and factors II, V, VII, or X; combined factors V and VIII deficiency; and α_2-antiplasmin deficiency
Bleeding from stump of umbilical cord and habitual abortions	Afibrinogenemia, hypofibrinogenemia, dysfibrinogenemia, or factor XIII deficiency
Impaired wound healing	Factor XIII deficiency
Facial purpura in newborns	Glanzmann thrombasthenia, severe thrombocytopenia
Recurrent severe epistaxis and chronic iron deficiency anemia	Hereditary hemorrhagic telangiectasias

Source: *Williams Hematology,* 8th ed, Chap. 118, Table 118–2, p. 1885.

- A history of bleeding involving one organ or system, such as hematuria, hematemesis, or hemoptysis suggests a local cause, such as a neoplasm. Bleeding from multiple sites may indicate a coagulation defect.
- Prolonged oozing of blood from sites of high fibrinolytic activity, such as the urinary tract, endometrium, or oral and nasal mucosa, may occur in patients with hemostatic abnormalities.
- Mucosal and cutaneous bleeding may also be caused by vascular disorders, such as hereditary hemorrhagic telangiectasia (Rendu-Osler-Weber syndrome) or scurvy.
- A detailed family history is particularly important, including all relatives going back at least one generation and specific inquiry on any consanguinity.
- A history of some bleeding problems may be suggestive of specific disorders:
- Epistaxis and gingival hemorrhage are the most common symptom of qualitative or quantitative platelet disorders, von Willebrand disease, and hereditary hemorrhagic telangiectasia.
- Cutaneous bruising may occur with a variety of hemostatic disorders.
- The frequency, size, location, color, and history of trauma are all relevant to evaluating the significance of the bruising.
- Dental extractions present severe hemostatic challenges that can be objectively evaluated by the need for suturing, packing, or transfusion.
- Prolonged bleeding from razor cuts inflicted while shaving often occur in patients with platelet disorders or von Willebrand disease.
- Hemoptysis, hematemesis, or hematuria is rarely the presenting symptom in patients with bleeding disorders.
- In patients who also have a local lesion, bleeding disorders may contribute to repeated episodes of hematochezia or melena.

- Menorrhagia occurs with platelet disorders and von Willebrand disease, but most often is not associated with a bleeding disorder.
- Excessive bleeding relating to pregnancy may occur with some bleeding disorders. Repeated spontaneous abortion may occur with factor XIII deficiency, hereditary disorders of fibrinogen, or the antiphospholipid syndrome.
- Hemarthroses occur with severe deficiencies of blood coagulation factors, especially the hemophilias, or with severe von Willebrand disease.
- Bleeding after circumcision occurs with hemophilia A and B. Delayed bleeding after circumcision may be a result of factor XIII deficiency.
- Bleeding from the umbilical cord in newborns is a typical symptom of factor XIII deficiency.
- Prolonged bleeding from sites of venipuncture or other invasive procedures is typical of disseminated intravascular coagulation.

Physical Examination

- The patients should be examined for petechiae, ecchymoses, telangiectases, and hematomas.
- Splenomegaly may occur in patients with thrombocytopenia.
- Venipuncture or other invasive sites should be examined for prolonged bleeding.
- Joints should be examined for deformity or restricted mobility.
- Throughout the examination, signs of underlying disorders that can cause hemostatic abnormalities should be sought (Table 73–2).

TABLE 73–2 CLASSIFICATION OF DISORDERS OF HEMOSTASIS

Major Types	Disorders	Examples
Acquired	Thrombocytopenias	Autoimmune and alloimmune, drug-induced, hypersplenism, hypoplastic (primary, suppressive, myelophthisic), DIC (see Chap. 74).
	Liver disease	Cirrhosis, acute hepatic failure, liver transplantation (see Chap. 84).
	Renal failure Vitamin K deficiency	Malabsorption syndrome, hemorrhagic disease of the newborn, prolonged antibiotic therapy, malnutrition, prolonged biliary obstruction (see Chap. 82).
	Hematologic disorders	Acute leukemias (particularly promyelocytic), myelodysplasias, monoclonal gammopathies, essential thrombocythemia (see Chaps. 42, 44, 46, 55, and 68).
	Acquired antibodies against coagulation factors	Neutralizing antibodies against factors V, VIII, and XIII; accelerated clearance of antibody-factor complexes, e.g., acquired von Willebrand disease, hypoprothrombinemia associated with antiphospholipid antibodies (see Chaps. 83 and 85).
	Disseminated intravascular coagulation	Acute (sepsis, malignancies, trauma, obstetric complications) and chronic (malignancies, giant hemangiomas, missed abortion) (see Chap. 86).
	Drugs	Antiplatelet agents, anticoagulants, anti-thrombin agents, and thrombolytic, myelosuppressive, hepatotoxic, and nephrotoxic agents (see Chap. 88).

(continued)

TABLE 73–2	(CONTINUED)	
Major Types	**Disorders**	**Examples**
	Vascular	Nonpalpable purpura ("senile," solar, and factitious purpura), use of corticosteroids, vitamin C deficiency, child abuse, purpura fulminans; palpable purpura (Henoch-Schönlein, vasculitis, dysproteinemias) (see Chap. 78).
Inherited	Deficiencies of coagulation factors	Hemophilia A (factor VIII deficiency), hemophilia B (factor IX deficiency), deficiencies of factors II, V, VII, X, XI, and XIII and von Willebrand disease (see Chaps. 79, 80, and 82).
	Platelet disorders	Glanzmann thrombasthenia, Bernard-Soulier syndrome, platelet granule disorders, etc. (see Chap. 76).
	Fibrinolytic disorders	α_2-Antiplasmin deficiency, plasminogen activator inhibitor-1 deficiency (see Chap. 87).
	Vascular	Hemorrhagic telangiectasias (see Chap. 78)
	Connective tissue disorders	Ehlers-Danlos syndrome (see Chap. 78).

Source: *Williams Hematology,* 8th ed, Chap. 118, Table 118–1, p. 1884.

EVALUATION BASED ON HISTORY AND INITIAL HEMOSTATIC TESTS

Initial Hemostatic Tests

- The initial evaluation should include a prothrombin time (PT), activated partial thromboplastin time (aPTT), and a platelet count.
- In Fig. 73–1, the results of these initial tests and the history of bleeding are integrated to suggest a tentative diagnosis of the hemostatic disorder.
- Prolongation of the PT, aPTT, or both may be a consequence of an inhibitor of one or more components of the coagulation scheme, as well as of a deficiency of an essential coagulation factor.
- It is possible to distinguish between an inhibitor and a deficiency by mixing equal parts of the patient's plasma with normal plasma, and repeating the test on the mixture. If a factor deficiency exists, the addition of normal plasma will lead to normal or nearly normal results, whereas if an inhibitor is present, the abnormality will persist.
- Some inhibitors, such as acquired antibodies to factor VIII, react slowly, and it is therefore necessary to incubate the mixture of normal and patient's plasma at 37 °C for 2 hours before performing the coagulation assay.
- If the PT, aPTT, and platelet count are all normal, but the patient has a history of bleeding, platelet function tests, measurement of von Willebrand factor, factor XIII, and α_2-antiplasmin should be performed (Fig. 73–2).

FIGURE 73–1 Measures for establishing a tentative diagnosis of a hemostatic disorder using basic tests of hemostasis and the patient's history of bleeding. aPTT, activated partial thromboplastin time; BT, bleeding time; DIC, disseminated intravascular coagulation; HK, high molecular weight kininogen; N, normal; PK, prekallikrein; PLT, platelets; PT, prothrombin time; vWd, von Willebrand disease.

(Source: *Williams Hematology,* 8th ed, Chap. 118, Fig. 118–1, p. 1887.)

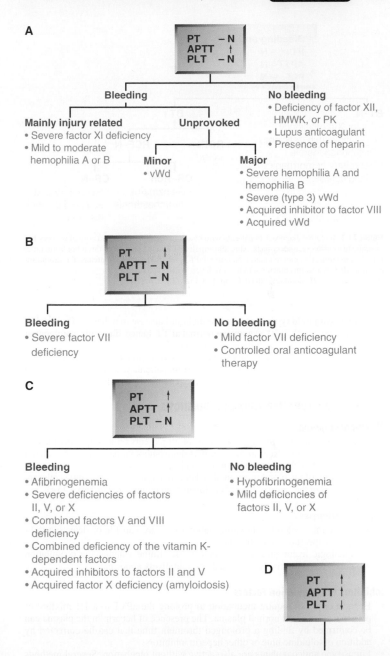

A

PT	– N
APTT	↑
PLT	– N

Bleeding

Mainly injury related
- Severe factor XI deficiency
- Mild to moderate hemophilia A or B

Unprovoked

Minor
- vWd

Major
- Severe hemophilia A and hemophilia B
- Severe (type 3) vWd
- Acquired inhibitor to factor VIII
- Acquired vWd

No bleeding
- Deficiency of factor XII, HMWK, or PK
- Lupus anticoagulant
- Presence of heparin

B

PT	↑
APTT	– N
PLT	– N

Bleeding
- Severe factor VII deficiency

No bleeding
- Mild factor VII deficiency
- Controlled oral anticoagulant therapy

C

PT	↑
APTT	↑
PLT	– N

Bleeding
- Afibrinogenemia
- Severe deficiencies of factors II, V, or X
- Combined factors V and VIII deficiency
- Combined deficiency of the vitamin K-dependent factors
- Acquired inhibitors to factors II and V
- Acquired factor X deficiency (amyloidosis)

No bleeding
- Hypofibrinogenemia
- Mild deficiencies of factors II, V, or X

D

PT	↑
APTT	↑
PLT	↓

Bleeding or no bleeding
- DIC
- Liver disease
- Lupus anticoagulant

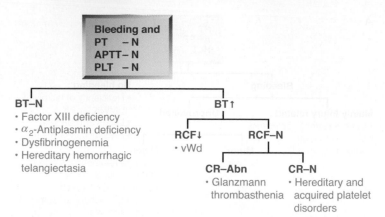

FIGURE 73–2 Tentative diagnoses in patients with bleeding manifestations and normal primary hemostatic tests using secondary tests. Abn, abnormal; aPTT, activated partial thromboplastin time; BT, bleeding time; CR, clot retraction; N, normal; PK, prekallikrein; PLT, platelets; PT, prothrombin time; RCF, ristocetin cofactor activity; vWd, von Willebrand disease. (Source: *Williams Hematology,* 8th ed, Chap. 118, Fig. 118–2, p. 1887.)

- Patients with mild types 1 or 2 von Willebrand disease may have sufficient factor VIII (greater than 30%) to give a normal aPTT, hence, direct measurement of von Willebrand factor activity is recommended.
- The thrombin time is prolonged by heparin; in disseminated intravascular coagulation; by an inhibitor present in plasma from patients with amyloidosis; and in patients with afibrinogenemia, hypofibrinogenemia, or dysfibrinogenemia.

SPECIFIC ASSAYS FOR ESTABLISHING THE DIAGNOSIS

Thrombocytopenia
- It is essential to examine the blood film of all patients on whom a low platelet count is reported in order to rule out pseudothrombocytopenia. Alternatively, a platelet count in blood drawn in citrate can be performed.
- Examination of the blood film can also detect a number of abnormalities relevant to diagnosis of the cause of thrombocytopenia, as summarized in Table 73–3.

Factor Deficiencies
- Modern clinical blood coagulation laboratories are capable of detecting deficiencies of specific coagulation factors.
- Immunologic techniques are available to determine whether the coagulation proteins are quantitatively decreased or qualitatively abnormal.

Inhibitors to Coagulation Factors
- Heparin does not require incubation to prolong the aPTT to a 1:1 mixture of patient's plasma and normal plasma. The presence of heparin in the plasma can be confirmed by finding a prolonged thrombin time that can be corrected by addition of toluidine blue or other heparin inhibitors.
- Lupus-type anticoagulants are also active without incubation. Several methods are available for specific detection of lupus-type anticoagulants.
- Antibodies to specific coagulation factors, such as factor VIII, are usually detected only after incubation of a mixture of normal and patient's plasma for 2 hours at 37 °C.

TABLE 73–3	**CONDITIONS THAT MAY BE SUGGESTED BY EXAMINATION OF THE BLOOD FILM FROM PATIENTS WITH THROMBOCYTOPENIA**
Disorder	Findings on Blood Film
Inherited thrombocytopenia	Giant platelets
May-Hegglin anomaly	Giant platelets and Döhle-like bodies in leukocytes
Diminished platelet survival (e.g., idiopathic thrombocytopenic purpura)	Moderately enlarged platelets
Wiskott-Aldrich syndrome	Small platelets
Thrombotic microangiopathy (e.g., thrombotic thrombocytopenic purpura, hemolytic uremic syndrome, malignant hypertension), disseminated intravascular coagulation	Schistocytes, burr cells
Rouleaux formation	Dysproteinemia
Neutrophil hypersegmentation and macrocytosis	Vitamin B_{12} or folic acid deficiency
Abnormal leukocytes	Leukemia, myeloproliferative disorders

- Some inhibitors form complexes with specific coagulation factors *in vivo*. These are rapidly cleared from the circulation, and severe deficiency of the factor results. Special testing methods are required to detect such inhibitors.

Platelet Function Disorders
- A flow diagram of the steps required for diagnosis of qualitative platelet disorders is given in Chap. 76, **Fig. 76-1**.

PREOPERATIVE ASSESSMENT OF HEMOSTASIS
- Preoperative assessment is based on the history of bleeding, any underlying disorder that compromises hemostasis, initial laboratory tests, and the type of surgery planned.

CLASSIFICATION OF HEMOSTATIC DISORDERS
- Hemostatic disorders can be conveniently classified as either hereditary or acquired, or according to the mechanism of the defect(s). **Table 73–2** classifies coagulation disorders as either "acquired" or "inherited."

For a more detailed discussion, see Uri Seligsohn and Kenneth Kaushansky: Classification, Clinical Manifestations and Evaluation of Disorders of Hemostasis. Chap. 118, p 1883 in *Williams Hematology*, 8th ed.

CHAPTER 74
Thrombocytopenia

- Thrombocytopenia is defined as a platelet count below the lower limit of normal for the specific method used; e.g., less than 150×10^9/L.
- The causes of thrombocytopenia are listed in **Table 74–1**.

SPURIOUS THROMBOCYTOPENIA (PSEUDOTHROMBOCYTOPENIA)

- A false diagnosis of thrombocytopenia can occur when laboratory conditions cause platelets to clump, resulting in artificially low platelet counts as determined by automated counters. This occurs in 0.1 to 0.2 percent of automated platelet counts. Occasionally, if a high proportion of platelets are unusually large, the automated count can be spuriously low.
- Blood films should always be carefully examined to confirm the presence of thrombocytopenia.

Etiology and Pathogenesis

- Falsely low platelet counts are caused by platelet clumping most often occurring in blood samples collected in EDTA anticoagulant. Blood collected in citrate will often confirm the spurious nature of the thrombocytopenia, although clumping may occur in any anticoagulant.
- Platelets may attach to each other to form clumps, or may form clumps with leukocytes, usually neutrophils.
- Platelet clumping is usually caused by a low-titer IgG antibody reacting with an epitope exposed on platelet GP IIb/IIIa by *in vitro* conditions.

Laboratory Features

- A film made from blood anticoagulated with EDTA demonstrates more platelets than expected from the platelet count, but many are in large pools or clumps. A blood film made directly from a fingerstick sample accurately reflects the true count.
- Pseudothrombocytopenia is often accompanied by a falsely elevated white count because some platelet clumps are sufficiently large to be detected as leukocytes by an automated counter.
- Correct platelet counts can be obtained by placing fingerstick blood directly into diluting fluid at 37 °C and performing counts by phase-contrast microscopy.

Clinical Features

- The platelet agglutinins causing spurious thrombocytopenia appear to have no other clinical significance.
- Platelet clumping is usually persistent.

THROMBOCYTOPENIA DUE TO SPLENIC POOLING (SEQUESTRATION) (SEE ALSO CHAP. 28)
Etiology and Pathogenesis

- The spleen normally sequesters about one-third of the platelet mass. Reversible pooling of up to 90 percent of the platelet mass occurs in patients with splenomegaly. A good example of this phenomenon is seen in patients with Gaucher disease.

TABLE 74–1   **CLASSIFICATION OF THROMBOCYTOPENIA**

Pseudothrombocytopenia
Platelet agglutination
Platelet satellitism
Antiphospholipid antibodies
GP IIa-IIIa antagonists
Giant platelets
Miscellaneous associations
Impaired platelet production
Congenital
   Autosomal dominant
   MYH9-related
   May-Hegglin anomaly
   Fechtner syndrome
   Epstein syndrome
   Sebastian syndrome
   Mediterranean macrothrombocytopenia
   Familial platelet syndrome with predisposition to acute myelogenous leukemia
   Thrombocytopenia with linkage to chromosome 10
   Paris-Trousseau syndrome
Thrombocytopenia with radial synostosis
   Autosomal recessive
   Congenital amegakaryocytic thrombocytopenia
Thrombocytopenia with absent radius (TAR) syndrome
   Bernard-Soulier syndrome
   Gray platelet syndrome
   X-linked thrombocytopenias
   Wiskott-Aldrich syndrome
   X-linked thrombocytopenia
   X-linked thrombocytopenia with dyserythrocytosis
Acquired
   Marrow infiltration
Infectious disease
   HIV
   Parvovirus
   Cytomegalovirus
Others
   Radiotherapy and chemotherapy
   Folic acid and vitamin B_{12} deficiency
   Paroxysmal nocturnal hemoglobinuria
   Acquired aplastic anemia
   Myelodysplastic syndromes
   Acquired pure megakaryocytic thrombocytopenia
   Accelerated platelet destruction
   Immune-mediated thrombocytopenia
   Autoimmune thrombocytopenic purpura
Idiopathic
   Secondary (infections, pregnancy-related, lymphoproliferative disorders, collagen vascular diseases)
   Alloimmune thrombocytopenia
   Neonatal thrombocytopenia
   Posttransfusion purpura
   Nonimmune thrombocytopenia

(continued)

TABLE 74–1	(CONTINUED)

Thrombotic microangiopathies
   Thrombotic thrombocytopenic purpura and hemolytic uremic syndrome
   Disseminated intravascular coagulopathy
   Kasabach-Merritt syndrome
   Platelet destruction by artificial surfaces
   Hemophagocytosis
   Abnormal platelet distribution or pooling
   Splenomegaly
   Hypersplenism
   Hypothermia
   Massive transfusion
Drug-induced thrombocytopenia
   Heparin-induced thrombocytopenia
   Other drug-induced thrombocytopenias

Source: *Williams Hematology*, 8th ed, Chap. 119, Table 119–1, p. 1892.

- Total platelet mass is normal, platelet production is usually normal but may be reduced, and platelet survival is often normal.
- Hypothermia can cause temporary thrombocytopenia in humans and animals, presumably because platelets are transiently sequestered in the spleen and other organs.

Clinical Features
- Thrombocytopenia caused by sequestration is often of no clinical importance. The degree of thrombocytopenia is moderate, the total body content of platelets is normal, and platelets can be mobilized from the spleen.
- In patients with liver disease and splenomegaly, bleeding is usually a result of blood-coagulation disorders, and the thrombocytopenia is worsened by thrombopoietin (TPO) deficiency.
- Hepatic cirrhosis with portal hypertension and congestive splenomegaly is the most common disorder causing platelet sequestration, but any disease with an enlarged congested spleen can be associated with thrombocytopenia.
- The spleen is usually palpable, and the degree of thrombocytopenia is correlated with the size of the spleen.
- Patients with very large spleens and severe thrombocytopenia usually have decreased platelet production because of a marrow infiltrative process or severe liver disease, as well as sequestration.
- Only a few patients with hypothermia develop thrombocytopenia.

Laboratory Features
- Rarely is the platelet count less than 50×10^9/L unless a second contributing fator is present. Marrow megakaryocytes are usually normal in number and morphology.

Treatment and Prognosis
- Because thrombocytopenia caused by sequestration is usually not a clinically significant problem, no treatment is indicated.
- Splenectomy for another reason usually results in return of the platelet count to normal or above normal (see Chap. 28). Platelet counts may also return to normal after portal-systemic shunting for cirrhosis.
- Therapy for thrombocytopenia of hypothermia is rewarming and documenting normalization of platelet count.

THROMBOCYTOPENIA ASSOCIATED WITH MASSIVE TRANSFUSION

- Patients receiving 15 or more units of red cells within 24 hours regularly develop thrombocytopenia with platelet counts as low as 25×10^9/L.
- The severity of the thrombocytopenia is related to the number of transfusions, but counts may be higher than predicted because of release from the splenic pool, or lower because of microvascular consumption.
- Management depends on the severity of the thrombocytopenia and the clinical condition of the patient.

HEREDITARY AND CONGENITAL THROMBOCYTOPENIAS

- Generally have a clear inheritance pattern. Because prenatal infection or developmental abnormalities may be implicated, some are congenital, but not hereditary.
- Thrombocytopenia may be the only abnormality, or it may be associated with well-defined abnormalities of platelet function, as in the Bernard-Soulier, Wiskott-Aldrich, and gray platelet syndromes (discussed in Chap. 76).
- Thrombocytopenia may be diagnosed at any age, including adulthood. In those cases discovered after infancy, a mistaken diagnosis of immune thrombocytopenia (ITP) may be made, particularly in children with moderate thrombocytopenia. Family studies can be helpful in such situations.

Fanconi Anemia (See Chap. 3)

- Autosomal recessive severe aplastic anemia usually beginning at age 8 to 9 years.
- Cells from homozygotes have increased sensitivity to chromosomal breakage by DNA cross-linking agents.
- Diverse congenital abnormalities may occur, including short stature, skin pigmentation, hypoplasia of the thumb and radius, and anomalies of the genitourinary, cardiac, and central nervous systems.
- Patients are at risk for acute leukemia and other malignancies.
- The condition is generally fatal unless corrected by allogeneic hematopoietic marrow transplantation with a reduced intensity conditioning regimen.

Thrombocytopenia with Absent Radius (TAR) Syndrome

- Inheritance pattern suggests autosomal recessive but may be more complex.
- Usually noted at birth because of absence of both radii. Both ulnas are often absent or abnormal, and the humeri, bones of the shoulder girdle and feet may also be abnormal.
- One-third of patients have congenital heart anomalies.
- Allergy to cow's milk is common.
- Platelet counts are typically 15,000 to 30,000/μL, lower during infancy and during periods of stress (surgery, infection). Thrombocytopenia may not be severe and may be overlooked until adulthood.
- Megakaryocytes are diminished or absent.
- Leukemoid reactions and eosinophilia are common.
- Treatments with glucocorticoids, splenectomy, and intravenous immunoglobulin (IVIG) are generally ineffective. Splenectomy may be effective in rare patients presenting as adults.
- Death is usually due to hemorrhage and usually occur within the first year.
- If patient can be sustained for the first 1 to 2 years of life, the platelet count usually recovers and survival is normal.
- Platelet counts vary during adulthood, but symptoms other than menorrhagia are unusual.

May-Hegglin Anomaly, Fechtner Syndrome, Sebastian Syndrome, and Epstein Syndrome

- May-Hegglin anomaly is characterized by autosomal dominant inheritance of giant platelets, and characteristic inclusion bodies in neutrophils, eosinophils, and monocytes. These resemble Döhle bodies seen with acute infections but have a different ultra-structure. Thrombocytopenia is common but may not be present and is rarely severe.

- Fechtner, Sebastian and Epstein syndromes are quite similar to May-Hegglin anomaly, but also manifest varying degrees of high-tone sensorineural deafness, nephritis, and cataracts.
- May-Hegglin anomaly, Fechtner syndrome, Sebastian syndrome, and Epstein syndrome are autosomal dominant macrothrombocytopenias with mutations in the *MYH9* gene, located on chromosome 22q12-13. This gene encodes non-muscle myosin heavy chain (NMMHC)-IIA, which is expressed in platelets, kidney, leukocytes, and the cochlea.
- Platelets are large, but ultrastructurally normal. Megakaryocytes are normal in appearance and number. Platelet survival and bleeding times are normal or slightly abnormal.
- The thrombocytopenia of most patients is well tolerated, and so usually no treatment is necessary, even for surgery or delivery, but platelet transfusions are commonly given.

X-linked Thrombocytopenia with Dyserythropoiesis

- A family of X-linked disorders of thrombocytopenia associated with dyserythropoiesis and thalassemia has been described, causing a modest bleeding diathesis proportionate to the degree of thrombocytopenia. These patients also have porphyria.
- GATA-1 is an erythroid and megakaryocyte specific transcription factor that drives gene expression essential for each of these two cell lineages.
- In several families, mutations in the amino terminal-finger are associated with macrothrombocytopenia and variable abnormalities in the erythroid lineage, whereas in other families mutations in the amino-terminal finger that disrupt the interaction of GATA-1 with a co-factor (FOG-1) lead to macrothrombocytopenia with dyserythropoietic anemia or β-thalassemia.
- Treatment is supportive, with platelet or erythrocyte transfusions if necessary.

Familial Platelet Syndrome with Predisposition to Myeloid Neoplasms

- Familial platelet syndrome with predisposition to acute myelogenous leukemia (FPS/AML) is a rare autosomal dominant condition characterized by qualitative and quantitative platelet defects resulting in pathologic bleeding and predisposition to the development of AML.
- Genetic analysis of several pedigrees linked the causative defect to a mutation in the transcription factor Runx-1 (also previously known as AML1 and CBFA2). Runx-1 binds to transcriptional complexes and regulates many genes important in hematopoiesis.
- Allogeneic hematopoietic stem cell transplantation is the only known, curative treatment.

Congenital Amegakaryocytic Thrombocytopenia

- Congenital amegakaryocytic thrombocytopenia (CAMT) is a rare autosomal recessive disease that in most cases presents with severe thrombocytopenia without physical abnormalities at birth.
- Bleeding complications usually are substantial because of the severe thrombocytopenia present in these children.
- The disorder progresses to aplastic anemia before age 3 to 5 years in most patients.
- CAMT results from mutations in the TPO receptor c-Mpl, rendering it deficient (type I CAMT) or of reduced function (type II CAMT).
- Treatment with allogeneic stem cell transplantation is essential for survival.

Thrombocytopenia with Radial-Ulnar Synostosis

- Patients with amegakaryocytic thrombocytopenia with radial-ulnar synostosis present at birth with severe normocytic thrombocytopenia with absent marrow

megakaryocytes, proximal radioulnar synostosis, and other skeletal anomalies such as clinodactyly and shallow acetabulae.
- Bleeding complications are proportional to the degree of thrombocytopenia.
- Subsequent development of hypoplastic anemia and pancytopenia occur in several patients, suggesting that the defect is not limited to megakaryocytic progenitors.
- Genetic analysis of patients with thrombocytopenia and radioulnar synostosis revealed a mutation in *HoxA11*, known to be expressed in hematopoietic stem cells.

Wiskott-Aldrich Syndrome

- Wiskott-Aldrich syndrome (WAS) is a rare X-linked immunodeficiency disorder characterized by microthrombocytopenia, eczema, recurrent infections, T cell deficiency, and increased risk for autoimmune and lymphoproliferative disorders (also see Chap. 51).
- The syndrome is caused by mutations of the *WASP* gene located on the short arm of the X chromosome (Xp11.22).
- The product of this gene, the WAS protein (WASP), is expressed in hematopoietic cells. WASP regulates actin polymerization and coordinates reorganization of the actin cytoskeleton and signal transduction pathways that occur during cell movement and cell–cell interaction.
- Supportive treatment during acute bleeding and disease complications consists of platelet transfusions, antibiotics, and systemic glucocorticoids when eczema is severe.
- Patients with mild phenotypes and severe thrombocytopenia may respond to splenectomy, but the risk of infection in these already immunocompromised patients may outweigh the benefit.
- If sufficiently severe, allogeneic hematopoietic stem cell transplantation is the only effective, curative treatment.

Paris-Trousseau Syndrome

- Paris-Trousseau syndrome and its variant Jacobsen syndrome are congenital dysmorphology syndromes in which affected individuals manifest trigonocephaly, facial dysmorphism, heart defects, and mental retardation.
- All affected patients have mild to moderate thrombocytopenia and dysfunctional platelets.
- The blood film shows a subpopulation of platelets containing giant α-granules. Marrow examination reveals two distinct subpopulations of megakaryocytes with expansion of immature megakaryocytic progenitors, dysmegakaryopoiesis, and many micromegakaryocytes.
- Pathologic bleeding usually is mild.
- Both disorders result from deletion of the long arm of chromosome 11 at 11q23, a region that includes the *FLI1* gene, the product of which is a transcription factor involved in megakaryopoiesis.
- The dominant inheritance pattern of Paris-Trousseau syndrome despite the presence of one normal allele seems to result from monoallelic expression of *FLI1* only during a brief window in megakaryocyte differentiation.

Autosomal Dominant Thrombocytopenia with Linkage to Chromosome 10

- This autosomal dominant thrombocytopenia displays variable degrees of thrombocytopenia, with bleeding proportionate to the degree of thrombocytopenia.
- Unlike familial platelet syndrome with predisposition to myeloid neoplasms, there is no risk of progression of the disease.
- Patients with this disorder have a genetic defect localized to 10p11-12 on the short arm of chromosome 10. In one large kindred with the disorder, a missense mutation was identified within the gene *FLJ14813*a, which encodes a putative tyrosine kinase of unknown function.

• Megakaryocyte precursors from affected individuals produce low numbers of polyploid cells *in vitro*, with delayed nuclear and cytoplasmic differentiation when analyzed by electron microscopy.

Kasabach-Merritt Syndrome

• Kasabach-Merritt syndrome is thrombocytopenia associated with giant cavernous angiomas. These lesions can infiltrate aggressively and require intensive treatment.
• The mechanism is platelet consumption in the tumor caused by intravascular coagulation.
• The hemangiomas are usually present at birth and neonatal thrombocytopenia may be present. The syndrome may develop in adults.
• Hemangiomas are usually solitary and superficial, but may involve any internal organ.
• A bruit may be heard over the hemangioma, and cardiac failure may develop as a consequence of arteriovenous shunting.
• Thrombocytopenia may be severe, with marked red cell fragmentation. Laboratory abnormalities consistent with disseminated intravascular coagulation (DIC) are often present.
• Treatment may be necessary because of bleeding or growth of the tumor. Surgery can eliminate accessible lesions, and radiation therapy may be effective.
• In some cases, hemostatic abnormalities have been corrected by local thrombosis induced by antifibrinolytic agents, and thrombocytopenia has been corrected by treatment with antiplatelet agents.

ACQUIRED THROMBOCYTOPENIAS DUE TO DECREASED PLATELET PRODUCTION

• A heterogeneous group of disorders, including those caused by marrow aplasia (see Chap. 3), infiltration with neoplasms (Chap. 12), treatment with chemotherapeutic agents (see Chap. 39), and radiotherapy.

Megakaryocytic Aplasia

• Pure megakaryocytic aplasia or hypoplasia with no associated abnormalities is a rare disorder.
• Amegakaryocytic thrombocytopenia associated with other abnormalities such as dyserythropoiesis is more often seen and is likely a prodrome for myelodysplastic syndrome or aplastic anemia.
• Pure megakaryocytic aplasia appears to be a result of autoimmune suppression of megakaryocytes.
• The natural history is unclear and treatment with immunosuppression is empiric.

Infection

• Thrombocytopenia has been reported with diverse viral infections, usually the result of cytomegalovirus, Epstein-Barr virus, and hantavirus, in children receiving live-attenuated measles vaccine, and with many other infectious agents, such as *Mycoplasma, Plasmodium, Mycobacterium,* and *Ehrlichia.* The thrombocytopenia appears usually to be a result of decreased platelet production, but in some cases, immune-mediated platelet destruction may occur.

Thrombocytopenia Associated with HIV Infection

• Thrombocytopenia has been reported to occur in up to approximately 40 percent of adults with HIV infection.

Etiology and Pathogenesis

- The principal cause is ineffective platelet production due to HIV infection of the stromal cells that facilitate hematopoiesis, such as macrophages and microvascular epithelial cells, and direct infection of megakaryocytes.
- Platelet survival is also decreased, possibly because of immune platelet injury.
- The occurrence of thrombocytopenia correlates with plasma viral load and CD4 cell depletion.
- Granulomatous infection or infiltration of the marrow with lymphoma may also contribute to the thrombocytopenia.

Clinical and Laboratory Features

- Platelet counts are rarely below 50×10^9/L, and thrombocytopenia frequently resolves spontaneously.
- The marrow contains normal or increased numbers of megakaryocytes, and may be infiltrated with lymphoma or granulomas.

Therapy, Course, and Prognosis

- Antiretroviral drug regimens are the principal treatment for thrombocytopenia.
- Severe and symptomatic thrombocytopenia should be treated with prednisone (1 mg/kg per day) or with short courses of dexamethasone.
- IVIG given weekly at a dose of 0.04 g/kg for up to five weeks may be effective. Anti-D reagent has also been used.
- Splenectomy may be the most effective therapy, and does not appear to influence the course of the HIV infection adversely.

Nutritional Deficiencies and Alcohol-Induced Thrombocytopenia

Alcohol

- In alcoholics, thrombocytopenia is usually the result of cirrhosis with congestive splenomegaly, or of folic acid deficiency.
- Acute thrombocytopenia may also occur, because of direct suppression of platelet production by alcohol.
- After withdrawal of alcohol, platelet counts return to normal in 5 to 21 days, and may rise above normal levels.

Nutritional Deficiencies

- Mild thrombocytopenia occurs in about 20 percent of patients with megaloblastic anemia caused by vitamin B_{12} deficiency. The frequency may be higher with folic acid deficiency because of the frequent association with alcoholism.
- Thrombocytopenia is caused primarily by ineffective platelet production.
- Iron deficiency typically causes thrombocytosis, but severe thrombocytopenia may occur, especially in children.

ACQUIRED THROMBOCYTOPENIA AS A RESULT PRIMARILY OF SHORTENED PLATELET SURVIVAL

Thrombotic Thrombocytopenic Purpura (TTP)

- TTP is a clinical syndrome of consumptive thrombocytopenia that left untreated results in a 95 percent mortality rate (See also Chap 91).

Etiology and Pathogenesis

- A well-documented mechanism for formation of platelet thrombi is disseminated platelet aggregation caused by increased plasma levels of high-molecular-weight multimers of von Willebrand factor (VWF) which appear to accumulate because of deficiency of a plasma VWF-cleaving metalloprotease (a disintegrin with thrombomodulin repeats 13 [ADAMTS13]).
- The deficiency may be inherited or may be a result of inhibition of the enzyme by an autoantibody.

Clinical Features

- Sixty to 70 percent of patients with TTP are female.
- Full clinical expression of the disease is the "classic" pentad: thrombocytopenia, microangiopathic hemolytic anemia, neurologic symptoms, renal involvement, and fever.
- Because current treatment depends on prompt plasma exchange, the diagnosis now requires only thrombocytopenia and microangiopathic hemolytic anemia without another clinically apparent cause. However, more than 50 percent of patients also have neurologic signs and renal abnormalities.
- The most common presenting symptoms are neurologic abnormalities (headache, confusion, seizure, dysphagia, paresis), hemorrhage (epistaxis, hematuria, gastrointestinal bleeding, menorrhagia), fatigue, and abdominal pain.

Laboratory Findings

- Thrombocytopenia is essential for the diagnosis and is usually found at presentation or develops rapidly thereafter.
- Anemia and red cell fragmentation may also be absent at presentation but develop rapidly during the course of the disease.
- Consistent with severe hemolysis, serum lactic acid dehydrogenase (LDH) values are often markedly elevated and serum indirect bilirubin levels are also increased.
- Most patients have microscopic hematuria and proteinuria; some have acute, oliguric renal failure.
- Tissue biopsy is usually not required for diagnosis, but may be necessary in difficult cases. The characteristic lesions are arteriolar and capillary thrombi composed primarily of platelets but also containing VWF and fibrin. Morphologically identical lesions are found in preeclampsia, malignant hypertension, acute scleroderma, and renal allograft rejection.
- Based on increased understanding of pathophysiology, several tests of ADAMTS13 activity are available. Severe acquired ADAMTS13 deficiency appears to be specific for TTP, although the sensitivity of the association is debated and the frequency of severe ADAMTS13 deficiency in TTP depends on how patients are ascertained. If adult patients with thrombotic microangiopathy are selected with no plausible secondary cause, no diarrheal prodrome, and no features suggestive of hemolytic uremic syndrome (HUS; e.g., oliguria, severe hypertension, need for dialysis, serum creatinine >3.5 mg/dL), then at least 80 percent have undetectable ADAMTS13 activity and the majority will have easily detected autoantibodies that inhibit the protease.

Differential Diagnosis

- Sepsis and DIC may cause an acute illness with fever, chills, and multiple organ dysfunction. The distinction should be clear from coagulation studies, which in TTP are not usually severely abnormal.
- Bacterial endocarditis can present with anemia, thrombocytopenia, fever, neurologic symptoms, and renal abnormalities.
- Evans syndrome, a combination of autoimmune hemolytic anemia and ITP, may be confused with TTP. The direct red cell antiglobulin (Coombs) test is usually positive in Evans syndrome.
- Other considerations include systemic lupus erythematosus, catastrophic antiphospholipid syndrome, scleroderma, megaloblastic anemia, or myelodysplastic thrombocytopenia.

Treatment

- Plasma exchange is the most important treatment modality.
- Rapid initial therapy with plasma exchange is essential. If facilities are not immediately available for apheresis, plasma infusions should be administered until the patient can be transferred for exchange therapy.

- Plasma exchange is effective because of removal of the autoantibody and of large VWF multimers, and because of replacement of the ADAMTS13.
- Daily exchange of one plasma volume (40 mL/kg) is performed until the patient responds, as defined by correction of neurologic abnormalities, return to a normal platelet count, and normal or nearly normal serum LDH levels.
- Initial response typically occurs in the first week, and recovery is nearly complete in 3 weeks, but response may not occur for more than 1 month.
- If prompt response is not achieved, plasma exchange of 40 mL/kg should be done twice daily.
- After neurologic findings have resolved and the platelet count is normal, plasma exchange should be continued at increasing time intervals for another 1 to 2 weeks to avoid relapse, although solid evidence that such tapering of therapy reduces relapses is lacking.
- Renal function recovers more slowly than the neurologic and hematologic abnormalities. It is unknown if continued plasma exchange will affect recovery of renal function.
- With plasma exchange, mortality has been reduced from greater than 90 percent to less than 20 percent.
- With the realization that TTP represents an autoimmune disorder, treatment with glucocorticoids makes some sense.
- Prednisone at a dose of 200 mg/d orally may be effective in some patients with minimal symptoms and no neurologic changes, but is used almost always as an adjunct to plasma exchange.
- Therapy with antiplatelet agents has not been generally effective, and carries a significant risk of hemorrhage.
- In patients who have had a stroke or transient cerebral ischemic events, aspirin therapy is appropriate when severe thrombocytopenia has resolved.
- Prior to the plasma exchange era, splenectomy was extensively used with some success in combination with glucocorticoids and dextran infusion.
- Anecdotal reports of success have appeared for numerous agents, including IVIG, vincristine, azathioprine, cyclophosphamide, cyclosporine, and extracorporal immunoadsorption.
- Platelet transfusion has been reported to exacerbate TTP and has been suggested as a cause of death in some reports.
- However, cautious administration of platelet transfusions may be indicated in some patients with major bleeding associated with marked thrombocytopenia.

Course and Prognosis
- Most of the now rare deaths occur early in the course of the disease.
- Approximately 30 to 50 percent of patients have relapsing disease.
- Patients who relapse long after the initial episode predictably recover with retreatment.
- It is not known whether or not those with chronic thrombocytopenia are more likely to relapse.
- The frequency of long-term sequelae after recovery from acute TTP is not known. Some patients may continue to have mild thrombocytopenia or abnormal renal function. Permanent neurologic complications are uncommon.

Epidemic HUS in Children Caused By Shiga-Toxin–Producing *E. coli*
- Follows acute enteric infection with *Escherichia coli* or *Shigella dysenteriae* serotypes which produce the Shiga toxin, most often infection with *E. coli* serotype 0157:H7.
- Progression of *E. coli* 0157:H7 infection to HUS occurs in 2 to 7 percent of sporadic cases and in up to 30 percent of cases in some epidemics.
- Boys and girls are equally affected, and most cases occur between April and September.

- Most outbreaks are caused by undercooked beef, but other sources have been implicated including lettuce. Person-to-person transmission may also occur.

Clinical and Laboratory Features

- The major presenting symptom is diarrhea, which is bloody in most patients. The diarrhea may be sufficiently severe to require colectomy.
- Most patients are oliguric on admission, but average duration of symptoms before diagnosis of HUS is 6 days.
- Fever and hypertension are common. Pancreatitis and seizures may occur.
- Laboratory features are thrombocytopenia, microangiopathic hemolytic anemia, and the findings of acute renal failure.

Treatment, Course, and Prognosis

- Treatment is supportive. Approximately 50 percent of patients require dialysis.
- Plasma exchange appears to have minimal or no benefit.
- Mortality of epidemic childhood HUS is 3 to 10 percent, but HUS in the elderly may have mortality up to approximately 90 percent.
- Patients frequently have permanently impaired renal function after recovery.
- Relapses do not appear to occur.

TTP/HUS Associated with Infections Other than Shiga-Toxin–Producing *E. coli*

- A syndrome resembling TTP and HUS has been reported to occur sporadically after infection caused by rickettsia, viruses, or bacteria other than those producing Shiga toxin.
- None of these infections is as clearly associated with TTP-HUS as is infection with *E. coli* 0157:H7.
- It appears some infections may cause bona fide HUS; others may exacerbate existing TTP.
- Patients infected with HIV may develop a syndrome similar to TTP and HUS, but differ in having a gradual onset and a less predictable response to plasma exchange. Some patients survive for weeks or months without plasma exchange. These patients often have associated medical problems that could account for some of the findings interpreted as caused by TTP or HUS.

Drug-Induced TTP

- A syndrome resembling ADAMTS13 deficient TTP may be due to drug-dependent antibodies to platelets and other cells.

Quinine

- Quinine is a frequent offender. Patients may have quinine-dependent antiplatelet antibodies. Some patients also have antineutrophil antibodies and develop severe neutropenia.
- Abdominal pain and nausea are common presenting symptoms.
- Plasma exchange is ineffective. Most patients also require hemodialysis, but usually recover normal renal function.
- Reexposure to quinine, even in small amounts, can cause immediate recurrence.

Ticlopidine

- Acute, severe TTP-HUS has been reported to occur in some patients treated with short courses of ticlopidine.

Cancer Chemotherapy

- Nearly all chemotherapy patients who develop TTP have been treated with mitomycin C, most often for gastric cancer. Cisplatin, bleomycin, and pentostatin have also been reported to cause TTP.
- Induction of TTP by mitomycin C may be dose related, but less than 10 percent of patients receiving high doses develop the disease.

- Renal pathology is identical to that of other patients with TTP.
- The efficacy of plasma exchange is uncertain.
- Most patients die of their cancer or of renal failure.

Cyclosporine A

- A syndrome of severe renal failure, microangiopathic hemolytic anemia, and thrombocytopenia has been reported in patients receiving cyclosporine after allogeneic marrow transplantation, but the etiologic role of cyclosporine is uncertain.
- Tacrolimus has also been reported to cause TTP.

Other Drugs

- TTP has been associated with administration of metronidazole, cocaine, simvastatin, and ecstasy.

TTP Associated with Marrow Transplantation

- Most patients have had allogeneic transplants, but the disorder has also occurred with transplantation of autologous marrow or peripheral blood stem cells.
- The diagnosis of TTP may be difficult to establish because of the severe, multiorgan dysfunction accompanying allogeneic hematopoietic stem cell transplantation.
- All features of TTP in these patients could be caused by graft-versus-host disease, radiation toxicity, and systemic infection.
- Most patients do not respond to plasma exchange, and even in responsive patients plasma exchange may not affect outcome.

TTP Associated with Cancer

- TTP may develop rarely in patients with metastatic carcinoma of various types, but more than half of such patients have had gastric cancer.
- Laboratory evidence of DIC is found in a minority of these patients.
- Therapy, course, and prognosis depend on the response of the tumor to chemotherapy. Plasma exchange appears not to be effective.

TTP Associated with Autoimmune Disorders

- Systemic lupus erythematosus, acute scleroderma, and the catastrophic antiphospholipid syndrome may present with clinical and pathologic findings difficult or impossible to distinguish from TTP.
- Treatment with plasma exchange has been reported to be effective in the severe autoimmune disorders as well as in TTP.

TTP Associated with Pregnancy

- TTP occurs in about 1 in 25,000 pregnancies.
- The clinical and pathologic features of TTP are similar to those of preeclampsia, particularly the HELLP syndrome (microangiopathic *h*emolytic anemia, *e*levated *l*iver enzymes, *l*ow *p*latelet count), suggesting a relationship between these disorders and complicating differential diagnosis.
- TTP has recurred in successive pregnancies in some patients and during pregnancy in women who have recovered from previous episodes of TTP unrelated to pregnancy. Pregnancy is therefore considered a risk for recurrence of TTP.
- With severe disease and a viable fetus, delivery should be induced. This will resolve preeclampsia, but may or may not resolve platelet consumption. Some patients have delivered healthy term infants after developing TTP during the pregnancy.

THROMBOCYTOPENIA IN PREGNANCY

Gestational Thrombocytopenia

- Gestational thrombocytopenia, as defined by the following five criteria, occurs in approximately 5 percent of pregnancies: mild, asymptomatic thrombocytopenia; no past history of thrombocytopenia (except during a prior pregnancy); occurrence during late gestation; absence of fetal thrombocytopenia; and spontaneous resolution after delivery.
- Platelet counts are usually greater than 70×10^9/L and most are between 130 and 150×10^9/L. Lower platelet count or onset early in gestation suggest the diagnosis of immune thrombocytopenia (see ITP below).
- Usual obstetric care is appropriate for both mother and infant.

Preeclampsia

- Preeclampsia is defined by the presence of hypertension, proteinuria, and edema occurring during pregnancy and resolving after delivery. Eclampsia is preeclampsia plus neurologic abnormalities occurring peripartum.
- Thrombocytopenia develops in approximately 15 percent of women with preeclampsia, but platelet counts below 50×10^9/L occur in less than 5 percent.
- Some patients with severe preeclampsia may develop the HELLP syndrome, which may mimic TTP.
- Delivery of the fetus is the most effective approach to these disorders. Recovery usually begins promptly but may be delayed for several days.
- Plasma exchange is indicated for patients with severe thrombocytopenia and microangiopathic hemolytic anemia if the fetus cannot be delivered or prompt recovery does not occur after delivery. Earlier initiation of plasma exchange is indicated for severe clinical problems, such as acute, anuric renal failure or neurologic abnormalities.

IMMUNE THROMBOCYTOPENIA

- Immune thrombocytopenia is an acquired disease of children and adults that is defined as isolated thrombocytopenia with no clinically apparent associated condition or other causes of thrombocytopenia. No specific criteria establish the diagnosis of ITP; the diagnosis relies on exclusion of other causes of thrombocytopenia.
- Adult ITP typically has an insidious onset and rarely resolves spontaneously.
- Childhood ITP characteristically is acute in onset and resolves spontaneously within 6 months.

Adult ITP

Etiology and Pathogenesis

- The mechanism of thrombocytopenia appears to be shortened intravascular survival of platelets as a consequence of splenic sequestration and destruction caused by antiplatelet antibodies.
- Antiplatelet antibodies also appear to bind to megakaryocytes and interfere with thrombocytopoiesis, leading to normal or decreased rates of platelet production even with increased or normal numbers of megakaryocytes.
- Most patients with ITP have demonstrable antibodies to platelet membrane glycoproteins GP IIb/GP IIIa and/or GP Ib/IX, but their specific pathogenetic role is not clear because they are also demonstrable in other conditions.
- Bleeding times are usually shorter than expected from the platelet count, suggesting enhanced platelet function.
- In some patients, impaired platelet function is demonstrable, but its clinical significance is unknown.

- In some patients, it is likely that T cell-mediated immune dysfunction is responsible for thrombocytopenia, and such patients are less likely to respond to now standard immunosuppressive treatments (rituximab, immune globulin).

Clinical Features

- Adult ITP appears to be more common in young women than in young men, but among older patients, the sex incidence may be equal.
- Most adults present with a long history of purpura, but many patients are now asymptomatic at diagnosis because of the widespread inclusion of platelet enumeration in routine blood counts.
- Petcchiae are not palpable, and occur most often in dependent regions. Hemorrhagic bullae may appear on mucosal surfaces with severe thrombocytopenia.
- Purpura, menorrhagia, epistaxis, and gingival bleeding are common. Gastrointestinal bleeding and hematuria are less so. Intracerebral hemorrhage occurs in approximately 1 percent of patients but is the most common cause of death.
- Overt bleeding is rare unless thrombocytopenia is severe (less than 10×10^9/L), and even at this level most patients do not experience major hemorrhage.
- A palpable spleen strongly suggests that ITP is *not* the cause for thrombocytopenia.

Laboratory Features

- Thrombocytopenia is the essential abnormality. The blood films should be reviewed to rule out pseudothrombocytopenia (see above). The platelets are usually of normal size but may be enlarged.
- White blood cell count is usually normal, and the hemoglobin level is also normal unless significant hemorrhage has occurred.
- Coagulation studies are normal.
- The bleeding time does not provide useful information.
- Marrow megakaryocytes may be increased in number, with a shift to younger, less polypoid forms, but assessment of megakaryocyte morphology and number is not quantitative.

Differential Diagnosis

- The diagnosis is one of exclusion. Other conditions that can mimic ITP are acute infections, myelodysplasia, chronic DIC, drug-induced thrombocytopenia, and chronic liver disease with platelet sequestration.
- The distinction from congenital thrombocytopenia is especially important to avoid inappropriate treatment.

Treatment: Initial Management

- Patients who are incidentally discovered to have asymptomatic mild or moderate ITP can safely be followed with no treatment.
- Patients with platelet counts over 50×10^9/L usually do not have spontaneous, clinically important bleeding, and may undergo invasive procedures.

Emergency Treatment of Acute Bleeding Caused by Severe Thrombocytopenia

- Immediate platelet transfusion is indicated for patients with hemorrhagic emergencies. Despite having a presumably short platelet survival time, some patients have substantial posttransfusion increments in their platelet counts.
- IVIG may be given as a single infusion of 0.4 to 1.0 g/kg followed immediately by a platelet transfusion. IVIG, 1 g/kg per day for 2 days, increases the platelet count in most patients within 3 days.
- High doses of glucocorticoids, such as 1 g of methylprednisolone daily for 3 days, may cause a rapid increase in the platelet count.
- ε-Aminocaproic acid can be effective in controlling acute bleeding after failure of platelet transfusion and prednisone.

Glucocorticoids

- Glucocorticoid therapy likely decreases sequestration and destruction of antibody-sensitized platelets and may enhance platelet production.

- Prednisone, given in a dose of 1 mg/kg per day orally, is indicated for patients with symptomatic thrombocytopenia, and probably for all patients with platelet counts below 30,000 to 50,000/µL who may be at increased risk for hemorrhagic complications.
- Sixty percent of patients will increase their platelet count to greater than 50×10^9/L, and approximately 25 percent will achieve a complete recovery. Most relapse when the prednisone dose is tapered or discontinued.
- The duration of prednisone therapy prior to consideration of splenectomy depends on the severity of the bleeding, the dose of prednisone required to maintain a response, and the risks of surgery.
- Long-term therapy with glucocorticoids can lead to many important side effects, including immunosuppression and osteoporosis.
- Courses of high-dose dexamethasone (40 mg/d × 4 days) is being used increasingly frequently in an attempt to induce a more sustained remission than the rather poor results obtained with standard prednisone therapy. Randomized clinical trials are necessary to prove that this therapy is superior to standard doses of prednisone, or whether the addition of other immunosuppressive agents (e.g., rituximab) is of real value.

Intravenous Immunoglobulin

- IVIG is used in adults when a transient rise in platelet count is desired, or when glucocorticoids are contraindicated.
- Initial dose is 2 g/kg given over 2 to 5 days. Comparable responses may occur with half this dose, or with 0.8 g/kg given once.
- Typical response is an increase in platelet count 2 or 3 days after the infusions begin, with return to pretreatment levels within several weeks.
- Fever, headache, nausea, and vomiting occur in approximately 25 percent of recipients, and aseptic meningitis occurs in 10 percent. Acute renal failure may occur, and hemolysis because of alloantibodies is also a side effect. Such doses of IVIG are a large volume load for patients with borderline cardiac function.

Anti-Rh(D) Immune Globulin

- Approximately 70 percent of patients receiving infusions of anti-Rh(D) antiserum at a dose of 50 µg/kg will respond with an increase in platelet count greater than 20×10^9/L, and half will have an increase greater than 50×10^9/L.
- In most patients, the response lasts longer than 3 weeks.
- Anti-Rh(D) is ineffective in Rh(D)-negative patients or following splenectomy.
- Side effects include alloimmune hemolysis, which is usually no more severe than that encountered with IVIG, but several deaths have been reported due to massive hemolysis. Anti-Rh(D) is less expensive than a standard course of IVIG.
- Headache, nausea, chills, and fever are much less frequent than with therapeutic doses of IVIG.

Splenectomy

- Sustained remission occurs in about two-thirds of patients who undergo splenectomy.
- The risks of operative bleeding complications with splenectomy are low even with severe thrombocytopenia, but it is prudent to have platelet preparations available in case of excessive intraoperative bleeding.
- Intravenous IVIG can induce a transient remission of thrombocytopenia and may be used to prepare for the operation.
- Most responses to splenectomy occur within several days. Responses after 10 days are unusual. The rapidity and extent of the response appear to correlate with durability of response.
- Splenectomy is associated with a small but significantly increased risk for severe infectious complications. All patients should be immunized with polyvalent

pneumococcal, *Haemophilus influenzae* type b and meningococcal vaccines at least 2 weeks before surgery.

- One-half of patients who relapse after an initial response to splenectomy will do so within 6 months.

Removal of Accessory Spleens

- Accessory spleens are found at splenectomy in 15 to 20 percent of patients, and may be present in as many as 10 percent of those refractory to splenectomy or who relapse after splenectomy.
- Remission after removal of an accessory spleen is unpredictable.

Thrombopoietin Mimics

- Two small molecule mimics of TPO have been approved by the US Food and Drug Administration for the treatment of refractory chronic ITP: romiplostim (N-plate), a "peptibody" composed of four copies of a TPO receptor binding peptide on an Ig scaffold, and eltrombopag (Promacta), a small organic molecule that is orally bio-available. Several other mimics are currently undergoing clinical trials.
- Both drugs are potent stimulators of thrombopoiesis, and rapidly (3 to 5 days) lead to major, dose-dependent increases (into the normal range) in platelet levels in the majority of patients.
- While on TPO mimic therapy, hemorrhagic complications of thrombocytopenia occur less commonly, are less severe, and the use of coexistent ITP therapeutics and salvage agents are significantly reduced.
- While studied carefully during clinical trials, neither agent has been associated with a statistically significant increase in thrombotic complications, and in only a small number of patients have marrow reticulin fibrosis been noted. Eltrombopag has been associated with a low (approximately 4%) incidence of a modest rise in hepatic transaminases levels.
- Neither of the approved agents is disease modifying, so that the platelet count remains normal only so long as the drug is used. Abrupt discontinuation of these agents can lead to rebound thrombocytopenia more severe than the patient's baseline thrombocytopenia seen before institution of the drug.

Treatment: Chronic Refractory ITP

- Most other treatments available for patients with ITP who have relapsed after splenectomy have given inconsistent results, and are often of significant risk. Refractory ITP presents an unusually complex clinical problem.
- Observation may be appropriate for asymptomatic patients, even those with platelet counts of less than 30×10^9/L.
- The goal of treatment is to achieve a platelet count that ensures hemostasis, not necessarily a normal platelet count.

Treatment of ITP During Pregnancy and Delivery

- It is extremely important to attempt to differentiate ITP from gestational thrombocytopenia.
- Early in pregnancy, treatment of maternal ITP should be the same as if the patient were not pregnant, using glucocorticoids in those patients whose symptoms require intervention.
- Splenectomy should be deferred if possible because ITP may improve after delivery. Therapy with IVIG may help delay splenectomy.
- In infants born to mothers with ITP, there is a 10 percent risk of a platelet count less than 50×10^9/L, and a 4 percent risk of a platelet count less than 20×10^9/L.
- The severity of neonatal thrombocytopenia correlates with the severity of maternal thrombocytopenia. Treatment of the mother with glucocorticoids or with IVIG close to term has no effect on the platelet count of the infant.
- No satisfactory method is available to obtain accurate fetal platelet counts.

- Current practice is to recommend cesarean section only for obstetric indications.
- It is critical to monitor the newborn's platelet count during the first several days of life because severe thrombocytopenia may develop after delivery.

Childhood ITP

Clinical Features

- Peak incidence is from ages 2 to 4 years, and is the same in both sexes until age 10 years, when female predominance appears.
- Bruises and petechiae are nearly universal presenting symptoms, usually of less than 1 to 2 weeks duration.
- Epistaxis, gingival bleeding, and gastrointestinal bleeding are uncommon.
- The frequency of a palpable spleen is the same as in unaffected children (approximately 10%).

Laboratory Features

- Most children present with platelet counts less than $20 \times 10^9/L$.
- Marrow examination is usually performed to rule out acute lymphocytic leukemia.

Course and Prognosis

- About 85 percent of patients selected for no specific treatment (e.g., glucocorticoids or splenectomy) have a complete response within 6 months.
- Good prognostic features are abrupt onset, brief duration, and mild symptoms.
- Most responders develop no new purpura after the first week, and the platelet count is usually normal in 2 to 8 weeks.
- Purpura for more than 2 to 4 weeks before diagnosis is the most important predictor of chronic thrombocytopenia. Other factors are female sex, age greater than 10 years, and higher platelet count at presentation.
- Few children with ITP have critical complications, and even fewer die. Only 1 percent or less have intracerebral hemorrhage.

Treatment

- The need for treatment is controversial. No specific treatment is recommended by some for patients with bruising as the only symptom, regardless of the severity of the thrombocytopenia, but most patients receive treatment, more often with IVIG than with glucocorticoids.
- IVIG given 0.8 g/kg in a single dose or 2.0 g/kg in divided doses is expected to improve the platelet count significantly more rapidly than no treatment.
- Treatment has not been shown to decrease the risk of bleeding or death.
- Because of the risks of severe infection, splenectomy should be deferred for 6 to 12 months after diagnosis, and then recommended only for children with severe thrombocytopenia and significant bleeding symptoms.
- Splenectomy in children is associated with an increased risk of severe infection. In addition to all routine immunizations, polyvalent pneumococcal, *H. influenzae* type b, and meningococcal vaccines should be given more than 2 weeks prior to splenectomy. Penicillin prophylaxis is routinely given to splenectomized children up to the age of 5 years.
- Efficacy of measures for therapy of chronic ITP in childhood is uncertain. Because the mortality is low and spontaneous remissions occur even after many years, potentially harmful treatments should be used only when there is a substantial risk of death or morbidity from hemorrhage.

CYCLIC THROMBOCYTOPENIA

- A rare disorder that occurs predominantly in young women, usually related to the menstrual cycle, but also occurs in men and postmenopausal women. In some patients, there are parallel cycles of leukopenia.

- The pathogenesis may be autoimmune platelet destruction, increased platelet phagocytosis because of cyclic increments in macrophage colony-stimulating factor (M-CSF), or cyclic decreases in platelet production.
- Although spontaneous remissions may occur, cyclic thrombocytopenia is chronic in most patients and may be a prodrome for marrow failure.
- Numerous therapies for cyclic thrombocytopenia have been attempted, with inconsistent success at best.

HEPARIN-INDUCED THROMBOCYTOPENIA (HIT) (SEE ALSO CHAP. 91)

Etiology

- HIT is an immune-mediated disorder caused by antibodies that recognize a neoepitope in platelet factor 4 exposed when it binds heparin. The result is activation of platelets, monocytes, and the coagulation cascade and, ultimately, thrombosis.

Clinical Features

- It should be noted that the platelet count of many, if not most patients drop by approximately 10 percent following the institution of heparin therapy. This may begin soon after heparin is started, and may resolve even while heparin is continued. This form of thrombocytopenia is most frequent with full-dose therapy. It is not antibody-mediated and may be a result of platelet aggregation by heparin.
- Patients may present with a wide range of platelet counts, including levels close to or above normal, as long as the count has dropped by 50 percent from baseline.
- Unless recently exposed to heparin (<100 days), the platelet count begins to fall 4 to 5 days after heparin therapy is instituted.
- The disease can occur with any heparin preparation: unfractionated heparin, low-molecular-weight heparins, and heparin-like compounds such as pentosan and danaparoid, and with all doses and routes of administration. Higher-molecular-weight fractions of heparin may interact more readily with platelets and thereby cause thrombocytopenia more frequently.
- Affects up to 5 percent of patients exposed to heparin, and to lesser numbers of patients exposed to other forms of heparin.
- Thrombocytopenia may recur upon readministration of heparin.
- Regardless of the degree of thrombocytopenia, the disease is the most hypercoagulable condition known.
- Venous thromboembolism is more commonly seen than is arterial thrombosis, although the latter is usually more striking. Thrombosis usually appears the first week after diagnosis and has high morbidity and mortality.

Laboratory Features

- Two assay prototypes for confirming the diagnosis are available. One measures the Ig antibodies to the heparin/PF4 complex (antigen assay), and the other measures heparin-dependent antibodies that activate platelets (activation assay) in plasma or sera.
- Commercially available antigen assays measure either binding to PF4-heparin or PF4-polyvinylsulfate by enzyme-linked immunosorbent assay.
- Activation assays are not commercially established because specific platelet donors are needed each time, and donor platelets can vary greatly in their sensitivity to activation by HIT sera. One of the earliest and best-established activation assays, serotonin release assay, involves ^{14}C-serotonin release from platelets induced by HIT antibodies and heparin.
- In patients with a high clinical risk, heparin should be stopped and alternative treatment started even before laboratory results are available. A positive antigen test and particularly a progressive increase in the number of platelets over the following days are confirmatory.

- A negative antigen test does not rule out the diagnosis and should be repeated after 24 hours while the patient is undergoing alternative anticoagulant therapy. If the repeat assay is negative and platelet count does not increase, alternative diagnoses should be considered.

Prevention, Diagnosis, and Therapy

- The platelet counts of patients on heparin therapy should be obtained frequently.
- For patients requiring long-term anticoagulation, the best means of avoiding thrombocytopenia associated with thrombosis is to initiate oral anticoagulant therapy simultaneously with heparin so that therapeutic warfarin-anticoagulation will be achieved before HIT is likely to occur.
- A clinical suspicion of HIT should be made if the platelet count falls below 100×10^9/L, or decreases by more than 50 percent from baseline and the decrease is unexplained by any other cause, or if a thromboembolic episode develops that is unexplained by other causes.
- Heparin therapy should be stopped once a strong clinical suspicion of HIT arises, and especially once a diagnosis is made.
- Two drugs available for anticoagulation in patients with HIT are lepirudin and argatroban, which directly inhibit thrombin.
- Lepirudin prolongs the activated partial thromboplastin time (aPTT), so this test can be used to monitor effective dosing. Lepirudin induces anti-lepirudin antibodies in approximately half of patients who receive the drug. These antibodies rarely alter biologic activity but tend to prolong the drug's half-life, necessitating careful monitoring by aPTT.
- Argatroban is synthesized from arginine and is rapidly metabolized in the liver. It affects both the aPTT and prothrombin time.
- Use of lepirudin and argatroban is efficacious; the incidence of thrombotic complication is reduced, perhaps by half, and the time to platelet count recovery is shortened. However, bleeding complications can occur.
- Lepirudin or argatroban should be given until patients recover from thrombocytopenia before adding and then switching to a prolonged course of an oral anticoagulant.

OTHER DRUG-INDUCED IMMUNOLOGIC THROMBOCYTOPENIAS

Etiology and Pathogenesis

- In these patients, thrombocytopenia is assumed to be a consequence of immune platelet destruction by drug-dependent antibodies. The target of antibody attack is usually composed of a drug-platelet surface protein complex.
- A vast number of drugs have been implicated as causing thrombocytopenia. Drugs for which modestly rigorous criteria for a causal effect are presented in Chap. 119, Table 119–5, page 1914, of *Williams Hematology,* 8th ed.

Clinical and Laboratory Features

- Drug-induced thrombocytopenia typically produces profoundly low platelet counts.
- The time from initiating drug therapy to the development of thrombocytopenia averages 14 days, but may be as long as 3 years. With rechallenge, thrombocytopenia may appear within minutes, but almost always appears within 3 days.
- Patients may have nausea and vomiting, rash, fever, and abnormal liver function tests. Leukopenia may also develop.

Diagnosis

- A careful history is crucial. In addition to prescription medications, the patients should be asked about over-the-counter drugs, alternative therapies, soft drinks, mixers, and aperitifs that may contain quinine.
- Laboratory tests to detect drug-dependent antiplatelet antibodies remain largely investigational.

- The diagnosis can only be made by rechallenge with the drug after recovery from thrombocytopenia, but rechallenge can be dangerous because of the possibility of developing severe thrombocytopenia, even with very small doses of a drug.
- For patients who require therapy with multiple drugs, it may be appropriate to reintroduce each drug individually, and to observe the patient for several days before adding another drug.

Treatment
- Withdrawal of the offending drug is essential.
- Prednisone therapy is commonly given but may not influence recovery.
- Major bleeding requires urgent intervention as for severe ITP: platelet transfusion, high-dose parenteral methylprednisolone, and possibly IVIG.

NEONATAL ALLOIMMUNE THROMBOCYTOPENIA

Etiology and Pathogenesis
- Pathogenesis is similar to neonatal alloimmune hemolytic disease except that fetal platelets rather than erythrocytes provide the antigenic challenge.
- Destruction of fetal platelets is caused by transplacentally acquired maternal antibodies directed against fetal-platelet–specific antigen inherited from the father.
- The platelet antigen HPA-1a, found in approximately 98 percent of the general population, provides the most frequent immunogenic stimulus in persons of European ancestry. Other alloantigens are also implicated.

Clinical and Laboratory Features
- First-born children are often affected, indicating that fetal platelets cross the placenta during gestation. Recurrence with subsequent pregnancies is common.
- Because only 2 percent of the general population lacks the HPA-1a antigen, finding that the mother's platelets are HPA-1a-negative provides presumptive evidence of alloimmune origin. Neonatal alloimmune thrombocytopenia is in every respect more severe than thrombocytopenia in infants born to mothers with ITP, with death or neurologic impairment occurring in up to 25 percent of infants.
- Platelet counts usually recover in 1 to 2 weeks.

Prevention and Management
- Antenatal screening for neonatal alloimmune thrombocytopenia has been studied, but the cost-effectiveness of such a program has not been established.
- Management of neonatal alloimmune thrombocytopenia requires platelet transfusion, glucocorticoids, and IVIG.
- Maternal platelets are HPA-1a-negative, and should be effective in transfusion, but require washing to remove maternal plasma containing antibodies, and irradiated to prevent graft-versus-host disease.
- If HPA-1a-negative platelets are unavailable, random donor platelets plus IVIG treatment may be used.
- Management of subsequent pregnancies may require *in utero* sampling of fetal blood to obtain platelet counts and serial *in utero* platelet transfusions, procedures with significant risks for the fetus.
- Administration of IVIG and glucocorticoids to the mother may reduce the prevalence of *in utero* cerebral hemorrhage but is not effective in all patients.
- Delivery by scheduled cesarean section may reduce the risk of neonatal cerebral hemorrhage.

POSTTRANSFUSION PURPURA
- Acute, severe thrombocytopenia occurring 5 to 15 days after transfusion of a blood product and associated with high-titer, platelet-specific alloantibodies.

Etiology and Pathogenesis

- Platelet destruction is caused by an alloantibody to a platelet-specific antigen.
- Anti-HPA-1a is present in more than 80 percent of cases, but alloimmunization to most other platelet-specific antigens has been reported.
- The mechanism of formation of the antibody is well established, but it remains uncertain how anti-HPA-1a antibodies can cause destruction of HPA-1a-negative platelets.

Clinical and Laboratory Features

- Most patients are women, and most are multiparous.
- Severe thrombocytopenia (platelet counts less than 5×10^9/L) with major bleeding, occurs several days after transfusion of 1 or more units of blood product, usually packed red cells.
- Fever often accompanies the inciting transfusion and the initial presentation.
- Antibodies to a platelet-specific alloantigen can be detected by appropriate serologic methods.
- Only after recovery can the patient's platelet types be determined.

Treatment, Course, and Prognosis

- Platelet transfusions are essential if there is severe, active bleeding, but these frequently lead to systemic reactions and the platelet count may not be increased.
- Glucocorticoids and IVIG are usually effective.
- Plasma exchange may be effective in 80 percent of patients.
- Thrombocytopenia begins to resolve after several days in most patients, but may be persistent and severe in some.

For a more detailed discussion, see Reyhan Diz-Küçükkaya, Junmei Chen, Amy Geddis and José A. López: Thrombocytopenia. Chap. 119, p. 1891 in *Williams Hematology*, 8th ed.

CHAPTER 75
Reactive (Secondary) Thrombocytosis

- The upper limit of a normal platelet count is usually between 350×10^9/L and 450×10^9/L depending on the clinical laboratory and specific method used.
- Table 75–1 presents the major causes of elevation of the platelet count above the normal limit.
- Reactive thrombocytosis may persist for prolonged periods and resolve only with resolution of the underlying disorder.
- Thrombocytosis after recovery from thrombocytopenia ("rebound") usually peaks in 10 to 14 days.
- The platelet count after splenectomy may reach 1000×10^9/L or more within the first week and return to normal within about 2 months. Severe or persistent postsplenectomy thrombocytosis may be a result of persistent iron deficiency anemia or unmasking of primary thrombocythemia.
- There is no convincing evidence that therapy to reduce the platelet count or interfere with platelet function is of benefit in reactive thrombocytosis, with the possible exception of severe postsplenectomy thrombocytosis in patients with persistent hemolytic anemia.

For a more detailed discussion, see Kenneth Kaushansky: Reactive Thrombocytosis. Chap. 120, p. 1929 in *Williams Hematology*, 8th ed.

TABLE 75–1	**MAJOR CAUSES OF THROMBOCYTOSIS**

1. Clonal thrombocytosis
   a. Primary (essential) thrombocythemia
   b. Other myeloproliferative disorders (polycythemia vera, chronic myelogenous leukemia, primary myelofibrosis)
2. Familial thrombocytosis
3. Reactive (secondary) thrombocytosis
   a. Acute blood loss
   b. Iron deficiency
   c. Postsplenectomy, asplenic states
   d. Recovery from thrombocytopenia ("rebound")
   e. Malignancies
   f. Chronic inflammatory and infectious diseases (inflammatory bowel disease, connective tissue disorders, temporal arteritis, tuberculosis, chronic pneumonitis)
   g. Acute inflammatory and infectious diseases
   h. Response to exercise
   i. Response to drugs (vincristine, epinephrine, all-*trans*-retinoic acid, cytokines, and growth factors)
   j. Hemolytic anemia

CHAPTER 76
Hereditary Platelet Disorders

Abnormalities of platelet function are expressed primarily by mucocutaneous bleeding. The most frequent laboratory abnormality is prolongation of the bleeding time, although the clinical value of the bleeding time is questionable because of lack of reproducibility and poor correlation with clinical bleeding.

- Hereditary qualitative platelet disorders classified according to the responsible abnormalities are presented in **Table 76–1**.

ABNORMAL GLYCOPROTEIN (GP) IIb/IIIa (αIIBβ3, CD41/CD61): GLANZMANN THROMBASTHENIA

- Glanzmann thrombasthenia is characterized by severely reduced or absent platelet aggregation in response to many physiologic agonists because of abnormalities of platelet GP IIb and/or IIIa (see **Table 76–1**).

Etiology and Pathogenesis

- GPIIb/IIIa functions as receptor for fibrinogen and other adhesive glycoproteins.
- It is required for platelet aggregation induced by all agonists believed to function *in vivo*.
- Both GPIIb and GPIIIa are required for normal function, and defects in either component may cause thrombasthenia.
- Many different molecular biologic abnormalities have been described that affect expression or various functions of the two molecules.
- Inherited as an autosomal recessive disorder, but about 40 percent of patients are compound heterozygotes rather than homozygotes.

Clinical Features

- The most frequent bleeding symptoms in patients with Glanzmann thrombasthenia are menorrhagia, easy bruising, epistaxis, and gingival bleeding.
- Clinical expression does not correlate with the degree of abnormality of the laboratory findings, and the severity of bleeding symptoms can vary significantly during the life of an individual patient.
- Carriers are usually asymptomatic and have normal platelet function.

Laboratory Features

- Normal platelet count and morphology.
- Prolonged bleeding time.
- Decreased or absent clot retraction.
- Abnormal platelet aggregation to physiologic stimuli (e.g., to ADP).
- Many other abnormalities of platelet function of research interest.

Differential Diagnosis

- Bleeding with normal platelet count.
- Other qualitative platelet disorders: specific laboratory findings.
- von Willebrand disease, afibrinogenemia, hemophilia, and related disorders: specific laboratory findings.

TABLE 76–1	**INHERITED DISORDERS OF PLATELET FUNCTION**

I. Abnormalities of Glycoprotein Adhesion Receptors
  A. $\alpha_{IIb}\beta_3$ (Glycoprotein IIb/IIIa; CD41/CD61): Glanzmann thrombasthenia
  B. Glycoproteins Ib (CD42b,c)/IX(CD42a)/V: Bernard-Soulier syndrome
  C. Glycoprotein GPIbα (CD42b): platelet-type (pseudo-) von Willebrand disease
  D. $\alpha_2\beta_1$ (Glycoprotein Ia/IIa; very-late antigen [VLA]-2; CD49b/CD29)
  E. CD36 (Glycoprotein IV)
  F. Glycoprotein VI
II. Abnormalities of Platelet Granules
  A. δ-Storage pool deficiency
  B. Gray platelet syndrome (α-storage pool deficiency)
  C. α,δ-Storage pool deficiency
  D. Quebec platelet disorder
III. Abnormalities of Platelet Coagulant Activity (Scott syndrome)
IV. Abnormalities of Platelet Signaling and Secretion
  A. Defects in platelet agonist receptors or agonist-specific signal transduction (thromboxane A_2 receptor defect, adenosine diphosphate [ADP] receptor defects [$P2Y_{12}$, $P2Y_1$, $P2X_1$], epinephrine receptor defect, platelet-activating factor receptor defect)
  B. Defects in guanosine triphosphate (GTP)-binding proteins (Gαq deficiency, Gαs hyperfunction and genetic variation in extralarge Gαs, Gαi1 deficiency)
  C. Phospholipase C (PLC)-β_2 deficiency and defects in PLC activation
  D. Defects in protein phosphorylation: protein kinase C (PKC)-θ deficiency
  E. Defects in arachidonic acid metabolism and thromboxane production (phospholipase A_2 deficiency, cyclooxygenase [prostaglandin H_2 synthase] deficiency, thromboxane synthase deficiency)
V. Abnormalities of a Cytoskeletal Structural Protein: β_1 Tubulin
VI. Abnormalities in Cytoskeletal Linking Proteins
  A. Wiskott-Aldrich syndrome protein (WASP)
  B. Kindlin-3: Leukocyte adhesion defect-III (LAD-III); LAD-1 variant, integrin activation deficiency disease defect (IADD)
VII. Abnormalities of Transcription Factors Leading to Functional Defects
  A. RUNX1 (familial platelet dysfunction with predisposition to acute myelogenous leukemia)
  B. GATA-1
  C. FLI1 (dimorphic dysmorphic platelets with giant αgranules and thrombocytopenia; Paris-Trousseau/Jacobsen syndrome)

Source: *Williams Hematology*, 8th ed, Chap. 121, Table 121–1, p. 1934.

- Autoantibodies to GP IIa/IIIb: demonstrate inhibitor of platelet function by mixing studies using normal plasma and platelets.

Therapy

- Preventive measures: dental hygiene, avoid antiplatelet drugs, hepatitis vaccination early in life, hormone therapy to avoid menorrhagia.
- Iron and folic acid therapy may be required in patients with continued bleeding.
- For management of bleeding, local therapy is given as appropriate, such as pressure dressings, Gelfoam, dental splints, etc; antifibrinolytic therapy may be helpful.
- Epistaxis may be particularly difficult to control.

- Platelet transfusions are given for serious hemorrhage, and packed red cell transfusions are often needed to correct blood loss anemia. All transfusions should be delivered through leukocyte-depletion filters.
- Antifibrinolytic agents (e.g., ε-aminocaproic acid) are useful in patients with gingival bleeding or who are undergoing tooth extractions.
- Treatment of patients with Glanzmann thrombasthenia with recombinant factor VIIa (rFVIIa) has produced considerable, but not universal success, but rare thromboembolic complications have been reported in association with this therapy.
- With repeated platelet transfusion, alloimmunization occurs to platelet proteins such as HLA and GPIIb and/or GPIIIa.
- A few patients with severe bleeding have had allogeneic marrow hematopoietic stem cell transplantation, with some success.

Prognosis
- Bleeding problems may be severe and frequent, but prognosis for survival is good.

GLYCOPROTEIN Ib (CD42b, c), GP IX (CD42a), AND GP V: BERNARD-SOULIER SYNDROME

- Bernard-Soulier syndrome (BSS) is characterized by moderate thrombocytopenia, giant platelets, and failure of platelets to undergo selective von Willebrand factor (VWF) interactions as a result of abnormalities of the GP Ib/IX complex.
- The mechanisms leading to the thrombocytopenia and the giant platelets are not known.
- The abnormal platelet reactions with VWF and thrombin and the abnormalities of coagulant activity are related to the glycoprotein abnormalities.

Etiology and Pathogenesis
- Patients with BSS are deficient in GP Ib, GP IX, and GP V.
- Several qualitative abnormalities of GP Ib and GP IX have been identified. No defective forms of GP V have been identified.
- Inherited as an autosomal recessive trait; an autosomal dominant form and acquired forms have also been reported.
- Six features contribute to the hemorrhagic diathesis: thrombocytopenia, abnormal platelet interactions with VWF, abnormal platelet interactions with thrombin, abnormal platelet coagulant activity, abnormal platelet interactions with P-selectin, and abnormal platelet interactions with leukocyte integrin αMβ2.

Clinical Features
- Epistaxis is the most common symptom. Ecchymoses, menometrorrhagia, gingival bleeding, and gastrointestinal bleeding also occur frequently.
- Symptoms vary considerably among patients, even those in a single family.

Laboratory Features
- Thrombocytopenia is found in nearly all patients, ranging from about 20 × 10^9/L to nearly normal levels.
- More than one-third of platelets are large; some are larger than lymphocytes.
- The bleeding time is nearly always prolonged.
- Platelets do not aggregate in response to ristocetin. In contrast to von Willebrand disease, this abnormality is not corrected by addition of normal plasma.
- Platelet coagulant activity may be reduced, normal, or increased.

Differential Diagnosis

- This is discussed under Glanzmann thrombasthenia.

Treatment and Prognosis

- These are similar to Glanzmann thrombasthenia.
- Desmopressin (DDAVP) has been variably effective in decreasing the bleeding time.

ABNORMAL GP Ib (CD42b, c): PLATELET-TYPE OR PSEUDO-VON WILLEBRAND DISEASE

- A heterogenous group of patients with mild to moderate bleeding symptoms, variable thrombocytopenia, variably enlarged platelets, and diminished plasma levels of high-molecular-weight multimers of VWF.

Etiology and Pathogenesis

- GP Ib/IX is the receptor for VWF.
- Abnormal forms of GP Ib cause enhanced binding of VWF, leading to reduction in high-molecular-weight multimers in plasma, and perhaps reduction in platelet survival time.
- Specific mutations have been demonstrated in some patients.
- Inherited as an autosomal dominant trait.

Clinical Features

- Patients have mild to moderate mucocutaneous bleeding.

Laboratory Features

- Bleeding time usually prolonged.
- Some patients have thrombocytopenia and large platelets.
- Plasma VWF concentration is reduced, especially the high-molecular-weight multimers.
- Enhanced platelet aggregation in response to low concentrations of ristocetin is not corrected by normal plasma. (In type II von Willebrand disease, this abnormality is corrected by normal plasma.)

Therapy

- Administration of VWF, or DDAVP to increase endogenous release of VWF, may be beneficial in low doses but can cause thrombocytopenia because of increased binding to platelets.
- Patients should be specifically instructed to avoid aspirin or other antiplatelet agents.
- Platelet transfusion may be beneficial if thrombocytopenia is severe.

OTHER GLYCOPROTEIN DEFICIENCIES

- A mild bleeding disorder has been described in association with decreased platelet content of GP Ia and GP IIa.
- Deficiency of GP IV occurs in a small number of people who have no bleeding disorder.
- Deficiency of GP VI has been found in patients with mild bleeding disorders.

WISKOTT-ALDRICH SYNDROME

- Wiskott-Aldrich syndrome is characterized by small platelets, thrombocytopenia, recurrent infections and eczema, although only a minority of patients have all features of the disorder.

Etiology and Pathogenesis

- Wiskott-Aldrich syndrome is inherited as an X-linked trait. In fact, if the eczema and immunodeficiency are minimal, the condition is termed X-linked thrombocytopenia. Female carriers of Wiskott-Aldrich syndrome have normal platelet counts and normal platelet size as they select against mutant X-chromosome *WAS* gene.
- Mutations of a Wiskott-Aldrich syndrome protein (WASP) occur in many, but not all, patients with the Wiskott-Aldrich syndrome and X-linked thrombocytopenia.
- WASP is a cytoplasmic protein, expressed in all hematopoietic stem cell–derived lineages. It plays a major role in organization and regulation of the actin cytoskeleton.
- A defect has also been found in sialophorin (CD43), a glycoprotein found on lymphocytes, monocytes, neutrophils, and platelets, but its role in pathogenesis is not clear.
- Deficiencies in GP Ia, Ib, IIb/IIIa, and IV have been found in some, but not all, patients.
- Deficiency of the platelet storage pool of adenine nucleotides and abnormal platelet energy metabolism are found in some patients.
- The thrombocytopenia is believed to be a result of diminished platelet survival, but ineffective thrombopoiesis may also play a role.
- The cause of the small platelets is unknown.

Clinical Features

- Mucocutaneous bleeding.
- Recurrent infections.
- Eczema.
- Increased risk of development of lymphoma, even in childhood.
- Autoimmune diseases, including hemolytic anemia and thrombocytopenia, may occur.

Laboratory Features

- Thrombocytopenia, often with counts of 20×10^9/L or less, and with reduced platelet volume, may occur.
- The bleeding time is usually prolonged.
- Platelet aggregation and release of dense body contents are variably abnormal.
- Defects in both humoral and cellular immunity, especially deficiency in immune response to polysaccharide antigens.

Treatment

- Patients should be specifically instructed to avoid aspirin or other antiplatelet agents.
- Splenectomy improves thrombocytopenia, and may lead to increased platelet size and improved function.
- Marrow hematopoietic stem cell transplantation may be curative.

PLATELET GRANULE DEFICIENCY STATES

δ-Storage Pool Deficiency

- A usually mild bleeding disorder with abnormalities in the second wave of platelet aggregation and deficiencies in the contents of the dense granules of platelets.
- There is predisposition to hematologic malignancies in some families.
- It occurs as a primary disorder or in association with inherited multisystem disorders:
  — Hermansky-Pudlak syndrome.
  — Chédiak-Higashi syndrome.

— Wiskott-Aldrich syndrome (see above).
— Others less frequently.
- The mode of inheritance of the primary disorder is not well defined, but autosomal dominance has been reported. The forms associated with other disorders are inherited following the pattern of the primary disease.

Clinical Features
- Severe bleeding may occur in patients with Hermansky-Pudlak syndrome; in others bleeding is mild to moderate.
- Mucocutaneous bleeding, excessive bruising, and epistaxis are common.
- Excess bleeding after surgery or trauma also may occur.

Laboratory Features
- The results of platelet function tests vary from patient to patient, and may vary in the same patient over time.
- The bleeding time is usually prolonged.
- Variable abnormalities of second wave of platelet aggregation are characteristic.

Differential Diagnosis
- See "Glanzmann Thrombasthenia," above.

Treatment
- Avoid antiplatelet drugs.
- The bleeding associated with surgery may be decreased by therapy with glucocorticoids.
- Bleeding time may be decreased by therapy with DDAVP or cryoprecipitate.
- Platelet transfusion may be helpful if bleeding is severe.

Hermansky-Pudlak Syndrome
- Hermansky-Pudlak syndrome is unusually common in patients from northwest Puerto Rico, affecting 1 in 1800 individuals, causing variable oculocutaneous albinism and the absence of dense platelets.
- Linkage analysis of patients from areas where Hermansky-Pudlak syndrome is relatively common led to the identification of the abnormal gene in these patients, then termed *HPS1*.
- The *HPS1* gene encodes a 700 amino acid protein that, along with HPS4, comprises BLOC-3 component of the granule exocytosis machinery.

Gray Platelet Syndrome (α-Granule Deficiency)
- α-Granule membranes form abnormal vesicular structures rather than granules.
- Platelets are deficient in α-granule contents, including fibrinogen and VWF.
- α-Granule deficiency (gray platelet) may be diagnosed by measuring platelet factor-4 and/or β-thromboglobulin in platelets.

Clinical Features
- Mild hemorrhagic manifestations are usual, but severe bleeding has been reported.

Laboratory Features
- Platelets on blood films are pale, gray, ghost-like, oval, and larger than normal.
- Thrombocytopenia is common, and the platelet count may be below 50×10^9/L.
- Platelet aggregation is often normal or nearly so, but may be abnormal.

Differential Diagnosis

- See "Glanzmann Thrombasthenia," above.
- Degranulated platelets may also be seen in myelodysplastic and myeloprolifera-tive disorders.

Treatment

- General measures should be used as in Glanzmann thrombasthenia.
- DDAVP or antifibrinolytic therapy may be beneficial.
- Platelet transfusion is indicated for serious hemorrhage.
- Thrombocytopenia may be improved by glucocorticoid therapy.

α, δ-Storage Pool Deficiency

- There are moderate to severe defects in both α and δ granules.
- Clinical and laboratory features are similar to δ-storage pool deficiency.

Quebec Platelet Disorder

- The early description of this autosomal dominant disorder included severe bleeding after trauma, mild thrombocytopenia, decreased functional platelet factor V, and normal plasma factor V.
- The bleeding time is abnormal, as is epinephrine-induced platelet aggregation.
- Subsequent studies demonstrated that the platelets of these patients had mark-edly reduced levels of multimerin and thrombospondin, and both reduced levels and proteolysis of a number of α-granule proteins, including factor V, fibrino-gen, VWF, fibronectin, and osteonectin.
- The defect in these patients' platelets appears to be excessive plasmin gen-eration as a result of increased expression of urokinase-type plasminogen activator (uPA); increased megakaryocyte expression of the uPA gene due to an abnormality in a *cis* regulatory element may be the primary abnormality.

ABNORMALITIES OF PLATELET COAGULANT ACTIVITY (SCOTT SYNDROME)

- Patients whose platelets fail to facilitate thrombin generation are defined as hav-ing defects in platelet coagulant activity. Only a few patients with isolated defects in platelet coagulant activity have been described.
- There is decreased translocation of platelet phosphatidyl serine to the outer membrane leaflet, which results in decreased binding of factors Va-Xa and VIIIa-IXa and hence, a diminished rate of blood clotting.

Clinical Features

- Bleeding, sometimes severe, occurs after trauma, dental extractions, delivery, or surgery. Epistaxis and menorrhagia also occur.
- Bleeding is not primarily mucocutaneous, in contrast to other qualitative platelet disorders.

Laboratory Features

- Bleeding time is usually normal.
- *Serum* prothrombin time is abnormal.
- Assays for "platelet factor 3" are abnormal.

Differential Diagnosis

- The normal bleeding time and abnormal serum prothrombin time distinguish patients with abnormalities of platelet coagulant activity.

Therapy

- Platelet transfusions have been effective for prevention and treatment.
- Prothrombin complex concentrates may be effective but may induce thrombosis.

ABNORMALITIES OF PLATELET AGONIST RECEPTORS, SIGNAL TRANSDUCTION, AND SECRETION

- A number of defects in the complex process of platelet activation that cause usually mild hemostatic disorders with rare episodes of severe clinical expression have been described.
- The most common pattern is blunted platelet aggregation with absence of the second wave of aggregation on exposure to ADP, epinephrine, or collagen, and decreased release of dense granule contents. Such patients have been lumped together, more out of convenience than because of an understanding of the mechanism, under the rubric of primary secretion defects, activation defects, or signal transduction defects.
- Occasional patients demonstrate defects in the thromboxane receptor, one of the ADP receptors ($P2Y_{12}$, $P2Y_1$ and $P2X_1$), the epinephrine receptor or the GTP binding proteins that mediate signaling for these heptahelical G-protein coupled receptors, or the signaling intermediates that mediate these platelet activation pathways, such as cyclooxygenase, thromboxane synthase, phospholipase (PL) $C\beta$ or $PLC\theta$.

For a more detailed discussion, see Barry S. Coller, Deborah L. French, and A. Koneti Rao: Hereditary Qualitative Platelet Disorders. Chap. 121, p. 1933 in *Williams Hematology*, 8th ed.

CHAPTER 77
Acquired Platelet Disorders

- The clinical manifestations of bleeding disorders are usually mild but may be severe if there is an accompanying hemostatic abnormality or a local lesion that may be predisposed to bleed.
- The usual laboratory abnormalities are prolongation of the bleeding time and/or abnormal platelet aggregation, but these results do not necessarily predict the risk of clinical bleeding.
- Table 77–1 lists the principal causes of acquired qualitative platelet abnormalities.

DRUGS THAT AFFECT PLATELET FUNCTION

- Table 77–2 lists drugs known to interfere with platelet function. Drugs are the most common cause of abnormal platelet function.
- Some drugs can prolong the bleeding time and cause or exacerbate a bleeding disorder.
- Some drugs prolong the bleeding time or induce abnormal platelet function tests but do not cause bleeding.

Aspirin

- Two isoforms of cyclooxygenase have been identified (COX-1 and COX-2). COX-1 is constitutively expressed by many tissues, including platelets, the gastric mucosa, and endothelial cells. COX-2 is undetectable in most tissues, but its synthesis is rapidly induced in cells such as endothelial cells, fibroblasts, and monocytes by growth factors, cytokines, endotoxin, and hormones.
- Aspirin irreversibly inhibits both COX-1 and COX-2 and thereby interferes with normal platelet function, such as aggregation with ADP or epinephrine.
- Aspirin prolongs bleeding time in normal people to 1.2 to 2 times baseline values.
- The bleeding time is markedly prolonged by aspirin in patients with coagulopathies or platelet abnormalities.
- The bleeding time remains prolonged for up to 4 to 5 days after aspirin is discontinued.
- Abnormal platelet aggregation persists for up to 1 week.
- Patients taking aspirin may have increased bruising, epistaxis, and gastric erosions that may bleed.
- A meta-analysis of clinical trials indicates that aspirin doses varying from 50 to 1500 mg daily are equally efficacious in preventing adverse cardiovascular and cerebrovascular events. This has led many to suggest that the lowest effective doses should be prescribed to minimize gastrointestinal toxicity. Nonetheless, even low doses of aspirin can be associated with gastrointestinal hemorrhage.
- Desmopressin (DDAVP) infusion may correct the prolonged bleeding time.

Other Nonsteroidal Antiinflammatory Drugs (NSAIDs)

- These drugs inhibit COX reversibly and usually for less than 4 hours.
- Because ibuprofen, and probably other NSAIDs, binds to COX and blocks its acetylation by aspirin, coadministration of NSAIDs may impair the irreversible effects of aspirin on platelets. For this reason, patients who require both medications should ingest aspirin at least 2 hours before the ingestion of other NSAIDs.

TABLE 77–1   **ACQUIRED QUALITATIVE PLATELET DISORDERS**
Drugs that affect platelet function
Thienopyridines (ticlopidine, clopidogrel, and prasugrel)
$\alpha_{IIb}\beta_3$ receptor antagonists
Drugs that increase platelet cyclic adenosine monophosphate
Antibiotics
Anticoagulants and fibrinolytic agents
Cardiovascular drugs
Volume expanders
Psychotropic agents and anesthetics
Antineoplastic drugs
Foods and food additives
Hematologic disorders associated with abnormal platelet function
Chronic myeloproliferative disorders
Leukemias and myelodysplastic syndromes
Dysproteinemias
Acquired von Willebrand disease
Systemic disorders associated with abnormal platelet function
Uremia
Antiplatelet antibodies
Cardiopulmonary bypass
Liver disease
Disseminated intravascular coagulation

Source: *Williams Hematology*, 8th ed, Chap. 122, Table 122–1, p. 1972.

- The effect of piroxicam may last for days because of the long half-life of the drug.
- These drugs may cause transient prolongation of the bleeding time, but the clinical significance of this phenomenon is uncertain.

COX-2 Inhibitors (Coxibs)

- The coxibs, designed to be relatively more specific for COX-2 versus COX-1, were intended to reduce pain and inflammation with less gastric side effects than traditional NSAIDs. However, clinical trials revealed that administration of coxibs was associated with cardiovascular toxicity (myocardial infarction, stroke, edema, exacerbation of hypertension), due at least in part to inhibition of PGI_2 synthesis. On the basis of these results, rofecoxib and valdecoxib were withdrawn from the market (valdecoxib was also associated with cases of Stevens-Johnson syndrome) and a black box warning regarding serious cardiovascular events was added to prescribing information for celecoxib, the only coxib now available in the United States.
- Clinical evidence through 2008 suggests there is no excess cardiovascular risk from daily doses of celecoxib of 200 mg or less. Because traditional NSAIDs also inhibit COX-2 and several clinical trials have suggested excess cardiovascular events with the use of some of these agents, a warning has also been added to their prescribing information.

Antibiotics

- Most penicillins cause dose-dependent prolongation of the bleeding time, probably by binding to the platelet membrane and thereby interfering with platelet function.
- Platelet aggregation is frequently abnormal.
- Inhibition of platelet function is maximal after 1 to 3 days of therapy, and persists for several days after treatment is discontinued.

TABLE 77-2	**DRUGS THAT INHIBIT PLATELET FUNCTION**

Nonsteroidal Antiinflammatory Drugs
Aspirin, sulfinpyrazone, indomethacin, ibuprofen, sulindac, naproxen, phenylbutazone, meclofenamic acid, mefenamic acid, diflunisal, piroxicam, tolmetin, zomepirac

Antibiotics
Penicillins
Penicillin G, carbenicillin, ticarcillin, methicillin, ampicillin, piperacillin, azlocillin, mezlocillin, apalcillin, sulbenicillin, temocillin
Cephalosporins
Cephalothin, moxalactam, cefoxitin, cefotaxime, cefazolin
Nitrofurantoin
Miconazole

Thienopyridines
Ticlopidine, clopidogrel

GP IIb/IIIa Antagonists
Abciximab, tirofiban, eptifibatide

Drugs that Affect Platelet cAMP Levels or Function
Prostacyclin, iloprost, dipyridamole, cilostazol

Anticoagulants, Fibrinolytic Agents, and Antifibrinolytic Agents
Heparin
Streptokinase, tissue plasminogen activator, urokinase
ϵ-Aminocaproic acid

Cardiovascular Drugs
Nitroglycerin, isosorbide dinitrate, propranolol, nitroprusside, nifedipine, verapamil, diltiazem, quinidine

Volume Expanders
Dextran, hydroxyethyl starch

Psychotropic Drugs and Anesthetics
Psychotropic drugs
Imipramine, amitriptyline, nortriptyline, chlorpromazine, promethazine, flufenazine, trifluoperazine, haloperidol
Anesthetics
Local
Dibucaine, tetracaine, metycaine, cyclaine, butacaine, nupercaine, procaine, cocaine, plaquenil
General
Halothane

Oncologic Drugs
Mithramycin, daunorubicin, BCNU

Miscellaneous Drugs
Ketanserin
Antihistamines
Diphenhydramine, chlorpheniramine, mepyramine
Radiographic contrast agent
Iopamidol, iothalamate, ioxalate, meglumine diatrizoate, sodium diatrizoate

Foods and Food Additives
Omega-3 Fatty acids, ethanol, Chinese black tree fungus, onion extract, ajoene, cumin, turmeric

Source: *Williams Hematology*, 8th ed, Chap, 122, Table 122–2, p. 1972.

- Clinically significant bleeding occurs much less frequently than prolongation of bleeding time.
- Patients with coexisting hemostatic defects are particularly vulnerable.
- Some cephalosporins cause problems similar to those caused by the penicillins.

Thienopyridines

- These drugs (ticlopidine and clopidogrel) are used as antithrombotic agents in arterial disease. They are more effective than aspirin or other NSAIDs for secondary prevention of cardiovascular events.
- Both thienopyridines are prodrugs that depend on metabolites to competitively inhibit the platelet P2Y12 ADP receptor. Effects of ticlopidine and clopidogrel on platelet aggregation and the bleeding time may be seen within 24 to 48 hours of the first dose, but are not maximal for 4 to 6 days.
- At therapeutic doses, they inhibit platelet aggregation and prolong the bleeding time as much or more than aspirin, and the effects appear to be additive to those of aspirin.
- Ticlopidine administration has been associated with potentially serious hematologic complications, including neutropenia ($<1200/\mu L$ in 2.4% of individuals), and less commonly, aplastic anemia, and thrombocytopenia. In addition, at least 1 in 5000 patients treated with ticlopidine develop thrombotic thrombocytopenic purpura.
- Results from a large clinical trial suggest that hematologic complications may be less common with clopidogrel.
- A loading dose of 300 mg of clopidogrel followed by a daily dose of 75 mg per day shortens the time required for the maximal antiplatelet effect. The presence of the common polymorphism of cytochrome P450, termed CYP2C19, results in lower levels of the active metabolite in patients. This effect can lead to decreased inhibition of platelet function, and elevated risk for major adverse cardiovascular events.
- It appears that the added benefit of double antiplatelet therapy (e.g., addition of aspirin) for most patients is small, and at times dangerous.

GP IIb/IIIa Receptor Antagonists

- Abciximab, eptifibatide, and tirofiban are three FDA approved GP IIb/IIIa inhibitors that are structurally dissimilar, but all rapidly impair platelet aggregation. Abciximab is a human-murine chimeric Fab fragment, eptifibatide is a cyclic heptapeptide, and tirofiban is a nonpeptide mimetic.
- Inhibitors of GP IIb/IIIa interfere with platelet function and are used as antithrombotic agents in patients with coronary atherosclerosis, usually in combination with heparin. These drugs predispose to bleeding, which is more severe with higher doses of heparin.
- Platelet transfusions appear to reverse the platelet functional defect in patients receiving abciximab, the Fab fragment of a monoclonal antibody. The effectiveness of platelet transfusion in patients receiving low-molecular-weight antagonists (tirofiban, eptifibatide) is not established.
- Thrombocytopenia has occurred within 24 hours of initiating therapy with all types of GP IIb/IIIa antagonists as a result of preformed antibodies to a ligand induced epitope on the platelet GP IIb/IIIa. Platelet counts less than $50 \times 10^9/L$ have been reported in approximately 1 to 4 percent of patients.
- In most cases of profound thrombocytopenia, a platelet count obtained 2 to 4 hours after initiating therapy provides evidence of a significant decrease in platelet count, although cases of delayed thrombocytopenia have been observed after abciximab. Thrombocytopenia usually reverses when drug administration is stopped.

Anticoagulants, Fibrinolytic Agents, and Antifibrinolytic Agents

- Heparin inhibits platelet function under some circumstances, but predisposes to bleeding primarily because of its anticoagulant effect.

- Platelet function may be altered during fibrinolytic therapy, but this appears not to be primarily responsible for hemorrhagic complications.
- Antifibrinolytic therapy with large doses of ε-aminocaproic acid can cause prolongation of the bleeding time after several days.

Volume Expanders
- Dextran interferes with platelet function by adsorption to the platelet surface but does not increase the bleeding time nor predispose to bleeding, unless administered with low-dose heparin.
- Hydroxyethyl starch may prolong the bleeding time and predispose to bleeding, especially at doses exceeding 20 mL/kg of a 6 percent solution.

FOODS
- Diets rich in fish oils containing omega-3 fatty acids may interfere with platelet function and prolong the bleeding time.

ABNORMAL PLATELET FUNCTION IN UREMIA

Etiology and Pathogenesis
- Patients may have a modest bleeding diathesis because of defects in platelet adhesion, aggregation, or procoagulant activity because of poorly understood mechanisms. For example, uremic plasma can inhibit the adhesion of normal platelets to de-endothelialized human umbilical artery segments, whereas uremic platelets adhere normally in the presence of normal plasma, but for unknown reasons. Moreover, increased nitric oxide synthesis by endothelial cells or platelets is at least partially responsible for defective platelet function in uremia.
- Anemia appears to be a major contributor to the adhesion defect and the prolonged bleeding times of uremic patients because of vascular rheology; normal red cell numbers force platelets to the endothelial surface of a column of flowing blood. Correction of the hematocrit to approximately 30 percent normalizes this defect.
- Concurrent medications may add to the abnormalities, e.g., aspirin, heparin.
- Thrombocytopenia may contribute to the bleeding tendency. If the platelet count is less than $100 \times 10^9/L$, causes of thrombocytopenia other than uremia must be considered.

Clinical and Laboratory Features
- The hemostatic defect in uremia is usually mild.
- The most common bleeding sites are skin, gastrointestinal, and genitourinary tracts.
- Patients with gastrointestinal bleeding frequently have a predisposing anatomic lesion.
- Serious bleeding requiring surgical intervention after biopsy is uncommon, and usually is a result of factors other than uremia.
- If bleeding occurs, a search for the cause should be initiated without assuming uremia is responsible.
- The bleeding time is often prolonged but does not quantitate risk of hemorrhage.

Therapy
- Intensive dialysis can correct the bleeding time and abnormal bleeding in many patients.
- DDAVP given intravenously or subcutaneously shortens the bleeding time in most uremic patients. For patients who need repeated doses, intranasal administration can be attempted
- DDAVP is usually given at a dose of 0.3 μg/kg intravenously over 15 to 30 minutes (maximum dose 20 μg).

- Repeated administration at intervals of 12 to 24 hours has been reported, but tachyphylaxis may occur.
- Transfusion of red cells to achieve a hematocrit of greater than or equal to 32 percent may improve the bleeding time. Combined transfusion of red cells and DDAVP may offer added benefit.
- Conjugated estrogens shorten the bleeding time in most patients with uremia. The dose is usually 0.6 mg/kg intravenously for 5 days.
- Cryoprecipitate may diminish bleeding, but the results are uncertain and risks significant.

ANTIPLATELET ANTIBODIES

Etiology and Pathogenesis

- Nearly all cases occur in association with immune thrombocytopenia.
- Antiplatelet antibodies may interfere with platelet function by binding to functional membrane components; others may activate platelets and induce aggregation and secretion.

Clinical Features

- Platelet dysfunction should be considered if a patient with ITP or systemic lupus erythematosus develops mucocutaneous bleeding with a platelet count above the usual bleeding level.

Laboratory Features

- The bleeding time may be longer than expected for platelet count.
- Platelet aggregation abnormalities are found in most patients. The most frequent pattern is absence of aggregation response to a low dose of collagen, and absence of the second wave in response to ADP or epinephrine.

Therapy

- Treatment is directed to the underlying immune thrombocytopenia.

CARDIOPULMONARY BYPASS

Etiology and Pathogenesis

- Thrombocytopenia is a consistent feature of bypass surgery. Typically, platelet counts decrease to 50 percent of presurgical levels by 25 minutes after the initiation of bypass, but thrombocytopenia can occur within 5 minutes and may persist for as long as several days.
- Approximately 5 percent of patients experience excessive postoperative bleeding after extracorporeal bypass; roughly half of the bleeding is due to surgical causes; much of the remainder is due to qualitative platelet defects and hyperfibrinolysis.
- The platelet defect is probably caused by activation and fragmentation.
- Drugs such as heparin and protamine may interfere with platelet function.

Clinical Features

- Platelet dysfunction is a possible cause of excessive postoperative bleeding.

Laboratory Features

- The bleeding time may be prolonged.
- Platelet aggregation to several agonists is abnormal.
- The platelet count is typically reduced by 50 percent during bypass and may remain low for several days.

Therapy

- Surgical causes of bleeding, incomplete neutralization of heparin, and persistence of hypothermia must be considered.
- Patients with prolonged bleeding time and excessive postoperative blood loss may respond to DDAVP.
- Aprotinin has been demonstrated to be beneficial, possibly through an antifibrinolytic effect.
- Transfusion with appropriate blood components may be necessary.

CHRONIC MYELOPROLIFERATIVE DISORDERS

- Multiple functional platelet abnormalities have been demonstrated.
- The bleeding time is prolonged in a minority of patients.

Clinical Features

- Bleeding or thrombosis occurs in about one-third of patients.
- Bleeding usually involves the skin or mucous membranes but may occur after surgery or trauma.

Laboratory Features

- The bleeding time is prolonged in some patients.
- None of the platelet function abnormalities is unique to a particular myeloproliferative disorder, and none is predictive of bleeding or thrombosis.
- Thrombocytosis is common, but the degree is not predictive of bleeding or thrombosis unless greater than 1000×10^9/L, where an acquired von Willebrand disease can cause bleeding due to platelet adsorption of von Willebrand factor.

Therapy

- Treatment should be reserved for symptomatic patients or those about to undergo surgery.
- Treatment should be directed to the underlying disorder.
- DDAVP may benefit storage pool defects or acquired von Willebrand disease in these patients.
- Aspirin may be helpful in patients with thrombosis but predisposes to bleeding.

ACUTE LEUKEMIA AND MYELODYSPLASTIC SYNDROMES

- Thrombocytopenia is the most common cause of bleeding, but platelet dysfunction may also contribute.
- Platelets may be morphologically abnormal, aggregate abnormally, and have decreased procoagulant activity.
- Bleeding usually responds to platelet transfusion and treatment of underlying disease.

PARAPROTEINEMIAS

- Platelet dysfunction occurs commonly due to direct interaction of the monoclonal protein with the platelets.
- Treatment is to reduce plasma levels of abnormal immunoglobulins by cytoreductive therapy or plasmapheresis.

For a more detailed discussion, see Charles S. Abrams, Sanford J. Shattil, Joel S. Bennett: Acquired Qualitative Platelet Disorders. Chap. 122, p. 1971 in *Williams Hematology*, 8th ed.

CHAPTER 78
The Vascular Purpuras

DEFINITIONS

- *Purpura* is the extravasation of red cells from vasculature into the skin and/or subcutaneous tissues.
- *Petechiae* are lesions less than 2 mm in diameter.
- *Purpura* describes lesions 2 mm to 1 cm.
- *Ecchymoses* are lesions greater than 1 cm.
- *Erythema* is reddened skin due to increased capillary flow.
- *Telangiectasia* is dilated superficial capillaries.
- Erythema and telangiectasia blanch with pressure. This can be easily demonstrable with a glass microscope slide.

PATHOPHYSIOLOGY

- Hemostatic mechanisms may be unable to protect against minor vascular trauma.
- Vessels and surrounding tissues may be weakened structurally.
- Transmural pressure gradient may be too great.
- Palpability may result from:
  — Extravascular fibrin deposition.
  — Cellular infiltration due to inflammation or malignancy.

NONPALPABLE PURPURA

Increased Transmural Pressure Gradient

- Increased intrathoracic pressure caused by coughing, vomiting, weight lifting, etc., may cause petechiae of the face, neck, and upper thorax.
- Venous valvular incompetence or tight clothing may cause petechiae on the lower extremities.

Decreased Mechanical Integrity of the Microvasculature or Supporting Tissues

- Actinic (senile) purpura is red to purple irregular patches on the extensor surfaces of the forearm and hands.
- Glucocorticoid excess causes bright red purpuric lesions in thin, fragile skin on flexor and extensor surfaces of both arms and legs.
- Vitamin C deficiency (scurvy) causes loss of collagen and ground substance in the skin, which leads to follicular hyperkeratosis, petechiae, perifollicular purpura with entrapped corkscrew hairs. Large ecchymoses and hemorrhagic gingivitis, stomatitis, and conjunctivitis may occur.
- Ehlers-Danlos syndrome is characterized by easy bruising in types IV and V, but this may occur with other types as well.
- Pseudoxanthoma elasticum may be associated with recurrent mucosal hemorrhages.
- In amyloidosis, infiltration of blood vessel walls may lead to increased vascular fragility and petechiae or purpura.
- The female easy-bruising syndrome (purpura simplex) is purpura or ecchymoses occurring predominantly in women, frequently on the thighs. This may be

related to hormonal changes, and can be aggravated by nonsteroidal antiinflammatory drug (NSAID) ingestion.

TRAUMA

- Physical trauma can cause cutaneous bleeding. The history, shape, and location of the lesions may suggest the etiology.
- Factitial purpura usually presents as medium to large ecchymoses on the lower extremities of patients who appear unconcerned about the lesions.

SUNBURN

- Acute sunburn may be sufficiently severe to have a petechial component.

INFECTIONS

- Purpura may occur with bacterial, fungal, viral, or rickettsial infections, or with parasitic infestations, including protozoan, often as a consequence of a complex, multifactorial process. Special forms include:
  — Bacterial sepsis due to various organisms can cause petechiae or purpura, macules or papules, hemorrhagic bullae, erosions, ulcers, or widespread ecchymoses and cutaneous infarctions (purpura fulminans, see below).
  — Ecthyma gangrenosum may accompany infections with *Pseudomonas* sp., *Klebsiella* sp., *Aeromona hydrophilia,* or *Escherichia coli* in patients with severe granulocytopenia or immune compromise. Lesions begin as erythematous or purpuric macules and progress to hemorrhagic or necrotic vesicles or bullae, then to edematous, hemorrhagic plaques, and finally to indurated painless ulcers.
  — Meningococcemia may cause erythematous papules that progress to widespread petechiae, purpura, and ecchymoses. Acrocyanosis and peripheral gangrene may occur.
  — Scarlet fever is characterized by a diffuse, erythematous rash often with confluent petechiae in skin folds (Pastia lines). Streptococcal pharyngitis without scarlet fever may also be associated with petechiae.
  — Rickettsial infections cause cutaneous lesions, beginning as urticarial macules and progressing to petechiae, ecchymoses, hemorrhagic bullae, and extensive skin necrosis.
  — In Lyme disease, the characteristic cutaneous lesion is erythema migrans, an annular, expanding plaque that may contain a purpuric macule or papule, or a hemorrhagic bulla.

EMBOLIC PURPURA

- Cholesterol crystals that embolize from atheromata in the aorta and in the lower extremities may produce petechiae and purpura, livedo reticularis, nodules, ulcers, or cyanosis and gangrene.
- Fat emboli may occur after severe trauma or after liposuction and cause petechiae of the upper extremities, thorax, and/or conjunctivae.

HYPERCALCEMIA

- Chronic hypercalcemia may lead to hemorrhagic cutaneous necrosis because of subcutaneous and vascular calcifications.

NEOPLASIA

- Petechiae or purpura may occur because of infiltration of the skin with neoplastic cells from a variety of malignancies, including leukemias, myeloma, or macroglobulinemia.

PIGMENTED PURPURIC ERUPTIONS

- Schamberg and Majocchi diseases are characterized by petechiae and purpura on a background of red-brown or orange hyperpigmentation, usually on the lower extremities.
- Similar lesions may be produced by cutaneous T-cell lymphoma, drug or chemical hypersensitivity, allergic or irritant contact dermatitis, and hyperglobulinemic purpura.

PYODERMA GANGRENOSUM

- Presents as a nodule, pustule, or hemorrhagic bulla that rapidly becomes an ulcer with an erythematous base and violaceous or blue margin surrounded by erythema.
- Associated with a number of diseases, including inflammatory bowel disease, rheumatoid arthritis, and hematologic malignancies.

INTRAABDOMINAL HEMORRHAGE

- Purpura or ecchymoses may develop around the umbilicus (Cullen sign) or in the flanks (Grey-Turner sign) in patients with intraabdominal hemorrhage.

COUMARIN NECROSIS

- Coumarin necrosis occurs in about 1 in 500 patients receiving coumarin drugs.
- The onset is sudden after 2 to 14 days of drug therapy, with painful erythematous patches that progress to hemorrhagic and necrotic plaques, nodules, and bullae.
- Women are more commonly affected, and lesions most often involve thighs, buttocks, or breasts.
- Coumarin necrosis is more likely to occur in patients with protein C deficiency.

PURPURA FULMINANS

- May present with widespread ecchymoses, often involving the extremities, abdomen, or buttocks.
- Often seen in association with infection, but may be idiopathic or occur in infants with homozygous protein C or protein S deficiency.

PAROXYSMAL NOCTURNAL HEMOGLOBINURIA

- May be associated with erythematous cutaneous lesions with central necrosis, hemorrhagic bullae, petechiae, purpura, or ecchymoses, likely related to microvascular thrombosis.

ANTIPHOSPHOLIPID ANTIBODY SYNDROME

- Patients with this disease may develop a variety of cutaneous manifestations, including ecchymoses, subungual splinter hemorrhages, and extensive cutaneous necrosis, all likely related to microvascular thrombosis.

DRUG REACTIONS

- Reactions to any of a large number of drugs may lead to petechiae or purpura in the absence of thrombocytopenia.

AUTOERYTHROCYTE SENSITIZATION

- This disorder is characterized by painful ecchymoses appearing without explanatory trauma.
- The cause is not established, but in some patients hypersensitivity to some component of the erythrocyte membrane may be responsible.
- Many patients have underlying psychiatric disorders, and lesions have been factitial in some.

PALPABLE PURPURA

Henoch-Schönlein Purpura

- This syndrome is a leukocytoclastic vasculitis of unknown cause involving precapillary, capillary, and postcapillary vessels.
- Lesions may be palpable purpura, urticarial papules, plaques, or hemorrhagic vesicles or bullae which can progress to larger, stellate, reticulate, and necrotic lesions.
- Lesions are usually symmetric on legs and buttocks, and are often associated with fever.
- It is predominantly a disease of children between ages 2 and 20 years. Several environmental triggers precede onset, such as viral (upper respiratory infections, hepatitis B virus, HCV, parvovirus B19, and HIV) and bacterial (*Streptococcus* species, *Staphylococcus aureus*, and *Salmonella* species) infections in children. Adult disease is precipitated by medications (NSAIDs, angiotensin-converting enzyme [ACE] inhibitors, and antibiotics), food allergies, vaccinations, and insect bites.
- Arthralgias and abdominal pain usually accompany the rash, and melena and signs of peritoneal irritation are common.
- Proteinuria and hematuria occur in 40 percent. In older children and adults, renal disease may be progressive in 10 to 20 percent.
- IgA1 immunoglobulins and complement components may be deposited in involved cutaneous and renal vessels.
- Therapy is usually initiated with glucocorticoids, but the success rate is low. Ultimate prognosis is almost uniformly good.

Sweet Syndrome

- Also referred to as acute, febrile neutrophilic dermatosis, Sweet syndrome is characterized by the acute manifestation of painful erythematous and violaceous papules, nodules, and plaques accompanied by fever and elevated neutrophil count.
- These papules, which most commonly appear on face, neck, and upper extremities, present a central yellowish discoloration and tend to coalesce forming well circumscribed, irregularly bordered plaques. Classically more prominent in middle age women, this syndrome is associated with a complex cytokine dysregulation. Other manifestations include respiratory and urinary infections, and autoimmune disorders.

Behçet Disease

- Besides its classification as a neutrophilic dermatosis, Behçet disease is also an inflammatory disorder that affects multiple organ systems.
- Clinical features are chronic and relapsing cutaneous manifestations, such as palpable purpura, infiltrative erythema, and papulopustular lesions, as well as oral mucosal and genital ulcers, arthralgias, and gastrointestinal and central nervous system involvement.

Serum Sickness

- Serum sickness refers to the systemic manifestation of immune complex formation and deposition.
- Serum sickness associated with infection or medical therapy can result in characteristic lesions.
- The use of anti-thymocyte globulin for marrow failure results in 75 percent of patients developing serpiginous bands of erythema and purpura on the sides of their hands and feet.
- Cutaneous lesions such as urticarial and morbilliform eruptions predominate, though palpable purpura and erythema multiforme are also often seen.

Erythema Multiforme

- Erythema multiforme (EM) is a cutaneous disorder characterized by the development of crops of well demarcated, erythematous target lesions with central clearing, most commonly representing a hypersensitivity reaction triggered by infection or drug exposure.
- The severity of this disorder ranges from mild (EM minor), to severe, (EM major or Stevens-Johnson syndrome). EM has been reported to be triggered by a number of viruses (most common herpes simplex, but also adenovirus, cytomegalovirus, and HIV), and medications (sulfonamides, penicillins, bupropion, phenylbutazone, phenytoin, NSAIDs, adalimumab).
- A cellular allergic reaction coupled with impaired histamine metabolism due to decrease in histamine-N-methyltransferase activity may be causative. Treatment for mild cases is supportive, while glucocorticoid use is often warranted in severe cases.

Churg-Strauss Syndrome

- Churg-Strauss syndrome is characterized by granulomatous inflammation in the lungs associated with asthma and eosinophilia.
- Cutaneous findings such as ulcers, papules, palpable purpura, cutaneous nodules, and infarcts of fingers and toes are encountered in 50 to 80 percent of cases.
- It can be limited to the skin. Eosinophilia accompanies elevated IgE levels and a positive P-antineutrophil cytoplasmic antibody (ANCA). Granulomatous inflammation and necrotizing vasculitis of small to medium sized blood vessels are present histologically.

Acute Hemorrhagic Edema of Infancy

- This disorder is composed of a triad of fever; iris-like or medallion-like, large purpuric, painful cutaneous lesions; and edema appearing in children age 4 months to 2 years.
- The onset is sudden, with spontaneous recovery in 1 to 3 weeks.
- The cutaneous lesions are limited to cheeks, eyelids, ears, and extremities and genitalia.
- Pathology is leukocytoclastic vasculitis with vascular deposits of immunoglobulins and complement components.

Vasculitis Associated with Other Diseases

- Palpable purpura may occur in several other disorders characterized by vasculitis:
  - Collagen vascular diseases.
  - Systemic vasculitides, including polyarteritis nodosa, Wegener granulomatosis, and Churg-Strauss angiitis.
  - Hypersensitivity vasculitis, associated with drug reactions or infections or idiopathic.
  - Paraneoplastic, in association with any of a variety of neoplasms, including the hematologic malignancies.
  - Long-distance walkers may develop purpuric vasculitis lesions on the legs.

Cryoglobulinemia

- May be single component, IgA, IgG, or IgM, occurring in essential monoclonal gammopathy, macroglobulinemia, myeloma, or lymphoma.
- May be cold-insoluble complexes of IgG with IgM that has anti-IgG activity, or similar complexes containing other immunoglobulin components, occurring in association with a variety of diseases.
- Skin lesions occur with both types of cryoglobulin, including macular or palpable purpura, acral hemorrhagic necrosis, livedo reticularis, or hemorrhagic bullae.

Hyperglobulinemic Purpura of Waldenström

- Usually occurs in women between ages 18 and 40 years, often in association with another disease.
- Crops of petechiae appear on the lower legs and ankles, recurring at intervals of days to months.
- Patients have polyclonal hypergammaglobulinemia due to elevated levels of IgA, IgG, and IgM.

Cryofibrinogenemia

- Cold-insoluble fibrinogen may be found as a primary disorder or secondary to neoplastic, thromboembolic, or infectious disorders, usually with laboratory evidence of disseminated intravascular coagulation.
- Cutaneous manifestations are similar to those described for cryoglobulinemia, above.

Primary Cutaneous Diseases

- Primary cutaneous diseases, including allergic contact dermatitis, drug eruptions, acne vulgaris, insect bites, and dermatitis herpetiformis, may present with purpuric papules and vesicles that look like septic or vasculitis lesions.

DISORDERS SIMULATING PURPURA

Telangiectasias

- Hereditary hemorrhagic telangiectasia:
  - Autosomal dominant inheritance.
  - The disease is characterized by widespread dermal, mucosal, and visceral telangiectasias.
  - Recurrent epistaxis is the most common problem, but bleeding may occur from any site.
  - Arteriovenous fistulae may occur, especially in the lungs, and may require surgical resection.
  - Treatment involves local therapy to accessible lesions. Hormonal therapy may be used for epistaxis or gastrointestinal bleeding. ε-Aminocaproic acid has been beneficial in some cases.
- Spider angiomata are telangiectasias that occur in chronic liver disease, a limited form of scleroderma (CREST syndrome: calcinosis, Raynaud syndrome, esophageal dysmotility, sclerodactyly, telangiectasia), and AIDS have a prominent central feeding vessel which is easily occluded, leading to blanching of the lesion.
  - They may be confused with lesions of hereditary hemorrhagic telangiectasia.

Kaposi Sarcoma

- Kaposi lesions may mimic petechiae, purpura, or ecchymoses on either skin or mucosae.

Extramedullary Hematopoiesis

- Cutaneous sites of extramedullary hematopoiesis appear as dark red, blue, or blue-gray macules in infants with congenital viral infections, hemolysis associated with Rh incompatibility, hereditary spherocytosis or twin transfusion syndrome, and in adults with primary myelofibrosis.

For more detailed information, see Doru T. Alexandrescu and Richard L. Gallo: The Vascular Purpuras. Chap. 123, p. 1993 in *Williams Hematology*, 8th ed.

PART X

DISORDERS OF COAGULATION PROTEINS

CHAPTER 79
Hemophilia A and B

GENERAL ASPECTS

- Hemophilia A and hemophilia B are caused by inherited deficiencies of factor VIII and factor IX, respectively.
- Both result from decreased production of the deficient factor, production of a factor with decreased functional activity, or a combination of these two abnormalities.
- The activated form of factor IX, factor IXa, is a serine protease that functions to activate factor X.
- Activated factor VIII, factor VIIIa, serves as a cofactor, forming a complex with factor IXa on the platelet surface and dramatically accelerating the rate of factor X activation by factor IXa.
- In patients with hemophilia, clot formation is delayed because thrombin generation is markedly decreased. The clot that does form is hemostatically ineffective, leading to excessive bleeding.
- Because deficiency of either factor VIII or factor IX causes an inability to activate factor X, the clinical characteristics and approach to treatment of hemophilia A and hemophilia B are similar.
- Both hemophilia A and B are X-linked recessive disorders, affecting only males, with rare exceptions (Fig. 79–1). Approximately 30 percent of mutations arise *de novo*.
- Hemophilia is found worldwide in all ethnic groups. Hemophilia A is estimated to occur in 1 of 10,000 male births and hemophilia B in 1 of 25,000 to 30,000 male births.

HEMOPHILIA A

Clinical Features

- Table 79–1 shows a clinical classification of hemophilia A based on factor VIII levels.
- Hemostasis is generally normal with levels in excess of 30 percent.
- The factor VIII level remains constant throughout the patient's life, and is similar in other affected members of the kindred, but varies between kindreds.
- Hemarthrosis accounts for 75 percent of bleeding episodes in patients with severe hemophilia A.

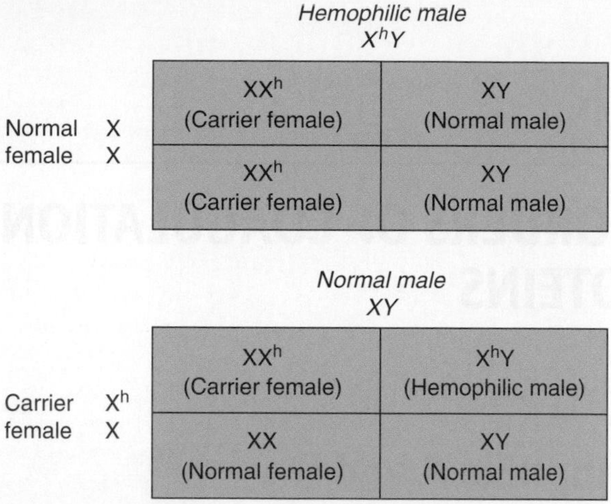

Hemophilic male
X^hY

		XX^h (Carrier female)	XY (Normal male)
Normal	X	XX^h (Carrier female)	XY (Normal male)
female	X		

Normal male
XY

		XX^h (Carrier female)	X^{h}Y (Hemophilic male)
Carrier	X^h	XX (Normal female)	XY (Normal male)
female	X		

FIGURE 79–1 Inheritance pattern of hemophilia A. X is normal; X^h has an abnormal X chromosome with the hemophilic gene; Y is normal; XX is a normal female; XY is a normal male; XX^h is a carrier female; X^{h}Y is a hemophilic male.
(Source: *Williams Hematology,* 8th ed, Chap. 124, Fig. 124–1, p. 2010.)

- The most frequent sites are the knees, followed by the elbows, ankles, shoulders, wrists, and hips.
- The acute form is characterized by initial mild pain without physical findings, followed by more intense pain, swelling and warmth of the joint, and decreased range of motion.

TABLE 79–1   CLINICAL CLASSIFICATION OF HEMOPHILIA A AND B

Classification	Hemophilia A Factor VIII Level	Hemophilia B Factor IX Level	Clinical Features
Severe	≤ 1% of normal (≤ 0.01 U/mL)	≤ 1% of normal. (≤ 0.01 U/mL)	1. Spontaneous hemorrhage from early infancy. 2. Frequent spontaneous hemarthroses and other hemorrhages requiring clotting factor replacement.
Moderate	1–5% of normal (0.01–0.05 U/mL)	1–5% of normal (0.01–0.05 U/mL)	1. Hemorrhage secondary to trauma or surgery. 2. Occasional spontaneous hemarthroses.
Mild	6–30% of normal (0.06–0.30 U/mL)	6–40% of normal (0.06–0.40 U/mL)	1. Hemorrhage secondary to trauma or surgery. 2. Rare spontaneous hemorrhage.

Source: *Williams Hematology,* 8th ed, Chap. 124, Table 124–2, p. 2014.

- The patient may have mild fever. Significant or sustained fever suggests infection in the joint.
- When bleeding stops, the blood resorbs and symptoms subside over several days.
- Repeated bleeding into the joint results in synovial hypertrophy and inflammation, with limitation of motion and a tendency for more frequent bleeding in that joint (target joint).
- Eventually, repeated hemorrhage into the joints causes destruction of the articular cartilage, synovial hyperplasia, and joint deformity with muscle atrophy and soft tissue contractures (Fig. 79–2).
- Hematomas may develop after bleeding into muscles or subcutaneous tissues (Fig. 79–3).
- Intramuscular hematomas occur most often in thigh, buttocks, calf muscles, and forearm.
- Hematomas may stabilize and slowly resorb without treatment, but in individuals with moderate or severe hemophilia, they often enlarge progressively and dissect in all directions. This can cause compression of adjacent organs, nerves, or blood vessels, sometimes leading to permanent sequelae. Hematomas may obstruct the airway.
- Pseudotumors are large, organized, encapsulated hematomas that may slowly expand and compress surrounding structures.

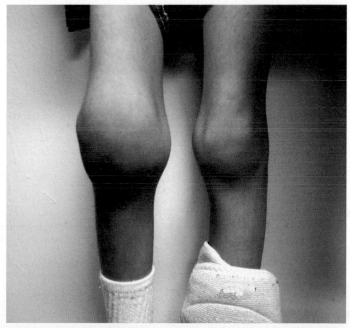

FIGURE 79-2 Hemophilic arthropathy. The chronic effects of repeated hemorrhage into the knee of a severely affected hemophilic patient are seen. Note swelling and deformity with atrophy of muscle tissue.
(Source: *Williams Hematology,* 8th ed, Chap. 124, Fig. 124–2, p. 2014.)

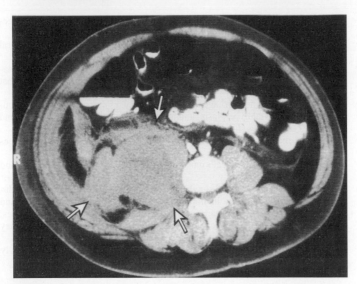

FIGURE 79-3 Computed tomography scan of a retroperitoneal hematoma in a patient with severe hemophilia A. Extent of the hematoma is indicated by the *arrows*.
(Source: *Williams Hematology,* 8th ed, Chap. 124, Fig. 124–11, p. 2015.)

- CNS hemorrhage, the most common cause of bleeding mortality, occurs spontaneously or after trauma. The onset of symptoms is usually prompt but may be delayed by several days.
- Virtually all patients with severe hemophilia have episodes of hematuria, which may cause renal colic because of clots in the ureters, but is seldom life-threatening.
- Postsurgical bleeding, often delayed by hours to several days, is associated with poor wound healing.
- Extraction of permanent teeth in patients with hemophilia may be followed by prolonged bleeding. Life-threatening pharyngeal or sublingual hematomas may follow extractions or regional block anesthesia.
- Inhibitory antibodies to factor VIII may develop in patients receiving replacement therapy (discussed below).

Laboratory Findings

- Hemophilia A causes prolongation of the activated partial thromboplastin time (aPTT) which is corrected by the addition of an equal volume of normal plasma. The prothrombin time is normal.
- A specific assay for factor VIII activity is required for definitive diagnosis.
- Immunologic assays coupled with clotting assays permit detection of dysfunctional factor VIII molecules.

Carrier Detection and Prenatal Diagnosis

- The average factor VIII level of carrier females is 50 percent, but occasional carriers have levels less than 30 percent and may have excessive bleeding with trauma or surgery.
- The family history is important for carrier detection (see Fig. 79–1).
- Molecular genetics techniques are available to identify carriers.
- Prenatal diagnosis can be made from fetal cells obtained by amniocentesis or by chorionic villus biopsy.

Differential Diagnosis

- Hemophilia A must be distinguished from hemophilia B and from other congenital disorders of coagulation that prolong the aPTT, such as factor XI and XII deficiencies.
- Hemophilia A must be distinguished from von Willebrand disease (especially the Normandy variant), an acquired inhibitor of factor VIII, and combined congenital deficiency of factor VIII and factor V.

Treatment

General

- Avoid aspirin, other antiplatelet agents, and intramuscular injections.
- Treat bleeding episodes promptly.
- Consider prophylaxis in severely affected patients.
- Home treatment should be available to all patients.
- Plan surgical procedures carefully.
- Hemophilia should preferably be treated in a designated Hemophilia Treatment Center.

Desmopressin (DDAVP)

- Deamino-8-D-Arginine Vasopressin (DDAVP) is often useful in the treatment of mild to moderate hemophilia A and symptomatic carrier females. Administration of 0.3 μg/kg intravenously can increase factor VIII levels of most of these patients two- to three-fold.
- The peak effect is in 30 to 60 minutes.
- Adverse reactions include flushing, rarely hyponatremia (mostly in children, can be prevented by water restriction), and angina in patients with coronary disease.
- Tachyphylaxis occurs with repeated doses.
- An intranasal preparation is also available.

Replacement with Factor Concentrates

- Bleeding episodes in patients with hemophilia A can be managed by replacing factor VIII (see Table 79–2).
- Commercial concentrates prepared from human plasma have been treated to inactivate viruses, including HIV and hepatitis B and C viruses. Hepatitis A and parvovirus are not inactivated by the treatment, and infection with these viruses has been transmitted.
- Recombinant factor VIII concentrates appear to be both safe and effective. These may be formulated with human plasma albumin, and are more expensive.
- The various available concentrates appear to differ little in safety, efficacy, or convenience.

Factor VIII Dosage (see Table 79–3)

- The dose of factor VIII can be determined by multiplying the patient's weight in kilograms by half the needed percent correction of the factor level. For example, for a 70-kg patient with a less than 1 percent factor VIII level who needs a 100 percent correction, the dose would be 70 (kg) $\times$ 100 percent/2 $-$ 3500 U. The full contents of mixed factor vials should be infused.
- The half-life of factor VIII is 8 to 12 hours. Factor levels may be maintained between 50 and 100 percent by giving half the loading dose every 8 to 12 hours.
- Reconstituted factor VIII concentrates may be administered by continuous intravenous infusion. After an initial loading dose to raise factor VIII to the desired level, 150 to 200 U per hour are administered.

TABLE 79–2	CURRENTLY AVAILABLE FACTOR VIII PRODUCTS [a]	
	Origin	Viral Inactivation
Intermediate purity		
Humate P [b]	Plasma	Pasteurization[c]
High purity		
Koate DVI [b]	Plasma	Solvent-detergent [d], heat treated [i]
Alphanate [b]	Plasma	Solvent-detergent, heat treated [i]
Ultrapure [e]		
Hemofil M	Plasma	Solvent-detergent [d]
Monoclate P	Plasma	Pasteurization[c]
Recombinant		
Advate [h]	CHO cells [f]	Solvent-detergent [d]
Recombinate [e]	CHO cells [f]	
Kogenate FS[e]	BHK cells [g]	Solvent-detergent
Helixate FS[e]	BHK cells [g]	Solvent-detergent
Xyntha [h]	CHO cells [f]	Solvent-detergent, nanofiltration

[a]Additional concentrates are available in Europe.
[b]Contains VWF.
[c]Pasteurization at 60 °C (140 °F) for 10 h.
[d]Solvent-detergent: tri-n-butyl phosphate (TNBP) + polysorbate 80.
[e]Human albumin added; insignificant VWF.
[f]Chinese hamster ovarian cells.
[g]Baby hamster kidney cells.
[h]Not exposed to human or animal protein during manufacture.
[i]Heat treated at 80 °C (176 °F) for 72 h.
Source: *Williams Hematology*, 8th ed, Chap. 124, Table 124–3, p. 2018.

Antifibrinolytic Agents

- Antifibrinolytic agents are useful adjunctive therapy for mucosal bleeding, and particularly so for dental extractions, but are contraindicated if the patient has hematuria.
- ε-Aminocaproic acid (EACA) can be given orally in a loading dose of 4 to 5 g followed by 1 g/h, or 4 g every 4 to 6 hours for 2 to 8 days, depending on the severity of the bleeding episodes.
- Tranexamic acid is given at an oral dose of 0.5 to 1 g four times daily but is not available for oral use in the United States.
- Fibrin glue, a mixture of fibrinogen and factor XIII applied locally to a bleeding site and then clotted with thrombin, may be useful adjunctive therapy for bleeding from circumcision, dental, or orthopedic procedures, including removal of large pseudotumors.

Treatment of Specific Types of Bleeding Episodes (Table 79–2)

- Superficial cuts and abrasions are managed with local pressure.
- Epistaxis may require replacement of factor VIII to levels of 50 percent of normal.
- Hematuria is often mild and needs no replacement therapy but may persist and require replacement to levels greater than 50 percent, with replacement continuing until the bleeding stops. Patients should be advised to drink a lot of fluids, to avoid obstructing clots in the urinary tract.
- Prior to endoscopy, factor VIII should be replaced to at least the 50 percent level. A single infusion may suffice, but if the procedure is complicated by bleeding, replacement must be continued until the bleeding stops.

TABLE 79–3   DOSES OF FACTOR VIII FOR TREATMENT OF HEMORRHAGE*

Site of Hemorrhage	Desired Factor VIII Level (% of normal)	Factor VIII Dose[†] (U/kg body weight)	Frequency of Dose[‡] (every no. of hours)	Duration (days)
Hemarthroses	30–50	~25	12–24	1–2
Superficial intramuscular hematoma	30–50	~25	12–24	1–2
Gastrointestinal tract	~50	~25	12	7–10
Epistaxis	30–50	~25	12	Until resolved
Oral mucosa	30–50	~25	12	Until resolved
Hematuria	30–100	~25–50	12	Until resolved
Central nervous system	50–100	50	12	At least 7–10 days
Retropharyngeal	50–100	50	12	At least 7–10 days
Retroperitoneal	50–100	50	12	At least 7–10 days

*Mild or moderately affected patients may respond to 1-deamino-8-D-arginine vasopressin (DDAVP), which should be used in lieu of blood or blood products whenever possible.
[†]Factor VIII may be administered in a continuous infusion if the patient is hospitalized. After initial bolus, approximately 150 U of factor VIII per hour usually are sufficient in an average-size adult. Doses are given every 12 to 24 hours.
[‡]The frequency of dosing and duration of therapy can be adjusted, depending on the severity and duration of the patient's bleeding episode.
Source: *Williams Hematology*, 8th ed, Chap. 124, Table 124–4, p. 2019.

603

- For expanding soft-tissue hematomas, replacement therapy should be started immediately and continued until the hematoma begins to resolve.
- Hemarthroses should be treated promptly to minimize degenerative changes, deformity, and muscle wasting. For chronic bleeding into a "target" joint, replacement to 100 percent for 6 to 8 weeks may be indicated.
- Retropharyngeal and retroperitoneal hematomas and any central nervous system bleeding require replacement of factor VIII to normal (100%), or nearly normal, levels for 7 to 10 days.
- Major surgical procedures require factor VIII replacement to normal levels before operation and maintenance of normal levels for 7 to 10 days, or until healing is well underway.
- The patient's factor VIII levels should be measured during surgery and once or twice daily postoperatively and the dose of factor VIII adjusted accordingly.
- Home therapy has facilitated prompt treatment of hematomas and hemarthroses and markedly improved the morbidity and mortality of the disease.
- Severely afflicted patients who receive prophylactic therapy with 50 units of factor VIII/kg body weight three times a week have markedly decreased frequency of arthropathy and other long-term complications of hemophilia.
- Transplantation of a normal liver can result in cure of hemophilia, but this has been done rarely.
- Gene therapy for hemophilia is being extensively investigated.

Course and Prognosis

- Unless treated properly, patients develop complications of recurrent bleeding, as noted under "Clinical Features," above.
- The introduction of replacement therapy with factor VIII concentrates in the 1960s led to a significant reduction in the morbidity and mortality from bleeding in hemophilia, but introduced serious complications such as infection with HIV, liver disease from hepatitis B and C, and the development of anti-factor VIII antibodies.
- Since 1985, factor VIII concentrates have been treated to destroy HIV and hepatitis viruses, with virtual elimination of infection with these agents. However, HIV infection and chronic liver disease from hepatitis B and C are still prevalent in older patients with hemophilia.

Factor VIII Inhibitors in Patients with Hemophilia A

- Factor VIII inhibitors are antibodies, most often IgG, usually IgG4 subclass, that interfere with the interaction of factor VIII with its cofactors and activators.
- Factor VIII inhibitors react slowly, and inactivation of factor VIII requires incubation with the inhibitor for 1 to 2 hours at 37 °C.
- Laboratory diagnosis of a factor VIII inhibitor requires that an appropriate dilution of the patient's plasma when mixed with normal plasma will neutralize only factor VIII and no other factor that influences the aPTT (factors IX, X, XI, XII, prekallikrien, or high-molecular-weight kininogen).
- Patients with factor VIII inhibitors are classified as "high" responders if their baseline inhibitor levels are above 10 Bethesda units (BU) or if their inhibitor level rises above 10 BU after receiving factor VIII replacement. "Low" responders have factor VIII inhibitor levels below 10 BU even after receiving factor VIII replacement.
- High-responder patients with major bleeding and initial inhibitors below 10 BU can be treated with high doses of human or porcine factor VIII concentrates in efforts to neutralize the inhibitor and still provide enough factor VIII for hemostasis.
- High-responder patients with initial inhibitor levels greater than 10 BU usually will not respond to any doses of human factor VIII, nor to porcine factor VIII if the inhibitor is cross-reactive.

TABLE 79–4	TREATMENT OF INHIBITORS IN HEMOPHILIA A PATIENTS		
Type of Patient	Initial Titer	Minor Hemorrhage*	Major Hemorrhage*
High responder	< 5 BU	Recombinant factor VIIa; FEIBA; prothrombin complex concentrates	Human factor VIII[†]; recombinant factor VIIa; FEIBA; prothrombin complex concentrates
High responder	> 5 BU	Recombinant factor VIIa; FEIBA; prothrombin complex concentrates	Recombinant factor VIIa; FEIBA; plasma exchange
Low responder	< 5 BU	Recombinant factor VIIa; FEIBA; prothrombin complex concentrates	High-dose human factor VIII; recombinant factor VIIa; FEIBA

BU, Bethesda unit; FEIBA, factor VIII inhibitor bypassing activity.
*Choices of agents for treatment of major and minor hemorrhage are listed. Some physicians will choose the first product listed as the agent of choice, but the choice varies among physicians.
[†]High dose of factor VIII may overcome an initial low-titer inhibitor, although an anamnestic response can be expected in high responders.
Source: *Williams Hematology*, 8th ed, Chap. 124, Table 124–6, p. 2022.

- High-responders should be treated with recombinant factor VIIa or another factor VIII inhibitor-bypassing agent for minor bleeding episodes or for major bleeding if the inhibitor level is high or if factor VIII replacement is ineffective (Table 79–4).
- Low-responders can be treated with recombinant factor VIIa or another factor VIII inhibitor-bypassing agent for major or minor bleeding. In addition, they can be treated with high dose human or porcine factor VIII for major bleeding (Table 79–4).
- Recombinant factor VIIa is the preferred factor VIII inhibitor-bypassing agent. Factor VIIa is believed to activate factor X on the surfaces of activated platelets, and factor Xa can then interact with factor Va, and convert prothrombin to thrombin. The effects of factor VIIa may be localized because activated platelets are found principally at sites of injury. Prothrombin complex preparations are probably of benefit also because of similar effects of activated coagulation factors in these products.
- In some patients, administration of daily doses of factor VIII can reduce the inhibitor titer to undetectable levels, and such immune tolerance regimens offer a promising approach to eradication of factor VIII inhibitors. Bleeding episodes that occur during induction of tolerance can be treated with inhibitor-bypassing agents.
- Details of treatment of patients with inhibitors are presented in Chap. 124 of *Williams Hematology*, 8th ed.

Spontaneous Factor VIII Inhibitors

- Autoantibodies against factor VIII may appear in patients without hemophilia. This occurs idiopathically in older adults, in pregnant and postpartum women, and in patients with immunologic disorders (e.g., systemic lupus erythematosus and rheumatoid arthritis).

- Clinical manifestations include spontaneous ecchymoses and intramuscular hemorrhages, which often cause compartment syndromes. Hemarthrosis is rare.
- Patients with acquired inhibitors are low responders.
- Transfusion therapy to achieve hemostasis is identical to the treatment of hemophiliacs with inhibitors.
- In contrast to hemophiliacs, most patients with spontaneous inhibitors respond to treatment to eradicate the inhibitor.
- Prednisone 1 mg/kg and oral cyclophosphamide 1 to 2 mg/kg daily have been used separately or in combination with high response rates.
- Intravenous immune globulin 1 g/kg daily for 2 days has also been shown to decrease inhibitor titers in some of these patients. Anecdotal successes after treatment with rituximab have been reported.

HEMOPHILIA B

Clinical Features
- Table 79–1 shows a clinical classification of hemophilia B based on factor IX levels.
- Bleeding episodes are clinically identical to those in hemophilia A.
- Factor IX inhibitors develop infrequently.

Laboratory Features
- In most cases, the aPTT is prolonged.
- Specific assay of factor IX levels is necessary for diagnosis.

Carrier Detection and Prenatal Diagnosis
- As with hemophilia A, molecular genetic techniques are available for carrier detection and prenatal diagnosis.

Differential Diagnosis
- Hemophilia B must be distinguished from hemophilia A, inherited or acquired deficiencies of other vitamin K–dependent coagulation factors, liver disease, or warfarin overdosage.

Therapy
- General treatment should be the same as for hemophilia A (see above).
- Replacement with factor IX concentrates (Table 79–5):
  — All currently available factor IX concentrates are treated to inactivate viruses.
  — Intermediate purity products ("prothrombin complex concentrates") contain prothrombin; factors VII, IX, and X; and proteins C and S. They may also contain small amounts of activated factors VII, IX, and X, which predispose to thrombosis, especially if large doses are given or the patient has liver disease.
  — Highly purified factor IX concentrates contain only traces of other prothrombin complex factors, and recombinant factor IX contains none. These are the currently preferred preparations for clinical use.
  — Intravascular recovery of factor IX from concentrates is about 50 percent, and is even less with the recombinant product.
  — Initial dosage can be calculated assuming 1 unit of highly purified factor IX per kg body weight will increase the plasma level of factor IX by 1 percent or 0.01 U/mL. Thus, to replace factor IX to 100 percent requires 100 U/kg body weight as a bolus. The half-life of factor IX is 18 to 24 hours. Continued dosage should be one-half of the initial dosage given every 12 to 18 hours. Larger doses are required with recombinant factor IX.
  — Factor IX may also be given by continuous infusion.
  — Factor IX levels should be monitored during therapy and doses adjusted appropriately.

TABLE 79–5	CURRENTLY AVAILABLE FACTOR IX PRODUCTS*	
	Origin	Viral Inactivation
Intermediate purity (prothrombin complex concentrates)		
Profilnine SD	Plasma	Solvent-detergent
Bebulin VH	Plasma	Vapor heating
High purity		
Mononine	Plasma	Ultra filtration; chemical
AlphaNine	Plasma	Solvent-detergent; virus filtered
Recombinant		
BeneFIX	CHO cells	Nanofiltration

*Additional factor IX concentrates are available in Europe.
Source: *Williams Hematology*, 8th ed, Chap. 124, Table 124–9, p. 2018.

- Prophylactic therapy may also be given for hemophilia B. The recommended dose is 25 to 40 U/kg twice weekly.
- Gene therapy for hemophilia B is being actively investigated.

Course and Prognosis

- Patients with hemophilia B are vulnerable to the same complications of recurrent bleeding that occur with hemophilia A.
- HIV infection and chronic liver disease are common in patients treated before viral inactivation of factor IX concentrates was introduced.

Factor IX Inhibitors

- Factor IX inhibitors at levels less than 10 BU can sometimes be overcome with large doses of purified factor IX concentrates.
- If the factor IX inhibitor level is greater than 10 BU, inhibitor-bypassing products (recombinant factor VIIa or prothrombin complex concentrates) should be used.
- Attempts to induce immune tolerance by administering daily infusions of factor IX concentrates have led to significant adverse reactions, including anaphylaxis and the nephrotic syndrome. Factor VIIa concentrates should be used for treatment of any patient who has developed anaphylaxis.

For a more detailed discussion, see Harold R. Roberts, Nigel S. Key, Miguel A. Escobar: Hemophilia A and Hemophilia B. Chap. 124, p. 2009 in *Williams Hematology*, 8th ed.

CHAPTER 80
von Willebrand Disease

von Willebrand disease (VWD) is a result of quantitative and qualitative abnormalities in von Willebrand factor (VWF), a plasma protein serving as a carrier for factor VIII and as an adhesive link between platelets and damaged blood vessel walls. Table 80–1 presents the nomenclature used in discussing the functions of VWF.

ETIOLOGY AND PATHOGENESIS

- VWF is synthesized in endothelial cells and megakaryocytes.
- Posttranslational modification of the molecule involves glycosylation, sulfation, and multimer formation through extensive disulfide bond formation.
- VWF is stored in platelets and in Weibel-Palade bodies in endothelial cells.
- Secretion of VWF from Weibel-Palade bodies is both constitutive and regulated. High-molecular-weight multimers with the greatest activity are released in response to agents such as thrombin *in vitro* or desmopressin (DDAVP) *in vivo*.
- A specific VWF processing protease can reduce the size of high-molecular-weight multimers in plasma.
- VWF plays an important role in platelet aggregation at sites of vessel injury.
- VWF stabilizes factor VIII through formation of a noncovalent complex between the two proteins.
- A large number of mutations of the VWF gene have been discovered and more than 20 distinct subtypes of VWD have been described. Table 80–2 presents a simplified classification of VWD.

TABLE 80–1　von WILLEBRAND FACTOR AND FACTOR VIII TERMINOLOGY
Factor VIII
Antihemophilic factor, the protein that is reduced in plasma of patients with classic hemophilia A and VWD and is measured in standard coagulation assays
Factor VIII activity (factor VIII:C)
The coagulant property of the factor VIII protein (this term is sometimes used interchangeably with factor VIII)
Factor VIII antigen (VIII:Ag)
The antigenic determinant(s) on factor VIII measured by immunoassays, which may employ polyclonal or monoclonal antibodies
von Willebrand factor (VWF)
The large multimeric glycoprotein that is necessary for normal platelet adhesion, a normal bleeding time, and stabilizing factor VIII
von Willebrand factor antigen (VWF:Ag)
The antigenic determinant(s) on VWF measured by immunoassays, which may employ polyclonal or monoclonal antibodies; *inaccurate designations of historical interest only* include factor VIII-related antigen (VIIIR:Ag), factor VIII antigen, AHF antigen, and AHF-like antigen
Ristocetin cofactor activity (or: von Willebrand factor activity; VWF:act)
The property of VWF that supports ristocetin-induced agglutination of washed or fixed normal platelets

Source: *Williams Hematology*, 8th ed, Chap. 127, Table 127–1, p. 2070.

TABLE 80–2 CLASSIFICATION OF VON WILLEBRAND DISEASE

Type	Inheritance	Frequency	Factor VIII Activity	VWF Antigen	Ristocetin Cofactor Activity	RIPA	Plasma VWF Multimer Structure	Previous Nomenclature
Type I	Autosomal dominant	1–30:1000; most common (>70% of VWD)	Decreased	Decreased	Decreased	Decreased or normal	Normal	Type I
Type 3	Autosomal recessive (or codominant)	$1–5:10^6$	Markedly decreased	Very low or absent	Very low or absent	Absent	Usually absent	Type III
Type 2A	Usually autosomal dominant	≈10–15% of clinically significant VWD	Decreased to normal	Usually low	Markedly decreased	Decreased	Largest and intermediate multimers absent	Type IIA, IB, I "platelet discordant," IIC-H
Type 2B	Autosomal dominant	Uncommon variant (<5% of clinical VWD)	Decreased to normal	Usually low	Decreased to normal	Increased to low concentrations of ristocetin	Largest multimers absent	Type IIB
Type 2M	Usually autosomal dominant	Rare (case reports)	Variably decreased	Variably decreased	Decreased	Variably decreased	Normal	Type B, IC, ID, Vicenza
Type 2N	Autosomal recessive	Uncommon: heterozygotes may be prevalent in some populations	Decreased	Normal	Normal	Normal	Normal	VWD Normandy
Platelet-type (pseudo-)	Autosomal dominant	Rare	Decreased to normal	Decreased to normal	Decreased	Increased to low concentrations of ristocetin	Largest multimers absent	

Source: *Williams Hematology*, 8th ed, Chap. 127, Table 127–2, p. 2071.

- Types 1 and 3 are deficiencies of normal VWF, either partial (type 1) or complete (type 3).
- Type 2 includes the qualitative abnormalities of VWF structure and/or function. The quantity of VWF (VWF antigen) in type 2 disease may be normal but is usually reduced.
- Platelet-type VWD is an inherited platelet abnormality due to a mutation in glycoprotein Ib (CD42b, c). It is discussed in Chap. 76.

CLINICAL FEATURES

Type 1
- Type 1 accounts for 70 percent of cases.
- It is usually transmitted as an autosomal dominant trait with variable expression and incomplete penetrance (heterozygous defect).
- Symptoms vary considerably in families. In two families, only 65 percent of individuals with both an affected parent and descendent had significant symptoms.
- Symptoms may vary in the same patient over time.
- The most common bleeding problems are epistaxis (60%), easy bruising and hematomas (40%), menorrhagia (35%), gingival bleeding (35%), and gastrointestinal bleeding (10%).
- In some families, there may be an association with hereditary hemorrhagic telangiectasia.
- Bleeding after trauma is common.
- Hemarthroses are rare except in association with trauma.
- In patients with mild to moderate disease, symptoms may ameliorate by the second or third decade of life.
- During pregnancy in patients with type 1 VWD, levels of factor VIII and ristocetin cofactor activities usually rise above 50 percent.

Type 2
- Types 2A and 2B are the most common qualitative VWF disorders. In type 2A, VWF function is impaired. In type 2B, the interaction between VWF and platelets is dysfunctional.
- Type 2 variants are usually transmitted as autosomal dominant traits. They account for 20 to 30 percent of cases.
- Thrombocytopenia occurs in type 2B but is usually not sufficiently severe to contribute to clinical bleeding.
- Infants with type 2B may have neonatal thrombocytopenia.
- Type 2N patients (with impaired factor VIII binding to VWF) usually have moderately decreased levels of factor VIII but may have low levels compatible with severe hemophilia A.

Type 3
- Inheritance may be autosomal recessive (homozygous or compound heterozygous defect).
- Major clinical bleeding, including hemarthroses and muscle hematomas, occurs as in severe hemophilia.

LABORATORY FEATURES

- In a patient suspected of having VWD, initial laboratory tests should include assay of VWF activity, VWF antigen, and factor VIII activity.
- Additional tests commonly performed are bleeding time, ristocetin-induced platelet agglutination, and VWF multimer analysis (Fig. 80–1).
- Great care must be exercised in interpreting these laboratory results. The bleeding time may be prolonged in normal people by drugs, such as aspirin or other nonsteroidal antiinflammatory agents.

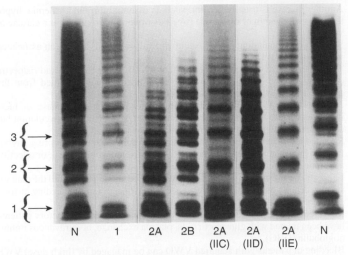

FIGURE 80–1 Agarose gel electrophoresis of plasma VWF. VWF multimers from plasma of patients with various subtypes of VWD are shown. The brackets to the left encompass three individual multimer subunits, including the main band and its associate satellite bands. N indicates normal control lanes. Lanes 5 through 7 are rare variants of type 2A VWD. The former designations for these variants are indicated in parentheses below the lanes (IIC through IIE).
(Reproduced with permission from Zimmerman TS, Dent JA, Ruggeri ZM, Nannini LH: Subunit composition of plasma von Willebrand factor. Cleavage is present in normal individuals, increased in IIA and IIB von Willebrand disease, but minimal in variants with aberrant structure of individual oligomers (types IIC, IID, and IIE). J Clin Invest Mar;77(3):947–51, 1986.)
(Source: *Williams Hematology,* 8th ed, Chap. 127, Fig. 127–4, p. 2075.)

- Factor VIII activity, VWF antigen, and ristocetin cofactor activity may all be increased to normal by many minor illnesses.
- VWF levels may vary with blood group. Carriers of blood group O typically have lower VWF levels.
- Wide variation is found in the results of repeated assays for VWF or ristocetin cofactor activity in the same subjects.
- Repeated studies are usually necessary, and the diagnosis or exclusion of VWD usually requires more than one set of laboratory data.

DIFFERENTIAL DIAGNOSIS

Prenatal Diagnosis

- In most instances, the clinical phenotype of VWD is mild and prenatal diagnosis is rarely sought.
- Prenatal diagnosis has been successful using DNA techniques in families with type 3 VWD.

Platelet-Type (Pseudo-) VWD

- This is a platelet defect discussed in Chap. 76. It can be differentiated from VWD by special laboratory tests.

Acquired VWD

- Acquired VWD usually appears later in life in a patient with no personal or family history of abnormal bleeding.

- Another disease is usually present, such as essential thrombocythemia, hypothyroidism, a benign or malignant B-cell disorder, a solid tumor, or a cardiac or vascular defect.
- Several drugs, including ciprofloxacin and valproic acid, have been associated with acquired VWD.
- The patients have decreased levels of factor VIII, VWF antigen, and ristocetin cofactor activity. Large multimers of VWF are relatively depleted from the plasma. The bleeding time is usually prolonged.
- Autoantibodies to VWF appear to be responsible for the disease in most instances, usually by causing rapid clearance of VWF from the circulation but sometimes by interfering with VWF function.
- Reduced levels of VWF may also be caused by decreased synthesis (e.g., hypothyroidism), increased destruction (e.g., heart disease, some drugs), or selective adsorption to tumor cells.
- Laboratory confirmation of acquired VWD can be very difficult, and the diagnosis may depend on the late onset, absence of personal or family bleeding history, and identification of the underlying disease.
- Management is usually directed to the underlying disorder. Refractory patients have been treated with glucocorticoids, plasma exchange, or intravenous immunoglobulin (IVIG).
- Bleeding in patients with acquired VWD can be managed by (high dose) VWF concentrate, DDAVP, or by recombinant factor VIIa.

THERAPY, COURSE, PROGNOSIS

- The goals of therapy are to correct the VWF deficiency and shorten or correct the bleeding time.

Desmopressin

- Patients with type 1 VWD release unusually high-molecular-weight multimers of VWF into the circulation for 1 to 3 hours after infusion of DDAVP.
- Therapy with DDAVP increases the baseline levels of factor VIII activity, VWF antigen, and ristocetin cofactor activity two- to five-fold in patients with type 1 VWD, and in many instances also corrects the abnormal bleeding time.
- Approximately 80 percent of type 1 patients have excellent responses to DDAVP. Many type 2 patients and nearly all type 3 do not respond adequately.
- DDAVP is regularly used in patients with type 1 VWD to treat mild to moderate bleeding, or as prophylaxis prior to surgery.
- Patients being considered for DDAVP therapy should, if possible, have factor VIII and ristocetin cofactor levels determined 1 to 2 hours following a preliminary dose.
- For patients undergoing surgery, DDAVP can be given 1 hour prior to the operation and repeated every 12 hours.
- The usual dose is 0.3 μg/kg in 100 mL saline over 30 to 45 minutes intravenously.
- Mild cutaneous vasodilatation is common, leading to facial flushing, tingling, warmth, and headaches.
- Fluid restriction may be necessary because of the potential for dilutional hyponatremia, in particular in children and perioperative patients.
- There have been isolated reports of arterial thrombosis (including myocardial infarction and unstable angina) with DDAVP therapy.
- Response to DDAVP may be reduced in patients receiving doses more frequently than every 24 to 48 hours (tachyphylaxis).
- The response of factor VIII level and ristocetin cofactor activity should be measured regularly in patients receiving frequent doses of DDAVP.
- VWF-containing concentrates and/or cryoprecipitate should be available for use in the event that DDAVP becomes ineffective.

- DDAVP has been successfully used to treat type 2B patients, but there is concern that the release of high-molecular-weight multimers could cause platelet aggregation and worsening thrombocytopenia in some patients.
- An intranasal form of DDAVP is available and appears to be effective, but with greater variability of response.

VWF Replacement

- Patients unresponsive to DDAVP may be treated with virus-inactivated, VWF-containing factor VIII concentrates, such as Humate P.
- Replacement therapy is largely empiric, with the initial goal normalization of factor VIII levels and shortening or normalization of the bleeding time.
- If clinical bleeding continues, additional replacement should be given and the patient evaluated for other causes of bleeding that may require additional intervention.
- Patients should be treated for 7 to 10 days after major surgical procedures and 3 to 5 days after minor.
- Postpartum bleeding may occur for more than a month after delivery, and may require prolonged treatment in some severe cases.
- Patients with type 3 VWD may develop an autoantibody against VWF, requiring treatment similar to that of factor VIII inhibitors in hemophilia A.

Other Therapies

- Estrogens or oral contraceptives have been used empirically for menorrhagia.
- Fibrinolytic inhibitors, such as ε-aminocaproic acid and tranexamic acid, may be useful adjuncts to prophylactic therapy for dental procedures, and have also been used empirically in menorrhagia or recurrent epistaxis.

 For a more detailed discussion, see Jill Johnsen and David Ginsburg: von Willebrand Disease. Chap. 127, p. 2069 in *Williams Hematology,* 8th ed.

CHAPTER 81
Hereditary Disorders of Fibrinogen

AFIBRINOGENEMIA AND HYPOFIBRINOGENEMIA

- Quantitative disorders of fibrinogen may be afibrinogenemia or hypofibrinogenemia, depending on the severity.
- Normal fibrinogen levels range from 150 to 350 mg/dL. In afibrinogenemia, the fibrinogen concentration is less than 20 mg/dL. In hypofibrinogenemia, the level is less than normal.
- Mutations resulting in afibrinogenemia or hypofibrinogenemia are presented in Chap. 126, Table 126–1, p. 2055 in *Williams Hematology*, 8th ed.

Clinical Features

- Congenital afibrinogenemia is a rare disorder of hepatic biosynthesis of fibrinogen, inherited as an autosomal recessive trait, with low levels of fibrinogen typically found in both parents.
- Bleeding varies from minimal to severe. Umbilical cord bleeding may occur at birth. Later, bleeding may be from mucosal surfaces, into muscles, or into joints.
- Spontaneous abortions are frequent.
- Death is most often a result of intracranial hemorrhage.
- Hereditary hypofibrinogenemia appears to be caused by abnormal intracellular hepatic storage of fibrinogen.

Laboratory Features

- All laboratory tests depending on formation of a clot are abnormal in afibrinogenemia or hypofibrinogenemia but can be corrected by mixing with normal plasma or fibrinogen solutions.
- The diagnosis is established by demonstrating a reduced fibrinogen concentration by immunologic testing.
- The bleeding time is prolonged and platelet aggregation is abnormal; both can be corrected by infusion of plasma or fibrinogen.

Therapy, Course, and Prognosis

- Replacement therapy with cryoprecipitate (if available) or fibrinogen concentrate may be required.
- Cryoprecipitate typically contains 300 mg of fibrinogen per unit. Approximately 50 to 70 percent of the administered fibrinogen circulates posttransfusion, and the biologic half-life of fibrinogen is 3 to 5 days. The recommended initial dose is 1 unit of cryoprecipitate (300 mg of fibrinogen) per 5 kg of body weight to reach hemostatic levels of fibrinogen.
- Fibrinogen concentrate should be given to increase the plasma concentrations by at least 150 mg/dL. One gram of fibrinogen concentrate raises the plasma fibrinogen level by 20 mg/dL.
- Patients should receive one-third of the initial loading dose daily as long as is necessary to sustain the fibrinogen level.
- Cryoprecipitate or fibrinogen concentrate may be given during pregnancy to prevent spontaneous abortion or premature birth.
- Thrombosis can occur after administration of fibrinogen, and antifibrinogen antibodies may develop.

DYSFIBRINOGENEMIA

- Inherited dysfibrinogenemia is the production of structurally abnormal fibrinogen molecules with altered functional properties. At least 300 families with this fibrinogenemia have been described thus far.
- Hypodysfibrinogenemia refers to patients with low levels of circulating abnormal fibrinogen.

Etiology and Pathogenesis

- Dysfibrinogenemia is inherited as an autosomal dominant trait. Most patients are heterozygous but some are homozygous.
- Fibrinogen abnormalities usually affect one or more phases of fibrin formation:
  — Impaired fibrinopeptide release.
  — Defective fibrin polymerization.
  — Defective cross-linking by factor XIIIa.
- Biochemical abnormalities do not correlate with clinical expression. For example, the same amino acid substitution can lead to either a familial bleeding tendency or to a familial thrombophilia.
- Hereditary renal amyloidosis is an autosomal dominant trait in which there is progressive extracellular deposition of "amyloid" protein in the kidneys, due in some instances, to deposition of fragments of a structurally abnormal fibrinogen.
- Dysfibrinogens with known structural defects or with defined functional characteristics are presented in Table 126–2, p. 2064, of *Williams Hematology,* 8th ed.

Clinical Features

- Most patients are asymptomatic. About 25 percent have abnormal bleeding, and 20 percent have thrombophilia. Some patients have both thrombophilia and bleeding.
- Bleeding is usually not severe; e.g., epistaxis, menorrhagia, mild to moderate postoperative hemorrhage.
- Spontaneous abortion may occur, and excessive bleeding or thromboembolism may be seen postpartum.
- Defective wound healing occurs with several variants.
- Thrombosis is usually venous but may be arterial.
- Renal amyloidosis occurs in some families.
- Thrombophilia caused by dysfibrinogenemia is discussed in Chap. 89 under "Hereditary Thrombotic Dysfibrinogenemia."

Laboratory Features

- Coagulation tests requiring the formation of a fibrin clot are usually prolonged (e.g., prothrombin time, activated partial thromboblastin time, thrombin time).
- Some variants may be detected only by abnormalities of the thrombin and/or reptilase times. It is essential to compare fibrinogen concentrations determined by different methods: functional, immunologic, and chemical. The diagnosis is based on an abnormally low functional fibrinogen level, with a normal level by immunologic or chemical methods. In hypodysfibrinogenemia, reduced levels are found by all three methods. Here the diagnosis must be made from abnormal thrombin and reptilase times.
- Impaired platelet aggregation and clot retraction have been reported in some families. In one family, enhanced platelet aggregation has been described.

Therapy

- Patients with bleeding or undergoing surgery may require replacement therapy with cryoprecipitate or fibrinogen concentrate as outlined for afibrinogenemia.
- Thromboembolism is treated with anticoagulants following standard protocols.

- Administration of cryoprecipitate or fibrinogen concentrate prior to surgery may be beneficial both to increase the level of normal fibrinogen and to dilute the prothrombotic fibrinogen. In patients with life-threatening thromboembolic disease undergoing surgery, plasma exchange has been effective.

 For a more detailed discussion, see Marguerite Neerman-Arbez and Phillipe de Moerloose: Hereditary Fibrinogen Abnormalities. Chap. 126, p. 2051 in *Williams Hematology*, 8th ed.

CHAPTER 82
Inherited Deficiencies of Coagulation Factors II, V, VII, X, XI, and XIII and the Combined Deficiencies of Factors V and VIII and of the Vitamin K–Dependent Factors

- Inherited deficiencies of coagulation factors other than factor VIII (hemophilia A) and factor IX (hemophilia B) are rare bleeding disorders that occur in most populations.
- Patients are usually homozygotes or compound heterozygotes.
- Factor XI and factor VII deficiency occur relatively frequently, other deficiencies are relatively rare (Table 82–1).
- The severity of the bleeding disorder usually relates to the severity of the factor deficiency.
- All may be caused by decreased synthesis of a specific coagulation factor, by synthesis of a dysfunctional form of the coagulation factor, or both.
- Inherited deficiency of a coagulation factor does not protect patients from thrombosis.

PROTHROMBIN (FACTOR II) DEFICIENCY

Pathogenesis
- May be hypoprothrombinemia or dysprothrombinemia.
- Both are inherited as autosomal recessive disorders.
- Both interfere with hemostasis by impairing thrombin generation.

Clinical Features
- The disorders are characterized by mucocutaneous and soft tissue bleeding, usually in proportion to the severity of the functional prothrombin deficiency.
- Bleeding may be spontaneous if prothrombin levels are less than 1 percent. Hemarthroses may occur.
- Individuals with higher prothrombin levels have a variable bleeding tendency, and some may be asymptomatic.

Laboratory Features
- The activated partial thromboplastin time (aPTT) and prothrombin time (PT) are prolonged. The thrombin time (TT) is normal.
- Diagnosis is established by demonstrating reduced levels of functional prothrombin.
- Both functional and antigen assays are required to identify dysprothrombinemia. Immunoelectrophoretic studies may demonstrate some forms of dysprothrombinemia.

TABLE 82–1	RELATIVE PREVALENCE OF RARE BLEEDING DISORDERS*							
Deficiency	WFH Survey (2002)[†]		Six National Registries (2007)[†]		UK Data (Oct. 2008)[‡]		Survey of 64 Centers (Aug. 2008)[†]	
	N	%	N	%	N	%	N	%
Factor XI	2446	35.3	1947	39.4	1762	59.5	770	23.5
Factor VII	1689	24.4	1050	21.3	580	19.6	927	28.3
Afibrinogenemia	644	9.3	496	10.0	203	6.9	241	7.4
Factor X	597	8.6	446	9.0	190	6.4	339	10.4
Factor V	769	11.1	415	8.4	129	4.4	233	7.1
Factor XIII	434	6.3	282	5.7	60	2.0	211	6.5
Factor V/ Factor VIII	188	2.7	203	4.1	25	0.8	495	15.1
Factor II	167	2.4	101	2.0	13	0.4	55	1.7
Total	6934	100	4940	100	2962	100	3271	100

*Patients with partial deficiency were included.
[†]Data courtesy of Professor Flora Peyvandi, Milan, Italy.
[‡]Data courtesy of Professor Paula Bolton-Maggs, Manchester, UK.
Source: *Williams Hematology*, 8th ed, Chap. 125, Table 125–1, p. 2032.

Differential Diagnosis

- Differential diagnosis includes inherited factor V or factor X deficiency, acquired deficiency of the vitamin K–dependent factors, or lupus anticoagulant.

Treatment

- Prothrombin deficiency may be corrected with intravenous prothrombin complex concentrates, but with risk of transmission of viruses not inactivated by solvent detergent treatment and/or nanofiltration and induction of intravascular coagulation.
- Fresh-frozen plasma is also effective but carries a risk of transmitting infectious agents. Solvent detergent treatment of pooled plasma reduces this risk, but viruses that are not inactivated in the pooled plasma source may still be transmitted, e.g., parvovirus, hepatitis A virus.
- Bruises and mild superficial bleeding do not require treatment.
- The biologic half-life of prothrombin is 3 days, and a single treatment for a bleeding episode may suffice.
- Prothrombin levels of 10 to 25 percent are usually sufficient for hemostasis.

FACTOR VII DEFICIENCY

Pathogenesis

- Factor VII deficiency is inherited as an autosomal recessive trait.
- The disorder is symptomatic only in homozygotes or compound heterozygotes.
- The disease may be caused by decreased production of factor VII, production of a factor VII with decreased functional activity, or both. Levels of factor VII antigen may be normal, reduced, or zero.
- Three polymorphisms of the factor VII gene that lead to reduced levels of factor VII but do not lead to abnormal bleeding have been described. These reduced levels of factor VII may be of benefit by lowering the risk of myocardial infarction.

Clinical Features

- Patients with factor VII levels below 1 percent may have a severe bleeding disorder indistinguishable from severe hemophilia A or B.

- Most patients with levels of factor VII of 5 percent or more have disease characterized by easy bruising, gingival bleeding, epistaxis, and menorrhagia.
- Dental extractions, tonsillectomy, and genitourinary tract surgery may induce excessive bleeding if no preoperative replacement therapy is given, but operations such as laparotomy and herniorrhaphy may not lead to excessive bleeding.
- Postpartum hemorrhage is unusual in women with factor VII deficiency.

Laboratory Features
- The diagnosis is suggested by a prolonged PT with a normal aPTT.
- Diagnosis requires demonstration of isolated factor VII deficiency by specific assay.
- Factor VII antigen can be detected by radioimmunoassay.
- The mutant gene can be detected by molecular biology techniques.

Differential Diagnosis
- Acquired factor VII deficiency occurs in patients with liver disease, vitamin K deficiency, and those receiving vitamin K antagonists.
- Rarely, patients may have an inherited deficiency of factor VII and X, factor VII and IX, or of all vitamin K–dependent factors.

Therapy
- Skin lacerations require only local hemostasis. Antifibrinolytic therapy is usually effective in patients with menorrhagia, epistaxis, and/or gingival bleeding.
- Replacement therapy is necessary in patients with severe bleeding, such as hemarthroses or intracerebral hemorrhage, and may be required with surgery, depending on the severity of the deficiency, bleeding history, and the operative site.
- Replacement may be achieved with plasma, prothrombin complex concentrates, specific factor VII concentrates, or recombinant human factor VIIa.
- The possibilities for transmission of viral infection and induction of thrombosis must be considered when selecting a therapeutic agent.
- The half-life of factor VII is approximately 5 hours. Hemostasis is achieved with levels between 10 and 25 percent.
- If plasma is used for major surgery, the recommended initial dose is 15 mL/kg, followed by 4 mL/kg every 6 hours for 7 to 10 days.
- Replacement therapy with plasma may lead to fluid overload requiring diuretic therapy or plasmapheresis.

FACTOR X DEFICIENCY

Pathogenesis
- Factory X deficiency is inherited as an autosomal recessive trait.
- Heterozygotes have factor X levels about 50 percent of normal and are usually asymptomatic.
- The disease may be caused by decreased production of factor X, production of factor X with decreased functional activity, or both.

Clinical Features
- Patients with factor X levels of less than 1 percent have severe bleeding, primarily in the joints, soft tissues, and from mucous membranes. Menorrhagia may be a major problem.
- In patients with mild to moderate factor X deficiency, bleeding usually occurs after trauma or surgery.

Laboratory Features
- The PT and aPTT are both prolonged, as is the Russell viper venom time. The TT is normal.

- Diagnosis requires demonstration of isolated factor X deficiency by specific assay.
- Factor X antigen can be detected by immunologic techniques.

Differential Diagnosis

- Laboratory testing will differentiate inherited factor X deficiency from deficiency of prothrombin, factor V, factor VII, multiple factor deficiencies, vitamin K deficiency, liver disease, or the lupus anticoagulants.
- Acquired factor X deficiency may occur in patients with primary amyloidosis due to selective binding of factor X to amyloid fibrils or to the presence of an abnormal form of factor X.
- Acquired isolated factor X deficiency has been reported to be associated with a number of other disorders. Acquired inhibitors of factor X also occur.

Treatment

- Factor X deficiency may be treated with prothrombin complex concentrates that contain factor X. Because of the (theoretical) risk of thrombosis with these concentrates, it is recommended that divided doses be used if more than 2000 units are required.
- For soft tissue, mucosal, or joint hemorrhages, replacement of factor X to 30 percent of normal is recommended. More serious bleeding requires replacement to 50 to 100 percent.
- The biologic half-life of factor X is 24 to 40 hours. Continuing therapy should be given every 24 hours.
- Fresh-frozen plasma may also be used to replace factor X deficiency but carries the risks of viral infection and fluid overload.

COMBINED DEFICIENCY OF THE VITAMIN K–DEPENDENT FACTORS

- This is a rare autosomal recessive disorder in which there is deficiency of prothrombin and factors VII, IX, and X. Proteins C and S may also be deficient. The precise pathogenesis is unclear but a defect in vitamin K carboxylation of coagulation factors is suspected.
- In some cases, hemostasis may be improved by administration of large doses of vitamin K.
- Replacement therapy with fresh-frozen plasma may be necessary.

FACTOR V DEFICIENCY

Pathogenesis

- Inherited factor V deficiency is transmitted as an autosomal recessive disorder.
- Homozygotes have a moderate bleeding tendency that is usually due to a true deficiency but the disorder may also be caused by dysfunctional factor V.
- Heterozygotes are usually asymptomatic.

Clinical Features

- Patients with 1 to 10 percent factor V activity have lifelong bleeding, usually expressed as ecchymoses, epistaxis, gingival bleeding, excessive bleeding from minor lacerations, and menorrhagia.
- Hemarthroses or intracranial hemorrhage has been reported.
- Severe bleeding may occur after trauma, dental extraction, or surgery.

Laboratory Features

- Factor V deficiency is characterized by prolongation of both the aPTT and the PT, and sometimes the bleeding time.
- Diagnosis requires specific demonstration of a factor V deficiency.

Differential Diagnosis

- The clinical and laboratory features of hereditary combined factor V and factor VIII deficiency are the same as those of factor V deficiency. Specific assay for factor VIII deficiency is needed to differentiate these diseases.
- The clinical features of severe liver disease or DIC are usually sufficient to permit diagnosis of this cause of acquired factor V deficiency.
- Acquired inhibitors of factor V may appear rarely after surgery or during therapy with antibiotics or other drugs, and can cause severe bleeding. These inhibitors often disappear spontaneously.

Therapy

- Severe or continuing mild bleeding is treated with replacement therapy using fresh-frozen plasma. A factor V level of 25 percent is usually sufficient for hemostasis. The plasma factor V half-life is 12 to 14 hours.
- Infusion of a loading dose of 20 mL/kg of fresh-frozen plasma followed by 5 to 10 mL/kg every 12 hours for 7 to 10 days is usually adequate to ensure hemostasis.
- Minor lacerations may be treated with local measures.
- Antifibrinolytic therapy may be effective in epistaxis or gingival bleeding.

COMBINED DEFICIENCY OF FACTORS V AND VIII

- A rare, autosomal recessive trait with reduced levels of both factor V and factor VIII expressed as a moderately severe lifelong bleeding disorder. The exact pathogenesis is not clear.
- Diagnosis requires specific assays of both factor V and factor VIII.
- Minor bleeding may respond to antifibrinolytic therapy.
- For severe bleeding or prophylaxis before surgery or dental extraction, replacement of both factor V, using fresh-frozen plasma, and factor VIII, using a factor VIII concentrate, is required.

FACTOR XI DEFICIENCY

Pathogenesis

- Factor XI deficiency is an autosomal recessive disorder caused by deficient production of factor XI in almost all instances.
- Homozygotes or compound heterozygotes have factor XI levels of less than 15 percent of normal.
- Factor XI is essential for the activation by thrombin of thrombin-activatable fibrinolysis inhibitor (TAFI) or carboxypeptidase B, an enzyme that inhibits fibrinolysis. This may result in increased fibrinolytic activity, with consequent increase in bleeding.

Clinical Features

- Most patients with factor XI deficiency are Jewish.
- Bleeding is usually related to trauma or surgery.
- Excessive bleeding may begin at the time of injury or be delayed for several hours.
- There appears to be a greater bleeding tendency in genotypes with lower levels of factor XI, and with surgery or injury at sites of high fibrinolytic activity, such as the urinary tract, tonsils, nose, or tooth sockets.
- Some patients who are heterozygous for factor XI deficiency may have excessive bleeding.
- Inhibitors of factor XI may develop in deficient patients who have received replacement therapy, but these do not appear to increase the risk of bleeding in most such patients.

Laboratory Features

- The aPTT is prolonged; the PT is normal.
- Diagnosis requires specific demonstration of a factor XI deficiency.
- The patient's genotype can be determined by molecular biology techniques.

Therapy

- Patients with severe factor XI deficiency may be given replacement therapy with fresh-frozen plasma, recognizing the attendant risk of transmission of infectious agents or allergic reactions. Alternatively, in some countries (plasma-derived) purified and virus-inactivated factor XI concentrates are available.
- The mean half-life of factor XI is about 48 hours.
- Trough levels of factor XI of 45 percent maintained for 10 to 14 days provide adequate hemostasis after major surgery or surgery at sites with high fibrinolytic activity.
- Surgery in areas of lower fibrinolytic activity requires factor XI trough levels of 30 percent maintained for 5 to 7 days.
- Antifibrinolytic therapy may be effective in achieving hemostasis after dental extraction, and is a similarly useful adjunct for treating patients after operation on sites with high local fibrinolytic activity.
- Heterozygous patients with a negative bleeding history, no associated hemostatic abnormality, and a factor XI level above 45 percent probably do not need treatment when undergoing surgery.
- Such individuals with a positive bleeding history and requiring surgery should have appropriate treatment of any associated disorder and replacement of factor XI to trough levels of 45 percent for 5 days.

FACTOR XIII DEFICIENCY

Pathogenesis

- Factor XIII deficiency is a lifelong bleeding disorder transmitted as an autosomal recessive trait.
- Factor XIII deficiency leads to clots that are less stable mechanically and more susceptible to fibrinolysis, resulting in the bleeding disorder.

Clinical Features

- Ecchymoses, hematomas, and prolonged posttraumatic bleeding are common.
- Bleeding from the umbilical cord of newborns occurs frequently.
- Intracranial hemorrhage occurs more often with factor XIII deficiency than with the other coagulation factor deficiencies when matched for the level of coagulation factor.
- Habitual abortion and poor wound healing also occur.

Laboratory Features

- Screening tests for coagulation abnormalities are all usually normal in factor XIII deficiency, although in some cases, the thrombin time may be minimally prolonged. The diagnosis is established by demonstrating increased clot solubility in 5-molar urea or by chemical assays for factor XIIIa activity.
- Deficiency of α_2-antiplasmin gives a similar pattern as factor XIII deficiency but can be diagnosed by specific assay.
- Acquired factor XIII deficiency may occur in DIC, primary fibrinolysis, or if an inhibitor develops to factor XIII. Factor XIII levels may also be decreased after major surgery, during chronic inflammatory conditions (e.g., inflammatory bowel disease), and major trauma.

Therapy

- Replacement therapy may be achieved with plasma or cryoprecipitate, with attendant risks of transmission of infectious agents, or with virus-inactivated concentrates of factor XIII from plasma, if available.
- Factor XIII levels of less than 5 percent will achieve hemostasis.
- The half-life of factor XIII is 19 days.
- Prophylactic therapy using plasma infusions every 4 weeks can achieve normal hemostasis and prevent habitual abortions.

For a more detailed discussion, see Uri Seligsohn, Ariella Zivelin, and Ophira Salomon: Inherited Deficiencies of Coagulation Factors II, V, VII, X, XI and XIII and Combined Deficiencies of Factors V and VIII and of the Vitamin K-Dependent Factors. Chap. 125, p. 2031 in *Williams Hematology*, 8th ed.

CHAPTER 83
Antibody-Mediated Coagulation Factor Deficiencies

- Clinically significant autoantibodies to coagulation factors are uncommon but can produce life-threatening bleeding and death.
- The most commonly targeted coagulation factor by an autoantibody is factor VIII (acquired hemophilia A) but also any other coagulation factor may be inhibited by an autoantibody.

ACQUIRED HEMOPHILIA A

- Acquired hemophilia A can either be idiopathic or associated with other autoimmune disorders, malignancy, the postpartum period, and the use of drugs (such as penicillin and sulfonamides).
- The incidence of autoantibodies to factor VIII is 0.2 to 1 per 1 million persons per year.
- Acquired hemophilia A patients usually present with spontaneous bleeding, which often is severe and life- or limb-threatening. These patients are more likely to have a more severe bleeding diathesis than patients with hemophilia A and an inhibitor.
- Common bleeding sites are soft tissues, skin, and mucous membranes. In contrast to patients with congenital hemophilia A, hemarthroses, intramuscular, and central nervous system bleeding are rare.
- Patients with acquired hemophilia A have a prolonged activated partial thromboplastin time (aPTT) and a normal prothrombin time (PT). The presence of a prolonged aPTT in a 1:1 mixture between patient and normal plasma establishes the diagnosis of a circulating anticoagulant. Specific assays for factor VIII activity and/or antigen will confirm the diagnosis.
- Once the identity of an inhibitor has been established, its titer is determined using the Bethesda assay. The inhibitor titer is defined as the dilution of patient plasma that produces 50 percent inhibition of the factor VIII activity and is expressed as Bethesda units per mL (BU/mL). Inhibitors are classified as low titer or high titer when the titers are less than 5 BU/mL or greater than 5 BU/mL, respectively.
- Acquired factor VIII inhibitors sometimes resolve spontaneously. However, it is not possible to predict in which subset of patients this will occur.
- Patients with a factor VIII inhibitor titer of less than 5 BU/mL often are treated successfully with sufficient doses of recombinant or plasma-derived factor VIII concentrates to neutralize the inhibitor. Patients with titers between 5 and 10 BU/mL also may respond to factor VIII concentrates, whereas those with titers greater than 10 BU/mL generally do not respond.
- Factor VIII bypassing agents, which drive the coagulation mechanism through the extrinsic pathway, are the mainstays of management of patients with a high titer of an inhibitor. Two agents, recombinant activated factor VII and plasma-derived factor eight-inhibitor bypassing agent (FEIBA, also called activated prothrombin complex concentrate) are approved by the U.S. Food and Drug Administration for treatment of acquired hemophilia A.
- The recommended dose range of rFVIIa for the treatment of patients with acquired hemophilia is 70 to 90 μg/kg repeated every 2 to 3 hours until hemostasis is achieved. The minimum effective dose in acquired hemophilia has not been determined.

- Recommended doses of activated prothrombin complex concentrate (FEIBA) depend on the type of bleeding.
  - In joint hemorrhage, 50 U/kg is recommended at 12-hour intervals, which may be increased to doses of 100 U/kg. Treatment should be continued until clear signs of clinical improvement appear, such as relief of pain, reduction of swelling, or mobilization of the joint.
  - For mucous membrane bleeding, 50 U/kg is recommended at 6-hour intervals under careful monitoring. If hemorrhage does not stop, the dose may be increased to 100 U/kg at 6-hour intervals.
  - For severe soft-tissue bleeding, such as retroperitoneal bleeding, 100 U/kg at 12-hour intervals is recommended.
  - Central nervous system bleeding has been effectively treated with doses of 100 U/kg at 6- to 12-hour intervals. One should not exceed a daily dose of FEIBA of 200 U/kg.
- The response to bypassing agents is variable and does not correlate with the inhibitor titer. A major concern with the use of rFVIIa and AICC is that there is no laboratory method available for predicting response to therapy or monitoring patients on therapy.
- The major serious adverse event associated with bypassing agents is thrombosis. However, this risk is considered low when used for approved indications at the recommended doses.
- A commercial plasma-derived porcine factor VIII concentrate was useful in the treatment of factor VIII inhibitor patients for approximately 20 years, but was discontinued in 2004 because of viral contamination of the product. Porcine factor VIII has the advantage of potentially being guided by laboratory monitoring of recovery of factor VIII activity in plasma. However, the development of antiporcine factor VIII antibodies may preclude its long-term use.
- Although acquired inhibitors may remit spontaneously, initiation of immunosuppressive therapy at the time of diagnosis to eradicate the inhibitor is recommended because of the serious course of this condition. A variety of immunosuppressive agents have been used, including cyclophosphamide, azathioprine, cyclosporine A, intravenous immunoglobulin, and rituximab. Plasmapheresis and immunoadsorption of the inhibitory antibody have been used. Finally, immune tolerance induction using human factor VIII has been used successfully.

ANTI-FACTOR V AND ANTITHROMBIN ANTIBODIES

- Antibodies inhibiting thrombin and factor V frequently coexist in immune responses to commercial products that contain thrombin. Thrombin products have been used widely in surgical and endoscopic procedures.
- Thrombin is used either alone or as a component of fibrin sealants, which consist of fibrinogen and thrombin preparations that are mixed together at the wound site to form a topical fibrin clot. Both types of products are heavily contaminated with other plasma proteins, including factor V and prothrombin. Almost all patients exposed to bovine proteins develop a detectable immune response. In half of these patients, antibovine antibodies crossreact with human thrombin, factor V, or prothrombin.
- Usually, these antibodies cause no clinical problems. However, mild to life-threatening hemorrhage can occur, especially if the titer of antihuman factor V antibodies is high. The risk of bleeding is higher in patients who receive bovine thrombin products more than once because of the development of a secondary immune response.
- β-Lactam antibiotics also have been associated with anti-factor V autoantibodies and may partly explain the increased incidence with surgery. Anti-factor V autoantibodies have been identified rarely in patients with autoimmune diseases, solid tumors, and monoclonal gammopathies. In approximately 20 percent of cases of factor V autoantibody formation, no underlying disease was identified.

- Patients with inhibitory antibodies to factor V have prolonged PT and aPTT, low factor V levels and a normal thrombin time. The diagnosis of a factor V inhibitor is based on the specific loss of factor V coagulant activity when patient and normal plasma are mixed in a coagulation assay.
- In case of bleeding, patients may be treated with (high dose) fresh frozen plasma or with a bypassing agent, such as recombinant factor VIIa.

ANTIPROTHROMBIN ANTIBODIES

- Antiprothrombin antibodies are most commonly associated with the antiphospholipid syndrome (see Chap. 85). The antiphospholipid syndrome is caused by lupus anticoagulants, which are defined as antibodies that produce phospholipid-dependent prolongation of *in vitro* coagulation assays.
- However, most patients with lupus anticoagulants have demonstrable antiprothrombin antibodies or a hypoprothrombinemia but no bleeding diathesis.

ACQUIRED ANTIBODIES TO OTHER COAGULATION FACTORS

- Clinically significant antibodies to coagulation factors other than factor VIII, factor V, and prothrombin that produce acquired bleeding disorders are rare. In contrast to acquired hemophilia A, acquired hemophilia B is extremely rare.
- An acquired inhibitor to protein C associated with a fatal thrombotic disorder has been reported, but evidently is rare.
- In contrast, there is a relatively high prevalence of pathogenic anti-protein S antibodies. Inhibitory antibodies to protein S were detected in 5 of 15 patients with acquired protein S deficiency. Anti-protein S antibodies appear to be a risk factor for venous thrombosis and can be manifested *in vitro* as activated protein C resistance.

For a more detailed discussion, see Pete Lollar: Antibody-Mediated Coagulation Factor Deficiencies. Chap. 128, p. 2089 in *Williams Hematology*, 8th ed.

CHAPTER 84
Hemostatic Dysfunction Related to Liver Diseases

PATHOGENESIS

- Loss of hepatic parenchymal cells leads to decreased plasma levels of all plasma coagulation factors except factor VIII and von Willebrand factor.
- Thrombocytopenia occurs frequently and is usually a result of splenic sequestration (see Chap. 74), but may also be caused by an autoimmune mechanism, disseminated intravascular coagulation (DIC), folic acid deficiency, and decreased platelet production. In some patients, thrombocytopenia due to thrombopoietin (TPO) deficiency and platelet dysfunction contribute to the hemostatic abnormalities.
- Enhanced fibrinolysis is common, and appears to be caused by complex pathogenetic mechanisms, including release and impaired clearance of plasminogen activators.
- Dysfibrinogenemia is relatively frequently found in patients with chronic liver disease.
- Patients with chronic liver disease may develop DIC.

CLINICAL FEATURES

- Patients with chronic liver disease may present with purpura, epistaxis, gingival bleeding, and/or menorrhagia.
- Bleeding may follow trauma or surgical procedures, especially in sites with high fibrinolytic activity, such as the urogenital tract or oral mucosa.
- Patients with acute viral or toxic hepatitis usually develop abnormal bleeding only if the disease is fulminant.
- Bleeding from esophageal varices requires primary attention to the bleeding site as well as efforts to correct the hemostatic abnormalities.
- The coagulopathy of liver disease may also predispose the patient to thromboembolic complications.

LABORATORY FEATURES

- Table 84–1 summarizes the laboratory abnormalities that can be found in patients with chronic liver disease. These abnormalities may both contribute to bleeding or thrombosis.
- Determination of plasma levels of factors V, VII, and VIII may help differentiate liver disease (factor VIII levels normal or increased; factors V and VII decreased), vitamin K deficiency (factor VII decreased; factors V and VIII normal), and DIC (all decreased).

THERAPY

- Correction of coagulation is only required in case of bleeding or when an invasive procedure has to be performed.
- Replacement of all the deficient coagulation factors may be attempted with fresh-frozen plasma, but large volumes of plasma are required and volume overload may occur. The risk of transmission of infectious agents can be minimized by using solvent-detergent–treated plasma.

TABLE 84–1	ALTERATIONS IN THE HEMOSTATIC SYSTEM IN PATIENTS WITH LIVER DISEASE THAT CONTRIBUTE TO BLEEDING (LEFT) OR COUNTERACT BLEEDING (RIGHT)
Changes That Impair Hemostasis	**Changes That Promote Hemostasis**
Thrombocytopenia	Elevated levels of VWF
Platelet function defects	Decreased levels of ADAMTS-13
Enhanced production of nitric oxide and prostacyclin	Elevated levels of factor VIII
Low levels of factors II, V, VII, IX, X, and XI	Decreased levels of protein C, protein S, antithrombin, and heparin cofactor II
Vitamin K deficiency	Low levels of plasminogen
Dysfibrinogenemia	
Low levels of α_2-antiplasmin, factor XIII, and TAFI	
Elevated t-PA levels	

VWF, von Willebrand factor; ADAMTS-13, a disintegrin-like and metalloprotease with thrombospondin domain 13; TAFI, thrombin-activatable fibrinolysis inhibitor; t-PA, tissue type plasminogen activator.
Source: *Williams Hematology*, 8th ed, Chap. 129, Table 129–1, p. 2096.

- Prothrombin complex concentrates may be used to correct deficiency of the vitamin K–dependent factors, but do not contain factor V. These preparations may (theoretically) result in thrombosis and can transmit blood-borne microorganisms.
- Vitamin K administration is effective in patients with vitamin K deficiency. Due to a relative resistance to vitamin K, high doses (10 mg) are advised.
- Platelet transfusion may be useful in correcting thrombocytopenia, but splenic sequestration may reduce the yield to ineffective levels.
- Antifibrinolytic agents may prevent bleeding in patients with mucosal bleeding or who require dental extraction, but enhance the risk of thrombosis in patients with DIC.

For a more detailed discussion, see Ton Lisman and Philip G. de Groot: Hemostatic Dysfunction Related to Liver Diseases and Liver Transplantation, Chap. 129, p. 2095 in *Williams Hematology*, 8th ed.

CHAPTER 85
The Antiphospholipid Syndrome (Lupus Anticoagulant and Related Disorders)

- The antiphospholipid syndrome is an acquired thrombotic disorder associated with circulating autoantibodies to anionic phospholipid-protein complexes.
- These antibodies were first detected as inhibitors of the partial thromboplastin time in patients with systemic lupus erythematosus (SLE) and, for this reason, were called "lupus anticoagulant," although this finding is not limited to patients with lupus.

PATHOGENESIS

- The disorder is generally considered to be autoimmune, although a direct causal relationship between antiphospholipid antibodies and thrombosis or pregnancy problems has not been demonstrated.
- The antiphospholipid antibodies found in the syndrome usually react with phospholipid bound to a plasma protein.
- A number of pathogenetic mechanisms have been proposed for the antiphospholipid syndrome, and it is possible that several of these act in concert to cause the disorder.

CLINICAL FEATURES

- Patients usually present with manifestations of thrombosis and/or pregnancy complications or loss.
- The disease usually presents in patients between ages 35 and 45 years. Both sexes are equally susceptible.
- The disorder is considered "secondary antiphospholipid syndrome" if the patient has a recognizable autoimmune disease, or "primary antiphospholipid syndrome" if there is no associated disorder.
- Table 85–1 summarizes the clinical manifestations of the antiphospholipid syndrome.
- The antiphospholipid syndrome should be considered in patients with recurrent thromboses in unusual locations.
- Venous and/or arterial thromboses may occur at any site but are most frequent in the lower extremities.
- Patients with concurrent inherited thrombophilia who develop antiphospholipid antibodies are at increased risk for thrombosis.
- Immune thrombocytopenia, usually of mild to moderate severity, occurs frequently in patients with antiphospholipid syndrome.
- Rarely, patients may develop a *catastrophic* form of the antiphospholipid syndrome, with severe, widespread vascular occlusions, despite intense anticoagulant treatment, often leading to death.
- Recurrent pregnancy loss occurs often in women with the antiphospholipid syndrome. About one-half of the abortions occur after the first trimester.
- Some patients develop a bleeding disorder because of a concurrent coagulopathy, such as acquired hypoprothrombinemia, or because of acquired inhibitors of factor VIII.

TABLE 85–1	CLINICAL MANIFESTATIONS OF THE ANTIPHOSPHOLIPID SYNDROME

Venous and arterial thromboembolism
Pregnancy losses and complications
Thrombocytopenia
Stroke
Livedo reticularis, necrotizing skin vasculitis
Coronary artery disease
Valvular heart disease
Pulmonary hypertension, acute respiratory distress syndrome
Atherosclerosis and peripheral artery disease
Retinal disease
Adrenal failure, hemorrhagic adrenal infarction
Gastrointestinal manifestations: Budd-Chiari syndrome, mesenteric and portal vein obstructions, hepatic infarction, esophageal necrosis, gastric and colonic ulceration, gallbladder necrosis.
Catastrophic antiphospholipid syndrome with microangiopathy

Source: *Williams Hematology*, 8th ed, Chap.132, Table 132–6, p. 2150.

LABORATORY FEATURES

- Diagnosis of the antiphospholipid syndrome requires demonstration of antibodies against phospholipids and/or relevant protein cofactors.
- No single test is sufficient for diagnosis, and usually a panel of tests is used, including assays for antibodies against cardiolipin, phosphatidylserine, and β_2-glycoprotein I (β_2-GPI), and coagulation tests for the lupus anticoagulant.

DIFFERENTIAL DIAGNOSIS

- The diagnosis of antiphospholipid syndrome is based on consensual (research) criteria, as presented in Table 85–2.
- Vasculitis may cause vascular occlusion in patients with autoimmune diseases.
- The catastrophic antiphospholipid syndrome should be differentiated from thrombotic microangiopathies (including thrombotic thrombocytopenic purpura (see Chaps. 21 and 91), disseminated vasculitis, or disseminated intravascular coagulation (see Chap. 86).
- The "lupus anticoagulant" as the cause of prolongation of the activated partial thromboplastin time should be differentiated from specific coagulation factor deficiencies or other inhibitors by using appropriate laboratory procedures.
- Antiphospholipid antibody levels may be elevated artifactually or because of specific infections, such as syphilis, Lyme disease, HIV, or hepatitis C.

THERAPY, COURSE, AND PROGNOSIS

Thrombosis

- Acute thrombosis in the antiphospholipid syndrome is treated the same as thrombosis from any cause.
- Patients with the antiphospholipid syndrome who develop spontaneous thromboembolism should receive long-term, possibly lifelong, oral anticoagulation. Clinical studies have not shown conclusive evidence that a higher intensity of anticoagulant therapy should be maintained.
- Hydroxychloroquine therapy appears to have an antithrombotic effect in patients with the antiphospholipid syndrome and SLE.
- Patients with the catastrophic antiphospholipid syndrome may benefit from treatment with anticoagulants, glucocorticoids, and plasma exchange or intravenous gamma-globulin. There is anecdotal successful experience with rituximab.

TABLE 85-2	**SYDNEY INVESTIGATIONAL CRITERIA FOR DIAGNOSIS OF ANTIPHOSPHOLIPID SYNDROME (APS)**

Clinical

Vascular thrombosis (one or more episodes of arterial, venous, or small vessel thrombosis). For histopathologic diagnosis, there should not be evidence of inflammation in the vessel wall.

Pregnancy morbidities attributable to placental insufficiency, including:

- Three or more otherwise unexplained recurrent spontaneous miscarriages, before 10 weeks of gestation.
- One or more fetal losses after the 10th week of gestation, stillbirth, episode of preeclampsia, preterm labor, placental abruption, intrauterine growth restriction or oligohydramnios that are otherwise unexplained.

Laboratory

aCL or anti-β_2GPI IgG and/or IgM antibody present in medium or high titer on two or more occasions, at least 12 weeks apart, measured by standard ELISAs.

Lupus anticoagulant in plasma, on two or more occasions, at least 12 weeks apart, detected according to the guidelines of the International Society of Thrombosis and Hemostasis Scientific Standardization Committee on Lupus Anticoagulants and Phospholipid-Dependent Antibodies.

"Definite APS" is considered to be present if at least one of the clinical criteria and one of the laboratory criteria are met.

---

aCL, anticardiolipin; aPL, antiphospholipid; β_2GPI, β_2-glycoprotein I; ELISA, enzyme-linked immunosorbent assay; Ig, immunoglobulin.
Source: *Williams Hematology*, 8th ed, Chap. 132, Table 132-3, p. 2147.

- Antiphospholipid antibodies may spontaneously disappear and its presence should be monitored.

Pregnancy Loss

- Pregnant patients who have antiphospholipid antibodies but have no history of clinical problems do not require treatment.
- Women who have antiphospholipid antibodies, and who have spontaneously lost three or more pregnancies should receive aspirin and heparin during the pregnancy and after delivery. For example, one suggested regimen calls for treatment with aspirin (80 mg) daily and unfractionated heparin (5000 U subcutaneously every 12 hours) beginning with diagnosis of the pregnancy and continuing until 1 month prior to the expected delivery date if no complications develop. Unfractionated heparin (5000 U subcutaneously every 12 hours) is then restarted 4 to 6 hours after delivery if bleeding has stopped, and is continued until the patient is fully ambulatory.
- Low-molecular-weight heparin is most probably as effective as unfractionated heparin in this setting and allows for once daily injection.
- Patients who have had systemic thromboembolism should be considered for oral anticoagulation for 6 to 12 weeks after delivery. Breastfeeding is possible if the baby is administered usual vitamin K treatment.

For a more detailed discussion, see Jacob H. Rand: The Antiphospholipid Syndrome. Chap. 132, p. 2145 in *Williams Hematology*, 8th ed.

CHAPTER 86
Disseminated Intravascular Coagulation

- Disseminated intravascular coagulation (DIC) is a syndrome that is characterized by systemic intravascular activation of coagulation, leading to fibrin deposition in the microvasculature and small-midsize vessels, thereby contributing to organ dysfunction. Simultaneously, ongoing consumption of platelets and coagulation factors lead to thrombocytopenia and impaired coagulation and may result in serious bleeding complications.
- DIC never occurs by itself but is always secondary to an underlying cause. Table 86–1 lists the most frequently occurring disorders know to be associated with DIC.

PATHOGENESIS

- The pathogenesis of DIC is diagrammed in Fig. 86–1.
- Exposure of blood to tissue factor appears to be the principal mechanism of activation of coagulation. Tissue factor may be expressed by mononuclear cells or by the endothelium.
- Other stimuli include activation of factor Xa by a cancer procoagulant, snake envenomation, and tissue/cellular debris in patients with massive trauma or pancreatitis.
- Activation of coagulation is insufficiently balanced by physiologic anticoagulant pathways (e.g., antithrombin, protein C system) and a downregulation of endogenous fibrinolysis due to high levels of the fibrinolysis inhibitor plasminogen activator inhibitor type 1 (PAI-1).

TABLE 86–1	**CLINICAL CONDITIONS THAT MAY BE COMPLICATED BY DIC**
Sepsis/severe infection	
Trauma	
Malignancy	
Solid tumors	
Acute leukemia	
Obstetrical conditions	
Amniotic fluid embolism	
Abruptio placentae	
HELLP syndrome	
Vascular abnormalities	
Kasabach-Merritt syndrome	
Other vascular malformations	
Aortic aneurysms	
Severe allergic/toxic reactions	
Severe immunologic reactions (e.g., transfusion reaction)	
Heatstroke	

HELLP, hemolysis, elevated liver enzymes, and low platelet count.
Source: *Williams Hematology,* 8th ed, Chap. 130, Table 130–1, p. 2105.

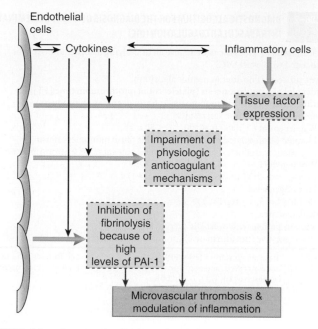

FIGURE 86-1 Schematic presentation of pathogenetic pathways involved in the activation of coagulation in DIC. In DIC, both perturbed endothelial cells and activated mononuclear cells may produce proinflammatory cytokines that mediate coagulation activation. Activation of coagulation is initiated by tissue factor expression on activated mononuclear cells and endothelial cells. In addition, downregulation of physiologic anticoagulant mechanisms and inhibition of fibrinolysis by endothelial cells further promote intravascular fibrin deposition. PAI-1, plasminogen-activator inhibitor type 1. Source: *Williams Hematology*, 8th ed, Chap. 130, Fig. 130–1, p. 2102.

CLINICAL FEATURES

- Clinical features are related to the underlying disorder, to the DIC, or both.
- Bleeding manifestations have been observed in about 25 percent of cases in several series.
- Persistent bleeding from venipuncture sites or other skin wounds occurs frequently.
- Hemorrhage may be life-threatening.
- Extensive organ dysfunction may be induced by microvascular thrombi, or by venous and/or arterial thromboembolism.
- Organ dysfunction may manifest as acute renal failure (renal cortical ischemia and acute tubular necrosis occur frequently), hepatic dysfunction, and respiratory insufficiency due to acute respiratory distress syndrome (ARDS).
- Coma, delirium, focal neurologic symptoms, and signs of meningeal irritation may occur because of thrombosis or hemorrhage in the cerebral vasculature.
- Mortality rates range from 30 to 85 percent. The presence of DIC is a strong predictor for mortality in sepsis, trauma, and other underlying conditions.

LABORATORY FEATURES

- The underlying disorders may influence the abnormalities expected in DIC and must be considered in interpretation of laboratory data.
- There is not a single laboratory test that is able to confirm or reject the diagnosis of DIC.

<table>
<tr><td>**TABLE 86–2**</td><td>**DIAGNOSTIC ALGORITHM FOR THE DIAGNOSIS OF OVERT DISSEMINATED INTRAVASCULAR COAGULATION (DIC)**</td></tr>
</table>

1. Risk assessment: Does the patient have an underlying disorder known to be associated with overt DIC?

   If yes, proceed. If no, do not use this algorithm.

2. Order global coagulation tests (platelet count, prothrombin time [PT], fibrinogen, soluble fibrin monomers, or fibrin degradation products).

3. Score global coagulation test results:
   • Platelet count ($>$100 = 0, $<$100 = 1, $<$50 = 2)
   • Elevated fibrin-related marker (e.g., soluble fibrin monomers/fibrin degradation products) (no increase: 0, moderate increase: 2, strong increase: 3)
   • Prolonged PT
     ($<$3 sec. = 0, $>$3 but $<$6 sec. = 1, $>$6 sec. = 2)
   • Fibrinogen level
     ($>$1.0 g/L = 0, $<$1.0 g/L = 1)

4. Calculate score.

5. If $\geq$5: compatible with overt DIC; repeat scoring daily.
   If $<$5: suggestive (not affirmative) for non-overt DIC; repeat next 1 to 2 days.

Reproduced with permissions from Taylor FBJ, Toh CH, Hoots WK, et al: Towards definition, clinical and laboratory criteria, and a scoring system for disseminated intravascular coagulation. Thromb Haemost Nov 86(5):1327–30, 2001.
Source: *Williams Hematology*, 8th ed, Chap. 130, Table 130–6, p. 2108.

• Typically, the platelet count is low, prothrombin time (PT) and activated partial thromboplastin time (aPTT) are prolonged, levels of coagulation factors and coagulation inhibitors are low, and fibrin related markers (fibrin degradation products, fibrin monomers, D-dimer) are elevated.

• A simple scoring algorithm, utilizing the platelet count, PT, D-dimer, and fibrinogen level has been proposed by the International Society on Thrombosis and Hemostasis and has been prospectively validated (see Table 86–2).

• Fibrinogen levels are rarely low as fibrinogen initially acts as an acute phase protein and levels may markedly increase due to the underlying cause.

• Primary fibrinogenolysis may be distinguished from DIC by finding a normal platelet count, greatly elevated fibrinogen degradation products, and very low levels of α_2- antiplasmin and plasminogen (see Chap. 87).

TREATMENT

• Rapid and appropriate treatment of the underlying disorder is of utmost importance, including antibiotics and source control for infection, anticancer treatment, surgical and medical management of trauma, or evacuation of a dead fetus.

• Because most patients with DIC are critically ill, appropriate supportive care including fluids, pressors, dialysis, and respiratory and ventilator management are essential.

• There is no convincing evidence that transfusion of blood components "fuels the fire," and patients with documented deficiencies who are bleeding or require surgical or invasive procedures should receive transfusion with platelets for thrombocytopenia, and fresh-frozen plasma or coagulation factor concentrates for coagulation factor depletion.

• Critically ill patients need prophylaxis for venous thromboembolism and therefore unfractionated or low-molecular-weight (LMW) heparin is recommended.

- The use of (therapeutic levels of) heparin to ameliorate DIC is a matter of debate. In general, in the absence of adequately controlled studies, there is no sound clinical evidence supporting the use of heparin in DIC.
- Heparin treatment may be beneficial in patients with purpura fulminans (overt hemorrhagic infarction of the skin and underlying tissue), overt thromboembolism, and when thrombosis is likely to cause irreversible tissue injury. In these cases, unfractionated heparin at a dose of 500 to 750 U/h via continuous infusion may be sufficient.
- The decision to use heparin must be individualized, and the risks and benefits considered carefully.
- Administration of recombinant human activated protein C (drotrecogin alfa 24 μg/kg/hr by continuous infusion for 4 days) was shown to reduce 28-day mortality in patients with severe sepsis, in particular when DIC was present.
- Recombinant human activated protein C may increase the risk of bleeding and should not be given when the platelet count is $< 30 \times 10^9$/L. The administration should be interrupted in case of a bleeding complication or when an invasive procedure need to be performed.
- Studies using antithrombin concentrates have not demonstrated unequivocal efficacy for this therapy.
- Antifibrinolytic therapy is generally contraindicated in DIC because it may provoke increased thrombosis and microvascular occlusion but may be considered in patients with severe bleeding when primary fibrin(ogen)olysis, rather than DIC, is the major process (see Chap. 87).

SPECIFIC UNDERLYING DISEASES

Infection

- Neonates, asplenic patients, and pregnant patients are more prone to development of infection-related DIC.
- All microorganisms, including gram-positive and gram-negative bacteria, viruses, parasites, and fungal infections may cause DIC.

Malignancy

- Solid tumors often produce a chronic DIC in which thrombosis is more prominent than bleeding. This syndrome may respond to heparin.
- Patients with acute promyelocytic leukemia (APL) frequently develop major bleeding. The pathogenesis of the hemostatic abnormalities in APL is complex and may involve both DIC and primary fibrin(ogen)olysis. With the use of modern treatment strategies, including all-*trans*-retinoic acid (ATRA), coagulopathy and bleeding has become a less prominent feature of APL (see Chap. 46).
- Acute lymphocytic leukemia has been associated with DIC, particularly with induction therapy.

Complications of Pregnancy

- Abruptio placentae causes acute DIC because of rapid entry of large quantities of placental tissue factor into the maternal circulation.
- Amniotic fluid embolism is a rare catastrophe that occurs most often in multiparous women undergoing difficult labors with postmature, large fetuses. DIC is caused by entry into the maternal circulation of amniotic fluid that contains tissue factor.
- The dead fetus syndrome occurs several weeks after intrauterine death and is caused by tissue factor from the fetus slowly entering the maternal circulation.
- Rapid volume replacement and evacuation of the uterus are treatments of choice. Replacement therapy with fresh-frozen plasma, coagulation factor concentrates, and platelets is given if severe bleeding occurs.

- The DIC usually rapidly resolves when the underlying cause has been handled properly.
- The syndrome of *h*emolysis, *e*levated *l*iver enzymes, and *l*ow *p*latelets (HELLP) occurs in the third trimester or postpartum. DIC appears to have a role in the pathogenesis of the HELLP syndrome. The HELLP syndrome may be confused with other forms of thrombotic microangiopathy (e.g., thrombotic thrombocytopenic purpura-hemolytic uremic syndrome [TTP-HUS]) (see Chap. 74).
- Patients should receive supportive care, careful monitoring, and blood component replacement therapy.

Trauma

- The initial coagulation defect after severe trauma is a dilutional coagulopathy due to blood loss and replacement therapy with red cells and plasma expanders.
- After 24 to 48 hours, a systemic inflammatory response syndrome may occur, leading to frank DIC.
- In the initial phase, restoration of coagulation factors and platelets by fresh frozen plasma and platelet transfusion, respectively, should be initiated. In the later phase, supportive treatment for DIC (see above) should be considered.

Newborns

- Laboratory evidence of DIC in newborns consists of progressive decline in hemostatic parameters, thrombocytopenia, and reduced levels of fibrinogen, factor V, and factor VIII.
- The most frequent underlying causes are sepsis, hyaline membrane disease, asphyxia, necrotizing enterocolitis, intravascular hemolysis, abruptio placentae, and eclampsia.
- Bleeding from multiple sites is the most frequent presentation, but in about 20 percent, no clinical manifestations of DIC are present.
- Management consists of treatment of the underlying disorder, support of vital functions, and replacement of blood components.

For a more detailed discussion, see Marcel Levi, Uri Seligsohn: Disseminated Intravascular Coagulation. Chap. 130, p. 2101 in *Williams Hematology*, 8th ed.

CHAPTER 87
Fibrinolysis and Thrombolysis

HYPERFIBRINOLYSIS

Pathophysiology

- Local activation of the fibrinolytic system accompanies the formation of the hemostatic plug and is important in repair of injury and reestablishment of blood flow.
- Excessive local or systemic fibrinolysis can prematurely degrade fibrin clots and lead to significant bleeding.

Systemic Hyperfibrin(ogen)olysis

- Endothelial cell plasminogen activator may be released in pathologic states in sufficient amounts to convert plasma plasminogen to plasmin.
- A hemorrhagic state may ensue with the following laboratory features:
  — Shortened euglobulin lysis time.
  — Decreased levels of fibrinogen, plasminogen and α_2-antiplasmin.
  — Elevated levels of fibrin(ogen) degradation products.
  — Normal platelet count.
  — Low levels of factor V and VIII (due to proteolytic degradation by plasmin).
- Localized fibrinolysis may also cause abnormal bleeding in patients with either normal or defective hemostasis.

THROMBOLYTIC TREATMENT

Principles

- All fibrinolytic drugs are enzymes that accelerate the conversion of plasminogen to plasmin, a serine protease that degrades the insoluble fibrin clot matrix into soluble derivatives.
- The basic principle of all fibrinolytic therapy is administration of pharmacologic amounts of plasminogen activator to achieve a high local concentration at the site of the thrombus and thereby accelerate conversion of plasminogen to plasmin and increase the rate of fibrin dissolution.
- If large amounts of plasminogen activator overwhelm the natural regulatory systems, plasmin may be formed in the blood resulting in degradation of susceptible proteins, the "lytic state." Additionally, because high concentrations of activator are not limited to the site of thrombosis, fibrin deposits at other sites, including physiologic hemostatic plugs needed at sites of injury, may also dissolve causing local bleeding, often exacerbated by the hypocoagulable state caused by proteolysis of other coagulation factors by plasmin.
- Several therapeutic agents are available and approved for thrombolytic use (see Table 87–1).

Streptokinase

- A single-chain polypeptide from β-hemolytic streptococci.
- It lacks intrinsic enzymatic activity but combines stoichiometrically with plasminogen to form a complex that possesses plasmin-like proteolytic activity.
- The streptokinase-plasminogen complex converts free plasminogen to plasmin.
- The activity of streptokinase is enhanced by fibrinogen, fibrin, and fibrin-degradation products.

TABLE 87–1　COMPARISON OF PLASMINOGEN ACTIVATORS

Agent (Regimen)	Source(Approved/Available)	Antigenic	Half-Life (min)
Streptokinase (infusion)	Streptococcus (Y/Y)	Yes	20
Urokinase (infusion)	Cell culture; recombinant (Y/N)	No	15
Alteplase (t-PA) (infusion)	Recombinant (Y/Y)	No	5
Anistreplase (bolus)	Streptococcus + plasma product (Y/N)	No	70
Reteplase (double bolus)	Recombinant (Y/Y)	No	15
Saruplase (scu-PA) (infusion)	Recombinant (N/N)	No	5
Staphylokinase (infusion)	Recombinant (N/N)	Yes	
Tenecteplase (bolus)	Recombinant (Y/Y)	No	15

Source: *Williams Hematology,* 8th ed, Chap. 136, Table 136–3, p. 2229.

- The streptokinase-plasmin(ogen) complex is itself proteolytically degraded by plasmin.
- Allergic reactions to streptokinase, including fever, hypotension, urticaria, and bronchospasm may occur.
- Neutralizing antibodies are commonly induced after treatment with streptokinase, which abrogates response to further streptokinase therapy at standard doses.

Urokinase

- A serine protease that directly activates plasminogen.
- *In vivo* is present in single-chain form (scu-PA) that possesses very low levels of activity and serves as a zymogen, a high-molecular-weight two-chain form (HMW-tcu-PA), and a low-molecular-weight two-chain form (LMW-tcu-PA).

Tissue Plasminogen Activator (t-PA)

- A serine protease synthesized by endothelial cells and commercially available as a recombinant product that activates plasminogen.
- t-PA binds to fibrin, which induces conformational changes in t-PA, in plasminogen, or in both that increase the catalytic efficiency of plasminogen activation several hundred-fold.
- The relative fibrin specificity of t-PA is a theoretical advantage over other fibrinolytic agents but may not be as clinically important as once believed. Effective treatment of arterial thrombosis entails rapid clot lysis, requiring t-PA doses high enough to provoke a systemic lytic state.
- t-PA does not provoke allergy or antibody formation but is relatively expensive.

Newer Plasminogen Activators
Staphylokinase

- Staphylokinase is a profibrinolytic protein produced by *Staphylococcus aureus.* Its mechanism of action is similar to that of streptokinase.
- A highly efficient fibrinolytic agent that produces high rates of clot lysis without significantly changing levels of fibrinogen, plasminogen, or α_2-antiplasmin levels.

- Effective in preliminary clinical trials on patients with acute myocardial infarction.
- Neutralizing antibodies may develop promptly following therapy.

Mutant Tissue-Type Plasminogen Activators

- Two mutant forms of t-PA, prepared by recombinant technology, t-PA∆ FEK-1 (reteplase) and TNK-t-PA, have been shown in clinical trials to be effective in restoring vessel patency.

CLINICAL USE OF THROMBOLYTIC AGENTS

- Thrombolysis, in particular recombinant tissue-type plasminogen activator, was shown to be effective for ST-elevation acute myocardial infarction. However, when primary percutaneous coronary intervention (with or without stent insertion) is readily available, this is superior to thrombolytic treatment.
- Thrombolysis in acute ischemic stroke is effective, when adhering to strict selection and exclusion criteria (see Table 87–2).
- Thrombolysis is accepted treatment in patients with severe pulmonary embolism and a compromised hemodynamic state and/or respiratory insufficiency. In less severe pulmonary embolism, thrombolytic treatment is effective but carries a high risk of major bleeding. Hence, in this circumstance thrombolysis is generally not recommended.
- Thrombolytic treatment may lead to more rapid resolution of deep venous thrombosis and possibly to a lower incidence of postthrombotic venous insufficiency; however, due to the high risk of major bleeding, this treatment is generally not recommended.

TABLE 87–2 GUIDELINES FOR t-PA THERAPY IN ISCHEMIC STROKE

Eligibility
Time from symptom onset to therapy ≤3 hours
Results from ECASS III trial suggest treatment within 4.5 h of onset is beneficial

Exclusions
Prior intracranial hemorrhage
Major surgery within 14 days
Gastrointestinal or urinary tract bleeding with 21 days
Arterial puncture in noncompressible site
Recent lumbar puncture
Intracranial surgery, serious head trauma, or prior stroke within 3 months
Minor neurologic deficit
Seizure at time of stroke onset
Clinical findings of subarachnoid hemorrhage
Active bleeding
Persistent systolic blood pressure (BP) >185 mm Hg and/or diastolic BP >110 mm Hg or requiring aggressive treatment
Arteriovenous malformation or aneurysm
Evidence of hemorrhage on computed tomography scan
Platelets <100 × 10^9/L
International normalized ratio >1.5 on warfarin
Elevated partial thromboplastin time on heparin
Blood glucose <40 or >400 mg/dL
ECASS III additionally excluded patients >80-years-old, patients with a combination of previous stroke and diabetes mellitus, and patients with an National Institutes of Health Stroke Scale score of >25.

Source: *Williams Hematology,* 8th ed, Chap.136, Table 136–6, p. 2233.

- Thrombolytic treatment is often used for local lysis of arterial thrombosis in peripheral arteries, dialysis shunts, or intravenous lines.
- Anecdotal reports document successful treatment of intraabdominal thrombosis including Budd-Chiari syndrome, portal vein thrombosis, and mesenteric vein thrombosis.

THERAPY WITH ANTIFIBRINOLYTIC AGENTS

- Table 87–3 lists disorders that have been treated with antifibrinolytic therapy.

Synthetic Lysine Analogues

- ϵ-Aminocaproic acid and tranexamic acid are synthetic lysine analogues that block the conversion of plasminogen to plasmin by occupying the lysine-binding site on plasminogen that is responsible for binding of plasminogen to fibrin, which accelerates its conversion to plasmin.

ϵ-Aminocaproic Acid

- Peak plasma levels achieved by 2 hours after oral dose.
- Eighty percent of intravenous dose cleared unchanged within 3 hours by the kidney.
- Excreted for 12 to 36 hours because of large volume of distribution.

TABLE 87–3	**ANTIFIBRINOLYTIC THERAPY WITH EACA OR TA IN BLEEDING STATES**	
Pathologic Process and Clinical Bleeding State	**Experience Using Antifibrinolytic Agents**	**Comment**
Systemic hyperfibrinolysis		
Inherited α^2-antiplasmin	Controlled with antifibrinolytic agents	Rare autosomal recessive trait; prophylactic treatment indicated only in severe cases
DIC	May aggravate DIC	Treatment indicated only in rare cases with excessive activation of fibrinolysis
Fibrinolytic therapy	Anecdotal	If bleeding is excessive, antifibrinolytic agents may be helpful
Malignancy (solid tumor)	Useful if bleeding is due to hyperfibrinolysis alone (rare)	Hypercoagulable state may be unmasked by antifibrinolytic treatment
Acute promyelocytic leukemia	May reduce bleeding manifestations	Coexistent thrombotic state may preclude use of antifibrinolytic agents
Liver disease and transplantation	Protracted oozing can be better controlled	An excessive hyperfibrinolytic state is present during the anhepatic and immediate postperfusion stages
Extracorporeal bypass surgery	Bleeding reduced	Intrapleural or intrapericardial clots resistant to lysis may occur with treatment

Pathologic Process and Clinical Bleeding State	Experience Using Antifibrinolytic Agents	Comment
Localized fibrinolysis with defective hemostasis		
Hemophilia A and B, von Willebrand disease, and factor XI deficiency	Proven use for dental extractions, probable usefulness after other surgical procedures	Antifibrinolytic agents not effective as prophylaxis for hemarthrosis
Anticoagulated patients	Dental surgery blood loss decreased with administration as mouthwash	
Thrombocytopenia	Controlled trials fail to show benefit	Antifibrinolytic agents may be useful in patients refractory to platelet transfusion
Kasabach-Merritt syndrome	Useful for shrinking hemangioma masses if properly used	Antifibrinolytic agents may trigger systemic DIC
Localized fibrinolysis with normal hemostasis		
Prostatectomy	Reduces postoperative bleeding	Treatment indicated only for cases with severe and prolonged bleeding
Menorrhagia	Effectively reduces blood loss	Evaluate for underlying pathology
Upper gastrointestinal	Useful adjunctive measure to reduce bleeding, studies were done in absence of endoscopic hemostasis	
Subarachnoid hemorrhage	Incidence of rebleeding reduced, but vasospasm is accentuated	No reduction in mortality with treatment
Hereditary hemorrhagic telangiectasia	May reduce severity and frequency of epistaxis and gastrointestinal bleeding	

DIC, disseminated intravascular coagulation; PAI-1, plasminogen activator inhibitor-1; EACA, ϵ-aminocaproic acid; TA, tranexamic acid.
Source: *Williams Hematology*, 8th ed, Chap. 136, Table 136–8, p. 2236.

- Administered as intravenous priming dose of about 0.1g/kg body weight over 20 to 30 minutes, followed by continuous intravenous infusion of 0.5 to 1g/h, or equivalent intermittent dose either intravenously or orally every 1, 2, or 4 hours.
- In patients receiving prolonged treatment with ϵ-aminocaproic acid, rhabdomyolysis has been described.

Tranexamic Acid
- Plasma half-life approximately 1 to 2 hours.
- More than 90 percent excreted unchanged in urine within 24 hours.

- Oral dosage is 5 to 10 mg/kg three or four times daily.
- Intravenous dose is 10 mg/kg three or four times daily.
- Side effects include infrequently thrombosis, myonecrosis, or hypersensitivity reaction.
- Thrombosis risk most significant when there is an associated thrombogenic process, such as occult disseminated intravascular coagulation.
- In patients with upper urinary tract bleeding, antifibrinolytic therapy can lead to obstructing clots in the urinary collecting system.

Aprotinin

- A polypeptide that inhibits serine proteases by forming a 1:1 complex with the enzyme.
- Administered intravenously because of gastric inactivation.
- Distributed in extracellular space and metabolized by the kidney.
- Potency expressed as "kallikrein inhibitor units" (KIU) where 10^6 KIU corresponds to 140 mg pure inhibitor.
- Most common side effects are nausea, vomiting, diarrhea, muscle pain, and hypotension.
- Allergic side effects are itching, rash, urticaria, and dyspnea. Cardiovascular collapse, bronchospasm, or anaphylactic shock is rare.
- Due to increased renal complications, cardiovascular morbidity and mortality in patients undergoing cardiac surgery, aprotinin is not available anymore in most countries.

For more detailed discussion, see Katherine A. Hajjar and Jian Ruar: Fibrinolysis and thrombolysis, Chap. 136, p. 2219; and Charles W. Francis and Mark Crowther: Principles of Antithrombotic Therapy. Chap. 23, p. 353 in *Williams Hematology*, 8th edition.

PART XI

THROMBOSIS AND ANTITHROMBOTIC THERAPY

CHAPTER 88
Principles of Antithrombotic Therapy

- Antithrombotic agents are characterized separately as anticoagulants (including vitamin K antagonists and heparin or heparin derivatives), antiplatelet agents, or fibrinolytic drugs (see Chap. 87), depending on their primary mechanism, although there is overlap in their activities.
- Anticoagulant therapy acts to decrease fibrin formation by inhibiting the formation and action of thrombin, and its most common use is in preventing systemic embolization in patients with atrial fibrillation, treatment of acute arterial thrombosis (e.g., myocardial infarction or peripheral arterial thrombosis) and for treatment or (secondary) prevention of venous thromboembolism.
- Anticoagulant therapy is often monitored using coagulation testing because of marked biologic variation in effect.
- Antiplatelet agents act to inhibit platelet function, and their primary uses are in preventing thrombotic complications of cerebrovascular and coronary artery disease. They also have a role in treatment of acute myocardial infarction. They have no effect in preventing or treating venous thromboembolism.
- For many agents, the risk-to-benefit ratio is narrow, with the result that bleeding complications occur.
- Bleeding is the most common adverse effect of anticoagulation (see Table 88–1). Consequently, the clinician should carefully weigh the risks and benefits for each patient when selecting treatment.
- The most common oral anticoagulants are vitamin K antagonists (coumarins). However, recently, new oral anticoagulants with specific antithrombin activity or anti-factor Xa activity have become available and are currently evaluated in clinical trials (see section, "Oral Antithrombin and Anti-factor Xa Agents" below).

VITAMIN K ANTAGONISTS

- Coumarins act by inhibiting vitamin K–dependent posttranslational γ-carboxylation of glutamic acid residues in the Gla domains of coagulation factors II, VII, IX, and X, and the anticoagulant proteins C and S.
- γ-Carboxylation requires the reduced form of vitamin K as a cofactor. During γ-carboxylation, vitamin K is oxidized. The enzymes, vitamin K epoxide reductase and vitamin K reductase, are required to recycle vitamin K back to its reduced form. Coumarins inhibit these reductases, thus depleting reduced vitamin K.

TABLE 88–1	**RISK FACTORS FOR HEMORRHAGIC COMPLICATIONS**

Too high intensity of anticoagulation
Simultaneous use of anticoagulants and antiplatelet agents
Old age
Initial phase of anticoagulation
Cerebrovascular disease
History of alcohol abuse
Renal insufficiency
Liver failure
Use of nonsteroidal antiinflammatory drugs (gastrointestinal bleeding)
Polymorphisms in cytochrome 450 CYP2C9 gene

- A decrease in the number of γ-carboxyglutamate residues results in coagulation factors with impaired activity because they are unable to bind calcium and undergo necessary conformation changes.
- The production of affected coagulation factors stops promptly, but the anticoagulant effect is delayed until the previously formed coagulation factors are removed from the circulation. Factor VII has the shortest half-life at 6 hours, while the others range from 24 to 72 hours.

Pharmacokinetics

- Warfarin, the most commonly used coumarin, has predictable oral absorption and a half-life of 35 to 45 hours. The pharmacokinetics appear to be dose-dependent.
- It is highly protein-bound and only the free compound is active.
- Warfarin is metabolized by hydroxylation in the liver and excretion of the hydroxylated derivative in the urine. Warfarin is not excreted in significant amounts in breast milk.
- Other frequently used coumarins are phenprocoumon (much longer half-life of 150 to 160 hours) or acenocoumarol (much shorter half-life of 8 to 12 hours).

Administration and Laboratory Monitoring

- Dosages required for adequate anticoagulation range from about 1 to 20 mg per day, probably a result of differences in hydroxylation rates and target-organ sensitivity.
- There is a significant negative correlation between age at start of therapy and dose. Requirement may decrease by 20 percent over 15 years.
- Warfarin resistance may be caused by impaired absorption, rapid clearance, or decreased affinity of the receptor, but poor compliance, excessive intake of vitamin K, and drug interactions must be ruled out.
- Many drugs interact with vitamin K antagonists, causing either an increased or decreased anticoagulant response (see Table 88–2). Several mechanisms have been described for these interactions.
- Vitamin K antagonist therapy is monitored by the prothrombin time (PT).
- The sensitivity of the PT to anticoagulation varies with the source of thromboplastin in the assay.
- Interlaboratory variation is corrected for by using the international normalized ratio (INR) instead of the PT ratio.
- The International Sensitivity Index (ISI) is a correction factor established for each thromboplastin. The INR is determined by the formula INR = (patient PT/control PT)^{ISI}.
- A target range of INR 2.0 to 3.0 has shown to be optimal for virtually all indications. Patients with prosthetic heart valves at high risk for thromboembolic complications may benefit from an INR range of 2.5 to 3.5. Also, in some patients with antiphospholipid syndrome and thrombosis, a higher range of 2.5 to 3.5 is recommended.

TABLE 88–2	**EFFECT OF COMMONLY USED DRUGS ON WARFARIN RESPONSE**

Potentiate Effect

α-Methyldopa	Indomethacin
Acetaminophen	Isoniazid
Acetohexamide	Ketoconazole
Allopurinol	Methimazole
Androgenic and anabolic steroids	Methotrexate
Antibiotics that disrupt intestinal flora	Methylphenidate
(tetracyclines, streptomycin,	Nalidixic acid
erythromycin, kanamycin, nalidixic	Nortriptyline
acid, neomycin)	Oxyphenbutazone
Cephaloridine	p-Aminosalicylic acid
Chloral hydrate	Paromomycin
Chloramphenicol	Phenylbutazone
Chlorpromazine	Phenyramidol
Chlorpropamide	Phenytoin
Cimetidine	Propylthiouracil
Clofibrate	Quinidine
Diazoxide	Salicylate
Disulfiram	Sulfinpyrazone
Fluconazole	Sulfonamides
Glucagon	Thyroid hormone
Guanethidine	Tolbutamide

Depress Effect

Antipyrine	Glutethimide
Azathioprine	Griseofulvin
Barbiturates	Haloperidol
Carbamazepine	Phenobarbital
Digitalis	Prednisone
Ethanol	Rifampin
Ethchlorvynol	Vitamin K

Source: *Williams Hematology*, 8th ed, Chap. 23, Table 23–2, p. 354.

- In established venous thromboembolism, vitamin K antagonist therapy is given concomitantly with heparin because the antithrombotic effect of vitamin K antagonists is achieved only after 3 to 4 days.
- Some studies have indicated that patients with mechanical heart valves may be effectively treated with a combination of vitamin K antagonists to achieve an INR of less than or equal to 2.5 and an antiplatelet agent, but such regimens carry an increased risk of bleeding complications.
- Bioprosthetic valves also may cause thromboembolism (in particular in the initial phase), and prophylaxis with vitamin K antagonists is recommended to an INR of 2.0 to 3.0 during the first 3 months and continued indefinitely if there is atrial fibrillation, atrial thrombi, or a prior embolism.
- The risk of thromboembolism from cardioversion may be reduced by vitamin K antagonist therapy to an INR of 2.0 to 3.0 for 3 weeks before the procedure and 4 weeks after.

Adverse Effects and Reversal
Bleeding
- The annual risk of major bleeding episodes has been estimated at between 1.2 and 7.0 per 100 patient-years. The wide variability is because of differences in intensity of anticoagulation and patient populations and in the definition of "major bleeding."

- The gastrointestinal tract is the most common site of bleeding. Gastrointestinal bleeding in anticoagulated patients may be caused by peptic ulcer or colon cancer. For this reason, detailed investigation to detect the source of bleeding should be carried out.
- Vitamin K antagonist treatment may be reversed by the administration of vitamin K (1 to 10 mg). However, it will take 6 to 8 hours after intravenous administration and 12 to 14 hours after oral administration of vitamin K before the effect is noticeable.
- Subcutaneous administration of vitamin K is less effective (more variable response) than oral administration. Intramuscular injections of vitamin K should be avoided in anticoagulated patients.
- In patients with major hemorrhage, rapid reversal of anticoagulation can be achieved with replacement therapy using fresh-frozen plasma or prothrombin-complex concentrates. It may be difficult to administer a sufficient volume of fresh-frozen plasma to replace the deficient coagulation factors, and therefore prothrombin-complex concentrates may be more convenient.
- Reversal of anticoagulant treatment with vitamin K antagonists is only required in case of serious bleeding. A too high INR in the absence of bleeding does not require vitamin K administration (see Table 88–3) and may make re-anticoagulation particularly difficult.
- Minor bleeding (e.g., epistaxis) may be managed by local measures if the INR is in the therapeutic range.

Warfarin-Induced Skin Necrosis
- A rare condition in which painful, discolored areas of skin, most often over fatty areas such as the buttocks, breasts, and thighs, appear, usually between the third and tenth day of warfarin therapy.
- Lesions progress to frank necrosis and eschar formation.
- The necrosis appears to be a result of more rapid decline of protein C and protein S levels than levels of factors II, IX, and X, thereby inducing a temporary hypercoagulable state.
- It may occur in patients with heparin-induced thrombocytopenia, in those with hereditary protein C or protein S deficiency, and in patients receiving large loading doses of warfarin.

TABLE 88–3	REVERSING WARFARIN THERAPY*
Indication	**Action**
INR <6	Lower the dose, consider withholding one or more doses Recheck in 3 to 7 days
INR 6–10	Lower the dose and withhold 1 to 3 doses Consider administering vitamin K, 1–2 mg orally Recheck INR in 24–48 hours
INR >10	Withhold doses until INR in desired range and cause of elevation ascertained Give vitamin K, 2–4 mg orally Recheck INR in 24 hours
Serious bleeding and major overdose	Consider fresh-frozen plasma or prothrombin complex concentrate, and give 5–10 mg vitamin K intravenously

*Only when there is bleeding or a high risk of bleeding.
Source: *Williams Hematology*, 8th ed, Chap. 23, Table 23–4, p. 356.

- Treatment with warfarin should be stopped immediately and the anticoagulation should be reversed by administration of plasma, or administration of protein C concentrate if protein C deficiency is present. Prompt administration of vitamin K may stop the progress of skin necrosis.
- Anticoagulation should be continued with an alternative anticoagulant until healing of the lesions.

Purple Toe Syndrome
- Patients receiving warfarin therapy may develop a syndrome of bilateral burning pain and dark blue discoloration of the toes and sides of the feet. The involved areas blanch with pressure.
- Occurs in patients with cardiac disease, diabetes mellitus, or peripheral vascular disease. It may be caused by cholesterol emboli.

Pregnancy
- Vitamin K antagonists are contraindicated in pregnancy because they may induce midface and nasal hypoplasia, stippled epiphysis, hypoplasia of the digits, optic atrophy, and mental impairment in the fetus. These teratogenic effects are mostly associated with use of vitamin K antagonists during the second trimester of pregnancy; however, many belief that vitamin K antagonist could be better avoided throughout pregnancy.
- Vitamin K antagonists are contraindicated in the last 4 weeks of pregnancy due to anticoagulation of the child and the risk of intracranial hemorrhage during vaginal delivery.

Perioperative Management of Anticoagulation
- It appears that full anticoagulant therapy can be safely continued with cutaneous surgery, soft-tissue aspirations or injections, and pacemaker surgery.
- Oral surgery is also safe at an INR <2.5, provided adequate local hemostasis and optionally use of tranexamic acid for irrigation at the time of the procedure and as a mouth rinse four times daily for a week postoperatively.
- For all other types of surgery on patients with high risk of thromboembolism, protocols have been developed for temporary discontinuation of vitamin K antagonists and sustained perioperative anticoagulation with (low-molecular-weight [LMW]) heparin.
- Spinal or epidural anesthesia as well as local nerve block should be avoided.

HEPARIN AND HEPARIN DERIVATIVES

Mechanism of Action
- Unfractionated heparin consists of a heterogeneous mixture of sulfated glycosaminoglycans of different chain length with an average molecular mass of 15,000 daltons and an average chain length of 50 sugar residues.
- LMW heparin is prepared by depolymerization of unfractionated heparin by chemical or enzymatic means. The average molecular mass is 4000 to 6000 daltons, with a range of 1000 to 10,000 daltons.
- Heparin enhances the inactivation by antithrombin of thrombin and factors Xa and IXa.
- Inhibition of thrombin by heparin-antithrombin involves formation of a ternary complex, with heparin binding both thrombin and antithrombin.
- Formation of the ternary complex requires a heparin chain of at least 18 saccharide units.
- Inhibition of factor Xa by heparin-antithrombin does not require direct binding of heparin to factor Xa and therefore LMW heparins have a relatively high anti-factor Xa over anti-factor IIa activity.
- Synthetic pentasaccharides (e.g., fondaparinux) highly selectively bind to antithrombin and have only anti-factor Xa activity.

- Danaparoid is a mixture of glycosaminoglycans, containing heparan sulfate, dermatan sulfate, and chondroitin sulfate. The predominant anticoagulant effect is on factor Xa.
- Danaparoid is used for therapeutic anticoagulation in patients with acute heparin-induced thrombocytopenia or prophylactic anticoagulation in patients with a history of heparin-induced thrombocytopenia.

Pharmacokinetics

- The pharmacokinetics of unfractionated heparin are compatible with saturable binding to endothelial cells and macrophages, combined with unsaturable renal excretion.
- The half-life of heparin increases with increased doses. In general, the half-life of unfractionated heparin at therapeutic dose is approximately 90 minutes.
- Therapeutic doses of unfractionated heparin are commonly administered by continuous intravenous infusion (after a single intravenous loading dose). Prophylactic unfractionated heparin can be given by twice daily subcutaneous injections.
- LMW heparins have a more predictable systemic bioavailability after subcutaneous administration and a much longer half-life (12 to 24 hours). Hence, they are administered by once or twice daily subcutaneous injections, both therapeutically or prophylactically.

Laboratory Monitoring of Therapy

- The activated partial thromboplastin time (aPTT) is the most frequently used test to monitor therapy with unfractionated heparin.
- In patients with venous thromboembolism and acute coronary syndromes, the aPTT response to a given heparin level is quite variable, and heparin dosages must be adjusted to achieve the desired aPTT range.
- Laboratory monitoring is not required for prophylactic subcutaneous heparin.
- LMW heparin does generally not require laboratory monitoring. However, in pregnant patients, critically ill patients, and patient with severe renal insufficiency (creatinine clearance <30 mL/min) measurement of the anti-factor Xa activity in plasma is useful. LMW heparin cannot be monitored by the aPTT.

Clinical Use
Venous Thromboembolism

- Unfractionated heparin administered at a dose of 5000 units every 8 to 12 hours is widely used for antithrombotic prophylaxis in patients undergoing surgery, in patients with ischemic stroke and leg paralysis, and in general medical patients.
- Alternatively, once daily subcutaneous low-dose LMW heparin is effective for antithrombotic prophylaxis as well (see Table 88–4).
- Fondaparinux is more effective and safe compared with (LMW) heparin in patients undergoing major orthopedic surgery.
- Randomized clinical trials demonstrate that patients may be effectively treated for venous thromboembolism by heparin given intravenously at an initial loading dose of 5000 units intravenously, followed by maintenance therapy with 750 to 1500 U/h adjusted to the aPTT (aim: 1.5 to 2-fold prolongation of baseline aPTT).
- Venous thromboembolism can also be effectively treated with LMW heparin or fondaparinux (see Table 88–4).
- Adequate initial infusion rates and frequent determination of the aPTT in the first 24 hours reduce the frequency of delayed adequate heparinization. Use of a validated heparin treatment protocol makes it more likely that adequate early heparinization will be achieved.

TABLE 88–4	LOW-MOLECULAR-WEIGHT HEPARIN REGIMENS*	
	Drug[†]	Regimen
Prophylaxis of VTE General surgery		
Low risk	Dalteparin	2500 U, 1 or 2 h preoperation and daily
	Enoxaparin	40 mg, 2 h preoperation and daily
	Fondaparinux	2.5 mg daily (start 6–8 h postoperation)
	Nadroparin	2850 anti-Xa U once daily
High risk	Dalteparin	5000 U, 10–14 preoperation and daily 2500 U 1–2 h preoperation and after 12 h; then 5000 U daily (with malignancy)
	Enoxaparin	40 mg, 2 h preoperation and daily
	Fondaparinux	2.5 mg daily (start 6–8 h postoperation)
Orthopedic surgery	Dalteparin	2500 U, 4–8 h postoperation and 5000 U daily; or 2500 U , 2 h preoperation and 2500 U 4–8 h postoperation and 5000 U daily; or 5000 U, 10–14 preoperation and 5000 U daily
	Enoxaparin	30 mg BID starting 12–24 h postoperation; 40 mg 9–15 h preoperation and once daily
	Fondaparinux	2.5 mg daily (start 6–8 h postoperation)
Medical patients	Enoxaparin	40 mg once daily
	Nadroparin	2850 anti-Xa U once daily
Treatment of VTE	Fondaparinux	weight <50 kg: 5 mg daily; 50–100 kg: 7.5 daily; >75 kg: 10 mg daily
	Dalteparin (VTE with cancer)	200 U/kg daily × 1 month; then, 150 U/kg daily for up to 6 months
	Enoxaparin	1 mg/kg q12h; 1.5 mg/kg daily
	Tinzaparin	175 U/kg daily
Acute coronary syndrome	Dalteparin	120 U/kg (max 10,000 U) q12h
	Enoxaparin	STEMI: 30 mg IV bolus plus 1mg/kg SQ q12h (older than age 75 y: initial 0.75 mg/kg with no IV bolus)
	Enoxaparin	Unstable angina and non-STEMI: 1 mg/kg 12 h

STEMI, ST-segment elevation myocardial infarction; VTE, venous thromboembolism.
*Consult package insert for more detailed dosing information. Only FDA approved-indications are included.
†Drug brand names: dalteparin, Fragmin; enoxaparin, Lovenox; fondaparinux, Arixtra; tinzaparin, Innohep; nadroparin, Fraxiparine.
Source: *Williams Hematology*, 8th ed, Chap. 23, Table 23–5, p. 358.

- Long-term treatment of venous thromboembolism in pregnant patients or for others for whom warfarin is unsatisfactory can be achieved by adjusted-dose subcutaneous heparin.

Acute Coronary Syndromes

- Heparin therapy is given to patients with acute coronary syndromes to reduce the risk of death, myocardial infarction, mural thrombosis, systemic embolism, and recurrent ischemia (see Table 88–4).

- In patients with unstable angina, combined use of intravenous heparin and aspirin is the preferred therapy.
- Low-dose, subcutaneous heparin is widely used in patients with acute myocardial infarction to prevent venous thromboembolism.
- Many patients with acute myocardial infarction receive more intensive heparin therapy either as an adjunct to fibrinolytic therapy or because they are at high risk for mural thrombosis and systemic thromboembolism.
- Patients requiring long-term anticoagulation because of high risk for mural thrombosis and systemic embolism are usually transferred to therapy with vitamin K antagonists.

Side Effects
- The principal side effects of heparin therapy are bleeding and thrombocytopenia.
- Heparin-induced thrombocytopenia is discussed in Chap. 74.
- Thrombocytopenia is less likely to occur with LMW heparin than with unfractionated heparin. However, LMW heparin is not recommended for patients who have developed thrombocytopenia while receiving unfractionated heparin.
- Long-term treatment with unfractionated heparin, usually for more than 3 months, may cause osteoporosis. Clinically significant osteoporosis may occur less frequently with LMW heparin than with unfractionated heparin.
- Heparin may cause elevation of serum transaminase levels, which return to normal when heparin treatment is discontinued.
- Rare side effects are hypersensitivity; skin reactions, including necrosis; alopecia; and hyperkalemia due to hypoaldosteronism.

Antidote to Heparin
- The anticoagulant effect of unfractionated heparin can be neutralized by intravenous administration of protamine sulfate, which should be considered for use in heparinized patients with major bleeding.
- Dosage is usually calculated assuming 1 mg of protamine sulfate will neutralize 100 units of heparin.
- The maximum recommended dose is 50 mg.
- Heparin is rapidly cleared from the plasma and calculation of the dose of protamine required must consider this important variable.
- LMW heparin is incompletely neutralized by protamine sulfate, but protamine may still be of benefit in treating bleeding caused by LMW heparin.

DIRECT THROMBIN AND FACTOR XA INHIBITORS

Hirudin and Derivatives
- Hirudin is a 65–amino acid peptide produced in the salivary gland of the leech. Hirudin is the most potent, naturally occurring, specific inhibitor of thrombin.
- Hirudin directly inactivates thrombin by forming a 1:1 complex.
- Hirudin for clinical use is produced by recombinant DNA technology. Recombinant hirudin is not sulfated on the tyrosine residue and consequently has markedly reduced affinity for thrombin, compared with native hirudin (see Table 88–5).
- Bivalirudin is a 20–amino acid peptide analog of hirudin that produces transient, albeit potent, inhibition of thrombin.
- Lepirudin is a recombinant form of hirudin approved for use in patients with heparin-induced thrombocytopenia.
- Hirudin has been clinically evaluated in patients with acute coronary syndromes, and does not appear to be a major advance. Bivalirudin has been compared with heparin in patients who have angina. It was not more effective than heparin in reducing the cluster outcome of death in the hospital, myocardial infarction, or abrupt vessel closure.

TABLE 88–5	CLINICAL INDICATIONS AND USE OF DIRECT THROMBIN INHIBITORS		
Agent	Clinical Indication	Regimen	Monitoring
Lepirudin	HIT	0.4 mg/kg bolus, then 0.15 mg/kg/h	aPTT
Bivalirudin	Angioplasty, PCI with HIT	0.75 mg/kg/bolus; then 1.75 mg/kg/h	ACT
Argatroban	HIT	2 μg/kg/min	aPTT
	IIIT with PCI	350 μg/kg/min bolus, then 15 to 400 μg/ kg/min	ACT

ACT, activated clotting time; aPTT, activated partial thromboplastin time; HIT, heparin-induced thrombocytopenia; PCI, percutaneous coronary intervention.
Source: *Williams Hematology,* 8th ed, Chap. 23, Table 23–6, p. 359.

- All hirudin derivatives are cleared by the kidney and have a markedly prolonged half-life in case of renal insufficiency.
- Hirudin derivatives carry a high risk of bleeding and currently there is no antidote available.

Argatroban
- Argatroban is a small-molecule arginine derivative that reversibly inhibits thrombin by binding directly to the active catalytic site.
- Argatroban is approved for treatment and prophylaxis of heparin-induced thrombocytopenia and for percutaneous interventions in patients with heparin-induced thrombocytopenia. It also shows some benefit in patients with thrombotic stroke in clinical trials (see Table 88–5).
- The anticoagulant effect can be assessed with the aPTT, which correlates well with plasma concentrations of the drug.
- Metabolism is primarily hepatic, and the clearance and half-life are prolonged in patients with hepatic functional abnormalities requiring dose reduction. Renal function has less effect on argatroban pharmacokinetics.
- As with other direct thrombin inhibitors, the main side effect is bleeding, and no specific agent is available to reverse its action.

ORAL ANTITHROMBIN AND ANTI-FACTOR XA AGENTS
- Recently, the oral antithrombin agent dabigatran has become available and was shown to be as effective or superior to vitamin K antagonists in patients with atrial fibrillation, and for prevention and treatment of venous thromboembolism.
- New oral anti-factor Xa agents include rivaroxaban and apixaban and are also effective antithrombotic agents.
- The new oral antithrombin and anti-factor Xa agents have been shown to be effective for the prevention venous thrombosis after orthopedic surgery, prevention of thromboembolic complications in patients with atrial fibrillation, and the treatment of venous thromboembolism.
- Dabigatran, rivaroxaban, and apixaban do not need laboratory monitoring, although data in elderly patients and patients with renal insufficiency are limited.
- Currently, there is no antidote against the anticoagulant effect of dabigatran, rivaroxaban, or apixaban.
- There are more new oral antithrombin and anti-factor Xa agents currently in clinical development.

ANTIPLATELET DRUGS

- The properties that make platelets useful in the arrest of hemorrhage also allow platelets to form thrombi in vessels, and on heart valves, artificial membranes, and prosthetic devices, in particular in situations with high shear stress.
- Drugs that inhibit platelet function may, therefore, have clinical application in the treatment and prevention of arterial thrombosis (Table 88–6 and Table 88–7).
- Drugs that inhibit platelet function include aspirin, nonsteroidal antiinflammatory drugs, dipyridamole, thienopyridine derivatives (ticlopidine, clopidogrel and prasugrel), and inhibitors of the platelet glycoprotein (GP) IIb/IIIa receptor.

Aspirin

- Inhibits prostaglandin synthesis by irreversibly acetylating a critical serine residue in cyclooxygenase, thereby blocking the formation of thromboxane A_2 ($T \times A_2$). Because platelets cannot synthesize new enzymes, the inhibition is permanent for the life span of the platelet.
- Inhibits collagen-induced platelet aggregation and secondary aggregation to weak agonists, such as ADP and epinephrine.
- Effects on aggregation and bleeding time last about 7 days after a single oral dose.
- Inhibits the synthesis of the potentially antithrombotic prostaglandin, PGI_2 (prostacyclin), in endothelial cells, but the inhibition is short-lived because endothelium can synthesize new enzyme.
- A dose of aspirin that inhibits TxA_2 but not PGI_2 production has not been found, nor has the optimal dose of aspirin been defined for any specific indication.
- The dose used for a specific indication should take into account efficacy, as determined by clinical trials, and adverse effects, which include, most importantly, gastrointestinal bleeding and hemorrhagic stroke.

TABLE 88–6	ANTIPLATELET AGENTS BY MECHANISM OF ACTION AND CLINICAL USE
Cyclooxygenase inhibitors	
Aspirin	Coronary, cerebrovascular, an peripheral arterial disease
	Very high platelet count (essential thrombocythemia, polycythemia vera)
Agents that increase cAMP	
Dipyridamole	Cerebrovascular, peripheral arterial disease
Pentoxifylline	Peripheral arterial disease
Cilostazol	Peripheral arterial disease
ADP receptor blockers (thienopyridine derivatives)	
Ticlopidine	Cerebrovascular disease
Clopidogrel	Coronary, cerebrovascular disease, PCI
Prasugrel	Coronary disease
ADP mimetic	
Cangrelor	Not approved in United States at time of this writing
Glycoprotein IIβ/IIIα ($\alpha_{IIb}\beta_3$) inhibitors	
Abciximab	ACS, PCI
Eptifibatide	ACS, PCI
Tirofiban	ACS, PCI

ACS, acute coronary syndrome; cAMP, cyclic adenosine monophosphate; PCI, percutaneous coronary intervention.
Source: *Williams Hematology*, 8th ed, Chap. 23, Table 23–7, p. 362.

TABLE 88–7	ANTIPLATELET AGENTS, APPROVED DOSING	
Agent	Usual Dose	Duration of Effect
Aspirin	80–100 mg daily	7–10 days (life of the platelet)
Dipyridamole	75–100 mg QID	$t_{1/2}$ 40 min
Pentoxifylline	400 mg BID	$t_{1/2}$ 1–1.6 h
Cilostazol	100 mg BID	$t_{1/2}$ 11–13 h
Ticlopidine	250 mg BID	7–10 days (life of the platelet)
Clopidogrel	75 mg daily, loading dose 300 mg*	7–10 days (life of the platelet)
Abciximab	0.25 mg/kg, then 10 μg/kg/min	<0 min and 30 min
Eptifibatide	ACS 180 μg/kg, then 2 μg/kg/min PCI 180 μg/kg, then 2 μg/kg/min with 180 μg/kg at 10 min†	$t_{1/2}$ 2.5 h
Tirofiban	0.4 μg/kg/min × 30 min, then 0.1 μg/kg/min*	$t_{1/2}$ 2 h

ACS, acute coronary syndrome; PCI, percutaneous coronary intervention; $t_{1/2}$, half-life.
*Larger loading and maintenance dosing is being studied.
†Decrease infusion rate by 50% for renal dysfunction.
Source: *Williams Hematology,* 8th ed, Chap. 23, Table 23–8, p. 362.

Nonsteroidal Antiinflammatory Drugs

- Appear to work by a mechanism similar to aspirin, but as the effect on cyclooxygenase is reversible, the effects are of much shorter duration.

Dipyridamole

- A phosphodiesterase inhibitor with vasodilator effects.
- Mechanisms of action may include increasing platelet cyclic AMP levels, or indirectly increasing the plasma levels of adenosine.
- Does not inhibit aggregation of platelets in platelet-rich plasma *in vitro,* but does inhibit aggregation of platelets in the presence of erythrocytes, as measured by whole-blood aggregometry.
- Other agents that increase cyclic adenosine monophosphate (cAMP) are pentoxifylline and cilostazol.

Thienopyridine Derivatives (Ticlopidine, Clopidogrel, and Prasugrel)

- Prolong the bleeding time and inhibit aggregation induced by ADP and low concentrations of collagen or thrombin.
- Antiplatelet effects are caused by metabolites. Appear to exert their antiplatelet effects by inhibiting the binding of ADP to platelets.
- Drugs are given orally and are fully effective only after 2 to 3 days. Loading doses may accelerate the onset of action.
- The usual dose of clopidogrel is 50 to 100 mg daily.
- Adverse effects include diarrhea and rash. Neutropenia may be severe but is usually reversible. Aplastic anemia and thrombotic thrombocytopenic purpura may occur, in particular with ticlopidine.

Inhibitors of the Platelet GP IIb/IIIa Receptor

- Platelets with absence or blockade of the receptor function of GP IIb/IIIa will not aggregate with any physiologic agonist.
- Blockade of GP IIb/IIIa can be achieved with monoclonal antibodies or with peptide or nonpeptide agonists.

- Abciximab is a human-mouse chimeric antibody fragment that inhibits platelet aggregation almost completely when 80 percent of GP IIb/IIIa receptors are blocked and that also inhibits the prothrombinase activity of platelets.
- The platelet count has been reported to be reduced to less than $100,000/\mu L$ in approximately 2 to 6 percent of patients, and to less than $50,000/\mu L$ in 1 to 2 percent.
- Cyclic peptides (eptifibatide) containing the arginine-glycine-aspartic acid (RGD) sequence or the lysine-glycine-aspartic acid (KGD) sequence bind with high affinity to GP IIb/IIIa and are relatively resistant to enzymatic breakdown.
- Nonpeptide agents (tirofiban) inhibit the binding of adhesive proteins to GP IIb/IIIa, presumably because they mimic the structural features of the RGD sequence.

ANTIPLATELET DRUGS IN CLINICAL MEDICINE

Ischemic Heart Disease
- Aspirin therapy is widely used for both primary and secondary prevention of acute coronary syndromes and other forms of ischemic heart disease.
- Aspirin is also useful alone, or in combination, in treating unstable angina and acute myocardial infarction, and as an adjunct in managing patients after thrombolytic therapy, percutaneous coronary interventions, or coronary artery bypass surgery.
- Thienopyridine derivatives are useful in combination with aspirin in unstable angina and in the prevention of acute occlusion after coronary stenting.
- GP IIb/GP IIa antagonists in combination with other drugs favorably influence unstable angina and evolving myocardial infarction, and prevent ischemic vascular complications following percutaneous coronary interventions.

Valvular Heart Disease
- Oral anticoagulant therapy is generally recommended for patients with prosthetic heart valves, but the addition of aspirin is recommended for patients who have systemic thromboembolism despite adequate anticoagulation.

Cerebrovascular Disease
- Antiplatelet therapy is effective in preventing cerebrovascular events in patients with either prior cerebrovascular events or prior cardiac events.
- In most studies, aspirin has been used in doses ranging from 38 to 100 mg per day, but the optimal dose has not been determined. Low doses appear to be as effective as higher doses but have less adverse effects.

Peripheral Vascular Disease
- Aspirin treatment may decrease the need for vascular surgery without affecting the pattern of stable intermittent claudication, suggesting that antiplatelet therapy decreases the incidence of thrombotic complications without affecting the basic disease process.
- The role of antiplatelet therapy in preventing graft occlusion after peripheral artery reconstruction is controversial.

For a more detailed discussion, see Charles W. Francis and Mark Crowther: Principles of Antithrombotic Therapy. Chap 23, p. 353 in *Williams Hematology*, 8th ed.

CHAPTER 89
Hereditary Thrombophilia

- Risk factors for thromboembolism may be genetic and acquired (Table 89–1).
- Hereditary thrombophilia is a genetically determined increased risk of thrombosis.
- Up to 50 percent of patients presenting with a first deep venous thrombosis will have an abnormal laboratory test suggesting a thrombophilic defect, and patients with recurrent thromboses or with a strong family history are even more likely to have laboratory evidence of a thrombophilic state (Table 89–2).
- Up to 16 percent of patients with thrombophilia have inherited more than one abnormality.
- These inherited defects also interact frequently with acquired risk factors, such as inactivity, trauma, malignancy, or oral contraceptive use, to lead to clinical thrombosis.

HEREDITARY RESISTANCE TO ACTIVATED PROTEIN C (APC)

Etiology and Pathogenesis

- APC resistance is an abnormally reduced anticoagulant response of a patient's plasma that, in more than 90 percent of cases, is caused by a genetic abnormality of factor V (substitution of glutamine for arginine at position 506), which significantly retards inactivation of factor Va by APC. The abnormal factor V is generally referred to as "factor V Leiden."

TABLE 89–1 **THROMBOPHILIAS AND PREDISPOSING RISK FACTORS FOR VENOUS THROMBOEMBOLISM**

Thrombophilias	Acquired Predisposing Risk Factors for Venous Thrombosis
Common	Increasing age
Factor V Leiden	Surgery or trauma
Prothrombin G20210A	Prolonged immobilization
Increased factor VIII level[x]	Obesity
Homozygous C677T polymorphism in methylenetetrahydrofolate reductase[†]	Smoking
	Malignant neoplasms
Rare	Myeloproliferative diseases
Protein C deficiency	Superficial vein thrombosis
Protein S deficiency	Previous venous thrombosis/Varicose veins
Antithrombin deficiency	Pregnancy and puerperium
Very rare	Use of female hormones
Dysfibrinogenemia	Antiphospholipid antibodies/Lupus anticoagulants
Homozygous homocystinuria	Hyperhomocysteinemia
	Activated protein C resistance unrelated to factor V Leiden

*Heritability is inferred. No gene alteration has been discerned.
†A questionable thrombophilia that can be associated with hyperhomocysteinemia in patients with deficiencies of folic acid or vitamin B_{12}.
Source: *William Hematology,* 8th ed, Chap. 131, Table 131–1, p. 2122.

| TABLE 89–2 | FREQUENCY OF THROMBOPHILIAS IN HEALTHY SUBJECTS AND UNSELECTED AND SELECTED PATIENTS WITH VENOUS THROMBOSIS |

	Healthy Subjects		Unselected Patients		Selected Patients	
Thrombophilia	No.	Percent Affected	No.	Percent Affected	No.	Percent Affected
Factor V Leiden	16,150* 2192†	4.8 0.05	1142	18.8	162	40
Prothrombin G20210A	11,932* 1811†	2.7 0.06	2884	7.1	551	16
Protein C deficiency	15,070	0.2–0.4	2008	3.7	767	4.8
Protein S deficiency	3788	0.16–0.21	2008	2.3	649	4.3
Antithrombin deficiency	9669	0.02	2008	1.9	649	4.3

*Whites.
†Africans and Orientals.
Adapted with permission from Seligsohn U, Lubetsky A: Genetic susceptibility to venous thrombosis. N Engl J Med Apr 19;344(16):1222-1231, 2001.
Source: *William Hematology*, 8th ed, Chap.131, Table 131–2, p. 2123.

Clinical Features

- The factor V Leiden mutation occurs in 3 to 12 percent of Caucasians but is rare in other ethnic groups.
- Deep and superficial venous thromboses are the most common manifestations of factor V Leiden, which has been reported to account for 20 to 25 percent of first thromboembolic events.
- Heterozygosity for factor V Leiden increases the relative risk of developing venous thrombosis 4 to 8 times. It is estimated that one-half of homozygous carriers will have a clinically significant thrombotic episode during their lives.
- The evidence regarding the role of factor V Leiden in recurrent thrombosis is conflicting.
- Factor V Leiden induces a relatively mild hypercoagulable state, but the risks of thrombosis are greatly increased by combination with other inherited disorders, such as antithrombin deficiency, or with acquired risk factors, such as immobility or use of oral contraceptives.
- A significantly increased risk of arterial thrombosis has been reported in patients with factor V Leiden and other vascular risk factors, such as smoking.

Laboratory Features

- Patients with APC resistance can be identified by special coagulation assays.
- DNA-based assays provide confirmation for positive coagulation tests and distinguish homozyotes and heterozygotes.

PROTHROMBIN G20210A GENE POLYMORPHISM

Etiology and Pathogenesis

- Substitution of guanylic acid (G) for adenylic acid (A) at nucleotide 20210 in the 3′-untranslated end of the prothrombin gene leads to an elevated plasma prothrombin level and predisposes to thrombosis.

Clinical Features

- This mutation is found primarily in Caucasians.
- The mutation is associated with venous thrombosis in all age groups, sometimes in unusual sites. Arterial thromboses also occur.

- The mutation increases the odds ratio for thrombosis by 2- to 5.5-fold.
- The risk of thrombosis in patients with the G20210A polymorphism is further increased by another inherited thrombophilic state or by other risk factors such as oral contraceptive use or smoking.

Laboratory Features

- Diagnosis depends on DNA analysis to identify the mutation in the prothrombin gene.

HYPERHOMOCYSTEINEMIA

Etiology and Pathogenesis

- Hyperhomocysteinemia is a plasma homocysteine level above the normal range.
- Severe hyperhomocysteinemia, or homocystinuria, is a rare autosomal recessive disorder with neurologic abnormalities, premature cardiovascular disease, stroke, and thromboses.
- Mild to moderate hyperhomocysteinemia is an independent risk factor for arteriosclerosis and arterial thrombosis and for venous thrombosis.
- Homocysteine appears to exert prothrombotic effects by interfering with endothelial cell function.
- Hyperhomocysteinemia may be the result of mutations of enzymes involved in metabolism of sulfur-containing amino acids, or may be the result of nutritional deficiency of vitamin B_6, vitamin B_{12}, or folic acid, or of a combination of these causes.

Clinical Features

- Hyperhomocysteinemia is commonly associated with both venous and arterial thromboses.
- Hyperhomocysteinemia increases the odds ratio for venous thrombosis to 2.5 to 3.0.
- The combination of hyperhomocysteinemia with another prethrombotic disorder, such as factor V Leiden, substantially increases the risk of thromboembolism.
- Hyperhomocysteinemia is a strong predictor of recurrent thrombosis.

Laboratory Features

- Homocysteine levels can be measured on properly collected plasma.
- Mutations in the genes for enzymes concerned with homocysteine metabolism (for example the *MTHFR* gene) can be determined using molecular biology techniques.

PROTEIN C DEFICIENCY

Etiology and Pathogenesis

- APC functions as an anticoagulant by inactivating activated factor V and activated factor VIII. Deficiency of protein C reduces this anticoagulant effect and leads to hypercoagulability.
- Protein C deficiency is inherited as an autosomal dominant trait.
- Affected heterozygotes have protein C levels of approximately 50 percent.
- Type I deficiency is caused by decreased synthesis of a normal protein.
- Type II deficiency is caused by production of an abnormally functioning protein.

Clinical Features

- Clinical expression of protein C deficiency is variable, perhaps because of coinheritance of other thrombophilic conditions.

- Most deficient patients are identified by screening apparently normal individuals who have no personal or family history of thrombosis.
- Deep and superficial venous thrombosis is the most common presentation. Venous thrombosis may occur in unusual sites. Arterial thrombosis is uncommon.
- By age 45 years, up to one-half of heterozygous persons from clinically affected families will have had venous thromboembolism.
- Homozygous patients with protein C levels less than 1 percent may develop severe thrombotic syndromes, such as neonatal purpura fulminans.
- Protein C deficiency may also be responsible for warfarin skin necrosis (see Chap. 83).

Laboratory Features

- Protein C deficiency may be detected by properly performed protein C assays.
- Immunoassays can distinguish type I deficiencies (decreased antigen, decreased activity) from type II (normal antigen, decreased activity).
- The large numbers of mutations make DNA analysis impractical.
- In patients who have been treated with warfarin, it is necessary to wait at least 2 weeks after stopping warfarin therapy before measuring protein C levels.

PROTEIN S DEFICIENCY

Etiology and Pathogenesis

- Protein S functions as an anticoagulant by enhancing the activity of APC and also may directly inhibit factors Va, VIIIa, and Xa.
- Plasma protein S circulates both unbound (free) and bound to C4b-binding protein. Only the free form is active.
- Protein S deficiency is inherited as an autosomal dominant trait.
- Protein S deficiency may be due to reduced synthesis of active protein (type I), normal synthesis of a defective protein (type II), or low levels of free protein S (the active form) combined with normal levels of bound protein S (type III).

Clinical Features

- The clinical features of inherited protein S deficiency are similar to those of protein C deficiency.
- Reduced levels of protein S occur in a number of clinical conditions, including oral contraceptive use, pregnancy, oral anticoagulant therapy, disseminated intravascular coagulation, liver disease, nephrotic syndrome, and inflammatory diseases.

Laboratory Features

- For screening purposes, estimation of free protein S antigen or APC-cofactor anticoagulant activity is better than determining total protein S antigen.
- Assessment of total and free protein S and of protein S activity permits classification into types I, II, and III.
- The high frequency of acquired protein S deficiency makes it difficult to identify hereditary defects.
- DNA techniques may be useful within a family with a previously established mutation, but the large number of mutations otherwise limit their value.

ANTITHROMBIN DEFICIENCY

Etiology and Pathogenesis

- Antithrombin is a protease inhibitor that forms irreversible, inactive complexes with thrombin and factors IXa, Xa, and XIa in reactions that are accelerated by heparin or heparan sulfate on endothelial surfaces.
- Antithrombin deficiency is inherited as an autosomal dominant trait.

- Type I deficiency is a result of reduced synthesis of the antithrombin protein.
- Type II deficiency is a result of production of an antithrombin protein with abnormal function.

Clinical Features

- Venous thrombosis of the lower extremities is the most common presentation. Venous thrombosis may also occur in unusual sites. Arterial thrombosis occurs infrequently.
- Antithrombin deficiency is found in about 1 percent of individuals younger than 70 years of age with a first documented venous thrombosis.
- The odds ratio for thrombosis in patients with antithrombin deficiency is 10 to 20.
- The occurrence of thrombosis peaks in the second decade of life.
- Coinheritance of another gene for thrombophilia or coexistence of prothrombotic environmental factors substantially increases the risk of thrombosis.
- Antithrombin deficiency with values less than 5 percent is extremely rare and causes severe arterial and venous thromboses.
- Resistance to heparin therapy occurs frequently in patients not deficient in antithrombin, and is not a useful indicator of the deficiency.

Laboratory Features

- Antithrombin deficiency can be detected using appropriate functional assays. Immunologic assays are needed to distinguish between type I and type II defects.
- Antithrombin activity levels usually range from 40 to 60 percent in deficient patients.
- Antithrombin activity may be reduced to similar levels by mild liver disease, thrombosis, or heparin therapy, and it may be necessary to repeat the assays and to perform family studies to establish the diagnosis.

ELEVATED LEVELS OF FACTOR VIII AND OTHER COAGULATION FACTORS

- Factor VIII levels above 150 percent of normal have been defined as an independent risk factor for thrombosis.
- Preliminary data suggest that elevation of levels of factors V, IX, X, and XI above 150 percent similarly predispose to thrombosis.
- The mechanism of elevation of coagulation factor levels is unknown. Pathogenesis of the thrombi may be increased thrombin generation.
- The clinical features of patients with elevated factor VIII levels are those of patients with other forms of thrombophilia.
- Levels of factor VIII antigen are increased corresponding to factor VIII procoagulation activity.

HEREDITARY THROMBOTIC DYSFIBRINOGENEMIA

- Dysfibrinogenemia is a qualitative defect in the molecule that can be asymptomatic (50%), or lead to either bleeding (30%) or thrombosis (20%). See Chap. 81.
- Dysfibrinogenemia is found in approximately 0.8 percent of patients presenting with thromboembolism.
- Patients with thrombotic dysfibrinogenemia usually present with venous thrombosis in the third to fourth decade of life.
- These patients have an increased rate of spontaneous abortion and stillbirth and may have postpartum hemorrhage.
- Prolongation of a dilute thrombin time or a reptilase time, and a disparity between levels of immunoreactive and clottable fibrinogen are common in dysfibrinogenemia.

OTHER POTENTIAL THROMBOPHILIC DISORDERS

- Hereditary defects of the fibrinolytic system or of thrombomodulin are potential causes of thrombophilia but are not yet clearly established.

DIAGNOSIS OF THROMBOPHILIA

- Comprehensive testing for patients with venous thromboembolism should include those assays listed in Table 89–1.
- Thrombophilic factors can be evaluated in patients receiving oral anticoagulants, except for protein C resistance, and protein C and protein S levels. Proteins C and S can be assayed in blood from patients who have received heparin therapy instead of oral anticoagulants for approximately 2 weeks before performing the tests. Factor V Leiden genotype can be performed instead of testing for APC resistance.
- Women with prior thromboembolism or with a strong family history of thromboembolism may be evaluated for thrombophilia before oral contraceptives are administered.
- Children with venous or arterial thrombosis are likely to have thrombophilia.
- Diagnostic studies for thrombophilia should be considered for women with recurrent midtrimester fetal loss or other adverse pregnancy outcomes.

THERAPY OF THROMBOPHILIA

- Patients with thrombophilia who develop thrombosis or pulmonary embolism should be treated according to standard protocols for treatment of venous thromboembolism, i.e., they should initially receive standard treatment with heparin followed by vitamin K antagonists to maintain the INR between 2 and 3.
- Warfarin therapy is usually continued for 6 months but may be prolonged if the risks of recurrent thrombosis appear to significantly outweigh the risks of complications of therapy.
- If oral anticoagulant therapy is not continued, antithrombotic prophylaxis with low-molecular-weight heparin can be initiated with high-risk events such as surgery, inflammation, or inactivity.
- B vitamins and folic acid are known to reduce plasma homocysteine levels, but their preventive value is not established. In clinical practice, however, this treatment is often prescribed.
- Prophylactic heparin therapy should be considered for pregnant women who have had previous thromboembolism, particularly if the prior event was pregnancy-related.
- Venous thromboembolism that occurs during pregnancy requires heparin throughout the pregnancy and anticoagulant therapy for 4 to 6 weeks postpartum (see Chap. 88).

 For a more detailed discussion, see Uri Seligsohn and Aharon Lubetsky: Hereditary Thrombophilia. Chap. 131, p. 2121, in *Williams Hematology,* 8th ed.

CHAPTER 90
Venous Thromboembolism

- Venous thromboembolism (deep venous thrombosis and/or pulmonary embolism) is a common disorder, which is estimated to affect 900,000 patients each year in the United States.
- Pulmonary embolism may cause sudden or abrupt death, underscoring the importance of prevention as the critical strategy for reducing death from pulmonary embolism.
- Of the estimated 600,000 cases of nonfatal venous thromboembolism in the United States each year, approximately 60 percent present clinically as deep venous thrombosis and 40 percent present as pulmonary embolism.
- Most clinically important pulmonary emboli arise from proximal deep venous thrombosis (thrombosis involving the popliteal, femoral, or iliac veins). Upper extremity deep venous thrombosis also may lead to clinically important pulmonary embolism. Other less common sources of pulmonary embolism include the deep pelvic veins, renal veins, inferior vena cava, right side of the heart, and axillary veins.
- Acquired and inherited risk factors for venous thromboembolism have been identified (for inherited thrombophilia see Chap. 89). The risk of thromboembolism increases when more than one predisposing factor is present.

CLINICAL FEATURES

- The clinical features of deep venous thrombosis and pulmonary embolism are nonspecific.

Venous Thrombosis

- The clinical features of venous thrombosis include leg pain, tenderness, and asymmetrical swelling, a palpable cord representing a thrombosed vessel, discoloration, venous distention, prominence of the superficial veins, and cyanosis.
- In exceptional cases, patients may present with phlegmasia cerulea dolens (occlusion of the whole venous circulation, extreme swelling of the leg, and compromised arterial flow).
- In 50 to 85 percent of patients, the clinical suspicion of deep venous thrombosis is not confirmed by objective testing. Conversely, patients with florid pain and swelling, suggesting extensive deep venous thrombosis, may have negative results by objective testing. Patients with minor symptoms and signs may have extensive deep venous thrombi.
- Although the clinical diagnosis is nonspecific, prospective studies have established that patients can be categorized as low, moderate, or high probability for deep venous thrombosis using clinical prediction rules that incorporates signs, symptoms, and risk factors.

Pulmonary Embolism

- The clinical features of acute pulmonary embolism include the following symptoms and signs that may overlap:
  — Transient dyspnea and tachypnea in the absence of other clinical features.
  — Pleuritic chest pain, cough, hemoptysis, pleural effusion, and pulmonary infiltrates noted on chest radiogram caused by pulmonary infarction or congestive atelectasis (also known as *ischemic pneumonitis* or *incomplete infarction*).
  — Severe dyspnea and tachypnea and right-side heart failure.

- — Cardiovascular collapse with hypotension, syncope, and coma (usually associated with massive pulmonary embolism).
- — Several less common and nonspecific clinical presentations, including unexplained tachycardia or arrhythmia, resistant cardiac failure, wheezing, cough, fever, anxiety/apprehension, and confusion.
- All of these clinical features are nonspecific and can be caused by a variety of cardiorespiratory disorders.
- Patients can be assigned to categories of pretest probability using implicit clinical judgment, or clinical decision rules.

DIAGNOSIS

- Objective diagnostic testing is required to confirm or exclude the presence of venous thromboembolism.
- An appropriately validated assay for plasma fibrin degradation product D-dimer, if available, provides a simple, rapid, and cost-effective first-line exclusion test in patients with low, unlikely, or intermediate clinical probability.
- Integrated diagnostic strategies for deep venous thrombosis and pulmonary embolism are presented in Fig. 90–1 and Fig. 90–2, respectively.

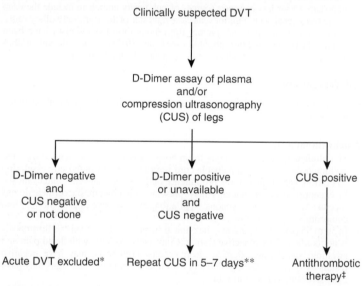

FIGURE 90–1 Diagnosis of patients with suspected first episode of deep venous thrombosis (DVT). *Negative D-dimer can be used to exclude acute DVT, without the need for further diagnostic testing with compression ultrasonography (CUS), if the patient has low, unlikely, moderate, or intermediate clinical probability. Ultrasonography should be performed in patients with a high clinical probability. A negative D-dimer can also be used with a negative CUS at presentation to exclude acute DVT without the need for a repeat CUS. **CUS is performed with imaging of the common femoral vein in the groin and of the popliteal vein in the popliteal fossa extending distally 10 cm from midpatella. A repeat CUS is required in 5 to 7 days to detect extending calf vein thrombi. In centers with the expertise, a single negative result of full-leg duplex ultrasonography (CUS plus flow evaluation) is sufficient to exclude acute DVT. ‡CUS that indicates noncompressibility of deep vein segments is highly predictive of DVT (>95%) and provides an indication for antithrombotic therapy in most patients. If CUS is positive at a single site isolated in the groin, additional testing with venography, computed tomography, or magnetic resonance imaging should be performed because of the potential for false-positive CUS results from disorders producing vein compression in the groin (e.g., tumor mass). (Source: *William Hematology,* 8th ed, Chap. 134, Fig. 134–1, p. 2188.)

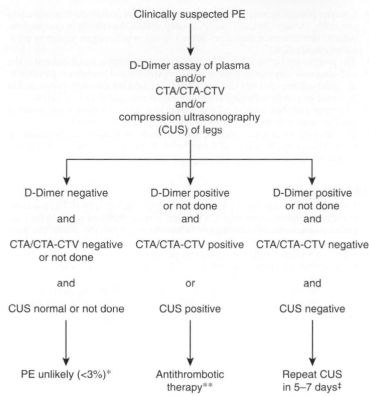

Clinically suspected PE

↓

D-Dimer assay of plasma
and/or
CTA/CTA-CTV
and/or
compression ultrasonography
(CUS) of legs

D-Dimer negative	D-Dimer positive or not done	D-Dimer positive or not done
and	and	and
CTA/CTA-CTV negative or not done	CTA/CTA-CTV positive	CTA/CTA-CTV negative
and	or	and
CUS normal or not done	CUS positive	CUS negative
PE unlikely (<3%)*	Antithrombotic therapy**	Repeat CUS in 5–7 days‡

FIGURE 90-2 Integrated strategy for diagnosis of patients with suspected pulmonary embolism (PE) using CT angiography (CTA) as the primary imaging test. *Negative D-dimer alone can be used as an exclusion test with high negative predictive value (>97%) in patients with low or moderate probability by the clinical assessment. Patients with a high clinical probability should undergo imaging with CTA or combined CTA-CT Venography (CTV). **Positive results on CTA or combined CTA-CTV, in patients with a high or moderate probability of pulmonary embolism by the clinical assessment, have positive predictive value of 90 percent or more for venous thromboembolism. Similarly, abnormal results by compression ultrasonography (CUS) of the proximal deep veins of the legs have high positive predictive value for proximal vein thrombosis and provide an indication to give antithrombotic therapy. If the patient has a low probability by the clinical assessment, positive results by CTA or CTA-CTV in the main or lobar pulmonary arteries are still highly predictive (97%) for the presence of pulmonary embolism; further testing is recommended for patients with a low clinical probability and positive CTA results only of segmental or subsegmental arteries, and the options include pulmonary arteriography or serial CUS. ‡Negative results by CTA or by combined CTA-CTV have high negative predictive value (96%) in patients with low probability by the clinical assessment. For patients with moderate clinical probability, the negative predictive value for combined CTA-CTV is also high (92%), but slightly lower for CTA alone (89%); in this latter group, and in patients with a high probability by the clinical assessment, serial CUS or pulmonary arteriography are recommended options.
Source: William Hematology, 8th ed., Chap. 134, Table 134–2, p. 2190.

Venous Thrombosis

- Enzyme-linked immunosorbent assay (ELISA) and quantitative rapid ELISA for D-dimer have high sensitivity (96%) and negative likelihood ratios of approximately 0.10 for deep venous thrombosis in symptomatic patients.

- Compression ultrasonography of the proximal veins performed at presentation can safely exclude clinically important deep venous thrombosis in symptomatic patients (with the exception of pelvic thrombosis, which may be missed by ultrasound examination).
- The positive predictive value of a positive ultrasonographic result isolated to the calf veins may vary among centers based on expertise and thrombosis prevalence. To detect calf vein thrombi that were initially missed but may have progressed to proximal venous thrombosis, ultrasonography is repeated after 5 to 7 days.
- In centers with the expertise, a single comprehensive evaluation of the proximal and calf veins with duplex (Doppler) ultrasonography is sufficient.
- Measurement of D-dimer using an appropriate assay method can be combined with ultrasonograph imaging of the leg veins. If the two tests are negative at presentation, repeat ultrasonograph imaging is unnecessary.

Pulmonary Embolism
- If capability for combined computed tomographic angiography (CTA) and computed tomographic venography (CTV) exists, it is the preferred approach for most patients with suspected pulmonary embolism because it provides a definitive basis to give or withhold antithrombotic therapy in more than 90 percent of patients.
- CTA is not inferior to using ventilation–perfusion lung scanning for excluding the diagnosis of pulmonary embolism when either test is used together with venous ultrasonography of the legs.
- Single-detector spiral CT is highly sensitive for large emboli (segmental or larger arteries) but is much less sensitive for emboli in subsegmental pulmonary arteries.
- Multidetector row CT, together with the use of contrast enhancement, has further improved the utility of CT for the diagnosis of pulmonary embolism, also in subsegmental pulmonary arteries.
- Contrast-enhanced CTA has the advantage of providing clear results (positive or negative), good characterization of nonvascular structures for alternate or associated diagnoses, and the ability to simultaneously evaluate the deep venous system of the legs (computed tomographic venography [CTV]).
- Ventilation-perfusion lung scanning is another imaging option for the diagnosis of pulmonary embolism. A normal perfusion lung scan excludes the diagnosis of clinically important pulmonary embolism.
- A high-probability lung scan result (i.e., large perfusion defects with ventilation mismatch) has a positive predictive value for pulmonary embolism of 85 percent and provides a diagnostic endpoint to give antithrombotic treatment in most patients.
- The major limitation of lung scanning is that the results are inconclusive in most patients, even when considered together with the pretest clinical probability. The nondiagnostic lung scan patterns are found in approximately 70 percent of patients with suspected pulmonary embolism.
- MRI appears to be highly sensitive for pulmonary embolism and is a promising diagnostic approach. However, clinically important interobserver variation exists in the sensitivity for pulmonary embolism, ranging from 70 to 100 percent.
- Pulmonary angiography using selective catheterization of the pulmonary arteries is a relatively safe technique for patients who do not have pulmonary hypertension or cardiac failure. If the expertise is available, pulmonary angiography should be used when other approaches are inconclusive and when definitive knowledge about the presence or absence of pulmonary embolism is required.
- Objective testing for nonsymptomatic deep venous thrombosis is useful in patients with suspected pulmonary embolism, particularly those with nondiagnostic lung scan results or inconclusive CT results. Detection of proximal venous thrombosis by objective testing provides an indication for anticoagulant treatment, regardless of the presence or absence of pulmonary embolism, and prevents the need for further testing.

LONG-TERM SEQUELAE OF VENOUS THROMBOEMBOLISM

- The postthrombotic syndrome is a frequent complication of deep venous thrombosis.
- Symptoms of the postthrombotic syndrome are pain, heaviness, swelling, cramps, and itching or tingling of the affected leg. Ulceration may occur. Symptoms usually are aggravated by standing or walking and improve with rest and elevation of the leg.
- Application of a properly fitted graded compression stocking, as soon after diagnosis as the patient's symptoms will allow and continued for at least 2 years, is effective in reducing the incidence of postthrombotic symptoms, including moderate-to-severe symptoms.
- Chronic thromboembolic pulmonary hypertension is a serious complication of pulmonary embolism and may occur in 1 to 3 percent of patients.
- Chronic thromboembolic pulmonary hypertension may be suspected if clinical signs and symptoms of pulmonary embolism persist over months despite adequate treatment and can be confirmed by echocardiography and ventilation-perfusion lung scanning.

TREATMENT

- The objectives of treatment in patients with established venous thromboembolism are to:
  - Prevent death from pulmonary embolism.
  - Prevent morbidity from recurrent venous thrombosis or pulmonary embolism.
  - Prevent or minimize the postthrombotic syndrome.
- Antithrombotic treatment is highly effective for venous thromboembolism. The principles of antithrombotic treatment are outlined in Chap. 88.
- Treatment is initiated with unfractionated or low molecular weight (LMW) heparin or a heparin derivative for 5 to 10 days (see Table 90–1).
- Long-term antithrombotic treatment is currently achieved by administration of vitamin K antagonists (e.g., warfarin). New oral anticoagulant agents are currently being evaluated.
- The appropriate duration of oral anticoagulant treatment for venous thromboembolism is at least 3 months in patients with a first episode of proximal venous thrombosis or pulmonary embolism secondary to a transient or reversible risk factor.
- Patients with a first episode of idiopathic (unprovoked) venous thromboembolism should be treated for at least 6 months
- The decision on the duration of antithrombotic treatment should be individualized, taking into consideration the estimated risk of recurrent venous thromboembolism, risk of bleeding, and patient compliance and preference.
- Patients with a first episode of venous thrombosis and a single thrombophilic risk factor (e.g., factor V Leiden) do not need prolonged antithrombotic treatment.
- Prolonged or even indefinite therapy is recommended for patients with recurrent thrombosis and/or persistent strong risk factors (e.g., active cancer or antiphospholipid antibodies) in whom risk factors for bleeding are absent and in whom good anticoagulant control can be achieved. If indefinite anticoagulant treatment is given, the risk-to-benefit ratio of continuing such treatment should be reassessed at periodic intervals.
- Long-term treatment with subcutaneous LMW heparin for 3 to 6 months is at least as effective as, and in cancer patients is more effective than, oral vitamin K antagonists. However, the repeated subcutaneous injections are not always well tolerated by patients.
- Insertion of an inferior vena cava filter is indicated for patients with acute venous thromboembolism and an absolute contraindication to anticoagulant therapy.

TABLE 90–1	REGIMENS OF LOW-MOLECULAR-WEIGHT HEPARIN AND FONDAPARINUX FOR TREATMENT OF VENOUS THROMBOEMBOLISM

Drug#	Regimen
Enoxaparin	1.0 mg/kg BID*
Dalteparin	200 IU/kg once daily[†]
Tinzaparin	175 IU/kg once daily[‡]
Nadroparin	5700 IU BID for 50–70 kg[§]
Reviparin	4200 IU BID for 46–60 kg[¶]
Fondaparinux	7.5 mg once daily for 50–100 kg**

*A once-daily regimen of 1.5 mg/kg can be used but probably is less effective in patients with cancer.
[†]After 1 month, can be followed by 150 IU/kg once daily as an alternative to an oral vitamin K antagonist for long-term treatment.
[‡]This regimen can also be used for long-term treatment as an alternative to an oral vitamin K antagonist.
[§]3800 IU BID if patient weighs <50 kg or 7600 IU BID if patient weighs >70 kg.
[¶]3500 IU BID if patient weighs 35–45 kg or 6300 IU BID if patient weighs >60 kg.
**5 mg once daily if patient weighs <50 kg or 10 mg once daily if patient weighs >100 kg.
#Drug brand names: dalteparin, Fragmin; enoxaparin, Lovenox; fondaparinux, Arixtra; tinzaparin, Innohep; nadroparin, Fraxiparine.
Source: *William Hematology,* 8th ed, Chap. 134, Table 134-2, p. 2192

- In patients with a temporary absolute contraindication to anticoagulant treatment (i.e., intercurrent bleeding or the need to undergo an invasive procedure), a retrievable inferior vena cava filter is preferable.
- The use of a permanent vena cava filter results in an increased incidence of recurrent deep venous thrombosis 1 to 2 years after insertion (increase in cumulative incidence at 2 years increases from 12% to 21%). If a permanent filter is placed, long-term anticoagulant treatment should be given as soon as safely possible to prevent morbidity from recurrent deep venous thrombosis.

Venous Thromboembolism in Pregnancy

- Adjusted-dose subcutaneous heparin is an appropriate long-term anticoagulant regimen for pregnant patients with venous thromboembolism (see also Chap. 88).
- LMW heparin does not cross the placenta, and initial experience suggests these agents are safe for treatment of venous thromboembolism in pregnant patients. With regard to safety advantages, LMW heparin causes less thrombocytopenia and potentially less osteoporosis than unfractionated heparin.
- An additional advantage is that LMW heparin is effective when given once daily, whereas unfractionated heparin requires twice-daily injection.
- Therapeutic LMW heparin in pregnancy should be monitored regularly with measurement of plasma anti-factor Xa activity.
- After delivery antithrombotic treatment may be switched to vitamin K antagonists. Breastfeeding while using vitamin K antagonists is possible, provided that the baby receives the usual vitamin K administration that is common in breastfed infants.

For more detailed discussion, see Gary E. Raskob, Russel D. Hull, Graham F. Pineo: Venous Thrombosis. Chap. 134, p. 2185 in *Williams Hematology,* 8th ed.

CHAPTER 91
Antibody-Mediated Thrombotic Disorders: Thrombotic Thrombocytopenic Purpura and Heparin-Induced Thrombocytopenia

- Thrombotic microangiopathies are characterized by thrombocytopenia, microangiopathic hemolytic anemia, and microvascular thrombosis, leading to variable injury of the central nervous system, kidney, and other organs.
- The classic form of thrombotic microangiopathy, i.e., thrombotic thrombocytopenic purpura (TTP) is usually associated with an acquired (autoimmune) deficiency of ADAMTS13, a metalloprotease that cleaves ultralarge multimers of von Willebrand factor.
- Hemolytic uremic syndrome (HUS) refers to the thrombotic microangiopathy that mainly affects the kidney and may be diarrhea-associated (caused by enteric infection with Shiga-toxin producing gram-negative microorganisms) or atypical.
- Secondary thrombotic microangiopathies occur in association with infections, certain drugs, metastatic cancer, malignant hypertension, or after stem cell transplantation.
- Heparin-induced thrombocytopenia (HIT) is a significant complication of heparin treatment, associated with mild to moderate thrombocytopenia and a high frequency of both arterial and venous thrombosis. HIT is caused by the formation of anti-heparin/platelet factor-4 antibodies that activate platelets, leukocytes and endothelial cells.

THROMBOTIC THROMBOCYTOPENIC PURPURA

Etiology and Pathogenesis
- Most cases of TTP are caused by autoantibodies that inhibit ADAMTS13. Congenital deficiency of ADAMTS13 (Upshaw-Schulman syndrome) is documented.
- The underlying mechanism causing TTP is unregulated von Willebrand factor-dependent platelet thrombosis.
- (Ultra)large von Willebrand factor multimers are released from endothelial cells of the vessel wall and mediate platelet adhesion by binding connective tissue at sites of vascular injury and to platelet glycoprotein Ib on the platelet surface. ADAMTS13 cleaves the von Willebrand factor multimers, thereby preventing platelet-vessel wall interactions in the absence of vascular injury.
- Deficiency of ADAMTS13 leads to spontaneous microvascular platelet thrombosis, causing microvascular obstruction and microangiopathic hemolytic anemia.

Epidemiology and Clinical Features
- The incidence of TTP in the United States has been estimated at approximately 4.5 per million per year.
- The peak incidence is between ages 30 and 50 years, the disease is rare before age 20 years. The female to male ratio averages approximately 2:1, but female preponderance is more pronounced at relatively younger age.
- Other risk factors for TTP include African ancestry and obesity, and genetic risk factors, such as a low frequency of HLA-DR53.

- The onset of TTP can be dramatically acute or insidious, developing over weeks.
- Approximately one-third of patients have symptoms of hemolytic anemia. Thrombocytopenia typically causes petechiae or purpura; oral, gastrointestinal or genitourinary bleeding is less common but can be severe.
- Systemic microvascular thrombosis can affect any organ, and the consequences are variable. Renal involvement is common, but acute renal failure occurs in fewer than 10 percent of cases. Neurologic findings can be transient or persistent and may include headache, visual disturbances, vertigo, personality change, confusion, lethargy, syncope, coma, seizures, aphasia, hemiparesis, and other focal sensory or motor deficits.
- Many patients have fever. The symptoms of TTP sometimes can be quite atypical, either at first presentation or upon relapse. Thrombocytopenia without hemolytic anemia may herald the onset of disease. In rare instances, visual disturbances, pancreatitis, stroke, or other thrombosis may precede overt thrombotic microangiopathy by days to months.
- Cardiac involvement may cause chest pain, myocardial infarction, congestive heart failure, or arrhythmias. Direct pulmonary involvement is uncommon but severe acute respiratory distress syndrome may occur, possibly secondary to cardiac failure.
- Gastrointestinal symptoms are common and can include abdominal pain, nausea, vomiting, and diarrhea. Physical examination may suggest acute pancreatitis or mesenteric ischemia.

Laboratory Features

- Because the symptoms and signs of TTP are nonspecific, the diagnosis depends on laboratory testing to document microangiopathic hemolytic anemia and thrombocytopenia, without another predisposing cause.
- Thrombocytopenia typically is severe, and one-half of patients have platelet counts below approximately 20×10^9/L. Signs of hemolysis are present and direct antiglobulin test (Coombs test) is almost always negative.
- The characteristic morphologic feature of TTP on the blood film is a marked increase in schistocytes. Patients with TTP often have markedly increased schistocytes; spherocytes also may be seen.
- Almost all patients have normal values for prothrombin time (PT), and activated partial thromboplastin time (aPTT), reflecting a minor role of intravascular coagulation in TTP. Mildly elevated fibrin degradation products have been reported in some patients.
- Severe congenital ADAMTS13 deficiency (level <5%) is characteristic of congenital TTP. Severe acquired ADAMTS13 deficiency appears to be specific for TTP, although the sensitivity of the association is debated and the frequency of severe ADAMTS13 deficiency in TTP depends on how patients are ascertained.

Differential Diagnosis

- Many diseases associated with secondary thrombotic microangiopathy can produce overlapping clinical and laboratory findings. As a consequence, making a diagnosis of TTP can be a challenge and a wide differential diagnosis often must be considered (Table 91–1).
- Schistocytes occur in a variety of conditions besides TTP, although the level seldom enters the 1 to 18 percent range typical of TTP. Severe Coombs-negative hemolysis and marked schistocytosis sometimes occur in patients with defective mechanical heart valves.
- Conditions resulting in disseminated intravascular coagulation sometimes cause microangiopathic changes and thrombocytopenia with little change in blood coagulation tests, which can suggest a diagnosis of TTP. Infections may trigger disease in patients with severe ADAMTS13 deficiency, but more commonly, infections cause secondary thrombotic microangiopathy by other mechanisms.

TABLE 91–1	CLASSIFICATION AND DIFFERENTIAL DIAGNOSIS OF THROMBOTIC MICROANGIOPATHY

Congenital TTP (Upshaw-Schulman Syndrome)
• Inherited ADAMTS13 deficiency

TTP
• With acquired ADAMTS13 deficiency
• Without acquired ADAMTS13 deficiency

Secondary thrombotic microangiopathy
• Infections and disseminated intravascular coagulation
• Tissue transplant associated
  — Chemotherapy or radiation injury
  — Tissue rejection
  — Graft-versus-host disease
• Cancer
  — Trousseau syndrome
  — Metastatic carcinoma
  — Erythroleukemia
• Pregnancy associated (preeclampsia, eclampsia, HELLP syndrome)
• Autoimmune disorders
  — Evans syndrome
  — Systemic lupus erythematosus and other vasculitides
  — Antiphospholipid syndrome
• Drugs (commonly implicated)
  — Autoimmune with anti–ADAMTS13 antibodies:
    • Ticlopidine
    • Clopidogrel (mechanism may be variable)
  — Autoimmune without anti–ADAMTS13 antibodies
    • Quinine
  — Dose-related toxicity
    • Mitomycin C
    • Gemcitabine
    • Cyclosporine
    • Tacrolimus
• Malignant hypertension

Hemolytic uremic syndrome
• Diarrhea positive (Infectious, Shiga-toxin associated)
  — Sporadic
  — Epidemic
• Diarrhea negative
  — Inherited complement regulatory protein deficiencies (factor H, MCP, factor I, factor B, C3, C4BP)

HELLP, hemolysis, elevated liver enzymes, and low platelet count.
Source: *Williams Hematology*, 8th ed, Chap.133, Table 133–1, p. 2167.

• Recipients of solid-organ transplantations can develop thrombotic microangiopathy, often dominated by renal involvement associated with immunosuppression by cyclosporine or tacrolimus. These drugs appear to damage renal endothelial cells directly and can cause neurotoxicity, adding another feature suggestive of TTP.
• Similarly, hematopoietic stem cell transplantation recipients may develop thrombotic microangiopathy associated with high-dose chemotherapy or radiation, immunosuppressive drugs, graft-versus-host disease, or infections.

- Thrombotic microangiopathy occurs in a small fraction of patients with almost any cancer but most commonly with adenocarcinoma of the pancreas, lung, prostate, stomach, colon, ovary, breast, or unknown primary site. In most cases, the cancer is widely metastatic.

- The differential diagnosis of thrombotic microangiopathy in pregnancy includes preeclampsia, eclampsia, HELLP (hemolysis, elevated liver enzymes, and low platelet count) syndrome, acute fatty liver of pregnancy, abruptio placenta, amniotic fluid embolism, and retained products of conception. In addition, pregnancy can sometimes trigger disease in patients with congenital or acquired ADAMTS13 deficiency; in most case series of TTP, between 12 and 31 percent of patients are pregnant women, usually in the third trimester or immediately postpartum.

- Autoimmune thrombocytopenia may be confused with TTP if other causes of microangiopathic hemolytic anemia are present. Asymptomatic thrombocytopenia also may sometimes be the only finding in TTP, as demonstrated by a previous or subsequent episode of disease. Patients have been described in whom TTP and autoimmune thrombocytopenia appeared to occur simultaneously or sequentially. Evans syndrome (autoimmune hemolytic anemia with autoimmune thrombocytopenia) usually can be distinguished from TTP by a positive Coombs test and the prominence of spherocytes relative to schistocytes in the blood film. HIT may sometimes resemble TTP, with thrombocytopenia and disseminated arterial and venous thrombosis (see "Heparin-Induced Thrombocytopenia" below).

- Systemic lupus erythematosus (SLE) can cause autoimmune hemolysis and thrombocytopenia, and lupus vasculitis can cause microangiopathic changes, renal insufficiency, and neurologic defects consistent with TTP. Vasculitis associated with other autoimmune disorders can pose a similar diagnostic problem.

- Thrombotic microangiopathy can develop in patients with antiphospholipid syndrome (APS), with or without concurrent SLE (see Chap. 85). The clinical features resemble HUS, catastrophic APS, malignant hypertension, TTP, or HELLP syndrome. One-third of patients present during pregnancy or in the postpartum period.

- Among the drugs that have been associated with thrombotic microangiopathy, the antiplatelet drugs ticlopidine and clopidogrel are unusual because they appear to induce autoantibody inhibitors of ADAMTS13, effectively causing TTP. Thrombotic microangiopathy occurs in 200 to 625 per 1 million users of ticlopidine, usually between 2 and 12 weeks after starting therapy. The incidence of TTP with clopidogrel is lower and is estimated to be 10 per 1 million users. A comprehensive list of other drugs causing TTP can be found in Table 91–2. Drugs commonly implicated include selected antineoplastic agents, cyclosporine A, tacrolimus, and quinine.

- Malignant hypertension is associated with microangiopathic hemolytic anemia, thrombocytopenia, neurologic symptoms, and renal insufficiency, and therefore may resemble TTP.

HEMOLYTIC UREMIC SYNDROME

- Diarrhea-associated HUS can occur at any age but affects mainly children younger than 10 years.

- The disease occurs sporadically and in epidemics, associated with ingestion of foods or other materials contaminated with Shiga toxin-producing bacteria. *Escherichia coli* O157:H7 accounts for at least 80 percent of cases in many series, but HUS can also be caused by other toxin-bearing *E. coli* serotypes or by *Shigella dysenteriae* type 1.

- Within 3 days of ingesting the bacteria, patients develop painful diarrhea, without fever, that usually evolves to bloody diarrhea within a few days. HUS may develop during the subsequent 2 weeks, with the acute onset of microangiopathic

| TABLE 91–2 | DRUGS AND TOXINS ASSOCIATED WITH SECONDARY MICROANGIOPATHY |

Immune-mediated:
Quinine
Ticlopidine
Clopidogrel

Antineoplastic agents:
All-*trans* retinoic acid
Bleomycin plus cisplatin
Carmustine
Chlorozotocin
Cytosine arabinoside
Daunorubicin
Deoxycoformycin
Estramustine
Gemcitabine
Lomustine (CCNU)
Mitomycin C
Tamoxifen (when combined with mitomycin C)

Antiangiogenic agents:
Bevacizumab
Sunitinib

Immunosuppressive and antiinflammatory agents:
Cyclosporine
Tacrolimus
Penicillamine
Muromonab-CD3 (OKT3)
Interferon-α
Interferon-β
Ibuprofen

Antibiotics:
Ciprofloxacin
Clarithromycin
Cephalosporin
Piperacillin
Rifampicin
Metronidazole
Pentostatin
Sulfonamides
Penicillin
Ampicillin
Oxophenarsine
Valacyclovir
Famciclovir
Mefloquine

Hormones:
Estrogen/progestogen oral contraceptives
Mestranol, norethindrone
17β-Estradiol transdermal patch
Conjugated estrogens

Illicit drugs:
Cocaine
Heroin
Ecstasy

Lipid-lowering agents:
Atorvastatin
Simvastatin

H_2-receptor antagonists:
Cimetidine
Famotidine

Vaccinations:
Polio vaccination
Measles/mumps/rubella vaccination
Bacillus Calmette-Guerin (intravesicular)
Influenza vaccination

Miscellaneous:
Bee sting
Bupropion
Chlorpropamide
Procainamide
Iodine
Carbon monoxide
Chloronaphthalene (in varnish)
Aminocaproic acid
Echinacea extract
Quetiapine

Source: *Williams Hematology*, 8th ed, Chap. 133, Table 133–3, p. 2169.

hemolytic anemia, thrombocytopenia, and renal injury. ADAMTS13 levels are normal in diarrhea-associated HUS.

- Diarrhea-negative HUS or atypical HUS is much less common than diarrhea-associated HUS. At least half of cases appear to be caused by inherited defects in complement regulatory proteins and activating components, including mutations in complement factor H, factor I, factor H-related proteins 1 and 3 (CFHR1, CFHR3), and C4 binding protein (C4BP). In addition, autoantibodies to factor H have been identified in some patients with atypical HUS, often in association with mutations in CFHR1 and CFHR3.

- The clinical presentation of diarrhea-negative HUS may be sporadic, recessive, or dominant. Many patients develop HUS in childhood, but some have their first episode in adulthood or remain asymptomatic. Occasional patients have long intervals between exacerbations, which may appear to be precipitated by infections, other illness, or pregnancy. The disease often recurs in patients with transplanted kidneys, probably because kidney transplantation does not alter the underlying complement defect.

TREATMENT OF THROMBOTIC MICROANGIOPATHIES

- The mainstay of therapy for TTP is plasma exchange (see **Table 91–3**), which removes antibody inhibitors and replenishes ADAMTS13.

- With the exception of factor H deficiency, and possibly APS and quinine-induced disease, no compelling evidence indicates that plasma therapy is effective for thrombotic microangiopathy caused by a mechanism other than ADAMTS13 deficiency. Regardless of mechanism, however, the clinical features are variable and overlapping. Consequently, plasma exchange may sometimes be used to treat apparent HUS or secondary thrombotic microangiopathy,

---

TABLE 91–3   **AN APPROACH TO THE TREATMENT AND MONITORING OF TTP**

Treatment:
Glucocorticoids (e.g., prednisone 2 mg/kg per day or equivalent)
Plasma exchange 1.5 volumes per day
Plasma infusion 15–30 mL/kg if plasma exchange will be delayed >12 hours
After the platelet count exceeds 50,000/μL, add aspirin 80 mg/day (optional) and routine thromboprophylaxis (e.g., low-molecular-weight heparin)
Continue until complete response for 3 days (platelets >150 × 10^9/L, LDH normal), then decrease plasma exchange to every other day for two more treatments and stop
If response is durable, taper glucocorticoids

Monitoring:
Neurologic status
Hemoglobin and platelet count
Blood film for schistocytes
LDH
Serum electrolytes, calcium, BUN, creatinine
Electrocardiogram, cardiac enzymes

Common complications:
Cardiac arrhythmias, infarction
Catheter-associated bleeding or thrombosis
Citrate toxicity (hypocalcemia, alkalosis)
Minor allergic reactions to plasma

TTP, thrombotic thrombocytopenic purpura; LDH, lactic acid dehydrogenase; BUN, blood urea nitrogen.
Source: *Williams Hematology*, 8th ed, Chap. 133, Table 133–4, p. 2171.

particularly in adults, based on the possibility that such patients may have an atypical presentation of TTP that will respond.

- After diagnosing TTP, or determining that the diagnosis is sufficiently likely to justify treatment, plasma exchange therapy should be started immediately. The optimal dose of plasma is not known, but a common practice is to perform plasma exchange once daily at a volume of 40 or 60 mL/kg, equivalent to 1 or 1.5 plasma volumes.
- Prompt treatment is essential and if plasma exchange must be delayed more than a few hours, plasma should be given by simple infusion at 20 to 40 mL/kg total dose per day, consistent with the patient's ability to tolerate the fluid load.
- Plasma exchange should be continued daily until the patient has a complete response, as shown by a platelet count greater than 150×10^9/L, lactic acid dehydrogenase (LDH) within the normal range, and resolution of nonfocal neurologic symptoms.
- The optimal schedule for tapering and discontinuing therapy has not been determined. A typical (however, not evidence-based) strategy is to continue plasma exchange until a complete response is sustained for a minimum of 2 days, and then reduce the frequency of plasma exchange to every other day (or twice per week) for several days. If the disease remains quiescent, then treatment can be stopped and the patient monitored closely for recurrence.
- The long-term mortality of TTP treated with plasma exchange ranges from 10 to 20 percent. Most deaths occur within a few days after presentation, and almost all occur within the first month.
- The duration of illness is quite variable. Complete response occurs after an average of 9 to 16 days of plasma exchange, and almost all responders are encompassed by a range of 2 to 40 days.
- Recurrences of disease more than 30 days after a complete response, occur in up to one-third of patients. Most relapses occur during the first year, but have been documented up to 13 years after diagnosis.
- TTP often is an autoimmune disease and the use of glucocorticoids is logical, although a beneficial effect has not been demonstrated conclusively. Common practice is to give prednisone or equivalent at a total daily dose of 1 or 2 mg/kg, in one or two doses, for the duration of plasma exchange, followed by tapering. An alternative regimen is methylprednisolone 1 g intravenously daily for 3 days.
- The use of antiplatelet agents in TTP is controversial. Aspirin and dipyridamole often are combined with plasma exchange but have not been shown conclusively to modify the course of TTP. Low-dose aspirin (e.g., 80 mg/day) has been suggested for thromboprophylaxis, once the platelet count exceeds 50×10^9/L.
- Transfusion of platelets may sometimes correlate with the acute deterioration and death in TTP, although direct harm is difficult to establish. Consequently, platelet transfusions are relatively contraindicated and should be reserved for the treatment of life-threatening hemorrhage, preferably after plasma exchange treatment has been initiated.
- TTP that is refractory to plasma exchange may respond to immunosuppression. Anecdotal experience suggests that vincristine may be beneficial, although its efficacy is difficult to assess. Dosing schedules have included 2 mg intravenously on day 1 followed by 1 mg on days 4 and 7, or 2 mg intravenously per week for 2 to 14 weeks. Cyclosporine has been used to treat TTP and may be effective in refractory disease. Apparent responses, with normalization of ADAMTS13 activity, have been observed with cyclosporine 2 to 3 mg/kg daily in two divided doses as an adjunct to plasma exchange, or without plasma exchange for early recurrences of TTP.
- Rituximab (375 mg/m^2 weekly for two to eight doses) resulted in an approximately 95 percent remission in patients with therapy-resistant TTP within 1 to 3 weeks of starting treatment, including a normal ADAMTS13 level and disappearance of anti–ADAMTS13 antibodies (if present).
- Other immunosuppressive regimens have included oral or intravenous cyclophosphamide, oral azathioprine, combination chemotherapy with cyclophosphamide,

doxorubicin, vincristine, and prednisone (CHOP), and autologous stem cell transplantation.
- Many reports suggest that splenectomy can result in lasting remissions or reduce the frequency of relapses for some patients with TTP who are refractory to plasma exchange or immunosuppressive therapy, presumably by removing a major site of anti–ADAMTS13 antibody production.
- The cornerstone for treatment of secondary thrombotic microangiopathy is management of the underlying disorder. In most cases, this is sufficient to ameliorate the manifestations of the thrombotic microangiopathy.

HEPARIN-INDUCED THROMBOCYTOPENIA

Epidemiology
- The frequency of HIT depends on the nature of the heparin used, dose and duration of heparin exposure, and clinical setting.
- The frequency of HIT in nonsurgical settings is clearly higher in patients treated with unfractionated, high-molecular-weight heparin (1–5%) than in patients treated with low-molecular-weight heparin (0.2–1%). Bovine-derived heparin may be associated with a higher incidence of HIT than porcine heparin. Newer, synthetic pentasaccharide anticoagulants may have a much lower or no risk of inducing HIT.
- HIT may be prevented by limiting the exposure time to heparin, and avoiding heparin flushes through intravenous lines. Heparin-bonded catheters can underlie the development of HIT.
- The greatest clinical risk factors for developing HIT are the patient's age and the nature of the patient's medical condition. HIT occurs rarely or never in pediatric patients, especially neonates. Patients being treated for medical conditions have a lower risk of developing HIT than do patients who are undergoing surgical procedures. Among surgical patients, those undergoing coronary artery bypass grafting, orthopedic procedures, or isolated limb perfusion are particularly vulnerable to developing HIT.
- Determination of the incidence of thrombosis in various settings has been hampered by the infrequency of HIT, and the need to carefully document both the diagnosis and the thrombotic complications. Nevertheless, some prospective studies suggest that the incidence of thrombosis is between 35 and 58 percent in patients with documented HIT. The ratio of arterial to venous thrombi is high (0.7:1).

Etiology and Pathogenesis
- HIT is an immune complex disorder of heparin therapy involving heparin–platelet factor (PF)-4 complexes. Such antibodies are not demonstrable in other forms of thrombocytopenia.
- Binding of these antibodies to platelets lead to platelet activation through the FcγRIIA and the formation of procoagulant platelet microparticles that contribute to the thrombosis.
- As part of this activation, HIT antibodies also bind to endothelial cells likely via PF4-surface glycosaminoglycan complexes. This binding may further increase vascular activation, augmenting local thrombosis.

Clinical Features
- The diagnosis of HIT is difficult to establish in a complicated patient who can have multiple causes for developing thrombocytopenia or thrombosis. A scoring system based on the severity of thrombocytopenia, timing of onset of symptoms, occurrence of thrombosis, and potential thrombocytopenia from other causes ("4 Ts") was developed to help maintain focus on potentially affected patients (Table 91–4).
- Typically, patients develop thrombocytopenia 5 to 10 days after the onset of heparin therapy unless exposure occurred within the preceding 3 months.

TABLE 91–4 THE 4 Ts

Clinical Sign	Points Per Category		
	0	1	2
Thrombocytopenia (acute)	Very low nadir (10 × 10⁹/L) or <30% fall	Low nadir (10–20 × 10⁹/L) or 30–50% fall	Moderate nadir (20–100 × 10⁹/L) or >50% fall
Timing of 1st event (thrombocytopenia or thrombosis)	≤4 days (unless prior heparin exposure in last 3 months)	Within 5–10 days (but not well documented) or ≤1 day (with exposure in last 3 months)	Documented occurrence in 5–10 days or ≤1 day with recent prior exposure
Thrombotic-related event	None	Common thrombi (DVT or line thrombus) or recurrent thrombus; erythematous skin lesion or not suspected thrombus	Major vessel thrombus or skin necrosis or skin lesion at site of heparin infusion
Thrombocytopenia (other causes)	Definite other cause is present	Possible other cause is present	No other strong explanation for thrombocytopenia

A score of 6–8 is high risk for HIT, 4–5 is intermediate risk, and 0–3 is low risk.
DVT, deep venous thrombosis.
Adapted with permission from Reilly MP, et al: Blood Oct 15;98(8):2442-2447, 2001.
Source: *Williams Hematology*, 8th ed, Chap. 133, Table 133–5, p. 2176.

- Bleeding manifestations secondary to the thrombocytopenia, such as petechiae, nosebleeds, and oozing from catheter sites, are not seen in HIT.
- Symptoms of venous thrombosis include those related to deep venous thrombosis of the lower or upper extremity and pulmonary embolism, adrenal infarctions, and cerebral venous thrombosis. Major venous obstruction can lead to limb gangrene.
- Arterial thrombi in this disease can be striking and were the first feature that led to the recognition of HIT as a distinct clinical entity. Common thrombotic complications include stroke, myocardial infarction, bowel infarction from mesenteric artery thrombosis, and renal infarction.

Laboratory Features
- Thrombocytopenia is the key laboratory finding in HIT. Most often it is moderate, ranging from 20 to 100 × 10⁹/L, or is represented by a 50 to 70 percent decline in platelet count. Rarely is the thrombocytopenia more severe or absent, as observed in some cases with skin necrosis.
- Although thrombin generation increases in HIT, patients rarely have decompensated disseminated intravascular coagulation.
- Two assay prototypes for confirming the diagnosis of HIT are available. One measures the Ig antibodies to the heparin–PF4 complex (antigen assay), and the other measures heparin-dependent antibodies that activate platelets (activation assay) in plasma or sera.
- Antigen assays are easily established in the laboratory and have a rapid turn-around time. The specificity of this test for the diagnosis of HIT is, however, limited. A recently described cause for a false-positive antigen test is the presence of anti-PF4 rather than anti-PF4/heparin antibodies.

- The activation assays are not commercially established because specific platelet donors are needed each time. Donor platelets can vary greatly in their sensitivity to activation by HIT sera. One of the earliest and best-established activation assays, serotonin-release assay, involves ^{14}C-serotonin release from platelets induced by HIT antibodies and heparin. An activation assay will have greater specificity than the antigen assay, although specificity may vary based on the experience of the reference center. Its major usefulness is in *post factum* documentation of the cause of thrombocytopenia.
- Other activation tests include platelet activation in a heparin-induced platelet activation assay (HIPA), luminography, and microparticle generation.
- A practical approach is that in patients with a high clinical risk of having HIT, heparin should be stopped and alternative treatment is started even before laboratory results are available. A positive antigen test and particularly a progressive increase in the number of platelets over the following days are confirmatory for HIT. A negative antigen test does not rule out HIT and should be repeated after 24 hours while the patient is undergoing alternative anticoagulant therapy. If the repeat assay is negative and platelet count does not increase, alternative diagnoses should be considered.
- Many patients with HIT often have complicated medical and surgical conditions, many of which can also cause thrombocytopenia. A differential diagnosis is listed in Table 91–5.

TABLE 91–5   **ALTERNATIVE CAUSES OF CLINICAL CONDITIONS SIMULATING HIT**

Thrombocytopenia
Increased destruction
- Acute immune thrombocytopenic purpura
- Dilutional thrombocytopenia
- Posttransfusion purpura
- Drug-induced thrombocytopenia
- Quinidine, quinine, trimethoprim-sulfamethoxazole, rifampicin, carbamazepine, diclofenac, ibuprofen
- Integrin $\alpha_{IIb}\beta b_3$ inhibitors: abciximab, tirofiban, eptifibatide
Decreased production
- Chemotherapy
- Malignancy
- Drug-related
- Thrombocytopenia and thrombosis
- Consumptive thrombohemorrhagic disorders
- Sepsis and disseminated intravascular coagulation
- Malignancies
- Disseminated intravascular coagulation in pregnancy or after snake bite
- Thrombotic thrombocytopenic purpura
- Hemolytic uremic syndrome
- Systemic lupus erythematosus

Thrombosis alone
- Venous stasis
- Central catheters
- Drugs
- Coumadin
- Vasculitis
- Antiphospholipid syndrome

Source: *Williams Hematology*, 8th ed, Chap. 133, Table 133–6, p. 2177.

Treatment of HIT

- An established diagnosis or high clinical suspicion of HIT should lead to immediate termination of heparin treatment. Since patients remain at high risk for thrombotic complications, alternative anticoagulant treatment should be instituted.
- Coumadin should not be used as the sole initial treatment of HIT because of the increased risk of untoward thrombosis, in particular skin gangrene. Low-molecular-weight heparin should not replace high-molecular-weight heparin because of cross-reactivity. Synthetic pentasaccharides may be considered as alternative anticoagulant treatment, although there is a single publication describing cross-reactivity with HIT antibodies.
- Other accepted drugs that are used in the treatment of patients with HIT are danaparoid sodium (no longer available in the United States), recombinant hirudin (lepirudin), and argatroban.
- Danaparoid is a mixture of low-molecular-weight heparanoids consisting of heparan sulfate, dermatan sulfate, and chondroitin sulfate. It has much greater anti-factor Xa activity than anti-factor IIa activity. Danaparoid is an effective anticoagulant that inhibits HIT antibody-induced platelet aggregation *in vitro*. Studies suggest danaparoid use improves platelet count recovery and decreases the incidence of serious thrombosis and death in patients with HIT.
- Lepirudin and argatroban directly inhibit thrombin. Both drugs are given intravenously and have rapid onset of action. Lepirudin binds to two sites on thrombin, the catalytic site and a fibrinogen-binding site, whereas argatroban binds only to the active site. Lepirudin prolongs the aPTT, so this test can be used to monitor effective dosing.
- Lepirudin is excreted in the urine, and its half life is dramatically increased in patients with renal failure. Lepirudin induces antilepirudin antibodies in approximately half of patients who receive the drug. These antibodies rarely alter biologic activity, but do tend to prolong the drug's half-life, necessitating careful monitoring by aPTT.
- Argatroban is synthesized from arginine and is rapidly metabolized in the liver. It affects both the aPTT and PT.
- Use of lepirudin and argatroban in HIT is efficacious; the incidence of thrombotic complication is reduced, perhaps by half, and the time to platelet count recovery is shortened. However, bleeding complications can occur.
- As with danaparoid, lepirudin or argatroban should be given until patients recover from thrombocytopenia before adding and then switching to a prolonged course of an oral anticoagulant.

For a more detailed discussion, see J. Evan Sadler and Mortimer Poncz: Antibody-Mediated Thrombotic Disorders: Thrombotic Thrombocytopenic Purpura and Heparin-Induced Thrombocytopenia. Chap. 133, p. 2163 in *Williams Hematology*, 8th ed.

PART XII

TRANSFUSION AND HEMAPHERESIS

CHAPTER 92
Red Cell Transfusion

STORAGE AND PRESERVATION OF BLOOD

- Erythrocytes are preserved by liquid storage at 4 °C or by frozen storage at either −80 °C or −150 °C.
- Preservative solutions for liquid storage all contain glucose, to provide energy, and citrate buffer at an acid pH to prevent coagulation by binding calcium and to counter the marked rise in pH that occurs when blood is cooled to 4 °C.
- CPD-adenine is the preservative solution most used now in the United States. It contains adenine, citrate, phosphate, and dextrose (glucose).
- Adenine is added to help maintain intracellular levels of ATP.
- Erythrocytes are then separated and stored in an additive solution that contains glucose, adenine, and mannitol.
- The remainder of the blood collection is separated into plasma and platelets.
- Stored erythrocytes develop the so-called storage lesion, characterized in part by reduced levels of ATP, which interfere with glucose metabolism and reduce cell viability. 2,3-Bisphosphoglycerate levels also rapidly fall during storage, which increase the oxygen affinity of hemoglobin and thereby decreases the initial effectiveness of reinfused red cells. Potassium also leaks rapidly from stored cells.
- Frozen storage requires a cryoprotective agent to avoid hemolysis during freezing and thawing. Glycerol is the most frequently used agent. With proper technique, more than 80 percent of erythrocytes will survive frozen storage and function normally after transfusion.

WHOLE-BLOOD PREPARATIONS

- A unit of whole blood contains 435 to 500 mL of blood and 14 to 15 mL of preservative-anticoagulant solution for each 100 mL. Thus, if 450 mL of blood is collected, stored, and transfused, the patient will receive about 515 mL of total fluid.
- Blood collected in CDPA-1 (CDP with adenine) may be used after storage up to 35 days.
- There are very few, if any, indications for whole blood, and it is rarely used in modern transfusion practice.

FRESH BLOOD

- When blood is stored, viable platelets are depleted within 48 hours, and the activity of coagulation factors V, VIII, and IX falls significantly.
- Thrombocytopenia and deficiency of the labile coagulation factors may occur in patients who receive transfusions of banked blood equal to their total blood volume in 24 hours.
- Fresh blood is often requested in an effort to avoid administration of blood deficient in these hemostatic components.
- It is better to treat such patients with a combination of packed red cells, fresh-frozen plasma, and platelet concentrates.
- Whole blood less than 5 to 7 days old may be transfused to patients with severe renal or hepatic disease, or in newborns receiving exchange transfusion, in order to avoid infusing excess free potassium.
- Patients who require massive transfusion should be given at least part of the transfusion as blood less than a few days old in order to avoid oxygen release problems caused by depletion of red cell 2,3-bisphosphoglycerate and to prevent replacing with platelet poor blood.
- Patients with chronic transfusion-dependent anemia should probably receive blood less than 10 days old in order to maximize the interval between transfusions and to minimize iron accumulation.

PACKED RED BLOOD CELLS

- Packed red blood cells can be prepared from stored blood any time before the expiration date by centrifugation and removal of plasma to give a hematocrit of 60 to 90 percent.
- Red cells packed to a hematocrit of less than 80 percent can be stored until the expiration date of the original blood.
- Red cells, rather than whole blood, should be used for replacement of a red cell deficit.
- Packed red cells and electrolyte solutions are as effective as whole blood in replacing surgical blood loss.

LEUKOCYTE-POOR BLOOD

- Best prepared by passing blood or packed cells through a special filter that removes leukocytes.
- Used to prevent or avoid febrile reactions to leukocytes or platelets in previously sensitized patients; to minimize transmission of viral diseases, such as HIV or cytomegalovirus infections; and perhaps in patients awaiting kidney transplant.

WASHED RED CELLS

- Obtained from whole blood by centrifugation techniques.
- Must be used within 24 hours of preparation because of the danger of bacterial contamination.
- Indicated for patients who are hypersensitive to plasma.
- Sometimes used in neonatal transfusions to reduce the amount of anticoagulant, extracellular potassium, etc., infused.

FROZEN RED CELLS

- May be stored for years but cost two to three times as much as stored liquid blood.
- Somewhat leukocyte poor and almost free of plasma.
- May be used for autotransfusion, to ensure a supply of rare blood, or to reduce sensitization to histocompatibility antigens in potential transplant patients.

INDICATIONS FOR TRANSFUSION THERAPY

- Informed consent should be obtained and documented before transfusion therapy is given.

Hemorrhage and Shock

- Volume support is of primary concern, but replacement of red cells is also necessary with larger losses of blood.
- Packed red cells with crystalloids or albumin are as effective as whole blood in replacing volume loss.

Surgery

- Blood loss (even greater than 1000 mL) may be safely replaced with crystalloids.
- Because of the hazards of blood transfusion (see below) every effort should be made to minimize the use of blood for volume replacement in surgery.

Burns

- Severe burns require extensive volume replacement in the first 24 hours.
- Plasma loss occurs over the next 5 days and can be replaced with plasma and colloids.
- Anemia can be treated with packed red cells.

Anemia

- Patients with stable anemia with a hemoglobin level above 7 g/dL should not be transfused unless they are elderly or have cardiac or pulmonary disease.
- Attempts to improve the efficiency of transfusion with longer circulation times at end of line by using young red cells ("neocytes") have had limited success.

MODE OF ADMINISTRATION

- It is essential that the person administering blood or a blood component read the label to ensure that the unit to be used was selected by the laboratory for the particular patient.
- Usually blood does not need to be warmed unless amounts greater than 3 liters are to be given at greater than 100 mL/min. At the usual rate of administration, the aggregates that may develop in patients with high-titer cold agglutinins are dispersed when the blood reaches body temperature.
- Blood being given to patients with cold agglutinins or cryoglobulinemia should be warmed to prevent further vascular damage.
- Blood should be given slowly in the first 30 minutes to minimize an adverse reaction.
- Drugs or medications should not be added to blood or blood components.

SPECIAL SITUATIONS

Autologous Transfusion

- Minimizes the probability of adverse reactions to transfusion, such as transmission of disease or alloimmunization.
- May be achieved by preoperative collection and storage of blood, immediate preoperative phlebotomy and hemodilution with postoperative return of the blood, or reinfusion of blood collected intraoperatively.
- In some patients, erythropoietin has been given to permit increasing the amount of blood taken preoperatively. Approximately one additional unit of blood can be collected if the patient is supplemented with erythropoietin, making the actual benefit questionable.
- Autologous donation is ideal for patients with rare blood types or with antibodies that make cross-matching difficult or impossible.

Directed or Designated Donations

- Donors recruited from among family or friends are no safer than volunteer blood donors. Graft-versus-host disease is a greater risk if blood is donated by family members.

TRANSFUSION REACTIONS

- Majority of fatal transfusion reactions are due to management-clerical errors.
- Up to 20 percent of all transfusions may lead to some type of adverse reaction.

Immediate Reactions

Acute Hemolytic Reactions

- May occur intravascularly, usually because of ABO incompatibility, or extravascularly.
- Intravascular hemolysis may lead to disseminated intravascular coagulation (DIC) or to ischemic necrosis of tissues, particularly the kidney.
- Patients may develop fever, low-back pain, sensation of chest compression, hypotension, nausea, or vomiting.
- The transfusion should be terminated immediately when an acute reaction is suspected, and measures to control hemorrhage, if present, and to prevent renal damage instituted promptly.
- Laboratory diagnosis is based on evidence of hemolysis (hemoglobinemia, methemalbuminemia, hemoglobinuria) and detection of a blood group incompatibility.
- Renal damage may be prevented by hydration with addition of a diuretic if necessary to maintain urinary flow greater than 100 mL/h. Mannitol may be used at an initial dose of 100 mL of a 20 percent solution given intravenously over 5 minutes. Furosemide in a dose of 40 to 80 mg intravenously may be more effective.
- If oliguria occurs, standard measures for acute renal failure should be instituted.
- The risk of sequelae is dependent on the amount of incompatible blood given. Severe complications rarely occur if less than 200 mL of red cells have been transfused.

Febrile Reactions

- Fever may be caused by a hemolytic reaction, sensitivity to leukocytes or platelets, bacterial pyrogens, cytokines released by stored leukocytes or unidentified causes.
- Thirty percent of all transfusion reactions are nonhemolytic, febrile reactions.
- A febrile reaction of itself is not an indication for termination of the transfusion, but one should not hesitate to stop if there is any doubt about the cause.
- Chills may indicate a more serious situation, but there are no reliable guidelines.
- Sensitization to leukocyte or platelet antigens is a common cause of febrile reactions.
- At least seven transfusions are usually required for sensitization, but previously pregnant women may be sensitized after only one or two.
- Clinical findings are primarily fever, which may continue to rise for 2 to 6 hours after the transfusion is stopped and may continue for 12 hours.
- Diagnosis depends on demonstration of antibodies to leukocyte or platelet antigens. Most reactions are a result of antibodies to granulocytes.
- Treatment is supportive.
- Many reactions can be prevented by use of a leukocyte filter, especially if applied to the unit of blood shortly after collection.

Transfusion-Related Acute Lung Injury (TRALI)

- TRALI is a syndrome of acute hypoxia as a result of noncardiogenic pulmonary edema that follows transfusion. All blood components have been implicated in TRALI, but most frequent are plasma-containing products, which account for 50 to 63 percent of TRALI fatalities.

- The precise mechanisms of the capillary leak syndrome in TRALI have not been fully determined, but two main hypotheses have been proposed. One involves white cell antibody-mediated TRALI and the other cytokine-mediated TRALI.
- It is often impossible to distinguish TRALI from acute respiratory distress syndrome. The typical presentation of TRALI is the sudden development of dyspnea, severe hypoxemia (O_2 saturation <90% in room air), hypotension, and fever that develop within 6 hours after transfusion and usually resolve with supportive care within 48 to 96 hours. Although hypotension is considered one of the important signs in diagnosing TRALI, hypertension can occur in some cases.

Pulmonary Hypersensitivity Reaction (Noncardiogenic Pulmonary Edema)

- Leukocyte incompatibility may also cause acute respiratory distress, chills, fever, and tachycardia as a consequence of pulmonary edema.
- Donor leukocytes may react with recipient antibodies, or donor antibodies may react with recipient leukocytes.
- Almost 25 percent of multiparous women have antibodies that can cause this reaction.
- Can occur with transfusion of platelets, plasma, whole blood, or packed red cells.
- Onset is usually within 4 hours of transfusion.
- Chest films show bilateral diffuse, patchy pulmonary densities without cardiac enlargement.
- Treatment is supportive.
- In a healthy individual, symptoms subside in less than 24 hours, and the pulmonary infiltrates disappear within 4 days.

Allergic Reactions

- Transfusion may result in generalized pruritus and urticaria, and occasionally there may be bronchospasm, angioedema, or anaphylaxis.
- The cause is poorly understood, but may be hypersensitivity to plasma proteins or other substances in the administered product.
- These reactions are usually mild and respond to antihistamine drugs, but epinephrine may be required in some cases.

Anti-IgA in IgA-Deficient Recipient

- Severe anaphylactic reactions may occur in IgA-deficient patients who have formed anti-IgA antibodies.
- Deficiency or absence of IgA occurs in about 1 in 800 people.
- IgA in the transfused product reacts with circulating antibody in the recipient. Less than 10 mL plasma can cause a reaction.
- Symptoms are dyspnea, nausea, chills, abdominal cramps, emesis, diarrhea, and profound hypotension. There is no fever.
- Diagnosis depends on demonstration of IgA deficiency and anti-IgA antibodies in the recipient.
- Reactions can usually be prevented by using washed red cells. Platelet or granulocyte transfusions for sensitized patients should be from donors with absent IgA.

Bacterial Contamination

- Blood may be contaminated by cold-growing organisms (*Pseudomonas* or coli-aerogenes group) that utilize citrate and may therefore lead to formation of visible clots.
- Infusion of blood containing large numbers of gram-negative organisms leads to endotoxin shock, with fever, hypotension, abdominal pain, vomiting, diarrhea, and vascular collapse, beginning immediately after infusion is started or 30 minutes or more after the infusion.
- Diagnosis may be made by examining a Gram stain of plasma obtained by low-speed centrifugation of some of the transfused blood. If the blood is heavily contaminated, organisms should be seen in every oil immersion field.

- Bacterial contamination of blood is uncommon if disposable plastic blood bags are used, but contamination may be a significant hazard with platelet concentrates stored at room temperature.

Circulatory Overload

- Congestive heart failure with pulmonary edema may develop following transfusion in patients with cardiovascular compromise. Treatment is primarily with diuretics.
- Patients with severe chronic anemia may also develop congestive heart failure if transfused rapidly. Diuretics should be given and the transfusion limited to 2 mL/kg/h.

Microaggregates in Blood

- Particles of 13 to 100 microns in size ("microaggregates") and consisting largely of platelets and fibrin in banked blood are not removed by the usual filters in transfusion sets.
- Such particles can cause pulmonary insufficiency when massive transfusion of banked blood is given using standard filters, but this can be prevented with microaggregate filters.

Citrate Intoxication

- Blood transfused into adults at a rate greater than 1 liter in 10 minutes will cause significant reduction in ionized calcium concentrations and lead to myocardial depression and ECG changes.
- Can be prevented by giving 10 mL of 10 percent calcium gluconate intravenously for every liter of citrated blood administered.

Delayed Reactions

Delayed Hemolytic Reaction

- Previously undetected alloantibodies may appear 4 to 14 days after transfusion and cause destruction of the transfused cells.
- Usually an anamnestic response to a previous immunization from prior transfusion or pregnancy.
- Clinical findings are jaundice, falling hemoglobin level, and a positive direct antiglobulin reaction (Coombs test).
- Delayed hemolytic reactions may be mild and probably are frequently undetected.

Posttransfusion Purpura

- Thrombocytopenia caused by antibodies to a platelet-specific antigen may develop shortly after transfusion (see Chap. 74).

Transmission of Disease

- The greatest risks are viral agents such as hepatitis B or C or HIV.

Other Adverse Effects

- Graft-versus-host disease is an uncommon complication of transfusion, preventable by administering irradiated blood.
- Iron overload may occur in patients who require chronic transfusion therapy.
- Alloimmunization to antigens not included in routine cross-matching occurs in immunocompetent patients receiving multiple transfusions and creates a major problem in obtaining blood for some patients with chronic anemia.

For a more detailed discussion, see Norma B. Lerner, Majed A. Rafaai, and Neil Blumberg: Red Cell Transfusion. Chap. 140, p. 2287 in *Williams Hematology*, 8th ed.

CHAPTER 93
Transfusion of Platelets

PLATELET PRODUCTS FOR TRANSFUSION

- Random donor platelets are prepared by centrifugation techniques that yield from 7 to 10×10^{10} platelets per unit of blood.
- Platelets so obtained are suspended in citrated autologous plasma and are significantly contaminated with leukocytes. Several units of platelets are pooled to provide sufficient platelets for transfusion (4 to 6 U for an adult).
- Single-donor platelets are prepared from a single individual by plateletpheresis. Each plateletpheresis contains approximately 3 to 4×10^{11} platelets, significantly contaminated with leukocytes.
- Fresh whole blood is used for platelet transfusion in children younger than 2-years-old who have undergone open-heart surgery.

STORAGE OF PLATELET CONCENTRATES

- Platelet suspensions may be stored with continuous agitation for 5 days at 20 °C to 24 °C in plastic containers, which allow for adequate diffusion of oxygen.
- *In vivo* function of stored platelets is nearly normal.
- Platelets may be stored frozen in plasma containing dimethyl sulfoxide (DMSO).
- Viability of thawed platelets is 50 percent that of fresh platelets.
- Frozen storage is usually used to provide autologous platelets for use in patients who are refractory to allogeneic platelet transfusions.

CHOICE OF A PLATELET PREPARATION

- Platelet transfusion may begin with random-donor pooled platelets. However, single-donor platelets are a better product with less risk of transmission of infectious agents. As such, whole blood–derived platelet use has fallen to 15 to 20 percent of the platelet doses transfused in the United States because of blood center convenience (no need to separate from whole blood) and the superiority of single donor platelets.
- ABO-compatible platelets should be used whenever possible.

CLINICAL RESPONSE AND COMPLICATIONS OF PLATELET TRANSFUSION

- The response to infusion of random donor platelets can be evaluated by calculating the *corrected count increment (P)*:

$$P = C \times S/U \ (platelets/L)$$

Where C = measured platelet increase (platelets/L)
S = body surface area in square meters
U = number of units of platelet given
- Average corrected count increment is 10×10^9/L.
- In a single-donor plateletpheresis product, there are about the same number of platelets as in five random-donor units.

- The 20-hour increment is two-thirds of the 1-hour increment under normal conditions (absence of alloimmunization, ongoing hyperconsumption of disseminated intravascular coagulation or bleeding, or pooling in an enlarged spleen).
- Additional factors that lower the corrected count increment are loss of platelet viability in storage, stem cell transplantation, or drug therapies (e.g., amphotericin).

Alloimmunization

- Frequently develops in patients receiving random-donor platelet transfusions.
- Should be considered if two to three consecutive random donor transfusions produce a corrected count increment of less than 3×10^9/L.
- Usually caused by development of antibody against HLA antigen on the platelet surface. Leukocyte depletion of platelet products may reduce alloimmunization.
- Patients may respond to single-donor platelets from either family members or unrelated individuals selected by matching for the HLA-A and -B antigens.
- Rh-negative recipients may become sensitized to Rh-positive red cells contaminating infused platelets.
- During and after platelet transfusion chills and fever may occur from alloantibodies against contaminating leukocytes.
- Leukocyte depletion reduces the frequency of chills and fever.
- Febrile reactions may be caused by allergic reactions to some component(s) of the suspending plasma.
- Graft-versus-host disease may occur in immunosuppressed patients given unirradiated platelet transfusions.

Transmission of Microorganisms

- Chills immediately upon infusion of platelets suggest bacterial contamination of the unit.
- Contamination of stored platelets by bacteria is much more common than contamination of other blood products, because they are stored at room temperature and because of their normally turbid appearance, an infected platelet unit may not appear physically different from a normal unit.
- Platelet transfusion can transmit viruses, e.g., hepatitis B and C, HIV, and cytomegalovirus.

INDICATIONS FOR PLATELET TRANSFUSION

- Platelet counts of greater than 5 to 10×10^9/L are adequate to protect patients against life-threatening spontaneous bleeding.
- Invasive procedures may require raising the platelet count to approximately 60×10^9/L.
- ϵ-Aminocaproic acid (3 to 5 g orally q 6 h) can reduce mucosal bleeding in thrombocytopenic patients.

Thrombocytopenia As a Result of Underproduction

- Platelets should be transfused prophylactically for a platelet count of 5×10^9/L or less, unless the patient has little hope of significant recovery from the underlying cause of thrombocytopenia, in which case bleeding should inform the decision to transfuse.
- Transfusion to maintain platelet counts greater than 20×10^9/L without regard to special circumstances has no support from clinical studies and results in waste of platelets and unnecessary risks to patients.
- The decision whether to transfuse platelets in the range of 5 to 20×10^9/L must be made on an individual basis using clinical considerations such as the presence of fever and sepsis, the presence of gastrointestinal ulceration or bleeding, the administration of drugs that interfere with platelet function, abnormalities of coagulation factors and/or a very high leukocyte count.

Thrombocytopenia Caused by Platelet Loss, Sequestration, or Destruction

- Massive red blood cell transfusion only rarely requires prophylactic platelet transfusion unless there is abnormal bleeding.
- Prophylactic platelet transfusion is not indicated for the thrombocytopenia that develops after cardiopulmonary bypass unless there is abnormal bleeding.
- Thrombocytopenia from splenomegaly and sequestration of platelets does not usually require prophylactic platelet transfusion unless an invasive procedure is to be done.
- Patients with immune thrombocytopenia do not usually require platelet transfusion.
- If bleeding is life-threatening, 3 to 6 units of random-donor platelets per square meter of body surface area may raise the platelet count for 12 to 48 hours.
- The same considerations apply for other disorders with accelerated destruction of platelets, e.g., thrombotic thrombocytopenic purpura, disseminated intravascular coagulation.
- Transfusion of washed maternal platelets to an infant is indicated in neonatal alloimmune thrombocytopenia. Unfortunately, arranging for apheresis of the mother often is difficult, so transfusion of platelet concentrates to neonates who are severely thrombocytopenic or bleeding is appropriate and lifesaving. It is not appropriate to wait for the laboratory confirmation of the diagnosis in suspected cases.

Qualitative Platelet Disorders

- Platelet transfusion is not indicated for extrinsic platelet disorders, e.g., uremia, von Willebrand disease, hyperglobulinemia.
- Inherited intrinsic platelet disorders are often mild and do not require platelet transfusion except for severe bleeding and surgery.
- Acquired intrinsic platelet disorders usually do not require platelet transfusion unless the patient is also thrombocytopenic.

 For a more detailed discussion, see Mike Murphy and Ralph Vassallo: Preservation and Clinical Use of Platelets, Chap. 141, p. 2301 in *Williams Hematology*, 8th ed.

CHAPTER 94
Therapeutic Hemapheresis

- Therapeutic apheresis is the application of blood cell separation techniques to treat certain clinical conditions.
- A continuous-flow blood separator is usually used.
- Table 94–1 contains the principal applications of the technique.
- Hemapheresis is usually used in hematologic therapy for acute problems.
- Adverse effects infrequent and mild: hypotension, urticaria, hypocalcemia.
- Cytapheresis refers to removal or exchange of a blood cell element, e.g., leukapheresis, plateletpheresis, erythrocytapheresis.
- Plasmapheresis refers to removal or exchange of plasma.

PLATELETPHERESIS

- Thrombocythemia or extreme thrombocytosis can usually be managed pharmacologically.
- Plateletpheresis is useful for those who need rapid, temporary reduction of the platelet count in emergent conditions (e.g., ongoing thrombosis) or for patients who cannot tolerate drug therapy (e.g., early pregnancy).
- If plateletpheresis is required in patients with thrombocythemia requiring urgent platelet reduction, pharmacologic therapy should be administered simultaneously for long-term control.
- Reduction in the platelet count of about 50 percent may be achieved with each procedure, but the platelet count returns to pretreatment value in a few days.

LEUKAPHERESIS

- Leukostasis may be ameliorated by leukapheresis with rapid cytoreduction in patients with acute myelogenous leukemia whose leukocyte count is greater than 50 to 100×10^9/L; patients with acute lymphocytic leukemia whose leukocyte count is greater than 75 to 100×10^9/L; or patients with chronic myelogenous leukemia (CML) whose leukocyte count is greater than 300×10^9/L, or who have $> 50 \times 10^9$/L blasts.
- Unfortunately, there are no clearly established thresholds, so that patients with any blast count who have signs of leukostasis should undergo leukapheresis.
- Therapeutic leukapheresis prior to chemotherapy reduces tumor burden and may minimize metabolic abnormalities due to tumor lysis.
- Therapeutic leukapheresis can lower the white cell counts, reduce organomegaly, and reduce tumor burden in chronic lymphocytic leukemia, but cytotoxic therapy is required for disease control.
- Therapeutic leukapheresis may be used in lieu of chemotherapy to treat CML, e.g., in pregnancy, to allow for delay in starting chemotherapy until after the first trimester or longer.
- In acute or chronic leukemia, a single therapeutic leukapheresis will reduce the leukocyte count by 25 to 50 percent.
- The rate of mobilization of cells and the rate of cell proliferation dictate the frequency of therapeutic leukapheresis required to achieve goal.
- Photopheresis, extracorporeal photochemotherapy, can improve erythroderma in cutaneous T-cell lymphoma (Sézary syndrome). Leukocytes removed by cytapheresis are treated with 8-methoxypsoralen and ultraviolet light and returned to patient.

TABLE 94–1	THERAPEUTIC HEMAPHERESIS TECHNIQUES

Cell depletion
  Plateletpheresis
  Leukapheresis
Blood component exchange
  Plasma exchange (plasmapheresis)
  Red cell exchange
Blood component modification
  Selective extraction of a plasma constituent
  Photopheresis

Source: *Williams Hematology*, 8th ed, Chap. 26, Table 26–1.

- Leukapheresis can be used to harvest lymphocytes, dendritic cells, or allogeneic or autologous blood stem cells for immunotherapy or stem cell transplantation.

ERYTHROCYTAPHERESIS (RED CELL EXCHANGE)

- Red cell exchange carries the same potential hazards as blood transfusion.
- Indications for red cell exchange in sickle cell disease include priapism, unremitting painful crises, acute chest syndrome, stroke, and prior to radiographic studies requiring hyperosmolar contrast medium. Its use during pregnancy, for chronic painful crises, and prior to surgery is controversial.
- Acute neurologic symptoms have occurred in sickle cell anemia patients undergoing red cell exchange for priapism.
- Red cell exchange has been used to decrease parasite load in severe falciparum malaria and extreme polycythemia.

PLASMA EXCHANGE THERAPY

- Plasma exchange is used in disorders in which there is a known or presumed abnormal plasma constituent to remove pathologic material in the plasma (e.g., thrombotic thrombocytopenic purpura or hyperviscosity syndrome in Waldenstrom macroglobulinemia).
- An exchange of 1 plasma volume reduces the abnormal plasma constituent by approximately 65 percent and an exchange of 2 plasma volumes reduces the abnormal plasma constituent by approximately 88 percent.
- Alterations in plasma components after plasma exchange include reduced levels of coagulation factors after large volume exchange and replacement with albumin and crystalloid, but bleeding is rare. Factor levels are restored over next 72 hours; serum immunoglobulin levels are decreased after repeated 1-volume plasma exchanges and replacement with albumin. It takes several weeks for levels to return to normal.
- Mortality associated with the procedure of plasma exchange is less than 3 in 10,000 procedures with today's technology.
- Table 94–2 lists disorders for which plasma exchange may be useful, and include thrombotic thrombocytopenic purpura, renal failure associated with multiple myeloma, hyperviscosity syndrome due to paraproteins (esp. macroglobulinemia, cold agglutinin disease with severe hemolysis not responding to other measures, cryoglobulinemia with vasculitis, glomerulonephritis, severe Raynaud syndrome, removal of coagulation factor inhibitors, recipients of ABO-incompatible marrow transplants prior to transplantation, posttransfusion purpura).
- See Table 94–3 for other antibody-mediated disease indications.

TABLE 94–2	INDICATION CATEGORIES FOR PLASMA EXCHANGE
Goal	Example
Immunoglobulin removal	
Abnormal physical properties	Hyperviscosity syndrome
Specific antibody	Goodpasture syndrome
Nonimmunoglobulin constituent removal	Familial hypercholesterolemia
Factor replacement	Thrombotic thrombocytopenic purpura

Source: *Williams Hematology*, 8th ed, Chap. 26, Table 26–3, p. 385.

TABLE 94–3	EXAMPLES OF SPECIFIC ANTIBODIES IN DISEASES TREATED WITH PLASMA EXCHANGE
Antibody Specificity	Disease
Autoantibodies	
Motor endplate acetylcholine receptor	Myasthenia gravis
Nerve ending calcium channel active zone	Lambert-Eaton myasthenic syndrome
Peripheral nerve myelin	Guillain-Barré syndrome, chronic inflammatory demyelinating polyneuropathy
Red cell I/i	Cold agglutinin disease
Factor VIII	Acquired hemophilia
a3 Chain of type IV collagen	Goodpasture syndrome
Alloantibodies	
HPA-1a or other platelet antigen	Posttransfusion purpura
Anti-A, anti-B	ABO-incompatible transplant
Anti-D	Hydrops fetalis
Factor VIII	Hemophilia A inhibitor

Source: *Williams Hematology*, 8th ed, Chap. 26, Table 26–4, p. 386.

For a more detailed discussion, see Bruce C. McLeod: Principles of Therapeutic Apheresis: Indications, Efficacy, and Complications. Chap. 26, p. 383 in *Williams Hematology*, 8th ed.

Table of Normal Values

Laboratory Variables Relevant to Hematologic Diagnosis (Normal Adult Values)

BLOOD CELLS

Variable (Common Abbreviations)	Units	Values
Hematocrit (HCT) or Packed cell volume (PCV)	mL red cells/dL blood or %	M = 42–51 F = 36–46
Hemoglobin (Hb, Hgb)	g/dL blood	M = 14–18 F = 12–16
Red cell count (RBC, RCC)	$10^6/\mu L$ or $10^{12}/L$	M = 4.5–6.0 F = 4.1–5.1
Mean cell volume (MCV)	fL/cell	M = 80–96 F = 79–94
Mean cell hemoglobin (MCH)	pg/cell	27–33
Mean cell hemoglobin concentration (MCHC)	g/dL red cells	33–36
Red cell distribution width (RDW)	percent	<15
Reticulocyte count	percent of red cells	0.5–1.5
Reticulocyte count, absolute	$\times 10^{12}/L$	M = 35,000–75,000 F = 25,000–65,000
Reticulocyte hemoglobin (CHr)	pg/cell	27–33
Total blood volume (TBV)	mL/kg	65–85[+]; 55–75[#]
Plasma volume (PV)	mL/kg	39–44
Red cell mass (RCM)	mL/kg	25–35
Platelet count	$10^3/\mu L$ or $10^9/L$	175–450
White cell count (WBC, WCC)	$10^3/\mu L$ or $10^9/L$	4.8–10.8
Absolute monocyte count	$10^3/\mu L$ or $10^9/L$	0.3–0.8
Absolute neutrophil count	$10^3/\mu L$ or $10^9/L$	1.8–7.7
Absolute lymphocyte count	$10^3/\mu L$ or $10^9/L$	1.0–4.8
CD3-positive lymphocytes	$10^3/\mu L$ or $10^9/L$	700–1900
CD4-positive lymphocytes	$10^3/\mu L$ or $10^9/L$	400–1400
CD8-positive lymphocytes	$10^3/\mu L$ or $10^9/L$	200–700
CD19-positive lymphocytes	$10^3/\mu L$ or $10^9/L$	50–375

HEMOGLOBIN ELECTROPHORESIS*

Hemoglobin A1	Percent of total hemoglobin	96.1–98.3
Hemoglobin A2	Percent of total hemoglobin	1.2–3.9
Hemoglobin F	Percent of total hemoglobin	0.1–1.2

COAGULATION TESTS

Prothrombin time (PT)	Seconds to clot	12–14
International Normalized Ratio (INR)	None	0.8–1.2
Partial thromboplastin time (PTT)	Seconds to clot	19–30
Thrombin time	Seconds to clot	10–15

(continued)

COAGULATION TESTS (CONTINUED)

Variable (Common Abbreviations)	Units	Values
Bleeding time		
Ivy	Minutes	3–6
Template	Minutes	6–10
Closure time (PFA-100)	Seconds	<175
Collagen/epinephrine (CEPI)		
Clot retraction	Percent in 1 hour	>40
Fibrinogen	mg/dL plasma	188–381
D-Dimer	ng/mL	<400
Factor II, V, and VII	Percent of normal mean	50–150
Factor VIII: c activity	Percent of normal mean	50–200
Willebrand factor activity	Percent of normal mean	60–200§
Willebrand factor antigen	Percent of normal mean	50–160§
	mg/L	~100
Factor VIII-inhibitor	Bethesda units	0–0.5
Factor IX	Percent of normal mean	50–150
	Mg/L	~4.0
Factor X	Percent of normal mean	50–150
	mg/L	~10
Factor XI	Percent of normal mean	50–150
	mg/L	~7.0
Factor XII	Percent of normal mean	50–150
Factor XIII	Percent of normal mean	70–130
α2- antiplasmin	Percent of normal mean	80–120
Plasminogen	Percent of normal mean	80–120
Antithrombin:		
Functional assay	Percent of normal mean	80–120
Immunologic assay	mg/dl	22–33
Protein C	Percent of normal mean	70–140
	μg/mL	3.0–5.0
Activated protein C resistance	APC ratio	>1.5
Protein S	Percent of normal mean	65–140
Total	μg/mL	20–25
Free	μg/mL	6–10
Free/total ratio	Unitless	~0.4
Fibrin degradation products	μg/mL	<20
(latex particles)		
Platelet Aggregation (in		
platelet-rich plasma)		
With collagen (2 μg/mL)	Percent of control	70–95
With arachidonic acid	Percent of control	70–100
(0.5 mM)		
With ADP 5 μM	Percent of control	70–90
With ADP 10 μM	Percent of control	70–90
With epinephrine (5 μM)	Percent of control	75–90
With ristocetin (1.0 mg/mL)	Percent of control	60–80
Platelet ATP release (in blood)		
With thrombin (1 unit)	nmoles of ATP	>0.5
With collagen (2 mg/mL)	nmoles of ATP	0.5–1.7
(5 mg/mL)	nmoles of ATP	0.9–1.7
With arachidonic acid (0.5 mM)	nmoles of ATP	0.56–1.4
ADP (5 mM)	nmoles of ATP	0–0.7
ADP (19 mM)	nmoles of ATP	0.38–1.71

RELEVANT BLOOD CHEMISTRIES

Variable (Common Abbreviations)	Units	Values
Serum haptoglobin	mg/dL	30–200
Serum iron	μg/dL	M = 75–175
	μmol/L	M = 13–31
	μg/dL	F = 65–165
	μmol/L	F = 11–29
Serum total iron	μg/dL	260–420
binding capacity	μmol/L	44–80
Saturation of total iron binding capacity	Percent	15–45
Serum ferritin	ng/mL or μg/L	M = 15–250
		F = 11–125
		F >40 yrs = 12–250
Serum soluble truncated transferrin	mg/L	1.0–3.7
receptor (sTfR)	nmol/L	9–28
Serum folate	nmol/L	7–45
Red cell folate	nmol/L	300–1000
	ng/mL	130–475
Serum Vitamin B_{12}	pg/mL	200–1000

Abbreviations: kg = kilograms, g = grams, mg = milligrams, μg = micrograms, pg = picograms, ng = nanograms, L = liter, dL = deciliter, mL = milliliters, μL = microliter, fL = femtaliter, nmol = nanomoles, ADP = adenosine diphosphate, ATP = adenosine triphosphate.
*Adult levels reached by about 1 year. Newborns have 60–80% HbF and 20 to 40% of Hb A1.
+TBV derived from measurement of plasma volume.
#TBV derived from measurement of red cell mass.
§May be as much as 20% lower in Blood type O individuals.

Values in infancy and childhood are not included (see Chap. 1 of this Manual and Chap. 7 of *Williams Hematology,* 8th Edition, 2011). The normal ranges described here are guidelines. They may vary from laboratory to laboratory and some lower and upper limits are still disputed. They vary based on reagents, assay and instruments used. Normal values should be established in the laboratory of record. This requirement is especially true of determinations such as prothrombin and thromboplastin time, D-dimer assay, platelet aggregometry, platelet ATP release, and others.

See also: Jacobs DS, Oxley DK, DeMott WR,: *Laboratory Test Handbook: Concise with Disease Index,* Lexi-Comp, Inc, 2004; Sacher RA, McPherson RA: *Widmann's Clinical Interpretation of Laboratory Tests,* 11th Edition, F.A. Davis, Co., 2000; Burtis CA, Ashwood ER, Bruns DE: *Tietz Textbook of Clinical Chemistry:* 4th Edition, W.B. Saunders Co., 2005.

INDEX

Page numbers followed by the letters f and t indicate figures and tables, respectively.